# Acute Care Handbook for Physical Therapists

# Acute Care Handbook for Physical Therapists
Second Edition

## Jaime C. Paz, M.S., P.T.

*Assistant Clinical Specialist, Department of Physical Therapy, Northeastern University, Boston; Adjunct Faculty Member, Department of Physical Therapy, Simmons College, Boston; Adjunct Physical Therapist, Care Group Home Care, Belmont, Massachusetts*

## Michele P. West, M.S., P.T.

*Physical Therapist, Inpatient Rehabilitation, Rehabilitation Services, Lahey Clinic, Burlington, Massachusetts*

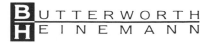

Boston Oxford Auckland Johannesburg Melbourne New Delhi

**Library of Congress Cataloging-in-Publication Data**

Paz, Jaime C., 1966–
  Acute care handbook for physical therapists / Jaime C. Paz, Michele P. West.—2nd ed.
    p. ; cm.
  Includes bibliographical references and index.
  ISBN 0-7506-7300-1
    1. Medicine—Handbooks, manuals, etc. 2. Hospital care—Handbooks, manuals, etc.
  I. West, Michele P., 1969– II. Title.
  [DNLM: 1. Acute Disease—therapy—Handbooks. 2. Intensive Care—Handbooks.
  WB 39 P348a 2002]
  RC55 .P375 2001
  616—dc21

                                        2001043457

**British Library Cataloguing-in-Publication Data**
A catalogue record for this book is available from the British Library.

The publisher offers special discounts on bulk orders of this book.
For information, please contact:

Manager of Special Sales
Butterworth–Heinemann
225 Wildwood Avenue
Woburn, MA 01801-2041
Tel: 781-904-2500
Fax: 781-904-2620

For information on all Butterworth–Heinemann publications available,
contact our World Wide Web home page at: http://www.bh.com

10 9 8 7 6 5 4 3 2 1

Printed in the United States of America

# Contents

# Contributing Authors

**Sean M. Collins, M.S., P.T., C.C.S.**
Department of Physical Therapy, University of Massachusetts, Lowell; Adjunct Physical Therapist, Department of Rehabilitation Services, Lowell General Hospital, Lowell, Massachusetts

**James J. Gaydos, M.S., P.T.**
Senior Physical Therapist, Department of Inpatient Acute Care, New England Baptist Hospital, Boston

**Marie Jarrell-Gracious, P.T.**
Owner, Specialty Care, Mokena, Illinois

**Jennifer Lee Hunt, M.S., P.T.**
Physical Therapist, Rehabilitation Services, Lahey Clinic, Burlington, Massachusetts

**Kimberly Knowlton, P.T.**
Clinical Lead Physical Therapist, Rehabilitation Services, University of Massachusetts Memorial Medical Center, Worcester

**Eileen F. Lang, P.T.**
Senior Physical Therapist, Rehabilitation Services, Lahey Clinic, Burlington, Massachusetts

**V. Nicole Lombard, M.S., P.T.**
Staff Physical Therapist, Department of Physical Therapy, New England Baptist Hospital, Boston

**Jaime C. Paz, M.S., P.T.**
Assistant Clinical Specialist, Department of Physical Therapy, Northeastern University, Boston; Adjunct Faculty Member, Department of Physical Therapy, Simmons College, Boston; Adjunct Physical Therapist, Care Group Home Care, Belmont, Massachusetts

**Susan Polich, P.T., M.T.(A.S.C.P.), M.Ed.**
Assistant Clinical Specialist, Department of Physical Therapy, Northeastern University, Boston; Adjunct Instructor, Physical Therapist Assistant Program, Community College of Rhode Island, Newport; Physical Therapist, Sturdy Memorial Hospital, Attleboro, Massachusetts

**Jason D. Rand, P.T.**
Physical Therapist, Inpatient Physical Therapy Services, Winthrop University Hospital, Mineola, New York

**Jennifer A. Silva, M.S., P.T.**
Physical Therapist, Outpatient Rehabilitation Center, South Shore Hospital, South Weymouth, Massachusetts

**Michele P. West, M.S., P.T.**
Physical Therapist, Inpatient Rehabilitation, Rehabilitation Services, Lahey Clinic, Burlington, Massachusetts

# Contributing Artists

Sean M. Collins, M.S., P.T., C.C.S.
Department of Physical Therapy, University of Massachusetts, Lowell;
Adjunct Physical Therapist, Department of Rehabilitation Services,
Lowell General Hospital, Lowell, Massachusetts

Barbara Cocanour, Ph.D.
Department of Physical Therapy, University of Massachusetts, Lowell

Marybeth Cuaycong
Graduate Student, Department of Physical Therapy, Northeastern
University, Boston

Peter L. Scotch, M.A.
English Teacher, Byram Hills High School, Armonk, New York

Michele P. West, M.S., P.T.
Physical Therapist, Rehabilitation Services, Lahey Clinic, Burlington,
Massachusetts

Peter P. Wu
Graduate Student, Department of Physical Therapy, Northeastern
University, Boston

# Preface

*Acute Care Handbook for Physical Therapists* was originally developed to provide clinicians with a handy reference for patient care in the hospital setting. It was created primarily for physical therapy students and clinicians unfamiliar with acute care. Because of the positive comments and feedback to the first edition, this second edition was written to serve the same purpose with updated information, including the following:

- A revision of all chapters and appendices with expanded information on new technologies, medical-surgical innovations, clinical tips, and guidelines to physical therapy management

- A new chapter on organ transplantation

- Updated information on common medications, including a new pharmacologic agents appendix

- New appendices, such as Acute Care Setting and Functional Tests

Additionally, the talents of new contributors have given this edition a broader perspective on clinical practice in the acute care setting. Last, language that is consistent with the *Guide to Physical Therapist Practice* is used throughout all the chapters and appendices.

As a member of the health care team, the physical therapist is often expected to understand hospital protocol, safety, medical-surgical "lingo," and the many aspects of patient care from the emergency room setting, to the intensive care unit, to the general ward. This handbook is therefore intended to be a resource to aid in the interpretation and understanding of the medical-surgical aspects of acute care.

Each chapter in this edition of *Acute Care Handbook for Physical Therapists* discusses a major body system. The chapters include the following:

- A review of basic structure and function

- An overview of the medical-surgical evaluation of a patient admitted to the hospital, including diagnostic procedures and laboratory tests

- A review of pathophysiology that emphasizes signs and symptoms of specific diseases and disorders

- Guidelines for physical therapy intervention

Clinical Tips appear throughout each chapter. These helpful hints are intended to maximize safety, quality, and efficiency of care. These clinical tips are suggestions from the editors and contributors that, from clinical experience, have proved to be valuable in acclimating therapists to the acute care setting.

Appendices provide information to complement topics presented in the chapters.

It is important to remember that all of the information presented in this book is intended to serve as a guide to stimulate independent critical thinking within the spectrum of medical-surgical techniques and trends. Developing and maintaining a rapport with the medical-surgical team is highly recommended, as the open exchange of information among professionals is invaluable. We believe this new edition of *Acute Care Handbook for Physical Therapists* can enhance the clinical experience by providing valuable information while reviewing charts, preparing for therapy intervention, and making clinical decisions in the acute care setting.

*J. P.*
*M. P. W.*

# Acknowledgments

We offer sincere gratitude to the following people:

Leslie Forman and Butterworth–Heinemann for their confidence in creating a second edition of this work.

Jennifer Rhuda for her editorial expertise and resourcefulness.

Shannon Riley at Silverchair for her graceful editing down the home stretch.

The contributors—we couldn't have completed this project without you.

The many patients, whose lives have enriched ours, both clinically and personally.

Personal thanks from Jaime to the following:

Tallie, for all your love, support and continuous encouragement. I couldn't have made it without you. Mahal kita.

The students, both at Northeastern University and Simmons College, who give me one of the best reasons to get up in the morning.

Jennifer Katz and Cindy Dubois for your research assistance.

My colleagues and mentors, who continually inspire me to become a better educator and clinician.

And to my extended family, whom I need to see a lot more of now that this is all over: Rory and Jane; John and Alex; Vic, Karen, Anna, and Little Vic; Steve, Jennifer, Christopher, and Aidan; Peter, Sally, and Hannah; Rick, Cheryl, Andrew, and Lauren; Mark, Gina, Benjamin, and Nicholas.

Personal thanks from Michele to the following:

My family and friends, who offered encouragement throughout the publishing process, including Mom and Dad, Marie, Heather, Tracee, Lynn, Kim J., Betsy, Kelly, Kelli, Kim P., Julie, and Bill.

Nana and Cookie, for reminding me to find the grandparent in each patient.

My husband, Jim, for teaching me more computer skills than I ever wanted to know.

My laser printer/fax/copier, I couldn't have done this without you!

My colleagues and patients, who inspire me to become a better clinician.

My fellow Lahey inpatient physical therapists, for bearing with me through the completion of this manuscript.

Lena, for cooking me dinner when I didn't have time.

Heather Hayden, M.S., P.T., and Kelly Madden, M.S., P.T., for your helpful suggestions and manuscript review.

Carol Spencer, Medical Librarian, Cattell Memorial Library, Lahey Clinic, for your research assistance.

# Acute Care
# Handbook for
# Physical Therapists

# 1

# Cardiac System
*Sean M. Collins*

## Introduction

Physical therapists in acute care facilities commonly encounter patients with cardiac system dysfunction as either a primary morbidity or comorbidity. Based on current estimates, 59,700,000 Americans have one or more types of cardiovascular disease (CVD), making the prevalence rate for men and women 20%.[1] In 1997, CVD ranked first among all disease categories and accounted for 6,145,000 inpatient admissions.[1] In the acute care setting, the role of the physical therapist with this diverse group of patients remains founded in examination, evaluation, intervention, and discharge planning, for the purpose of improving functional capacity and minimizing disability. The physical therapist must be prepared to safely accommodate for the effects of dynamic (pathologic, physiologic, medical, and surgical intervention) changes into his or her evaluation and intervention.

The normal cardiovascular system provides the necessary pumping force to circulate blood through the coronary, pulmonary, cerebral, and systemic circulation. To perform work, such as during functional tasks, energy demands of the body increase, therefore increasing the oxygen demands of the heart. A variety of pathologic states can create impairments in the cardiac system's ability to successfully meet these demands, ultimately leading to functional limitations. To fully address these functional limitations, the physical therapist must understand normal and abnormal cardiac function, clinical tests, and medical and surgical management of the cardiovascular system.

The objectives of this chapter are to provide the following:

1.   A brief overview of the structure and function of the cardiovascular system

2.   An overview of cardiac evaluation, including physical examination and diagnostic testing

3.   A description of cardiac diseases and disorders, including clinical findings and medical and surgical management

4.   A framework on which to base physical therapy evaluation and intervention in patients with CVD

## Structure

The heart and the roots of the great vessels (Figure 1-1) occupy the pericardium, which is located in the *mediastinum.* The sternum, the costal cartilages, and the medial ends of the third to fifth ribs on the left side of the thorax create the anterior border of the mediastinum. It is bordered inferiorly by the diaphragm, posteriorly by the vertebral column and ribs, and laterally by the pleural cavity (which contains the lungs).[2] Specific cardiac structures and vessels and their respective functions are outlined in Tables 1-1 and 1-2.

Note: The mediastinum and the heart can be displaced from their normal positions with changes in the lungs secondary to various disorders. For example, a tension pneumothorax will shift the mediastinum away from the side of dysfunction (see Chapter 2 for further description of pneumothorax).

## Function

The cardiovascular system must adjust the amount of nutrient and oxygen rich blood pumped out of the heart (cardiac output [CO]) to meet the wide spectrum of daily energy (metabolic) demands of the body.

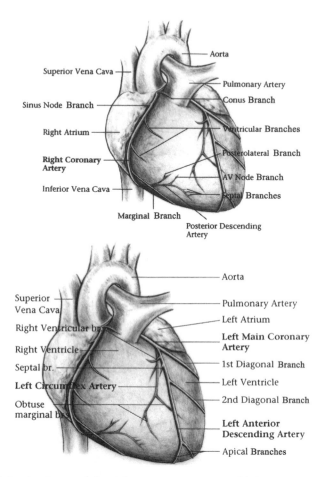

**Figure 1-1.** *Anatomy of the right coronary artery and left coronary artery, including left main, left anterior descending, and left circumflex coronary arteries. (Reprinted with permission from RC Becker. Chest Pain: The Most Common Complaints Series. Boston: Butterworth–Heinemann, 2000;26–28.)*

The heart's ability to pump blood depends on the following characteristics[3]:

- Automaticity—the ability to initiate its own electrical impulse

- Excitability—the ability to respond to electrical stimulus

**Table 1-1.** Primary Structures of the Heart

| Structure | Description | Function |
|---|---|---|
| Pericardium | Double-walled sac of elastic connective tissue, a fibrous outer layer and serous inner layer | Protects against infection and trauma |
| Epicardium | Outermost layer of cardiac wall, covers surface of heart and great vessels | Protects against infection and trauma |
| Myocardium | Central layer of thick muscular tissue | Provides major pumping force of the ventricles |
| Endocardium | Thin layer of endothelium and connective tissue | Lines the inner surface of heart, valves, chordae tendineae, and papillary muscles |
| Right atrium | Heart chamber | Receives blood from venous system and is a primer pump for the right ventricle |
| Tricuspid valve | Atrioventricular valve between right atrium and ventricle | Prevents backflow of blood from right ventricle to atrium during ventricular systole |
| Right ventricle | Heart chamber | Pumps blood to pulmonary circulation |
| Pulmonic valve | Semilunar valve between right ventricle and pulmonary artery | Prevents backflow of blood from pulmonary artery to right ventricle during diastole |
| Left atrium | Heart chamber | Acts as a reservoir for blood and primer pump for left ventricle |
| Mitral valve | Atrioventricular valve between left atrium and ventricle | Prevents backflow of blood from left ventricle to atrium during ventricular systole |
| Left ventricle | Heart chamber | Pumps blood to systemic circulation |
| Aortic valve | Semilunar valve between left ventricle and aorta | Prevents backflow of blood from aorta to left ventricle during ventricular diastole |

**Table 1-1.** *Continued*

| Structure | Description | Function |
| --- | --- | --- |
| Chordae tendineae | Tendinous attachment of atrioventricular valve cusps to papillary muscles | Prevents valves from everting into atria during ventricular systole |
| Papillary muscle | Muscle that connects chordae tendineae to floor of ventricle wall | Constricts and pulls on chordae tendineae to prevent eversion of valve cusps during ventricular systole |

- Conductivity—the ability to transmit electrical impulse from cell to cell within the heart

- Contractility—the ability to stretch as a single unit and then passively recoil while actively contracting

- Rhythmicity—the ability to repeat the cycle in synchrony with regularity

**Table 1-2.** Great Vessels of the Heart and Their Function

| Structure | Description | Function |
| --- | --- | --- |
| Aorta | Primary artery from the left ventricle that ascends and then descends after exiting the heart | Ascending aorta delivers blood to neck, head, and arms. Descending aorta delivers blood to visceral and lower body tissues. |
| Superior vena cava | Primary vein that drains into the right atrium | Drains venous blood from head, neck, and upper body. |
| Inferior vena cava | Primary vein that drains into the right atrium | Drains venous blood from viscera and lower body. |
| Pulmonary artery | Primary artery from right ventricle | Carries blood to lungs. |

## Cardiac Cycle

Blood flow throughout the cardiac cycle depends on circulatory and cardiac pressure gradients. The right side of the heart is a low-pressure system with little vascular resistance in the pulmonary arteries, whereas the left side of the heart is a high-pressure system with high vascular resistance from the systemic circulation. The cardiac cycle is the period from the beginning of one contraction, starting with sinoatrial (SA) node depolarization, to the beginning of the next contraction. *Systole* is the period of contraction, whereas *diastole* is the period of relaxation. Systole and diastole can also be categorized into atrial and ventricular components:

1.   *Atrial diastole* is the period of atrial filling. The flow of blood is directed by the higher pressure in the venous circulatory system.

2.   *Atrial systole* is the period of atrial emptying and contraction. Initial emptying of approximately 70% of blood occurs as a result of the initial pressure gradient between the atria and the ventricles. Atrial contraction then follows, squeezing out the remaining 30%.[3] This is commonly referred to as the *atrial kick*.

3.   *Ventricular diastole* is the period of ventricular filling. It initially occurs with ease; then, as the ventricle is filled, atrial contraction is necessary to squeeze the remaining blood volume into the ventricle. The amount of stretch placed on the ventricular walls during diastole, referred to as *left ventricular end diastolic pressure* (LVEDP), influences the force of contraction during systole. (Refer to description of preload in the section Factors Affecting Cardiac Output.)

4.   *Ventricular systole* is the period of ventricular contraction. The initial contraction is isovolumic (meaning it does not eject blood), which generates pressure necessary to serve as the catalyst for rapid ejection of ventricular blood. The left ventricular *ejection fraction* (EF) represents the percent of end diastolic volume ejected during systole and is normally approximately 60%.[3]

### Cardiac Output

CO is the quantity of blood pumped by the heart in 1 minute. It can also be described relative to body mass as the *cardiac index*, the amount of blood pumped per minute per square meter of body mass. Regional demands for tissue perfusion (based on local metabolic needs) compete for systemic circulation, and total CO adjusts to meet these demands. Adjustment to CO occurs with changes in heart rate (HR) (*chronotropic*) or stroke volume (SV) (*inotropic*).[4] Normal resting CO is approximately 4–8 liters per minute, and normal cardiac index is approximately 2.5–4.0 liters per minute per meter[2,3] (with a resting HR of 70 beats per minute [bpm], resting SV is approximately 71 ml/beat). The maximum value of CO represents the functional capacity of the circulatory system to meet the demands of physical activity.

$$CO \text{ (liters per minute)} = HR \text{ (bpm)} \times SV \text{ (liters)}$$

**Factors Affecting Cardiac Output**

*Preload*
*Preload* is the amount of tension on the ventricular wall before it con-tracts. It is related to venous return and affects SV by increasing left ventricular end diastolic volume as well as pressure and therefore con-traction.[3] This relationship is explained by the *Frank-Starling Mechanism* and is demonstrated in Figure 1-2.

*Frank-Starling Mechanism*
The Frank-Starling mechanism defines the normal relationship between length and tension of the myocardium.[5] The greater the stretch on the myocardium before systole (preload), the stronger the ventricular contraction. The length-tension relationship in skeletal muscle is based on the response of individual muscle fibers; however, relationships between cardiac muscle length and tension consist of the whole heart. Therefore, length is considered in terms of volume; tension is considered in terms of pressure. A greater volume of blood returning to the heart during diastole equates to greater pressures generated initially by the heart's con-tractile elements. Ultimately facilitated by elastic recoil, a greater volume of blood is ejected during systole. The effectiveness of this mechanism can be reduced in pathologic situations.[4]

*Afterload*

*Afterload* is the force against which a muscle must contract to ini-tiate shortening.[5] Within the ventricular wall, this is equal to the

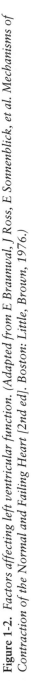

Sympathetic Tone
Catecholamines
Force-Frequency Relation
Inotropic Agents
Anoxia/Hypercapnia/Acidosis
Loss of Myocardium
Intrinsic Depression

**Systolic State of the Myocardium:**
The four lines provide an example of how the contractile state of the myocardium influences the relationship between LVEDV and ventricular performance.

Elasticity of Myocardium
Capacity of Ventricular Chamber

**Diastolic State of the Myocardium**

Total Blood Volume
Pump of Skeletal Muscles
Body Position
Intrathoracic Pressure
Intrapericardial Pressure
Venous Tone

Venous Return

Atrial Contribution to Ventricular Filling (Atrial Kick)

Stretching of Myocardium

**Left Ventricular End Diastolic Volume (LVEDV)**

Ventricular Performance

**Figure 1-2.** *Factors affecting left ventricular function. (Adapted from E Braunwal, J Ross, E Sonnenblick, et al. Mechanisms of Contraction of the Normal and Failing Heart [2nd ed]. Boston: Little, Brown, 1976.)*

tension developed across its wall during systole. The most prominent force contributing to afterload in the heart is BP, specifically
vascular compliance and resistance. BP affects aortic valve opening
and is the most obvious load encountered by the ejecting ventricle.
An example of afterload is the amount of pressure in the aorta at
the time of ventricular systole.[3]

## Cardiac Conduction System

A schematic of the cardiac conduction system and a normal electrocardiogram (ECG) are presented in Figure 1-3. Normal conduction begins
in the SA node and travels throughout the atrial myocardium (atrial
depolarization) via intranodal pathways to the atrioventricular (AV)
node, where it is delayed momentarily. It then travels to the bundle of
His, to the bundle branches, to the Purkinje fibers, and finally to the
myocardium, resulting in ventricular contraction.[6] Disturbances in con-

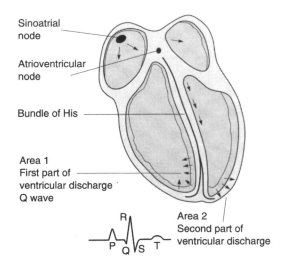

**Figure 1-3.** *Schematic representation of the sequence of excitation in the
heart. (With permission from M Walsh, A Crumbie, S Reveley. Nurse Practitioners: Clinical Skills and Professional Issues. Boston: Butterworth–Heine-
man, 1999;99.)*

duction can decrease CO (refer to the discussion of rhythm and conduction disturbances in the Pathophysiology section).[7]

### Neural Input

The SA node has its own inherent rate. Neural input can, however, influence HR, HRV, and contractility through the autonomic nervous system.[3,8]

Parasympathetic system (vagal) neural input generally decelerates cardiac function, thus decreasing HR and contractility. Parasympathetic input travels through the vagus nerves. The right vagus nerve primarily stimulates the SA node and affects rate, whereas the left vagus nerve primarily stimulates the AV node and affects AV conduction.[3,8]

Sympathetic system neural input is through the thoracolumbar sympathetic system and serves to increase HR and augment ventricular contractility, thus accelerating cardiac function.[3]

### Endocrine Input

In response to physical activity or stress, a release in catecholamines increases HR, contractility, and peripheral vascular resistance for a net effect of increased cardiac function.[3] Refer to Table 1-3 for the cardiac effects of hormones.

### Local Input

Tissue pH, concentration of carbon dioxide ($CO_2$), concentration of oxygen ($O_2$), and metabolic products (e.g., lactic acid) can affect vascular tone.[3] During exercise, increased levels of $CO_2$, decreased levels of $O_2$, decreased pH, and increased levels of lactic acid at the tissue level dilate local blood vessels and therefore increase CO distribution to that area.

### Cardiac Reflexes

Cardiac reflexes influence HR and contractility and can be divided into three general categories: baroreflex (or pressure), Bainbridge reflex (or stretch), and chemoreflex (or chemical reflexes).

Table 1-3. Cardiac Effects of Hormones

| Hormone | Primary Site | Stimulus | Cardiac Effect |
|---|---|---|---|
| Norepinephrine | Adrenal medulla | Stress/exercise | Vasoconstriction |
| Epinephrine | Adrenal medulla | Stress/exercise | Coronary artery vasodilation |
| Angiotensin | Kidney | Decreased arterial pressure | Vasoconstriction, increases blood volume |
| Vasopressin | Posterior pituitary | Decreased arterial pressure | Potent vasoconstrictor |
| Bradykinin | Formed by polypeptides in blood when activated | Tissue damage/ inflammation | Vasodilation, increased capillary permeability |
| Histamine | Throughout tissues of body | Tissue damage | Vasodilation, increased capillary permeability |
| Atrial natriuretic peptides | Atria of heart | Increased atrial stretch | Decreased blood volume |
| Aldosterone | Adrenal cortex | Angiotensin II (stimulated) by hypovolemia or decreased renal perfusion | Increases blood volume, kidneys excrete more potassium |

Source: Data from AC Guyton, JE Hall. Textbook of Medical Physiology (9th ed). Philadelphia: Saunders, 1996.

Baroreflexes are activated through a group of mechanoreceptors located in the heart, great vessels, and intrathoracic and cervical blood vessels. These mechanoreceptors are most plentiful in the walls of the internal carotid arteries.[3] Mechanoreceptors are sensory receptors that are sensitive to mechanical changes, such as pressure and stretch. Activation of the mechanoreceptors by high pressures results in an inhibition of the vasomotor center of the medulla that increases vagal stimulation. This chain of events is known as the *baroreflex* and results in vasodilation, decreased HR, and decreased contractility.

Mechanoreceptors located in the right atrial myocardium respond to stretch. With an increased volume in the right atrium, there is an increase in pressure on the atrial wall. This reflex, known as the *Bainbridge reflex*, stimulates the vasomotor center of the medulla, which in turn increases sympathetic input and increases HR and contractility.[3] *Respiratory sinus arrhythmia*, an increased HR during inspiration and decreased HR during expiration, may be facilitated by changes in venous return and SV caused by changes in thoracic pressure induced by the respiratory cycle. At the beginning of inspiration, when thoracic pressure is decreased, venous return is greater, and therefore there is a greater stretch on the atrial wall.[9]

Chemoreceptors located on the carotid and aortic bodies have a primary effect on increasing rate and depth of ventilation in response to $CO_2$ levels, but they also have a cardiac effect. Changes in $CO_2$ during the respiratory cycle may also result in sinus arrhythmia.[3]

## Coronary Perfusion

For a review of the major coronary arteries, refer to Figure 1-1. Blood is pumped to the large superficial coronary arteries during ventricular systole. At this time, myocardial contraction limits the flow of blood to the myocardium; therefore, myocardial tissue is actually perfused during diastole.

## Systemic Circulation

For review of the primary anatomic structures and distribution of the systemic circulation, refer to Figure 1-4. Systemic circulation is affected by total peripheral resistance (TPR), which is the resistance to blood flow by the force created by the aorta and arterial system. Two factors that contribute to resistance are (1) vasomotor tone, in which vessels dilate and constrict, and (2) blood viscosity, in which greater pressure is required to propel thicker blood. Also called *systemic vascular resistance*, TPR and CO influence blood pressure (BP).[3] This relationship is illustrated in the following equation:

$$BP = CO \times TPR$$

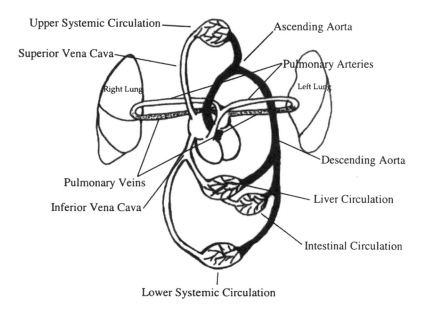

Upper Systemic Circulation

Superior Vena Cava

Right Lung

Ascending Aorta

Pulmonary Arteries

Left Lung

Descending Aorta

Pulmonary Veins

Inferior Vena Cava

Liver Circulation

Intestinal Circulation

Lower Systemic Circulation

**Figure 1-4.** *Schematic of systemic circulation. (Drawn by Barbara Cocanour, Ph.D., University of Massachusetts, Lowell, Department of Physical Therapy.)*

## Cardiac Evaluation

Cardiac evaluation consists of patient history, physical examination (which consists of observation, palpation, BP measurement, and heart sound auscultation), laboratory tests, and diagnostic procedures.

### Patient History

In addition to the general chart review presented in Appendix I-A, pertinent information about patients with cardiac dysfunction that should be obtained before physical examination includes the following[4,10–12]:

• Presence of chest pain (see Appendix X for an expanded description of characteristics and etiology of chest pain)

1. Location, radiation

2. Character and quality (crushing, burning, numbing, hot) and frequency

3. Angina equivalents (what the patient feels as angina, e.g., jaw pain, shortness of breath, dizziness, lightheadedness, diaphoresis, burping, nausea, or any combination of these)

4. Aggravating and alleviating factors

5. Precipitating factors

- Medical treatment sought and its outcome

- Presence of palpitations

- Presence of cardiac risk factors (Table 1-4)

- Family history of cardiac disease

Table 1-4. Cardiac Risk Factors

| Major Independent Risk Factors | Predisposing Risk Factors | Conditional Risk Factors |
|---|---|---|
| Smoking | Physical inactivity | Elevated triglycerides |
| Hypertension | Obesity | Small LDL particles |
| Elevated serum cholesterol, total (and LDL) | Body mass index >30 kg/m² | Elevated homocysteine Elevated lipoprotein (a) |
| | Abdominal obesity (waist-hip ratio) | |
| Decreased high-density lipoprotein cholesterol | Men >40 in. | Elevated inflammatory markers |
| Diabetes mellitus | Women >35 in. | C-reactive protein |
| Advancing age | Family history of premature heart disease | Fibrinogen |
| | Psychosocial factors | |
| | Ethnic characteristics | |

LDL = low-density lipoprotein.
Source: Data from SM Grundy, R Pasternak, P Greenland, et al. Assessment of cardiovascular risk by use of multiple-risk-factor assessment equations: a statement for healthcare professionals from the American Heart Association and the American College of Cardiology. Circulation 1999;100:1481–1492.

- History of dizziness or syncope

- Previous myocardial infarction (MI), cardiac studies, or procedures

---

**Clinical Tip**

- When discussing angina with a patient, use the patient's terminology. If the patient describes the angina as "crushing" pain, ask the patient if he or she experiences the crushing feeling during treatment as opposed to asking the patient if he or she has chest pain.
- The common medical record abbreviation for chest pain is *CP*.

---

*Physical Examination*

**Observation**
Key components of the observation portion of the physical examination include the following[4,7]:

1.   Facial color, skin color and tone, or the presence of diaphoresis

2.   Obvious signs of edema in the extremities

3.   Respiratory rate

4.   Signs of trauma (e.g., paddle burns or ecchymosis from cardiopulmonary resuscitation)

5.   Presence of jugular venous distention, which results from the backup of fluid into the venous system from right-sided CHF (Figure 1-5)

   a.  Make sure the patient is in a semirecumbent position (45 degrees).

   b.  Have the patient turn his or her head away from the side being evaluated.

   c.  Observe pulsations in the internal jugular neck region. Pulsations are normally seen 3–5 cm above the sternum. Pul-

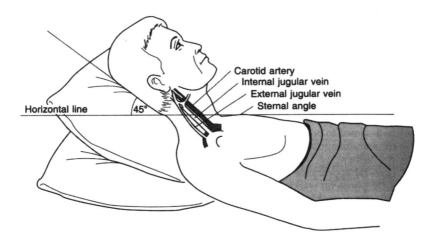

**Figure 1-5.** *Measurement of jugular venous distention (JVP). The JVP reading is the maximum height, in centimeters, above the sternal angle at which venous pulsations are visible.*

sations higher than this or absent pulsations indicate jugular venous distention.

**Palpation**

*Palpation* is the second component of the physical examination and is used to evaluate and identify the following:

- Pulses for circulation quality, HR, and rhythm (Table 1-5, Figure 1-6)

- Extremities for pitting edema bilaterally (Table 1-6)

---

Clinical Tip

- When palpating HR, counting pulses for 15 seconds and multiplying by 4 is sufficient with normal rates and rhythms. If rates are faster than 100 bpm or slower than 60 bpm, they should be palpated for 60 seconds. If the rhythm is irregularly irregular (e.g., during atrial fibrillation) or regularly irregular (e.g., premature ventricular contractions [PVCs]), auscultation of heart sounds should be performed to identify the apical HR for a full minute.

**Table 1-5.** Pulse Amplitude Classification and Pulse Abnormalities

Pulse Amplitude Classification

| Scale | Degree | Description |
|---|---|---|
| 0 | Absent pulse | No pulse—no circulation |
| 1+ | Diminished pulse | Reduced stroke volume and ejection fraction, increased vascular resistance |
| 2+ | Normal pulse | Normal resting conditions, no pathologies |
| 3+ | Moderately increased | Slightly increased stroke volume and ejection fraction |
| 4+ | Markedly increased (bounding)* | Increased stroke volume and ejection fraction, can be diminished with vasoconstriction |

Pulse Abnormalities

| Abnormality | Palpation | Description |
|---|---|---|
| Pulsus alternans | Regular rhythm with strong pulse waves alternating with weak pulse waves | Indicates left ventricular failure when present at normal heart rates |
| Bigeminal pulses | Every other pulse is weak and early | Due to preventricular contractions (bigeminy) |
| Pulsus paradoxus | Reduction in strength of the pulse with an abnormal decline in blood pressure during inspiration | May be caused by chronic obstructive lung disease, pericarditis, pulmonary emboli, restrictive cardiomyopathy, and cardiogenic shock |

*Corrigan's pulse is a bounding pulse visible in the carotid artery that occurs with aortic regurgitation.
Source: Data from SL Woods, ES Sivarajian-Froelicher, S Underhill-Motzer (eds). Cardiac Nursing (4th ed). Philadelphia: Lippincott, 2000.

In these cases, palpation of pulse cannot substitute for ECG analysis to monitor the patient's rhythm, but it may alert the therapist to the onset of these abnormalities.

• Use caution in palpating pulses, as manual pressure on the carotid sinus may cause reflexive drops in HR, BP, or both.

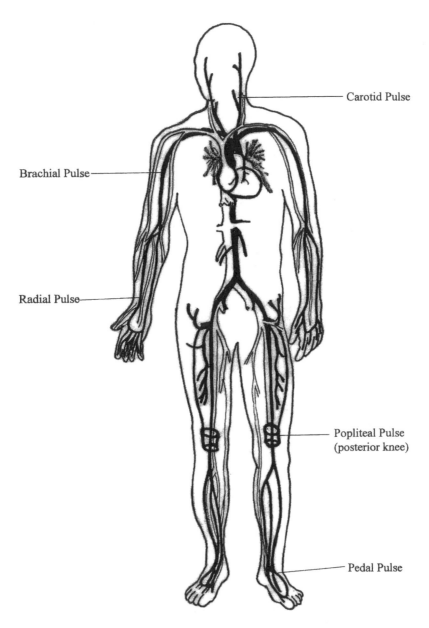

**Figure 1-6.** *Arterial pulses. (Drawn by Barbara Cocanour, Ph.D., University of Massachusetts, Lowell, Department of Physical Therapy.)*

**Table 1-6.** Pitting Edema Scale

| Scale | Degree | Description |
|-------|--------|-------------|
| 1+ Trace | Slight | Barely perceptible depression |
| 2+ Mild | 0–0.6 cm | Easily identified depression (EID) (skin rebounds in <15 secs) |
| 3+ Moderate | 0.6–1.3 cm | EID (rebound 15–30 secs) |
| 4+ Severe | 1.3–2.5 cm | EID (rebound >30 secs) |

EID = easily identified depression.
Sources: Data from SL Woods, ES Sivarajian Froelicher, S Underhill-Motzer (eds). Cardiac Nursing (4th ed). Philadelphia: Lippincott, 2000; and EA Hillegass, HS Sadowsky (eds). Essentials of Cardiopulmonary Physical Therapy (2nd ed). Philadelphia: Saunders, 2001.

## Blood Pressure

BP measurement with a sphygmomanometer (cuff) and auscultation is an indirect, noninvasive measurement of the force exerted against the arterial walls during ventricular systole (*systolic blood pressure [SBP]*) and during ventricular diastole (*diastolic blood pressure*). BP is affected by peripheral vascular resistance (blood volume and elasticity of arterial walls) and CO. Table 1-7 lists normal BP ranges. Occasionally, BP measurements can only be performed on certain limbs secondary to the presence of conditions such as a percutaneous inserted central catheter, arterio-

**Table 1-7.** Normal Blood Pressure Ranges

| | Systolic | Diastolic |
|---|----------|-----------|
| Age 8 yrs | 85–114 mm Hg | 52–85 mm Hg |
| Age 12 yrs | 95–135 mm Hg | 58–88 mm Hg |
| Adult | 100–140 mm Hg | 60–90 mm Hg |
| Borderline hypertension | 140–150 mm Hg | 90–100 mm Hg |
| Hypertension | >150 mm Hg | >100 mm Hg |
| Normal exercise | Increases during time and with increased load or intensity | ±10 mm Hg |

Sources: Data from SL Woods, ES Sivarajian Froelicher, S Underhill-Motzer (eds). Cardiac Nursing (4th ed). Philadelphia: Lippincott, 2000; and LS Bickley. Bate's Guide to Physical Examination and History Taking (7th ed). Philadelphia: Lippincott, 1999.

venous fistula for hemodialysis, blood clots, scarring from brachial artery cutdowns, or lymphedema (i.e., status-post mastectomy). BP of the upper extremity should be measured in the following manner:

1. Check for posted signs, if any, at the bedside that indicate which arm should be used in taking BP. BP variations of 5–10 mm Hg between the right and left upper extremity are considered normal. Patients with arterial compression or obstruction may have differences of more than 10–15 mm Hg.[12]

2. Use a properly fitting cuff. The inflatable bladder should have a width of approximately 40%, and length of approximately 80% of the upper arm circumference.[13]

3. Position the cuff 2.5 cm above the antecubital crease.

4. Rest the arm at the level of the heart.

5. To determine how high to inflate the cuff, palpate the radial pulse, inflate until no longer palpable, and note this cuff inflation value. Deflate the cuff.
Note: With a patient who is in circulatory shock, auscultation may be too difficult. In these cases, this method can be used to measure the SBP and is recorded as systolic BP/P (i.e., "BP is 90 over palp").[13]

6. Place the bell of the stethoscope gently over the brachial artery.

7. Re-inflate the cuff to 30–40 mm Hg greater than the value in step 5. Then slowly deflate the cuff. Cuff deflation should occur at approximately 2–3 mm Hg per second.[13]

8. Listen for the onset of tapping sounds, which represents blood flow returning to the brachial artery. This is the systolic pressure.

9. As the pressure approaches diastolic pressure, the sounds will become muffled and in 5–10 mm Hg will be completely absent. These sounds are referred to as *Korotkoff's sounds* (Table 1-8).[12,13]

---

### Clinical Tip

- Recording pre-, para-, and postexertion BP is important in identifying BP responses to activity. During recovery from exercise, blood vessels dilate to allow for greater blood flow to muscles. In cardiac-compromised or very

**Table 1-8.** Korotkoff's Sounds

| Phase | Sound | Indicates |
|---|---|---|
| 1 | First sound heard, faint tapping sound with increasing intensity | Systolic pressure (blood starts to flow through compressed artery). |
| 2 | Start swishing sound | Because of the compressed artery, blood flow continues to be heard while the sounds change due to the changing compression on the artery. |
| 3 | Sounds increase in intensity with a distinct tapping | — |
| 4 | Sounds become muffled | Diastolic pressure in children <13 yrs old and in adults who are exercising, pregnant, or hyperthyroid (see phase 5). |
| 5 | Disappearance | Diastolic pressure in adults—occurs 5–10 mm Hg below phase 4 in normal adults. In states of increased rate of blood flow, it may be greater than 10 mm Hg below phase 4. In these cases, the phase 4 sound should be used as diastolic pressure in adults. |

Sources: Data from SL Woods, ES Sivarajian-Froelicher, S Underhill-Motzer (eds). Cardiac Nursing (4th ed). Philadelphia: Lippincott, 2000; and LS Bickley. Bate's Guide to Physical Examination and History Taking (7th ed). Philadelphia: Lippincott, 1999.

deconditioned individuals, total CO may not be able to support this increased flow to the muscles and may lead to decreased output to vital areas, such as the brain.

• If unable to obtain BP on the arm, the thigh is an appropriate alternative, with auscultation at the popliteal artery.

• Falsely high readings will occur if the cuff is too small or applied loosely, or if the brachial artery is lower than the heart level.

• Evaluation of BP and HR in different postures can be used to monitor orthostatic hypotension with repeat measurements on the same arm 1–5 minutes after position changes. The symbols that represent patient position are shown in Figure 1-7.

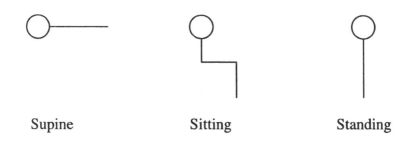

| Supine | Sitting | Standing |

**Figure 1-7.** *Orthostatic blood pressure symbols.*

- The same extremity should be used when serial BP recordings will be compared for an evaluation of hemodynamic response.
- A BP record is kept on the patient's vital sign flow sheet. This is a good place to check for BP trends throughout the day and, depending on your hospital's policy, to document BP changes during the therapy session.
- An auscultatory gap is the disappearance of sounds between phase 1 and phase 2 and is common in patients with high BP, venous distention, and severe aortic stenosis. Its presence can create falsely low systolic pressures if the cuff is not inflated high enough (which can be prevented by palpating for the disappearance of the pulse prior to measurement), or falsely high diastolic pressures if the therapist stops measurement during the gap (prevented by listening for the phase 3 to phase 5 transitions).[13]

**Auscultation**

Evaluation of heart sounds can yield information about the patient's condition and tolerance to medical treatment and physical therapy through the evaluation of valvular function, rate, rhythm, valvular compliance, and ventricular compliance.[4] To listen to heart sounds, a stethoscope with both a bell and a diaphragm is necessary. For a review of normal and abnormal heart sounds, refer to Table 1-9. The examination should follow a systematic pattern using both the bell (for low-pitched sounds) and diaphragm (for high-pitched sounds) and should cover all auscultatory areas, as illustrated in

**Table 1-9.** Normal and Abnormal Heart Sounds

| Sound | Location | Description |
|-------|----------|-------------|
| S1 (normal) | All areas | First heart sound, signifies closure of atrioventricular valves and corresponds to onset of ventricular systole. |
| S2 (normal) | All areas | Second heart sound, signifies closure of semilunar valves and corresponds with onset of ventricular diastole. |
| S3 (abnormal) | Best appreciated at apex | Immediately following S2, occurs early in diastole and represents filling of the ventricle. In young healthy individuals, it is considered normal and called a *physiologic third sound*. In the presence of heart disease, it results from decreased ventricular compliance (a classic sign of congestive heart failure). |
| S4 (abnormal) | Best appreciated at apex | Immediately preceding S1, occurs late in ventricular diastole, associated with increased resistance to ventricular filling; common in patients with hypertensive heart disease, coronary heart disease, pulmonary disease, or myocardial infarction, or following coronary artery bypass grafts. |
| Murmur (abnormal) | Over respective valves | Indicates regurgitation of blood through valves; can also be classified as systolic or diastolic murmurs. Common pathologies resulting in murmurs include mitral regurgitation and aortic stenosis. |
| Pericardial friction rub (abnormal) | Third or fourth intercostal space, anterior axillary line | Sign of pericardial inflammation (pericarditis), associated with each beat of the heart, sounds like a creak or leather being rubbed together. |

Source: Data from LS Bickley. Bate's Guide to Physical Examination and History Taking (7th ed). Philadelphia: Lippincott, 1999.

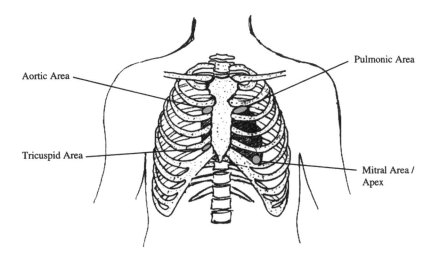

**Figure 1-8.** *Areas for heart sound auscultation. (Drawn by Barbara Cocanour, Ph.D., University of Massachusetts, Lowell, Department of Physical Therapy.)*

Figure 1-8. Abnormal sounds should be noted with a description of the conditions in which they were heard (e.g., after exercise or during exercise).

---

### Clinical Tip

- Always ensure proper function of stethoscope by tapping the diaphragm before applying the stethoscope to the patient.
- Rubbing the stethoscope on extraneous objects can add noise and detract from true examination.
- Auscultation of heart sounds over clothing should be avoided, because it muffles the intensity of both normal and abnormal sounds.
- If the patient has an irregular cardiac rhythm, HR should be determined through auscultation (apical HR). To save time, this can be done during a routine auscultatory examination with the stethoscope's bell or diaphragm in any location.

---

## Diagnostic and Laboratory Measures

The diagnostic and laboratory measures discussed in this section provide information that is used to determine medical diagnosis, guide interventions, and assist with determining prognosis. The clinical relevance of each test in serving this purpose varies according to the pathology. This section is organized across a spectrum of least invasive to most invasive measures. When appropriate, the test results most pertinent to the physical therapist are highlighted. Information that bears a direct impact on physical therapy clinical decision making usually includes that which helps the therapist identify indications for intervention, relative or absolute contraindications for intervention, possible complications during activity progression, and indicators of performance.

### Oximetry

Oximetry ($Sao_2$) is used to indirectly evaluate the oxygenation of a patient and can be used to titrate supplemental oxygen. Refer to Chapter 2 for a further description of oximetry.

### Electrocardiogram

ECG provides a graphic analysis of the heart's electrical activity. The ECG is commonly used to detect arrhythmias, heart blocks, and myocardial perfusion. It can also detect atrial or ventricular enlargement. ECG used for continuous monitoring of patients in the hospital typically involves a two- or three-lead system. A lead represents a particular portion or "view" of the heart. The patient's rhythm is usually displayed in his or her room, in the hall, and at the nurses' station. Diagnostic ECG involves a 12-lead analysis, the description of which is beyond the scope of this book. For a review of basic ECG rate and rhythm analysis, refer to Table 1-10 and Figure 1-3.

### Holter Monitoring

Holter monitoring is 24- or 48-hour ECG analysis. This is performed to detect cardiac arrhythmias and corresponding symptoms during a patient's daily activity.[12] Holter monitoring is different than telemetric monitoring because the ECG signal is recorded on a tape, and the subsequent analysis follows from this recording.

Indications for Holter monitoring include the evaluation of syncope, dizziness, shortness of breath with no other obvious cause, pal-

**Table 1-10.** Electrocardiograph Interpretation

| Wave/Segment | Duration (secs) | Amplitude (mm) | Indicates |
|---|---|---|---|
| P wave | <0.10 | 1–3 | Atrial depolarization |
| PR interval | 0.12–0.20 | Isoelectric line | Elapsed time between atrial depolarization and ventricular depolarization |
| QRS complex | 0.06–0.10 | 25–30 (maximum) | Ventricular depolarization and atrial repolarization |
| ST segment | 0.12 | −1/2 to +1 | Elapsed time between the end of ventricular depolarization and the beginning of repolarization |
| QT interval (QTc) | 0.42–0.47 | Varies | Elapsed time between the beginning of ventricular repolarization and the end of repolarization (QTc is corrected for heart rate) |
| T wave | 0.16 | 5–10 mm | Ventricular repolarization |

Sources: Data from RS Meyers (ed). Saunders Manual of Physical Therapy Practice. Philadelphia: Saunders, 1995; B Aehlert (ed). ACLS Quick Review Study Guide. St. Louis: Mosby, 1994; and D Davis (ed). How to Quickly and Accurately Master ECG Interpretation (2nd ed). Philadelphia: Lippincott, 1992.

pitations, antiarrhythmia therapy, pacemaker functioning, activity-induced silent ischemia, and risk of cardiac complications with the use of heart rate variability (HRV).

*Heart Rate Variability*
The most common measure of HRV is the standard deviation of all HR intervals during a 24-hour period (SDNN).[8] HRV has been used in clinical studies to test a variety of health outcomes.[8,14–16] In healthy populations, low HRV has been shown to be a risk factor for all causes of cardiac mortality,[17–19] as well as new onset of hypertension.[20] Low HRV is also a risk for mortality in patients who have had an MI,[21–23] have coronary artery disease,[24] or have CHF.[25] A classic study performed by Kleiger et al.[26] demonstrated a fivefold risk of re-infarction in post-MI patients with an SDNN (in

milliseconds) of less than 50, when compared to patients with an SDNN of greater than 100.

*Telemetric Electrocardiogram Monitoring*
Telemetric ECG monitoring provides real time ECG visualization via radiofrequency transmission of the ECG signal to a monitor. Telemetry has the benefit of Holter monitoring (because there is no hard wire connection of the patient to the visual display unit) as well as the benefit of the standard ECG monitor attachment, because there is a real-time graphic display of the ECG signal.

---

### Clinical Tip

- Some hospitals use an activity log with Holter monitoring. If so, be sure to document physical therapy intervention on the log. If there is no log, be sure to document time of day and intervention during physical therapy in the medical record.
- The use of cellular phones, although usually prohibited in any hospital, is especially prohibited on a telemetry unit. The cellular phone may interfere with the radio frequency transmission of the signal.

---

### Complete Blood Cell Count
Relevant values from the complete blood cell count are hematocrit, hemoglobin, and white blood cell counts. Hematocrit refers to the number of red blood cells per 100 ml of blood and therefore fluctuates with changes not only in the total red blood cell count (hemoglobin) but also with blood volume. Elevated levels of hematocrit (which may be related to dehydration) indicate increased viscosity of blood that can potentially impede blood flow to tissues.[12] Hemoglobin is essential for the adequate oxygen-carrying capacity of the blood. A decrease in hemoglobin and hematocrit levels (10% below normal is called anemia) may decrease activity tolerance or make patients more susceptible to ischemia secondary to decreased oxygen-carrying capacity.[11,27] Slight decreases in hematocrit due to adaptations to exercise (with no change in hemoglobin) are related to increases in blood volume. The concomitant exercise-related decreases in blood viscosity may be beneficial to post-MI patients.[28]

Elevated white blood cell counts can indicate that the body is fighting infection, or they can occur with inflammation caused by cell death, such as in MI. Erythocyte sedimentation rate (ESR), another hematologic test, is a nonspecific index of inflammation and is commonly elevated for 2–3 weeks after MI.[27] Refer to Chapter 6 for more information about these values.

### Coagulation Profiles

Coagulation profiles provide information about the clotting time of blood. Patients who undergo treatment with thrombolytic therapy after the initial stages of MI or who are receiving anticoagulant therapy owing to various cardiac arrhythmias require coagulation profiles to monitor anticoagulation in an attempt to prevent complications, such as bleeding. The physician determines the patient's therapeutic range of anticoagulation by using the prothrombin time (PT), partial thromboplastin time, and international normalized ratio.[27] Refer to Chapter 6 for details regarding these values and their significance to treatment.

Patients with low PT and partial thromboplastin time are at higher risk of thrombosis, especially if they have arrhythmias (e.g., atrial fibrillation) or valvular conditions (mitral regurgitation) that produce stasis of the blood. Patients with a PT greater than 2.5 times the reference range should not undergo physical therapy because of the potential for spontaneous bleeding. Likewise, an international normalized ratio of more than 3 warrants asking the physician if treatment should be withheld.[27]

### Blood Lipids

Elevated total cholesterol levels in the blood are a significant risk factor for atherosclerosis and therefore ischemic heart disease.[29] Measuring blood cholesterol level is necessary to determine the risk for development of atherosclerosis and to assist in patient education, dietary modification, and medical management. Normal values can be adjusted for age; however, levels of more than 240 mg/dl are generally considered high, and levels of less than 200 mg/dl are considered normal.

A blood lipid analysis categorizes cholesterol into *high-density lipoprotiens* (HDLs) and *low-density lipoproteins* (LDLs) and provides an analysis of *triglycerides*.

HDLs are formed by the liver and are considered beneficial because they are readily transportable and do not adhere to the intimal walls of the vascular system. People with higher amounts of HDLs are at lower risk for coronary artery disease.[27,29] HDL levels of less than 33 mg/dl carry an elevated risk of heart disease, and a more important risk for heart disease is an elevated ratio of total cholesterol to HDL. Normal total cholesterol to HDL ratios range from 3 to 5.[12]

LDLs are formed by a diet excessive in fat and are related to a higher incidence of coronary artery disease. Low-density lipoproteins are not as readily transportable, because they adhere to intimal walls in the vascular system.[27] Normal LDLs are below 100 mg/dl.[12]

Triglycerides are fat cells that are free floating in the blood. When not in use, they are stored in adipose tissue. Their levels increase after eating foods high in fat and decrease with exercise. High levels of triglycerides are associated with a risk of coronary heart disease.[27]

---

Clinical Tip

Cholesterol levels may be falsely elevated after an acute MI; therefore, pre-infarction levels (if known) are used to guide risk factor modification. Values will not return to normal until at least 6 weeks post-MI.

---

Biochemical Markers

After an initial myocardial insult, the presence of tissue necrosis can be determined by increased levels of biochemical markers. Levels of biochemical markers, such as serum enzymes (creatine kinase [CK], lactate dehydrogenase [LDH]) and proteins (myoglobin, troponin I and T), can also be used to determine the extent of myocardial death and the effectiveness of reperfusion therapy. In patients presenting with specific anginal symptoms and diagnostic ECG, these biochemical markers assist with confirmation of the diagnosis of an MI (Table 1-11). Enzymes play a more essential role in medical assessment of the many patients with nonspecific or vague symptoms and inconclusive ECG changes.[30] Such analysis also includes evaluation of isoenzyme levels as well.[31] *Isoenzymes* are different chemical forms of the same enzyme that are tissue specific and allow differentiation of damaged tissue (e.g., skeletal muscle vs. cardiac muscle).

*CK* (formally called *creatine phosphokinase*) is released after cell injury or cell death. CK has three isoenzymes. The CK-MB isoenzyme is related to cardiac muscle cell injury or death. The most widely used

**Table 1-11.** Biochemical Markers

| Enzyme or Marker | Isoenzyme | Normal Value | Onset of Rise (hrs) | Time of Peak Rise | Return to Normal |
|---|---|---|---|---|---|
| Creatine kinase (CK) | | 55–71 IU | 3–6 | 12–24 hrs | 24–48 hrs |
| | CK-MB | 0–3% | 4–8 | 18–24 hrs | 72 hrs |
| Lactate dehydrogenase | | 127 IU | 12–24 | 72 hrs | 5–14 days |
| | LDH-1 | 14–26% | 24–72 | 3–4 days | 10–14 days |
| Troponin T (cTnT) | — | <0.2 µg/ liter | 2–4 | 24–36 hrs | 10–14 days |
| Troponin I (cTnI) | — | <3.1 µg/ liter | 2–4 | 24–36 hrs | 10–14 days |
| Myoglobin | — | 31–80 ng/ml | 1–2 | 6–9 hrs | 24–36 hrs |

Sources: Data from RH Christenson, HME Azzazy. Biochemical markers of the acute coronary syndromes. Clin Chem 1998;44:1855–1864; and AK Kratz, KB Leqand–Rowski. Normal reference laboratory values. N Engl J Med 1998;339:1063–1072.

value is the *relative index* (100%[CK-MB/Total CK]).[30] Temporal measurements of the CK-MB relative index help physicians diagnose MI, estimate the size of infarction, evaluate the occurrence of reperfusion as well as possible infarct extension. An early CK-MB peak with rapid clearance is a good indication of reperfusion.[12] Values may increase from skeletal muscle trauma, cardiopulmonary resuscitation, defibrillation, and open-heart surgery. Postoperative coronary artery bypass surgery tends to elevate CK-MB levels secondary to cross-clamp time. Early postoperative peaks and rapid clearance seem to indicate reversible damage, whereas later peaks and longer clearance times with peak values exceeding 50 U/liter may indicate an MI.[12] Treatment with thrombolytic therapy, such as streptokinase or a tissue plasminogen activator (tPa), has been shown to falsely elevate the values and may create a second peak of CK-MB, which strongly suggests successful reperfusion.[12,30]

Troponins are essential contractile proteins found in both skeletal and cardiac muscle. *Troponin I* is an isotype found exclusively in the myocardium and is therefore 100% cardiac specific. *Troponin T* is another isotype, and although it is sensitive to cardiac damage, it also rises with muscle and renal failure.[30] These newer markers are emerging as sensitive and cardiac specific clinical indicators for diagnosis of MI and for risk stratification.

*Myoglobin* is an $O_2$-binding heme protein in both cardiac and skeletal muscle. Although myoglobin is good for identifying acute MI in the early stages, skeletal muscle origin needs to be ruled out. One mechanism of ruling out skeletal muscle damage is a rise in carbonic anhydrase. Carbonic anhydrase only rises with skeletal muscle damage, and its rise is early, very similar to myoglobin. Some have advocated a ratio of myoglobin and carbonic anhydrase to diagnose acute MI.[12]

*LDH* is also released after cell injury or death. LDH has five isoenzymes. LDH-1 is specific for cardiac muscle injury. Testing for LDH-1 is valuable for determining myocardial injury in patients admitted a few days after the initial onset of chest pain, because it takes approximately 3 days to peak and may stay elevated for 5–14 days.[27]

---

Clinical Tip

• Physical therapy geared toward testing functional capacity or increasing the patient's activity should be withheld until CK-MB levels have peaked and begun to fall.
• It is best to await the final diagnosis of location, size, and type of MI before active physical therapy treatment. This allows for rest and time for the control of possible post-MI complications.

---

**Arterial Blood Gas Measurements**

Arterial blood gas measurement may be used to evaluate the oxygenation ($Pao_2$), ventilation ($Paco_2$), and pH in patients during acute MI and exacerbations of congestive heart failure (CHF) in certain situations (i.e., obvious tachypnea, low $Sao_2$). These evaluations can help determine the need for supplemental oxygen therapy and mechanical ventilatory support in these patients. Oxygen is the first drug provided during a suspected MI. Refer to Chapter 2 and Appendix III-A for further description of arterial blood gas interpretation and supplemental oxygen, respectively.

**Chest Radiography**

Chest x-ray can be ordered for patients to assist in the diagnosis of CHF or cardiomegaly (enlarged heart). Patients in CHF have an increased density in pulmonary vasculature markings, giving the appearance of congestion in the vessels.[4,7] Refer to Chapter 2 for further description of chest x-rays.

## Echocardiography

Transthoracic echocardiography or "cardiac echo" is a noninvasive procedure that uses ultrasound to evaluate the function of the heart. Evaluation includes the size of the ventricular cavity, the thickness and integrity of the septum, valve integrity, and the motion of individual segments of the ventricular wall. Volumes of the ventricles are quantified, and EF can be estimated.[4]

Transesophageal echocardiography is a newer technique that provides a better view of the mediastinum in cases of pulmonary disease, chest wall abnormality, and obesity, which make standard echocardiography difficult.[12,32] For this test, the oropharynx is anesthesized and the patient is given enough sedation to be relaxed but still awake since he or she needs to cooperate by swallowing the catheter. The catheter, a piezoelectric crystal mounted on an endoscope, is passed into the esophagus. Specific indications for transthoracic echocardiography include bacterial endocarditis, aortic dissection, regurgitation through or around a prosthetic mitral or tricuspid valve, left atrial thrombus, intracardiac source of an embolus, and interarterial septal defect. Patients usually fast for at least 4 hours prior to the procedure.[32]

Principal indications for echocardiography are to assist in the diagnosis of pericardial effusion, cardiac tamponade, idiopathic or hypertrophic cardiomyopathy, a variety of valvular diseases, intracardiac masses, ischemic cardiac muscle, left ventricular aneurysm, ventricular thrombi, and a variety of congenital heart diseases.[12]

Transthoracic echocardiography can also be performed during or immediately following bicycle or treadmill exercise to identify ischemia-induced wall motion abnormalities or during a pharmacologically induced exercise stress test (e.g., a dobutamine stress echocardiograph [DSE]). This *stress echocardiograph* adds to the information obtained from standard stress tests (ECGs) and may be used as an alternative to nuclear scanning procedures. Transient depression of wall motion during or after stress suggests ischemia.[33]

### Contrast Echocardiograph

The ability of the echocardiograph to diagnose perfusion abnormalities and myocardial chambers is improved by using an intravenously injected contrast agent. The contrast allows greater visualization of wall motion and wall thickness, and calculation of EF.[34]

*Dobutamine Stress Echocardiograph*
Dobutamine is a potent alpha-1 ($\alpha_1$) agonist and a beta-receptor agonist with prominent inotropic and less-prominent chronotropic effects on the myocardium. Dobutamine (which—unlike persantine—increases contractility, HR, and BP in a manner similar to exercise) is injected in high doses into subjects as an alternative to exercise.[33] Dobutamine infusion is increased in a stepwise fashion similar to an exercise protocol. The initial infusion is 0.01 mg/kg and is increased 0.01 mg/kg every 3 minutes until a maximum infusion of 0.04 mg/kg is reached. This infusion is maintained for 5 minutes for a total dose of approximately 0.38 mg/kg. Typically, the echocardiograph image of wall motion is obtained during the final minute(s) of infusion. This image can then be compared to baseline recordings.[33] If needed, atropine is occasionally added to facilitate a greater HR response for the test.[33] Low-dose DSE has the capacity to evaluate the contractile response of the impaired myocardium. Bellardinelli et al.[35] have demonstrated that improvements in functional capacity after exercise can be predicted by low dose DSE. Patients with a positive contractile response to dobutamine were more likely to increase their $\dot{V}o_2$max after a 10-week exercise program. Having a positive contractile response on the low-dose DSE had a positive predictive value of 84% and a negative predictive value of 59%.[35] With research such as this study beginning to demonstrate the prognostic value of certain medical tests for determining functional prognosis, physical therapists will need to be prepared to critically assess this area of literature in order to assist the medical team in determining the level of rehabilitative care for a patient during his or her recovery.

## Exercise Testing
Exercise testing, or stress testing, is a noninvasive method of assessing cardiovascular responses to increased activity. The use of exercise testing in cardiac patients can serve multiple purposes, which are not mutually exclusive. The most widespread use of exercise testing is as a diagnostic tool for the presence of coronary artery disease. Other uses include determining prognosis and severity of disease, evaluating the effectiveness of treatment, early

detection of labile hypertension, evaluation of CHF, evaluation of arrhythmias, and evaluation of functional capacity.[33] Exercise testing involves the systematic and progressive increase in intensity of activity (e.g., treadmill walking, bicycling, stair climbing, arm ergometry). These tests are accompanied by simultaneous ECG analysis, BP measurements, and subjective reports, commonly using Borg's Rating of Perceived Exertion (RPE).[36,37] Occasionally, the use of expired gas analysis can provide useful information about pulmonary function and maximal oxygen consumption.[33] Submaximal tests, such as the 12- and 6-minute walk tests, can be performed to assess a patient's function. For further discussion of the 6-minute walk test, refer to Appendix IX.

*Submaximal tests* differ from *maximal tests* because the patient is not pushed to his or her maximum HR; instead, the test is terminated at a predetermined end point, usually at 75% of the patient's predicted maximum HR.[38] For a comparison of two widely used exercise test protocols and functional activities, refer to Table 1-12. For a more thorough description of submaximal exercise testing, the reader is referred to Noonan and Dean.[38]

Contraindications to exercise testing include the following[39]:

- Recent MI (less than 48 hours earlier)

- Acute pericarditis

- Unstable angina

- Ventricular or rapid arrhythmias

- Untreated second- or third-degree heart block

- Decompensated CHF

- Acute illness

Exercise test results can be used for the design of an exercise prescription. Based on the results, the patient's actual or extrapolated maximum HR can be used to determine the patient's target HR range and a safe activity intensity. RPE with symptoms during the exercise test can also be used to gauge exercise or activity intensity. (Especially in subjects on beta-blockers—please refer to the Physical Therapy Intervention section of this chapter for a discussion on the use of RPE.)

**Table 1-12.** Comparison of Exercise Test Protocols and Functional Tasks—
Energy Demands

| Oxygen Requirements (ml $O_2$/kg/min) | Metabolic Equivalents (METS) | Functional Tasks | Treadmill: Bruce Protocol 3-Min Stages (mph/elevation) | Bike Ergometer: for 70 kg of Body Weight (kg/min) |
|---|---|---|---|---|
| 52.5 | 15 | | | |
| 49.5 | 14 | | | |
| 45.5 | 13 | | 4.2/16.0 | 1,500 |
| 42.0 | 12 | | | 1,350 |
| 38.5 | 11 | | | 1,200 |
| 35.0 | 10 | Jogging ↑ | | |
| | | | 3.4/14.0 | 1,050 |
| 31.5 | 9 | ↓ | | |
| | | | | 900 |
| 28.0 | 8 | | | |
| | | | | 750 |
| 24.5 | 7 | ↑ | 2.5/12.0 | |
| 21.0 | 6 | Stair climbing | | 600 |
| 17.5 | 5 | ↓  ↑ | 1.7/10.0 | 450 |
| 14.0 | 4 | Walking (level surface) | | 300 |
| 10.5 | 3 | ↓ | | |
| | | | | 150 |
| 7.0 | 2 | Bed exercise (arm exercises in supine or sitting) | | |

Sources: Data from American Heart Association, Committee on Exercise. Exercise Testing and Training of Apparently Healthy Individuals: A Handbook for Physicians. Dallas, 1972; and GA Brooks, TD Fahey, TP White (eds). Exercise Physiology: Human Bioenergetics and Its Applications (2nd ed). Mountain View, CA: Mayfield Publishing, 1996.

---

**Clinical Tip**

Synonyms for exercise tests include exercise tolerance test and graded exercise test.

---

*Thallium Stress Testing*
*Thallium stress testing* is a stress test that involves the injection of a radioactive nuclear marker for the detection of myocardial perfusion. The injection is typically given (via an intravenous line) during peak exercise or when symptoms are reported during the stress test. After the test, the subject is passed under a nuclear scanner to be evaluated for myocardial perfusion by assessment of the distribution of thallium uptake. The subject then returns 3–4 hours later to be re-evaluated for myocardial reperfusion. This test appears to be more sensitive than stress tests without thallium for identifying patients with coronary artery disease.[12]

*Persantine Thallium Stress Testing*
*Persantine thallium stress testing* is the use of dipyridamole (Persantine) to dilate coronary arteries. Coronary arteries with atherosclerosis do not dilate; therefore, dipyridamole shunts blood away from these areas. It is typically used in patients who are very unstable, deconditioned, or unable to ambulate or cycle for exercise-based stress testing.[33] Patients are asked to avoid all food and drugs containing methylxanthines (e.g., coffee, tea, chocolate, cola drinks) for at least 6 hours prior to the test as well as phosphodiesterase drugs, such as aminophyline, for 24 hours. While the patient is supine, an infusion of dipyridamole (0.56 ml/kg diluted in saline) is given intravenously over 4 minutes (a large-vein intracatheter is used). Four minutes after the infusion is completed, the perfusion marker (thallium) is injected, and the patient is passed under a nuclear scanner to be evaluated for myocardial perfusion by assessment of the distribution of thallium uptake.[33]

**Cardiac Catheterization**
Cardiac catheterization, classified as either right or left, is an invasive procedure that involves passing a flexible, radiopaque catheter into the heart to visualize chambers, valves, coronary arteries, great vessels, cardiac pressures and volumes to evaluate cardiac function (estimate EF, CO).

The procedure is also used in the following diagnostic and therapeutic techniques[12]:

- Angiography
- Percutaneous transluminal coronary angioplasty (PTCA)
- Electrophysiologic studies (EPSs)
- Cardiac muscle biopsy

Right-sided catheterization involves entry through a sheath that is inserted into a vein (commonly subclavian) for evaluation of right heart pressures; calculation of CO; and angiography of the right atrium, right ventricle, tricuspid valve, pulmonic valve, and pulmonary artery.[12] It is also used for continuous hemodynamic monitoring in patients with present or very recent heart failure to monitor cardiac pressures (see Appendix III-A). Indications for right heart catheterization include an intracardiac shunt (blood flow between right and left atria or right and left ventricles), myocardial dysfunction, pericardial constriction, pulmonary vascular disease, valvular heart disease, and status post–heart transplant.

Left-sided catheterization involves entry through a sheath that is inserted into an artery (commonly femoral) to evaluate the aorta, left atrium, and left ventricle; left ventricular function; mitral and aortic valve function; and angiography of coronary arteries. Indications for left heart catheterization include aortic dissection, atypical angina, cardiomyopathy, congenital heart disease, coronary artery disease, status post MI, valvular heart disease, and status post heart transplant.

---

### Clinical Tip

- After catheterization, the patient is on bed rest for approximately 4–6 hours when venous access is performed or for 6–8 hours when arterial access is performed.[12]
- The sheaths are typically removed from the vessel 4–6 hours after the procedure, and pressure is applied constantly for 20 minutes following sheath removal.[12]
- The extremity should remain immobile with a sandbag over the access site to provide constant pressure to reduce the risk of vascular complications.[12]

- Some hospitals may use a knee immobilizer to assist with immobilizing the lower extremity.
- Physical therapy intervention should be deferred or limited to bedside treatment within the limitations of these precautions.
- During the precautionary period, physical therapy intervention, such as bronchopulmonary hygiene or education, may be necessary. Bronchopulmonary hygiene is indicated if there are pulmonary complications or if risk of these complications exists. Education is warranted when the patient is anxious and needs to have questions answered regarding his or her functional mobility.
- After the precautionary period, normal mobility can progress to the limit of the patient's cardiopulmonary impairments; however, the catheterization results should be incorporated into the physical therapy treatment plan.

## Angiography

Angiography involves the injection of radiopaque contrast material through a catheter to visualize vessels or chambers. Different techniques are used for different assessments[12]: *Aortography* is used to assess the aorta and aortic valve. *Coronary arteriography* is used to assess the coronary arteries. *Pulmonary angiography* is used to assess the pulmonary circulation. *Ventriculography* is used to assess the right or left ventricle and AV valves.

## Electrophysiologic Studies

EPSs are performed to evaluate the electrical conduction system of the heart.[12] An electrode catheter is inserted through the femoral vein into the right ventricle apex. Continuous ECG monitoring is performed both internally and externally. The electrode can deliver programmed electrical stimulation to evaluate conduction pathways, formation of arrhythmias, and the automaticity and refractoriness of cardiac muscle cells. EPSs evaluate the effectiveness of antiarrhythmic medication and can provide specific information about each segment of the conduction system.[12] In many hospitals, these studies may be combined with a therapeutic procedure, such as an ablation procedure (discussed later in this chapter, in the Management section). Indications for EPSs include the following[12]:

- Sinus node disorders
- AV or intraventricular block
- Previous cardiac arrest
- Tachycardia at greater than 200 bpm
- Unexplained syncope

---

**Clinical Tip**

Patients undergoing EPS should remain on bed rest for 4–6 hours after the test.

---

## Pathophysiology

When disease and degenerative changes impair the heart's capacity to perform work, a reduction in CO occurs. If cardiac, renal, or central nervous system perfusion is reduced, a vicious cycle resulting in heart failure can ensue. A variety of pathologic processes can impair the heart's capacity to perform work. These pathologic processes can be divided into four major categories: (1) myocardial ischemia and infarction, (2) rhythm and conduction disturbance, (3) valvular heart disease, and (4) myocardial and pericardial heart disease. CHF occurs when this failure to pump blood results in an increase in the fluid in the lungs, liver, subcutaneous tissues, and serous cavities.[5]

### Myocardial Ischemia and Infarction

When myocardial oxygen demand is higher than supply, the myocardium must use anaerobic metabolism to meet energy demands. This system can be maintained for only a short period of time before tissue ischemia will occur, which typically results in angina (chest pain). If the supply and demand are not balanced by rest, medical management, surgical intervention, or any combination of these, injury of the myocardial tissue will ensue, followed by infarction (cell death). This balance of supply and demand is achieved in individuals with normal coronary circulation; however, it is compromised in individuals with impaired coronary blood flow. The following pathologies can result in myocardial ischemia:

- Coronary arterial spasm is a disorder of transient spasm of coronary vessels that impairs blood flow to the myocardium. It can occur with or without the presence of atherosclerotic coronary disease. It results in variant angina (Prinzmetal's angina).[12]

- Coronary atherosclerotic disease (CAD) is a multistep process of the deposition of fatty streaks or plaques on artery walls (atherosis). The presence of these deposits eventually leads to arterial wall damage and platelet and macrophage aggregation that then leads to thrombus formation and hardening of the arterial walls (sclerosis). The net effect is a narrowing of coronary walls. It can result in stable or unstable angina (UA), or MI.[4,5,12]

Clinical syndromes caused by these pathologies are the following[7,12]: *Stable (exertional) angina* occurs with increased myocardial demand, such as during exercise, is relieved by reducing exercise intensity or terminating exercise, and responds well to nitroglycerin. *Variant angina (Prinzmetal's angina)* is a less-common form of angina caused by coronary artery spasm. This form of angina tends to be prolonged, severe, and not readily relieved by nitroglycerin.

*UA* is considered intermediate in severity between stable angina and MI. It usually has a sudden onset, occurs at rest or with activity below the patient's usual ischemic baseline, and may be different from the patient's usual anginal pattern. It is not induced by activity or increased myocardial demand that cannot be met. It can be induced at rest, when supply is cut down with no change in demand. A common cause of UA is believed to be a rupture of an atherosclerotic plaque.

*MI* occurs with prolonged or unmanaged ischemia. It is important to realize that there is an evolution from *ischemia* to *infarction.* Ischemia is the first phase of tissue response when the myocardium is deprived of oxygen. It is reversible if sufficient oxygen is provided in time. However, if oxygen deprivation continues, myocardial cells will become injured and eventually will die (infarct). The location and extent of cell death are determined by the coronary artery that is compromised and the amount of time that the cells are deprived. Refer to Table 1-13 for common types of MI and their complications. Figure 1-9 provides a schematic of possible clinical courses for patients admitted with chest pain.

Table 1-13.  Myocardial Infarctions (MIs)

| MI/Wall Affected | Possible Occluded Coronary Artery | Possible Complications |
|---|---|---|
| Anterior MI/ anterior left ventricle | Left coronary | Left-sided CHF, pulmonary edema, bundle branch block, AV block, and ventricular aneurysm (which can lead to CHF, dysrhythmias, and embolism) |
| Inferior MI/ inferior left ventricle | Right coronary (RCA) | AV blocks (which can result in bradycardia) and papillary muscle dysfunction (which can result in valvular insufficiency and eventually CHF) |
| Anterolateral MI/anterolateral left ventricle | Left anterior descending (LAD), circumflex | Brady or tachyarrhythmias, acute ventricular septal defect |
| Anteroseptal MI/septal region— between left and right ventricles | LAD | Brady or tachyarrhythmias, ventricular aneurysm |
| Posterior MI/ posterior heart | RCA, circumflex | Bradycardia, heart blocks |
| Right ventricular MI | RCA | Right ventricular failure (can lead to left ventricular failure and therefore cardiogenic shock), heart blocks, hepatomegaly, peripheral edema |
| Transmural MI (Q-wave MI) | Any artery | Full wall thickness MI, as above |
| Subendocardial MI (non–Q-wave MI) | Any artery | Partial wall thickness MI, as above, potential to extend to transmural MI |

AV = atrioventricular; CHF = congestive heart failure; LAD = left anterior descending; RCA = right coronary artery.

Source: Data from SL Woods, ES Sivarajian-Froelicher, S Underhill-Motzer (eds). Cardiac Nursing (4th ed). Philadelphia: Lippincott, 2000.

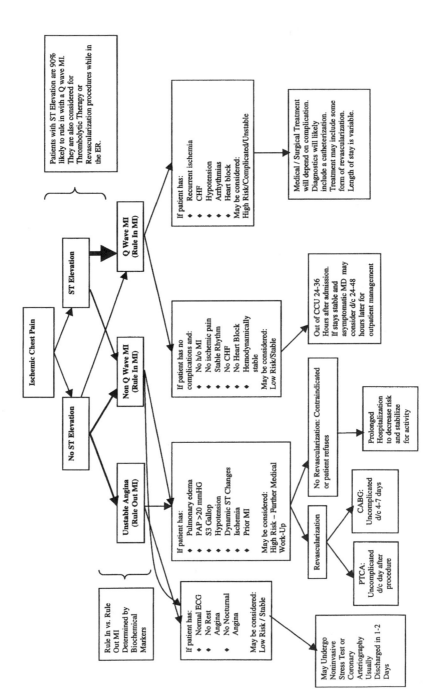

Clinical Tip

- (ST) depression, on a patient's ECG, of approximately 1–2 mm is generally indicative of ischemia.
- ST elevation is generally indicative of myocardial injury or infarction.

*Rhythm and Conduction Disturbance*

Rhythm and conduction disturbances can range from minor alterations with no hemodynamic effects to life-threatening episodes with rapid hemodynamic compromise.[4,5,7] Refer to Chapter Appendix 1-A for a description of atrial, ventricular, and junctional rhythms and AV blocks. Refer also to Chapter Appendix 1-B for examples of common rhythm disturbances. Physical therapists need to be able to identify abnormalities in the ECG to determine patient tolerance to activity. In particular, physical therapists should understand progressions of common ECG abnormalities so they can identify, early on, when the patient is not tolerating an intervention. (Refer to the Physical Therapy Intervention section for the ECG discussion.)

◀ **Figure 1-9.** *Possible clinical course of patients admitted with chest pain. (CABG = coronary artery bypass graft; CHF = congestive heart failure; CCU = coronary care unit; d/c = discharge; ECG = electrocardiogram; h/o = history of; MI = myocardial infarction; PAP = pulmonary arterial pressure; PTCA = percutaneous transluminal coronary angioplasty; ST Elevation = electrocardiogram that shows elevation of the ST segment.) (Data from American College of Cardiology/American Heart Association. 1999 Update: ACC/AHA guidelines for the management of patients with acute myocardial infarction: executive summary and recommendations. Circulation 1999;100:1016–1030; American College of Cardiology/American Heart Association. ACC/AHA guidelines for the management of patients with acute myocardial infarction. J Am Coll Cardiol 1996;28:1328–1428; and American College of Cardiology/ American Heart Association. ACC/AHA guidelines for the management of patients with unstable angina and non-ST segment elevation myocardial infarction. J Am Coll Cardiol 2000;36:971–1048.)*

A common form of rhythm disturbance is a *PVC*, which also can be referred to as a *ventricular premature beat*. These abnormalities originate from depolarization of a cluster of cells in the ventricle (an *ectopic foci*), which results in ventricular depolarization. From the term *ectopic foci*, PVCs may be refered to as *ventricular ectopy*.

### Valvular Heart Disease

Valvular heart disease encompasses valvular disorders of one or more of the four valves of the heart. The following three disorders can occur[4,5]:

1. *Stenosis* involves the narrowing of the valve.

2. *Regurgitation*, the back flow of blood through the valve, occurs with incomplete valve closure.

3. *Prolapse* involves enlarged valve cusps. The cusps can become floppy and bulge backward. This condition may progress to regurgitation.

Over time, these disorders can lead to pumping dysfunction and, ultimately, heart failure.

Refer to Table 1-14 for common valvular heart diseases and a description of their signs and symptoms.

### Myocardial and Pericardial Heart Disease

Myocardial heart disease affects the myocardial muscle tissue and can also be referred to as *cardiomyopathy*; pericardial heart diseases affect the pericardium. Refer to Tables 1-15 and 1-16 for common myocardial and pericardial diseases.

### Heart Failure

*Heart failure*, a decrease of CO, can be caused by a variety of cardiac pathologies. Because CO is not maintained, life cannot be sustained if heart failure continues without treatment. Heart failure results in the congestion of the pulmonary circulation and, in certain cases, even the systemic circulation. Therefore, it is commonly referred to as *CHF*. The

**Table 1-14.** Signs and Symptoms of Valvular Heart Diseases

| Disease | Symptoms | Signs |
|---|---|---|
| Aortic stenosis | Angina, syncope or near syncope, signs of left ventricle failure (dyspnea, orthopnea, cough). | Elevated left ventricular wall pressure, decreased subendocardial blood flow, systolic murmur, ventricular hypertrophy |
| Chronic aortic regurgitation | Angina, symptoms of left ventricular failure. | Dilated aortic root, dilated left ventricle, diastolic murmur, left ventricular hypertrophy |
| Acute aortic regurgitation | Rapid progression of symptoms of left ventricular failure, pulmonary edema, angina. | Sinus tachycardia to compensate for decreased stroke volume, loud S3, diastolic murmur, signs of ventricular failure |
| Mitral stenosis | Symptoms of pulmonary vascular congestion (dyspnea, orthopnea). If patient develops pulmonary hypertension (which can cause hypoxia, hypotension), he or she may have angina, syncope. | Left atrial hypertrophy, pulmonary hypertension, atrial fibrillation, can have embolus formation (especially if in atrial fibrillation), long diastolic murmur |
| Chronic mitral regurgitation | Symptoms of pulmonary vascular congestion, angina, syncope, fatigue. | Left atrial enlargement, atrial fibrillation, elevated left atrial pressure |
| Acute mitral regurgitation | Rapid progression of symptoms of pulmonary vascular congestion. | Sinus tachycardia, presence of S3 or S4, pulmonary edema |
| Mitral valve prolapse | Most commonly asymptomatic, fatigue, palpitation. | Systolic click, may have tachyarrhythmia syncope |

Sources: Data from SL Woods, ES Sivarajian-Froelicher, S Underhill-Motzer (eds). Cardiac Nursing (4th ed). Philadelphia: Lippincott, 2000; and MD Cheitlin, M Sokolow, MB McIlroy. Clinical Cardiology (6th ed). Norwalk, CT: Appleton & Lange, 1993.

Table 1-15.  Myocardial Diseases—Cardiomyopathies

**Functional Classification**

| Cardiomyopathy | Dysfunction | Description |
| --- | --- | --- |
| Dilated | Systolic | Ventricle is dilated, and there is marked contractile dysfunction of myocardium. |
| Hypertrophic | Diastolic | Thickened ventricular myocardium, less compliant to filling, and therefore decreased filling during diastole. |
| Restrictive | Systolic and diastolic | Endocardial scarring of ventricles, decreased compliance during diastole, and decreased contractile force during systole. |

**Etiologic Classification**

| Etiology | Examples | Etiology | Examples |
| --- | --- | --- | --- |
| Inflammatory | Viral infarction, bacterial infarction | Infiltrative | Sarcoidosis, neoplastic |
| | | Hematologic | Sickle cell anemia |
| Metabolic | Selenium deficiency, diabetes mellitus | Toxic | Alcohol, bleomycin |
| | | Physical agents | Heat stroke, hypothermia, radiation |
| Fibroplastic | Carcinoid fibrosis, endomyocardial fibrosis | Miscellaneous acquired | Postpartum cardiomyopathy, obesity |
| | | | Status post myocardial infarction |
| Hypersensitivity | Cardiac transplant rejection, methyldopa | Ischemic | |
| Genetic | Hypertrophic cardiomyopathy, Duchenne's muscular dystrophy | | |
| Idiopathic | Idiopathic hypertrophic cardiomyopathy | | |

Source: Adapted from L Cahalin. Cardiac Muscle Dysfunction. In EA Hillegass, HS Sadowsky (eds). Essentials of Cardiopulmonary Physical Therapy (2nd ed). Philadelphia: Saunders, 2001.

**Table 1-16.** Signs and Symptoms of Pericardial Heart Diseases

| Disease | Symptoms | Signs |
|---|---|---|
| Acute pericarditis | Retrosternal chest pain (worsened by supine and/or deep inspiration), dyspnea, cough, hoarseness, dysphagia, fever, chills, and weakness may occur. | Pericardial friction rub; diffuse ST segment elevation; decreased QRS voltage in all ECG leads if pericardial effusion also present |
| Constrictive pericarditis | Abdominal swelling, peripheral edema, fatigue, dyspnea, dizziness and/or syncope, signs of pulmonary venous congestion, vague non-specific retrosternal chest pain. | Jugular venous distention; QRS voltage diminished on ECG; occasionally atrial fibrillation |
| Chronic pericardial effusion (without tamponade) | May have vague fullness in anterior chest, cough, hoarseness, dysphagia. | Muffled heart sounds; may have pericardial friction rub; QRS voltage diminished on ECG; chest x-ray with cardiomegaly without pulmonary congestion |
| Pericardial tamponade | Symptoms of low cardiac output (dyspnea, fatigue, dizziness, syncope); may have retrosternal chest pain; may have cough, hiccoughs, hoarseness. | Jugular venous distention, cardiomegaly, diminished QRS voltage on ECG; becomes tamponade from effusion when right heart catheterization shows equal pressures in right atrium, ventricle, and capillary wedge (signifies left atria pressure), and left heart catheterization would show equal pressure on left side of heart to right side |

ECG = electrocardiogram.
Sources: Data from SL Woods, ES Sivarajian-Froelicher, S Underhill-Motzer (eds). Cardiac Nursing (4th ed). Philadelphia: Lippincott, 2000; and MD Cheitlin, M Sokolow, MB McIlroy. Clinical Cardiology (6th ed). Norwalk, CT: Appleton & Lange, 1993.

most common pathologic etiology of CHF is some type of cardiomyopathy (see Table 1-15).

The following terms are used to classify the types of cardiac impairment in CHF[42]:

*Left-sided heart failure* refers to failure of the left ventricle, resulting in back flow into the lungs.

*Right-sided failure* refers to failure of the right side of the heart, resulting in back flow into the systemic venous system.

*High-output failure* refers to heart failure that is secondary to renal system failure to filter off excess fluid. The renal system failure places a higher load on the heart that cannot be maintained.

*Low-output failure* refers to the condition in which the heart is not able to pump the minimal amount of blood to support circulation.

*Systolic dysfunction* refers to a problem with systole or the actual strength of myocardial contraction.

*Diastolic dysfunction* refers to a problem during diastole or the ability of the ventricle to allow the filling of blood.

Possible signs and symptoms of CHF are described in Table 1-17. The American Heart Association revised the New York Heart Association

Table 1-17. Signs and Symptoms of Congestive Heart Failure

| Symptoms | Signs |
| --- | --- |
| Dyspnea | Cold, pale possibly cyanotic extremities |
| Tachypnea | Weight gain |
| Paroxysmal nocturnal dyspnea | Peripheral edema |
| Orthopnea | Hepatomegaly |
| Cough | Jugular venous distention |
| Fatigue | Crackles (rales) |
| | Tubular breath sounds and consolidation |
| | S3 heart sound |
| | Sinus tachycardia |
| | Decreased exercise tolerance and physical work capacity |

Source: Adapted from LP Cahalin. Heart failure. Phys Ther 1996;76:520.

**Table 1-18.** American Heart Association's Functional Capacity and Objective Assessment of Patients with Diseases of the Heart

| Functional Capacity[a] | Objective Assessment[b] |
| --- | --- |
| Class I: Patients with cardiac disease but without resulting limitations of physical activity. Ordinary physical activity does not cause undue fatigue, palpitation, dyspnea, or anginal pain. | No objective evidence of cardiovascular disease |
| Class II: Patients with cardiac disease that results in a slight limitation of physical activity. Patients are comfortable at rest, but ordinary physical activity results in fatigue, palpitations, dyspnea, or anginal pain. | Objective evidence of minimal cardiovascular disease |
| Class III: Patients with cardiac disease that results in a marked limitation of physical activity. Patients are comfortable at rest, but less-than-ordinary activity causes fatigue, palpitations, dyspnea, or anginal pain. | Objective evidence of moderately severe cardiovascular disease |
| Class IV: Patients with cardiac disease that results in an inability to carry on any physical activity without discomfort. Fatigue, palpitations, dyspnea, or anginal pain may be present even at rest. If any physical activity is undertaken, symptoms increase. | Objective evidence of severe cardiovascular disease |

[a]*Functional capacity* refers to subjective symptoms of the patient. This aspect of the classification is identical to the New York Heart Association's Classification.
[b]*Objective assessment* was added to the classification system by the American Heart Association in 1994. It refers to measurements such as electrocardiograms, stress tests, echocardiograms, and radiologic images.[43]

Functional Classification of Heart Disease, and this new classification is described in Table 1-18. Activity progression for patients hospitalized with CHF is based on the ability of medical treatments (e.g., diuresis, inotropes) to keep the patient out of heart failure. When a patient with CHF is medically stabilized, the CHF is thought to be "compensated." Clinical examination findings allow the therapist to continuously evaluate the patient's tolerance to the activity progression. Although metabolic equivalent (MET) tables are not commonly used clinically, they do provide a method of progressively increasing a patient's activity level. As greater MET levels are achieved with an appropriate hemodynamic response, the next level of activity can be attempted. Table 1-12 provides MET levels for common activities that can be performed with patients.

## Management

The following section discusses surgical and nonsurgical procedures, pharmacologic interventions, and physical therapy interventions for patients with cardiac dysfunction.

### *Revascularization and Reperfusion of the Myocardium*

#### Thrombolytic Therapy

Thrombolytic therapy has been established as an acute management strategy for patients experiencing an MI because of the high prevalence of coronary artery thrombosis during acute MIs. Thrombolytic agents, characterized as fibrin-selective and nonselective agents, are administered to appropriate candidates via intravenous access. The most common agents include: streptokinase (nonselective), anisylated plasminogen streptokinase activator complex (nonselective), and tissue plasminogen activator (t-PA) (fibrin-selective).[12] Fibrin-selective agents have a high velocity of clot lysis, whereas the nonselective agents have a slower clot lysis and more prolonged systemic lytic state.

The indication for thrombolytic therapy includes chest pain that is suggestive of myocardial ischemia and is associated with acute ST segment elevation on a 12-lead ECG or a presumed new left ventricular bundle branch block. Hospital protocol regarding the time period to perform thrombolytic therapy usually varies, as clinical trials have led to some controversy.[12] Some studies show benefits only if treatment is conducted within 6 hours of symptoms, whereas others have demonstrated improvement with treatment up to 24 hours after onset of symptoms.[12]

The contraindications to thrombolytic therapy generally include patients who are at risk for excessive bleeding. Because of the variability that can occur among patients, many contraindications are considered relative cautions, and the potential benefits of therapy are weighed against the potential risks. Thrombolytic therapy is used in conjunction with other medical treatments such as aspirin, intravenous heparin, intravenous nitroglycerin, lidocaine, atropine, and a beta-blocker. As previously discussed, early peaking of CK-MB is associated with reperfusion.[12]

#### Percutaneous Revascularization Procedures

Percutaneous revascularization procedures are used to return blood flow through coronary arteries that have become occlusive secondary to atherosclerotic plaques. The following list briefly describes three percutaneous revascularization procedures[12]:

1.  *Percutaneous transluminal coronary angioplasty* (PTCA) is performed on small atherosclerotic lesions that do not completely occlude the vessel. PTCA can be performed at the time of an initial diagnostic catheterization, electively at some time after a catheterization, or urgently in the setting of an acute MI.

A sheath is inserted into the femoral, radial, or brachial artery, and a catheter is guided through the sheath into the coronary artery. A balloon system is then passed through the catheter to the lesion site. Inflations of variable pressure and duration may be attempted to reduce the lesion by at least 20% diameter with a residual narrowing of less than 50% in the vessel lumen.[12] Owing to some mild ischemia that can occur during the procedure, patients occasionally require temporary transvenous pacing, intra-aortic ballon counterpulsation, or femorofemoral cardiopulmonary bypass circulatory support during PTCA.

The use of coronary laser angioplasty, directional coronary atherectomy, and endoluminal stents was developed in response to the major limitations of PTCA, which include abrupt closure (in up to 7.3% of patients), restenosis, anatomically unsuitable lesions, chronic total occlusions, unsatisfactory results in patients with prior coronary artery bypass graft (CABG) surgery.[44]

2.  *Coronary laser angioplasty* uses laser energy to create precise ablation of plaques without thermal injury to the vessel. The laser treatment results in a more pliable lesion that responds better to balloon expansion. The use of laser angioplasty is limited owing to the expense of the equipment and a high restenosis rate (>40%).[45]

3.  *Directional coronary atherectomy* can be performed by inserting a catheter with a cutter housed at the distal end on one side of the catheter and a balloon on the other side.[12] The balloon inflates and presses the cutter against the atheroma (plaque). The cutter can then cut the atheroma and remove it from the arterial wall. This can also be performed with a laser on the tip of the catheter. Rotational ablation uses a high-speed rotating bur coated with diamond chips, creating an abrasive surface. This selectively removes atheroma due to its inelastic properties as opposed to the normal elastic tissue.[12] The debris emitted from this procedure is passed into the coronary circulation and is small enough to pass

through the capillary beds. Commonly, PTCA is used as an adjunct to this procedure to increase final coronary diameter or to allow for stent placement.

4. *Endoluminal stents* are tiny spring-like tubes that can be placed permanently into the coronary artery to increase the intraluminal diameter. Stents are occasionally necessary when initial attempts at revascularization (e.g., angioplasty) have failed.[12]

---

Clinical Tip

Refer to the Diagnostic and Laboratory Section's discussion for precautions after a catheterization procedure.

---

Transmyocardial Revascularization

In transmyocardial revascularization, a catheter with a laser tip creates transmural channels from patent coronary arteries into an area of the myocardium that is thought to be ischemic. It is intended for patients with chronic angina who, due to medical reasons, cannot have angioplasty or CABG. Theoretically, ischemia is reduced by increasing the amount of oxygenated blood in ischemic tissue. *Angiogenesis* (the growth of new blood vessels) has also been proposed as a mechanism of improvement after this procedure. Although therapists should expect improvements in functional capacity with decreased angina, the patient's risk status related to CAD or left ventricular dysfunction does not change.[46] Postcatheterization procedure precautions, as previously described, will apply after this procedure.

Coronary Artery Bypass Graft

A CABG is performed when the coronary artery has become completely occluded or when it cannot be corrected by PTCA, coronary arthrectomy, or stenting. A vascular graft is used to revascularize the myocardium. The saphenous vein and the left internal mammary artery are commonly used as vascular grafts. CABG can be performed either through a median sternotomy, which extends caudally from just inferior to the suprasternal notch to below the xiphoid process and splits the sternum longitudinally, or through a variety of minimally invasive incisions.[12]

A minimally invasive technique that is being used for CABG includes a CABG with a median sternotomy but without coronary bypass (off-pump CABG). This procedure eliminates the need for cross clamping the aorta and is desirable in patients with left ventricular dysfunction or with severe atherosclerosis.[12]

If a median sternotomy is performed instead of the minimally invasive incisions, then patients are placed on sternal precautions for at least 8 weeks. They should avoid lifting of moderate to heavy weights (e.g., greater than 10 lb) with the upper extremities.

---

### Clinical Tip

- To help patients understand this concept, inform them that a gallon of milk weighs approxminately 8.5 lb.
- Because of the sternal incision, patients are at risk of developing pulmonary complications after a CABG. The physical therapist should be aware of postoperative complication risk factors as well as postoperative indicators of poor pulmonary function. Refer to Chapter 2 and Appendix V for further description of postoperative pulmonary complications.

---

### Ablation Procedure

Catheter ablation procedures are indicated for supraventricular tachycardia, AV nodal re-entrant pathways, atrial fibrillation, atrial flutter, and some patients with certain types of ventricular tachycardia.[12] The procedure attempts to remove or isolate ectopic foci in an attempt to reduce the resultant rhythm disturbance. Radiofrequency ablation uses low-power, high-frequency AC current to destroy cardiac tissue and is the most effective technique for ablation.[12] After the ectopic foci are located under fluoroscopic guidance, the ablating catheter is positioned at the site to deliver a current for 10–60 seconds.

---

### Clinical Tip

- After an ablation procedure, the leg used for access (venous puncture site) must remain straight and immobile for 3–4 hours. If an artery was used, this time generally increases to 4–6 hours. (The exact time will depend on hospital policy.)
- Patients are sedated during the procedure and may require time after the procedure to recover.

• Most of the postintervention care is geared toward monitoring for complications. Possible complications include bleeding from the access site, cardiac tamponade from perforation, and arrhythmias.

• After a successful ablation procedure (and the initial immobility to prevent vascular complications at the access site), there are usually no activity restrictions.

### Cardiac Pacemaker Implantation and Automatic Implantable Cardiac Defibrillator

Cardiac pacemaker implantation involves the placement of a unipolar or bipolar electrode on the myocardium. This electrode is used to create an action potential in the management of certain arrhythmias. Indications for cardiac pacemaker implantation include the following[12,47,48]:

• Sinus node disorders (bradyarrhythmias [HR lower than 60 bpm])

• Atrioventricular disorders (complete heart block, Mobitz type II block)

• Tachyarrhythmias (supraventricular tachycardia, frequent ectopy)

Temporary pacing may be performed after an acute MI to help control transient arrhythmias and after a CABG. Table 1-19 classifies the various pacemakers.

One of the most critical aspects of pacer function for a physical therapist to understand is rate modulation. *Rate modulation* refers to the pacer's ability to modulate HR based on activity or physiologic demands. Not all pacers are equipped with rate modulation; therefore, some patients have HRs that may not change with activity. In pacers with rate modulation, a variety of sensors are available to allow adjustment of HR. The type of sensor used may impact the ability of the pacer to respond to various exercise modalities. For more detail, the reader is referred to the review by Sharp.[48]

### Clinical Tip

• If the pacemaker does not have rate modulation, low-level activity with small increases in metabolic demand is

**Table 1-19.** Pacemaker Classification

| First Symbol Pacing Location | Second Symbol Sensing Location | Third Symbol Response to Pacing | Fourth Symbol Programmability/ Modulation | Fifth Symbol Antitachyarrhythmia Function |
|---|---|---|---|---|
| O = None | N = None | O = None | O = None | O = None |
| A = Atrium | A = Atrium | I = Inhibited | S = Simple programmable | P = Pacing |
| V = Ventricle | V = Ventricle | T = Triggered | M = Multi- programmable | S = Shock |
| D = Dual | D = Dual | D = Dual | C = Communicating | D = Dual |
|  |  |  | R = Rate modulation |  |

Dual = atrium and ventricle can be sensed and/or paced independently; Inhibited = pending stimulus is inhibited when a spontaneous stimulation is detected; Triggered = detection of stimulus produces an immediate stimulus in the same chamber; Simple programmable = program either rate or output; Multiprogrammable = can be programmed more extensively; Communicating = has telemetry capabilities; Rate modulation = can adjust rate automatically based on one or more physiologic variables.

Source: Adapted from AD Bernstein, AJ Camm, RD Fletcher, et al. The NASPE/BPEG generic pacemaker code for antibradyarrhythmia and adaptive pacing and antitachyarrhythmia devices. PACE 1987;10:795.

preferred. Assessment of RPE, BP, and symptoms should be used to monitor tolerance.[48]

• If the pacemaker does have rate modulation, then the type of rate modulation used should be considered[48]:

• With activity sensors, HR may respond sluggishly to activities that are smooth—such as on the bicycle ergometer.

• For motion sensors, treadmill protocols should include increases in both speed and grade, as changes in grade alone may not trigger an increase in HR.

• QT sensors and ventilatory driven sensors may require longer warm-up periods owing to delayed responses to activity.

• Medication changes and electrolyte imbalance may impact responsiveness of HR with QT interval sensors.

• The upper limit of the rate modulation should be known. When HR is at the upper limit of rate modulation, BP needs to be monitored to be sure it is maintained.[48]

• In individuals who do not have rate modulated pacers, BP response can be used to gauge intensity, as shown in the following equation[48]:

$$\text{Training SBP} = (\text{SBP max} - \text{SBP rest}) \,(\text{intensity usually } 60\text{–}80\%) + \text{SBP rest}$$

• For example,

$$\text{Training SBP} = (180 - 120)([0.6 \text{ for lower limit}] \, [0.8 \text{ for upper limit}]) + 120$$

$$\text{Training SBP} = 156\text{–}168 \text{ mm Hg}$$

*Automatic implantable cardiac defibrillator* (AICD) is used to manage uncontrollable, life-threatening ventricular arrhythmias by sensing the heart rhythm and defibrillating the myocardium as necessary to return the heart to a normal rhythm. Indications for AICD include ventricular tachycardia and ventricular fibrillation.[12]

## Valve Replacement

Valve replacement is an acceptable method for treatment of valvular disease. Patients with mitral and aortic stenosis, regurgitation, or both are the primary candidates for this surgery. Like the CABG, a median sternotomy is the route of access to the heart. Common valve replacements include mitral valve replacements and aortic valve replacements. Prosthetic valves can be classified as mechanical (bileaflet and tilting disc valves are commonly used) as well as biological valves (derived from cadavers, porcine, or bovine tissue).

Mechanical valves are preferred if the patient is younger than 65 years and is already on anticoagulation therapy (commonly due to history of atrial fibrillation or embolic cerebral vascular accident). The benefit of mechanical valves is their durability and long life.[12] Mechanical valves also tend to be thrombogenic and, therefore, require lifelong adherence to anticoagulation. For this reason, they may be contraindicated in patients who have a history of previous bleeding-related problems, wish to become pregnant, or have a history of poor medication compliance. These patients may benefit from biological valves since there is no need for anticoagulation therapy. Biological valves may also be preferred in patients older than 65 years of age.[12] Postoperative procedures and recovery from mitral valve replacement and aortic valve replacement surgeries are very similar to CABG.[12]

## Dynamic Cardiomyoplasty

Dynamic cardiomyoplasty uses the latissimus dorsi muscle to provide a muscular assist to the left ventricle during systole for patients with dilated cardiomyopathies.[46] The latissimus dorsi is detached distally, moved forward, and wrapped around the left ventricle. The latissimus dorsi is mechanically paced to contract with cardiac contraction. It takes approximately 12 weeks for transformation of the latissimus dorsi's contractile structure to correspond to cardiac requirements, and patients may not receive benefit for 2–3 months.[46] Moving the latissimus dorsi may restrict the thorax and result in atelectasis, which needs to be addressed in postoperative physical therapy intervention. This procedure is reserved for patients with end-stage heart failure who have limited treatment options.[46] In light of the marginal benefits and high postoperative mortality rates, the continued use of dynamic cardiomyoplasty has recently been questioned.[49]

*Partial Left Ventriculectomy (Batista Procedure)*

The Batista procedure reduces the volume of the left ventricular chamber radius through surgical resection of a portion of the myocardium.[46] This in turn decreases wall tension and improves diastolic filling. To reduce the negative effects of mitral regurgitation, the mitral valve is repaired or replaced during the surgery. The initial study of patients receiving this procedure included individuals with New York Heart Association Class IV heart failure. Patients are generally discharged in 7 to 10 days, and low-level activity can begin as soon as the patient is hemodynamically stable, although vigorous exercise is deferred for 6 to 8 weeks postoperatively.[46] Like other relatively new, experimentally available procedures, this procedure has generally been reserved for patients with end-stage heart failure who have limited treatment options. The procedure requires a sternotomy and the concomitant sternal precautions, as discussed after CABG.

*Cardiac Transplantation*

Cardiac transplantation is an acceptable intervention for the treatment of end-stage heart disease. A growing number of facilities are performing heart transplantation, and a greater number of physical therapists are involved in the rehabilitation of pre- and post-transplant recipients. Physical therapy intervention is vital for the success of heart transplantation, as recipients have often survived a long period of convalescence both before and after surgery, rendering them deconditioned. In general, heart transplant patients are immunosuppressed and are without neurologic input to their heart. These patients rely first on the Frank-Starling mechanism to augment SV and then on the catecholamine response to augment both HR and SV. The reader is referred to Chapter 12 for information on heart and heart-lung transplantation.

*Cardiac Medications*

Cardiac medications are classified according to functional indications, drug classes, and mechanism of action. Cardiac drug classes are occasionally indicated for more than one clinical diagnosis.

The primary functional indications and descriptions are provided below. Appendix IV lists the functional indications, mechanisms of action, side effects, and the generic (trade names) of these cardiac medications.

### Anti-Ischemic Medications

Anti-ischemic drugs attempt to re-establish the balance between myocardial oxygen supply and demand.[4] To balance the supply and demand, medications can decrease HR or systemic BP or increase arterial lumen size by decreasing spasm or thrombus.

Medications that are successfully used for this task include the following[50]:

- Beta-blockers (see Appendix Table IV-12)

- Calcium channel blockers (see Appendix Table IV-14)

- Nitrates (smooth muscle cell selective) (see Appendix Table IV-24)

- Thrombolytic agents (see Appendix Table IV-29)

- Antiplatelet and anticoagulation agents (see Appendix Tables IV-10 and IV-4, respectively)

### Medications for Congestive Heart Failure

Heart failure treatment may include oral medications for a low-level chronic condition or intravenous medications for an acute and life-threatening condition. Medical management generally attempts to improve the pumping capability of the heart by reducing preload, increasing contractility, reducing afterload, or a combination of these.

Medication classes successful in achieving these goals include the following[50]:

- Diuretics (see Appendix Table IV-17)

- Positive inotropes (see Appendix Table IV-27.A,B)

- Vasodilators (see Appendix Table IV-30)

- Angiotensin-converting enzyme inhibitors (see Appendix Table IV-2)

Note: Digitalis toxicity can occur in patients taking digitalis as a positive inotrope. Refer to Table 1-20 for signs and symptoms of digitalis toxicity (digitalis level >2).

**Table 1-20.** Signs and Symptoms of Digitalis Toxicity

| System Affected | Effects |
| --- | --- |
| Central nervous system | Drowsiness, fatigue, confusion, visual disturbances |
| Cardiac system | Premature atrial and/or ventricular contractions, paroxysmal supraventricular tachycardia, ventricular tachycardia, high degrees of atrioventricular block, ventricular fibrillation |
| Gastrointestinal system | Nausea, vomiting, diarrhea |

Source: Data from SL Woods, ES Sivarajian-Froelicher, S Underhill-Motzer (eds). Cardiac Nursing (4th ed). Philadelphia: Lippincott, 2000.

## Antiarrhythmic Drugs

Antiarrhythmic drugs attempt to normalize conduction of the cardiac electrical system.[50] These drugs are classified in the following manner according to their mechanism of action:

- Class I (sodium channel blockers) (see Appendix Table IV-3)

- Class II (beta-blockers) (see Appendix Tables IV-3 and IV-13)

- Class III (refractory period alterations) (see Appendix Table IV-3)

- Class IV (calcium channel blockers) (see Appendix Tables IV-3 and IV-14)

## Antihypertensive Drugs

Antihypertensive drugs attempt to assist the body in maintenance of normotension by decreasing blood volume, dilating blood vessels, preventing constriction of blood vessels, preventing the retention of sodium, or a combination of these.

Medication classes successful in achieving these goals include the following[50]:

- Diuretics (see Appendix Table IV-17)

- Beta-blockers (see Appendix Table IV-12)

- Alpha-blockers (see Appendix Table IV-12)

- Calcium channel blockers (see Appendix Table IV-14)

- Angiotensin-converting enzyme inhibitors (see Appendix Table IV-2)
- Vasodilators (see Appendix Table IV-30)

**Lipid-Lowering Drugs**
Lipid-lowering drugs attempt to decrease lipid levels. They are usually prescribed in combination with a change in diet and exercise habits (see Appendix Table IV-22).[50] Medications successful in lowering lipid levels are the following:

- Anion exchange resin
- Fibric acid derivatives
- Hepatic 3-methylglutaryl coenzyme A reductase inhibitor
- Nicotinic acid
- Probucol
- Fish oils

*Physical Therapy Intervention*

In the acute care setting, physical therapy intervention is indicated for patients with cardiac impairments that result from CHF, MI, or status post CABG. However, a great majority of patients who receive physical therapy present with one or many other cardiac impairments or diagnoses. Given the high prevalence of cardiac disease in the elderly population and the hospital admissions for the elderly, the likelihood of working with a patient who has cardiac impairment is very high. This section discusses basic treatment guidelines for physical therapists working with patients who have present or past cardiac impairments.

*Goals*

The primary goals in treating patients with primary or secondary cardiac pathology are the following[51]:

- Assess hemodynamic response in conjunction with medical or surgical management during self-care activities and functional mobility
- Maximize activity tolerance

- Provide patient and family education regarding behavior modification and risk factor reduction (especially in patients with CAD, status post MI, PTCA, CABG, or cardiac transplant).

### Basic Concepts for the Treatment of Patients with Cardiac Dysfunction

The patient's medical or surgical status must be considered in intervention planning, because it is inappropriate to treat an unstable patient. An unstable patient is a patient who clearly requires medical intervention to stabilize a life-threatening condition. A patient's status may fluctuate on a daily or hourly basis. Table 1-21 provides general guidelines of when to withhold physical therapy (i.e., instances in which further medical care should precede physical therapy).[50] These are provided as absolute and relative indications of instability. Relative indications of instability should be considered on a case-by-case basis.

Once it is determined that a patient is stable at rest, the physical therapist is able to proceed with activity or an exercise program, or both. Figure 1-10 provides a general guide to determining whether a patient's response to activity is stable or unstable.

Everything the physical therapist asks a patient to do is an activity that requires energy and therefore needs to be supported by the cardiac system. Although an activity can be thought of in terms of absolute energy requirements (i.e., metabolic equivalents—refer to Table 1-12), an individual's response to that activity is relative to that individual's capacity. Therefore, although MET levels can be used to help guide the progression of activity, the physical therapist must be aware that even the lowest MET levels may represent near-maximal exertion for a patient or may result in an unstable physiologic response.

Unstable responses provide some indication that the patient is not able to meet physiologic demands owing to the pathologic process for the level of work that the patient is performing. In this situation, the physical therapist needs to consider the patient's response to other activities and determine whether these activities create a stable response. If it is stable, can the patient function independently doing that level of work?

For example, some patients may be stable walking 10 ft to the bathroom at one time, yet this activity may require maximal exertion for the patient and therefore should be considered too much for the patient to continue to do independently throughout the day.

If the patient's response is not stable, then the therapist should try to discern why it is not stable, along with finding out if anything can be

**Table 1-21.** Indications of Patient Instability

| Absolute Indications That the Patient Is Unstable and Treatment Should Be Withheld | Relative Indications That the Patient Is Unstable and Treatment Should Be Modified or Withheld |
|---|---|
| Decompensated congestive heart failure | Resting heart rate >100 bpm |
| Second-degree heart block coupled with premature ventricular contractions (PVCs) of ventricular tachycardia at rest | Hypertensive resting BP (systolic >160 mm Hg, diastolic >90 mm Hg) |
| Third-degree heart block | Hypotensive resting BP (systolic |
| More than 10 PVCs per min at rest | <80 mm Hg) |
| Multifocal PVCs | Myocardial infarction or exten- |
| Unstable angina pectoris with recent changes in symptoms (less than 24 hrs) and electrocardiographic changes associated with ischemia/injury | sion of infarction within the previous 2 days |
| Dissecting aortic aneurysm | Ventricular ectopy at rest |
| New onset (less than 24 hrs) of atrial fibrillation with rapid ventricular response at rest (HR >100 bpm) | Atrial fibrillation with rapid ventricular response at rest (HR >100 bpm) |
| Chest pain with new ST segment changes on ECG | Uncontrolled metabolic diseases |
|  | Psychosis or other unstable psychological condition |

BP = blood pressure; ECG = electrocardiogram; HR = heart rate.
Sources: Data from LP Cahalin. Heart failure. Phys Ther 1996;76:520; MH Ellestad. Stress Testing: Principles and Practice (4th ed) Philadelphia: FA Davis, 1996; and NK Wegener. Rehabilitation of the Patient with Coronary Heart Disease. In RC Schlant, RW Alexander (eds), Hurst's the Heart (8th ed). New York: McGraw-Hill, 1994;1227.

done to make the patient stable (i.e., medical treatment may stabilize this response). Additionally, the therapist should find the level of function that a patient could perform with a stable response. However, at times, patients will not be able to be stabilized to perform activity. In these cases, physical therapists need to determine whether a conditioning program would allow the patient to meet the necessary energy demands without becoming unstable. Proceeding with therapy at a lower level of activity is based on the premise that conditioning will improve the patient's response. The cardiac system supports the body in its attempt to provide enough energy to perform work. Often, becoming stronger—increased peripheral muscle strength and endurance—will reduce the demands on the heart at a certain absolute activity

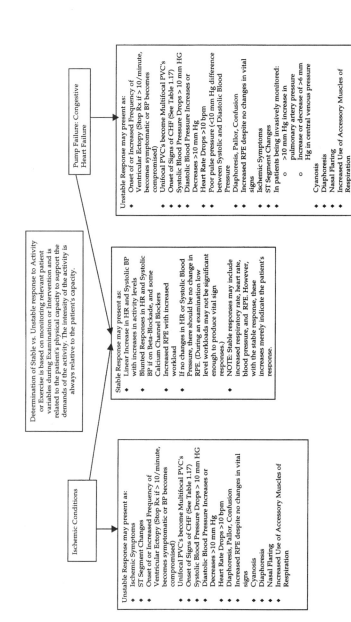

**Determination of Stable vs. Unstable response to Activity or Exercise** is based on monitoring relevant patient variables during Examination or Intervention and is related to the patient's physical capacity to support the demands of the activity. The intensity of the activity is always relative to the patient's capacity.

**Ischemic Conditions**

Unstable Response may present as:
- Ischemic Symptoms
- ST Segment Changes
- Onset of or Increased Frequency of Ventricular Ectopy (Stop Rx if > 10/minute, becomes symptomatic or BP becomes compromised)
- Unifocal PVC's become Multifocal PVC's
- Onset of Signs of CHF (See Table 1.17)
- Systolic Blood Pressure Drops > 10 mm HG
- Diastolic Blood Pressure Increases or Decreases >10 mm Hg
- Heart Rate Drops >10 bpm
- Diaphoresis, Pallor, Confusion
- Increased RPE despite no changes in vital signs
- Cyanosis
- Diaphoresis
- Nasal Flaring
- Increased Use of Accessory Muscles of Respiration

**Stable Response may present as:**
- Linear Increase in HR and Systolic BP with increases in activity levels
- Blunted Responses in HR and Systolic BP if on Beta-Blockade, and some Calcium Channel Blockers
- Increased RPE with increased workload
- If no changes in HR or Systolic Blood Pressure, there should be no change in RPE. (During an examination low level workloads may not be significant enough to produce vital sign responses.)
- NOTE: Stable responses may include increased respiratory rate, heart rate, blood pressure, and RPE. However, with the stable response, these increases merely indicate the patient's response.

**Pump Failure: Congestive Heart Failure**

Unstable Response may present as:
- Onset of or Increased Frequency of Ventricular Ectopy (Stop Rx if > 10/minute, becomes symptomatic or BP becomes compromised)
- Unifocal PVC's become Multifocal PVC's
- Onset of Signs of CHF (See Table 1.17)
- Systolic Blood Pressure Drops > 10 mm HG
- Diastolic Blood Pressure Increases or Decreases >10 mm Hg
- Heart Rate Drops >10 bpm
- Poor pulse pressure (<10 mm Hg difference between Systolic and Diastolic Blood Pressure
- Diaphoresis, Pallor, Confusion
- Increased RPE despite no changes in vital signs
- Ischemic Symptoms
- ST Segment Changes
- In patients being invasively monitored:
  - >10 mm Hg increase in pulmonary artery pressure
  - Increase or decrease of >6 mm Hg in central venous pressure
- Cyanosis
- Diaphoresis
- Nasal Flaring
- Increased Use of Accessory Muscles of Respiration

**Figure 1-10.** *Determination of stable vs. unstable responses to activity/exercise. (BP = blood pressure; CHF = congestive heart failure; HR = heart rate; PVC = premature ventricular contraction; RPE = rating of perceived exertion; Rx = treatment.)*

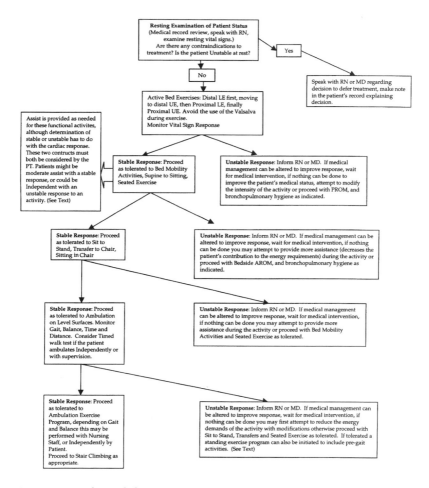

**Figure 1-11.** *Physical therapy activity examination algorithm. (AROM = active range of motion; LE = lower extremity; PROM = passive range of motion; UE= upper extremity.)*

(work) level. Figure 1-11 provides a general guide to advancing a patient's activity while considering his or her response to activity.

Physical therapy intervention should include a warm-up phase to prepare the patient for activity. This is usually performed at a level of activity that is lower than the expected exercise program. For example, it may consist of supine, seated, or standing exercises. A conditioning phase follows the warm-up period. Very often in the acute care hospital, this conditioning phase is part of the patient's functional mobility training. With patients who are independent with functional mobility, an aerobic-based conditioning program of walking or stationary cycling may be used for conditioning. Finally, a cool-down or relaxation phase of deep breathing and stretching ends the physical therapy session.

Listed below are various ways to monitor the patient's activity tolerance.

1. *HR*: HR is the primary means of determining the exercise intensity level for patients who are not taking beta-blockers or who have non–rate-responsive pacemakers.

- There is a linear relationship between HR and work.

- In general, a 20- to 30-beat increase from the resting value during activity is a safe intensity level in which a patient can exercise.

- If a patient has undergone an exercise stress test during the hospital stay, a percentage (e.g., 60–80%) of the maximum HR achieved during the test can be calculated to determine the exercise intensity.[52]

- An example of a disproportionate HR response to low-level activity (bed or seated exercises or ambulation in room) is an HR of more than 120 bpm or less than 50 bpm.[52]

- When prescribing activity intensity for a patient taking beta-blockers, the HR should not exceed 20 beats above resting HR.

- If prescribing activity intensity using HR for patients with an AICD, the exercise target HR should be 20–30 beats below the threshold rate on the defibrillator.[52]

- HR cannot be used to prescribe exercise status post heart transplant secondary to denervation of the heart during transplantation.

- Baseline HR and recent changes in medications should always be considered before beginning an exercise session.

2. *BP*: Refer to the cardiac assessment section regarding BP measurements and Table 1-6 for BP ranges. Examples of a disproportionate response to exercise are a systolic pressure decrease of 10 mm Hg below the resting value, a hypertensive systolic response of more than 180 mm Hg, or a hypertensive diastolic response of more than 110 mm Hg.[52]

- If the patient is on a pacemaker that does not have rate modulation, BP response can be used to gauge intensity. Please refer to the Procedures section for the discussion on pacemakers.

**Table 1-22.**  Borg's Rating of Perceived Exertion

| Original Scale | 10-Point Scale |
| --- | --- |
| 6 | 0  Nothing at all |
| 7  Very, very light | 0.5  Very, very slight |
| 8 | 1  Very slight |
| 9  Very light | 2  Slight |
| 10 | 3  Moderate |
| 11  Fairly light | 4  Somewhat severe |
| 12 | 5  Severe |
| 13  Somewhat hard | 6 |
| 14 | 7  Very severe |
| 15  Hard | 8 |
| 16 | 9  Very, very severe |
| 17  Very hard | (almost maximal) |
| 18 | 10  Maximal |
| 19  Very, very hard | |
| 20 | |

3.    *Borg's Rating of Perceived Exertion* (RPE) is depicted in Table 1-22. Borg's RPE scale was initially proposed in 1962 and has evolved today to be the classic means of objectively documenting subjective feelings of exercise intensity.

• This scale can be easily used to monitor exercise intensity for the purpose of exercise prescription in a variety of patient populations.

• It is the preferred method of prescribing exercise intensity for a patient taking beta-blockers.

• A general guideline for everyone is to exercise to a point no greater than 5 on the 10-point scale and no greater than 13 on the original scale.[52]

4.    *Rate pressure product* (RPP) is HR × SBP and is an indication of myocardial oxygen demand.

• If a patient undergoes maximal exercise testing and has myocardial ischemia, RPP can be calculated at the point when ischemia is occurring to establish the patient's ischemic threshold.

• This RPP value can then be used during exercise to provide a safe guideline of exercise intensity.

5.   *Heart sounds*: Refer to the section on Auscultation and Table 1-9 for normal and abnormal heart sounds.

- The onset of murmurs, S3 heart sounds, or S4 heart sounds during treatment may be detected and could indicate a decline in cardiac function during activity. This finding should be brought to the attention of the nurse and physician.

6.   *Breath sounds*: Refer to Chapter 2 for a discussion of lung auscultation and the interpretation of breath sounds.

- The presence of or increase in bibasilar crackles during activity may be indicative of acute CHF. Activity should be terminated and the nurse and physician notified.

7.   *ECG rhythm*: Refer to the section on ECG and the section Rhythm and Conduction Disturbance.

- When treating patients who are being continuously monitored by an ECG, it is important to know their baseline rhythm, the most recently observed rhythm, what lead is being monitored, and why they are being monitored.

- It is important to recognize their normal rhythm and any deviations from this norm. It is also important to recognize changes that could indicate a decline in cardiac status. Examples of declining cardiac status include the following:

- Onset of ST changes (elevation or depression of more than 1 mm) could indicate ischemia

- Increased frequency of PVCs (trigeminy to bigeminy or couplets)

- Unifocal PVCs to multifocal PVCs

- Premature atrial contractions to atrial flutter or atrial fibrillation

- Atrial flutter to atrial fibrillation

- Any progression in heart blocks (first degree to Mobitz I)

- Loss of pacer spike capturing (pacer spike without resultant QRS complex on ECG)

- The physical therapist should also be able to recognize signs and symptoms of cardiac decompensation and immediately notify the physician if any develop (see Figure 1-10). It is important to record any signs noted during activity and other objective data at that time. Other signs and symptoms include weakness, fatigue, dizziness, lightheadedness, angina, palpitations, and dyspnea. It is important to record any symptoms reported by the patient and any objective information at that time (ECG readings; BP, HR, and RPP measurements; breath sounds).

---

### Clinical Tip

Patients should be encouraged to report any symptom(s), even if they think it is trivial.

---

## References

1. American Heart Association. 2001 Heart and Stroke Statistical Update. Dallas: American Heart Association, 2000.
2. Moore K (ed). Clinically Oriented Anatomy (3rd ed). Baltimore: Williams & Wilkins, 1992.
3. Guyton AC (ed). Textbook of Medical Physiology (9th ed). Philadelphia: Saunders, 1996.
4. Cheitlin MD, Sokolow M, McIlroy MB (eds). Clinical Cardiology (6th ed). Norwalk, CT: Appleton & Lange, 1993.
5. Braunwald E (ed). Heart Disease: A Textbook of Cardiovascular Medicine (4th ed). Philadelphia: Saunders, 1992.
6. Davis D (ed). How to Quickly and Accurately Master ECG Interpretation (2nd ed). Philadelphia: Lippincott, 1992.
7. Hillis LD, Firth BG, Willerson JT (eds). Manual of Clinical Problems in Cardiology. Boston: Little, Brown, 1984.
8. Task Force of the European Society of Cardiology and the North American Society of Pacing and Electrophysiology. Heart rate variability: standards of measurement, physiological interpretation, and clinical use. Circulation 1996;93:1043–1065.
9. Bernston G, Cacioppo JT, Quigley KS. Autonomic determinism: the modes of autonomic control, the doctrine of autonomic space, and the laws of autonomic constraint. Psychol Rev 1991;98:459–487.
10. Urden LD, Davie JK, Thelan LA (eds). Essentials of Critical Care Nursing. St. Louis: Mosby, 1992.
11. Cohen M, Michel TH (eds). Cardiopulmonary Symptoms in Physical Therapy Practice. New York: Churchill Livingstone, 1988.
12. Woods SL, Sivarajian Froelicher ES, Underhill-Motzer S (eds). Cardiac Nursing (4th ed). Philadelphia: Lippincott, 2000.

13. Bickley LS (ed). Bate's Guide to Physical Examination and History Taking (7th ed). Philadelphia: Lippincott, 1999.
14. Fetsch T, Reinhart L, Wichter T, et al. Heart rate variability and electrical stability. Basic Res Cardiol 1998;93:S117–S124.
15. Kristal-Boneh E, Raifal M, Froom P, Ribak, J. Heart rate variability in health and disease. Scand J Work Environ Health 1995;21:85–95.
16. Stein PK, Kleiger RE. Insights from the study of heart rate variability. Annu Rev Med 1999;50:249–261.
17. Algra A. Heart rate variability from 24-hour holter ecg and the 2 year risk for sudden death. Circulation 1993;88:180–185.
18. Dekker JM. Heart rate variability from short electrocardiographic recordings predicts mortality from all causes in middle aged and elderly men. Am J Epidemiol 1997;145:899–908.
19. Tusji H, Larson MG. Impact of reduced HRV on risk for cardiac events. The Framingham Heart Study. Circulation 1996;94:2850–2855.
20. Singh JP, Larson MG, Tsuji H, et al. Reduced heart rate variability and new onset hypertension. Hypertension 1998;32:293–297.
21. Bigger JT, La Rovere RT, Marcus FI, et al. Baroreflex sensitivity and heart rate variability in prediction of total cardiac mortality after MI. Lancet 1998;351:478–484.
22. Bigger JT. Frequency domain measures of heart period variability and mortality after myocardial infarction. Circulation 1992;85:164–171.
23. Doulalas A, Flather MD, Pipilis A, Campbell S. Evolutionary pattern and prognostic importance of heart rate variability during the early phase of acute myocardial infarction. Int J Cardiol 2001;77: 169–179.
24. Van Boven AJ, Crijns H, Haaksma J, Zwinderman AH. Depressed heart rate variability is associated with events in patients with stable coronary artery disease and preserved left ventricular dysfunction. Am Heart J 1998;135:571–576.
25. Galinier M, Pathak A, Fourcade J, et al. Depressed low frequency power of heart rate variability as an independent predictor of sudden cardiac death in chronic heart failure. Eur Heart J 2000;21:475–482.
26. Kleiger RE, Miller JP, Bigger TJ, Moss A. Decreased heart rate variability and its association with increased mortality after acute myocardial infarction. Am J Cardiol 1987;59:256–262.
27. Polich S, Faynor SM. Interpreting lab test values. PT Magazine 1996;3:110.
28. Suzuki T, Yamauchi K, Yamada Y. Blood coaguability and fibrinolytic activity before and after physical training during the recovery phase of acute myocardial infarction. Clin Cardiol 1992;15:358–364.
29. Grundy SM, Pasternak R, Greenland P, et al. Assessment of cardiovascular risk by use of multiple-risk-factor assessment equations: a statement for healthcare professionals from the American Heart Association and the American College of Cardiology. Circulation 1999; 100:1481–1492.
30. Christenson RH, Azzazy HME. Biochemical markers of the acute coronary syndromes. Clin Chem 1998; 44:1855–1864.
31. Kratz AK, Leqand–Rowski KB. Normal reference laboratory values. N Engl J Med 1998;339:1063–1072.

32. Fisher EA, Stahl JA, Budd JH, Goldman ME. Transesophageal echocardiography: procedures and clinical application. J Am Coll Cardiol 1991;18:1333–1348.
33. Ellestad MH (ed). Stress Testing: Principles and Practice (4th ed). Philadelphia: FA Davis, 1996.
34. Perez JE. Current role of contrast echocardiography in the diagnosis of cardiovascular disease. Clin Cardiol 1997;20:I31–I38.
35. Bellardinelli R, Geordiou D, Prucaro A. Low dose dobutamine echocardiography predicts improvement in functional capacity after exercise training in patients with ischemic cardiomyopathy: prognostic implications. J Am Coll Cardiol 1998;31(5):1027–1034.
36. American Heart Association, Committee on Exercise. Exercise Testing and Training of Apparently Healthy Individuals: A Handbook for Physicians. Dallas, 1972.
37. Brooks GA, Fahey TD, White TP (eds). Exercise Physiology: Human Bioenergetics and Its Applications (2nd ed). Mountain View, CA: Mayfield Publishing, 1996.
38. Noonan V, Dean E. Submaximal exercise testing: clinical applications and interpretation. Phys Ther 2000;80:782–807.
39. American College of Cardiology/American Heart Association. 1999 update: ACC/AHA guidelines for the management of patients with acute myocardial infarction: executive summary and recommendations. Circulation 1999;100:1016–1030.
40. American College of Cardiology/American Heart Association. ACC/AHA guidelines for the management of patients with acute myocardial infarction. J Am Coll Cardiol 1996;28:1328–1428.
41. American College of Cardiology/American Heart Association. ACC/AHA guidelines for the management of patients with unstable angina and non-st segment elevation myocardial infarction. J Am Coll Cardiol 2000;36:971–1048.
42. Cahalin LP. Heart failure. Phys Ther 1996;76:520.
43. American Heart Association. AHA Medical/Scientific Statement. 1994 Revisions to Classification of Functional Capacity and Objective Assessment of Patients with Diseases of the Heart. Dallas: American Heart Association, 1994.
44. Detre KM, Holmes DR, Holudrov R, et al. Incidence and consequences of periprocedural occlusion. Circulation 1990;82:739.
45. Litzak F, Margilis J, Cumins R. Excimer laser coronary (ECLA) registry: report of the first 2080 patients. J Am Coll Cardiol 1992;19:276A.
46. Humphrey R, Arena R. Surgical innovations for chronic heart failure in the context of cardiopulmonary rehabilitation. Phys Ther 2000;80:61–69.
47. Bernstein AD, Camm AJ, Fletcher RD, et al. The NASPE/BPEG generic pacemaker code for antibradyarrhythmia and adaptive pacing and antitachyarrhythmia devices. PACE 1987;10:795.
48. Sharp CT, Busse EF, Burgess JJ, Haennel RG. Exercise prescription for patients with pacemakers. J Cardiopulm Rehabil 1998;18:421–431.
49. Hayward MP. Dynamic cardiomyoplasty: time to wrap it up? [Editorial]. Heart 1999;82:263.

50. Grimes K, Cohen M. Cardiac Medications. In EA Hillegass, HS Sadowsky (eds), Essentials of Cardiopulmonary Physical Therapy (2nd ed). Philadelphia: Saunders, 2001;537–585.
51. Cahalin LP, Ice RG, Irwin S. Program Planning and Implementation. In S Irwin, JS Tecklin (eds), Cardiopulmonary Physical Therapy (3rd ed). St Louis: Mosby, 1995;144.
52. Wegener NK. Rehabilitation of the Patient with Coronary Heart Disease. In RC Schlant, RW Alexander (eds), Hurst's The Heart (8th ed). New York: McGraw-Hill, 1994;1227.

# Appendix 1-A

**Table 1-A.1.** Electrocardiographic (ECG) Characteristics and Causes of Atrial Rhythms

| Name | ECG Characteristics | Common Causes | PT Consideration |
|---|---|---|---|
| Supraventricular tachycardia | Regular rhythm, rate = 160–250, may originate from any location above atrioventricular node, can be paroxysmal (comes and goes without reason). | Rheumatoid heart disease (RHD), mitral valve prolapse, cor pulmonale, digitalis toxicity. | May produce palpitations, chest tightness, dizziness, anxiety, apprehension, weakness; PT would not treat if in supraventricular tachycardia until controlled. |
| Atrial flutter | Rhythm can be regular or irregular, atrial rate of 250–350, ventricular rate is variable and depends on the conduction ratio (atrial:ventricular—i.e., atrial rate = 250, ventricular rate = 125; 2:1 classic saw tooth P waves.) | Mitral stenosis, CAD, hypertension. | Signs and symptoms depend on presence or absence of heart disease but can lead to CHF, palpitations, angina, and syncope if cardiac output decreases far enough to reduce myocardial and cerebral blood flow; PT treatment would depend on tolerance to the rhythm. |
| Atrial fibrillation (AF) | Irregular rhythm, atrial has no rate (just quivers) ventricular varies. | One of most commonly encountered rhythms, CHF, CAD, RHD, hypertension, cor pulmonale. | Can produce CHF, syncope secondary to no "atrial kick"; if new diagnosis, hold PT until medical treatment; if chronic and not in CHF, would treat with caution. |

| Premature atrial contractions | Irregular rhythm (can be regularly irregular, i.e., skip every third beat); rate normal 60–100. | Normal people with caffeine, smoking, emotional disturbances; abnormal with CAD, CHF, electrolyte disturbances. | Usually asymptomatic but needs to be considered with other cardiac issues at time of treatment; can proceed with treatment with close monitoring; if they are consistent and increasing can progress to AF. |

AF = atrial fibrillation; CAD = coronary artery disease; CHF = congestive heart failure; RHD = rheumatoid heart disease. Sources: Data from B Aehlert. ACLS Quick Review Study Guide. St. Louis: Mosby, 1993; and EK Chung. Manual of Cardiac Arrhythmias. Boston: Butterworth–Heinemann, 1986.

Table 1-A.2. Electrocardiographic (ECG) Characteristics and Causes of Ventricular Rhythms

| Name | ECG Characteristics | Common Causes | PT Considerations |
|---|---|---|---|
| Agonal rhythm | Irregular rhythm, rate <20, no P wave | Near death | Do not treat. |
| Ventricular tachycardia (VT) | Usually regular rhythm, rate >100, no P wave or with retrograde conduction and appears after the QRS complex | CAD most common after acute MI; may occur in rheumatoid heart disease, cardiomyopathy, hypertension | Do not treat; patient needs immediate medical assistance; patient may be stable (maintain CO) for short while but can progress quickly to unstable (no CO) called pulseless VT. |
| Multifocal VT (torsades de pointes) | Irregular rhythm, rate >150, no P waves | Drug induced with antiarrhythmic medicines (quinidine, procainamide); hypokalemia; hypomagnesemia; MI; hypothermia | Do not treat; patient needs immediate medical attention. |

| Premature ventricular contractions (PVCs) (*focal* = one ectopic foci and all look the same; *multifocal* = more than one ectopic foci and will have different wave forms) | Irregular rhythm, (can be regularly irregular, i.e., skipped beat every fourth beat); rate varies but is usually normal 60–100; *couplet* is 2 in a row; *bigeminy* is every other beat; *trigeminy* is every third beat | In normal individuals, secondary to caffeine, smoking, emotional disturbances; CAD, MI, cardiomyopathy, MVP, digitalis toxicity | Frequency will dictate effect on CO; need to monitor electrocardiograph with treatment; can progress to VT; and this is more likely if multifocal in nature or if >6 per min; stop treatment or rest if change in frequency or quality. |
|---|---|---|---|
| Ventricular fibrillation | Chaotic | Severe heart disease most common after acute MI, hyper- or hypokalemia, hypercalcemia, electrocution | Needs immediate medical assistance; no PT treatment. |
| Idioventricular rhythm | Essentially regular rhythm, rate 20–40 | Advanced heart disease; high degree of atrioventricular block; usually a terminal arrhythmia | CHF is common secondary to slow rates; hold treatment unless rhythm well tolerated. |

CAD = coronary artery disease; CHF = congestive heart failure; CO = cardiac output; MI = myocardial infarction; MVP = mitral valve prolapse; VT = ventricular tachycardia.

Sources: Data from B Aehlert. ACLS Quick Review Study Guide. St. Louis: Mosby, 1994; and EK Chung. Manual of Cardiac Arrhythmias. Boston: Butterworth–Heinemann, 1986.

**Table 1-A.3.** Electrocardiographic (ECG) Characteristics and Causes of Junctional Rhythms

| Name | ECG Characteristics | Common Causes | PT Considerations |
|---|---|---|---|
| Junctional escape rhythm | Regular rhythm, rate 20–40; inverted P wave before or after QRS complex; starts with ectopic foci in AV junction tissue | Usual cause is physiologic to control the ventricles in AV block, sinus bradycardia, AF, sinoatrial block, drug intoxication | If occasional and intermittent during bradycardia or chronic AF, usually insignificant and can treat (with close watch of possible worsening condition via symptoms and vital signs); if consistent and present secondary to AV block, acute myocardial infarction, or drug intoxication, can be symptomatic with CHF. (See Table 1-21.) |
| Junctional tachycardia | Regular rhythm; rate 100–180; P wave as above | Most common with chronic AF; also with coronary artery disease, rheumatoid heart disease, and cardiomyopathy | May produce or exacerbate symptoms of CHF or angina secondary to decreased cardiac output; PT treatment depends on patient tolerance—if new, onset should wait for medical treatment. |

AF = atrial fibrillation; AV = atrioventricular; CHF = congestive heart failure.
Sources: Data from B Aehlert. ACLS Quick Review Study Guide. St. Louis: Mosby, 1994; and EK Chung. Manual of Cardiac Arrhythmias. Boston: Butterworth–Heinemann, 1986.

**Table 1-A.4.** Electrocardiographic (ECG) Characteristics and Causes of Atrioventricular Blocks

| Name | ECG Characteristics | Common Causes | PT Considerations |
|---|---|---|---|
| First-degree AV block | Regular rhythm, rate normal 60–100, prolonged PR interval >0.2 (constant). | Elderly with heart disease, acute myocarditis, acute MI | If chronic, need to be more cautious of underlying heart disease; if new onset, monitor closely for progression to higher level block. |
| Second-degree AV block type I (Wenkebach, Mobitz I) | Irregular rhythm, atrial rate > ventricular rate, usually both 60–100; PR interval lengthens until P wave appears without a QRS complex. | Acute infection, acute MI | Symptoms are uncommon, as above. |
| Second-degree AV block type II (Mobitz II) | Irregular rhythm, atrial rate > ventricular rate, PR interval may be normal or prolonged but is constant for each conducted QRS. | Anteroseptal MI | CHF is common; can have dizziness, fainting, complete unconsciousness; may need pacing and PT treatment; should be held for medical management. |
| Third-degree AV block (complete heart block) | Regular rhythm, atrial rate > ventricular rate. | Anteroseptal MI, drug intoxication, infections, electrolyte imbalances, coronary artery disease, degenerative sclerotic process of AV conduction system | Severe CHF; patient will need medical management; a pacer (temporary or permanent depending on reversibility of etiology) is almost always necessary; |

AV = atrioventricular; CHF = congestive heart failure; MI = myocardial infarction.
Sources: Data from B Aehlert. ACLS Quick Review Study Guide. St. Louis: Mosby, 1994; and EK Chung. Manual of Cardiac Arrhythmias. Boston: Butterworth–Heinemann, 1986.

# Appendix 1-B

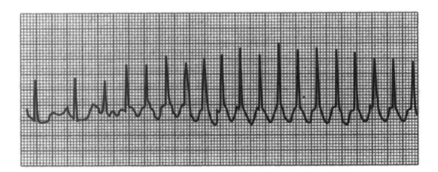

**Figure 1-B.1.** *Paroxysmal supraventricular tachycardia. Note development from normal sinus rhythm. (With permission from M Walsh, A Crumbie, S Reveley. Nurse Practitioners: Clinical Skills and Professional Issues. Boston: Butterworth–Heinemann, 1993;96.)*

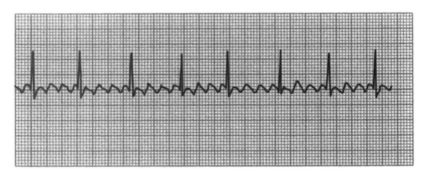

**Figure 1-B.2.** *Atrial flutter. Note regular rhythm (P waves) but ventricular rhythm depends on conduction pattern. (With permission from M Walsh, A Crumbie, S Reveley. Nurse Practitioners: Clinical Skills and Professional Issues. Boston: Butterworth–Heinemann, 1993;95.)*

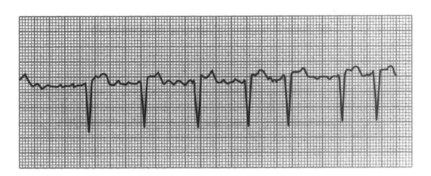

**Figure 1-B.3.** *Atrial fibrillation. Note the irregular rhythm and absence of normal P waves. (With permission from M Walsh, A Crumbie, S Reveley. Nurse Practitioners: Clinical Skills and Professional Issues. Boston: Butterworth–Heinemann, 1993;95.)*

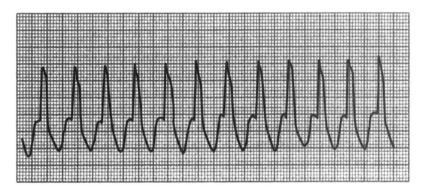

**Figure 1-B.4.** *Ventricular tachycardia. Rate 100–170 beats per minute. No P waves, broad electrocardiographic wave complexes. (Reprinted with permission from M Walsh, A Crumbie, S Reveley. Nurse Practitioners: Clinical Skills and Professional Issues. Boston: Butterworth–Heinemann, 1993;98.)*

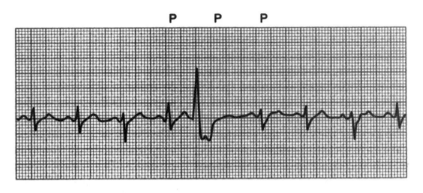

**Figure 1-B.5.** *Ventricular ectopy with refractory period afterward. (With permission from M Walsh, A Crumbie, S Reveley. Nurse Practitioners: Clinical Skills and Professional Issues. Boston: Butterworth–Heinemann, 1993;97.)*

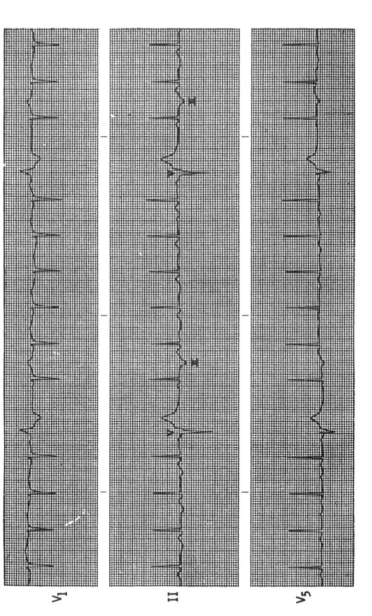

Figure 1-B.6. *Sinus rhythm with premature ventricular contractions. (With permission from EK Chung. Manual of Cardiac Arrhythmias. Boston: Butterworth–Heinemann, 1986;102.)*

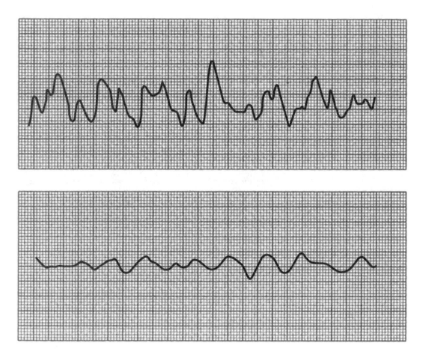

Figure 1-B.7. *Ventricular fibrillation. (With permission from M Walsh, A Crumbie, S Reveley. Nurse Practitioners: Clinical Skills and Professional Issues. Boston: Butterworth–Heinemann, 1993;97.)*

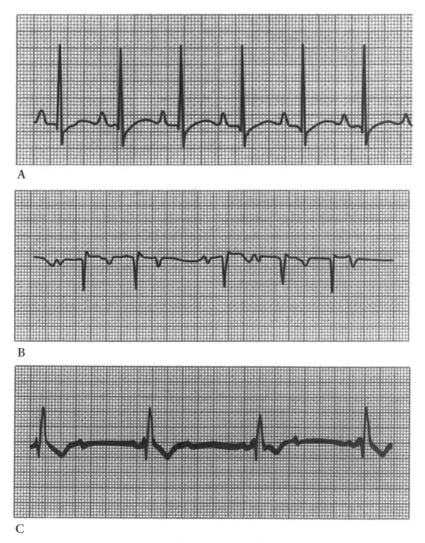

**Figure 1-B.8 (A–D).** *Degrees of heart block. (With permission from M Walsh, A Crumbie, S Reveley. Nurse Practitioners: Clinical Skills and Professional Issues. Boston: Butterworth–Heinemann, 1993;96.)*

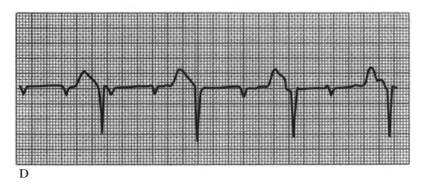

D

**Figure 1-B.8 (A–D).** *Continued.*

# 2

# Respiratory System
*Michele P. West and Jaime C. Paz*

## Introduction

To safely and effectively provide exercise, bronchopulmonary hygiene program(s), or both to patients with respiratory dysfunction, physical therapists require an understanding of the respiratory system and of the principles of gas exchange. The objectives of this chapter are to provide the following:

1.   A brief review of the structure and function of the respiratory system

2.   An overview of respiratory evaluation, including physical examination and diagnostic testing

3.   A description of respiratory diseases and disorders, including clinical findings, medical-surgical management, and physical therapy intervention

Note: *Ventilation* is defined as gas (oxygen [$O_2$] and carbon dioxide [$CO_2$]) transport into and out of lungs, and *respiration* is defined as gas exchange across the alveolar-capillary and capillary-tissue interfaces. The term *pulmonary* primarily refers to the lungs, their airways, and their vascular system.[1]

## Structure

The primary organs and muscles of the respiratory system are outlined in Tables 2-1 and 2-2, respectively. A schematic of the pulmonary system within the thorax is presented in Figure 2-1.

## Function

To accomplish ventilation and respiration, the respiratory system is regulated by many neural, chemical, and nonchemical mechanisms, which are discussed below.

### Neural Control

Respiration is regulated by two separate neural mechanisms: One controls automatic respiration, and the other controls voluntary respiration. Automatic respiration is controlled by the medullary respiratory center in the brain stem, which is responsible for the rhythmicity of breathing. The pneumotaxic center located in the pons controls respiratory rate and depth. Voluntary respiration is mediated by the cerebral cortex, which sends impulses directly to the motor neurons of respiratory muscles.[2]

### Chemical Control

Arterial levels of $CO_2$ ($Pco_2$), hydrogen ions ($H^+$), and $O_2$ ($Po_2$) can modify the rate and depth of respiration. To maintain homeostasis in the body, specialized chemoreceptors on the carotid arteries and aortic arch (carotid and aortic bodies, respectively) will either respond to a rise in $Pco_2$ and $H^+$ or to a fall in $Po_2$. Stimulation of these chemoreceptors results in transmission of impulses to the respiratory centers to increase or decrease the rate or depth, or both, of respiration. For example, an increase in $Pco_2$ would increase the respiratory rate to help increase the amount of $CO_2$ exhaled and ultimately lower the $Pco_2$ levels in arterial blood. Chemoreceptors are also found in the medulla and will respond to a rise in $Pco_2$ and $H^+$ as well.[2,3]

### Nonchemical Influences

Coughing, bronchoconstriction, and mucus secretion occur in the lungs as protective reflexes to irritants such as smoke or dust. Emo-

**Table 2-1.** Structure and Function of Primary Organs of the Respiratory System

| Structure | Description | Function |
|---|---|---|
| Nose | Paired mucosal-lined nasal cavities supported by bone and cartilage. | Conduit that filters, warms, and humidifies air entering lungs. |
| Pharynx | Passageway connecting nasal and oral cavities to larynx, and oral cavity to esophagus. Subdivisions naso-, oro-, and laryngopharynx. | Conduit for air and food. Facilitates exposure of immune system to inhaled antigens. |
| Larynx | Connects pharynx to trachea. Opening (glottis) is covered by vocal folds or by the epiglottis during swallowing. | Passageway that prevents food from entering the lower respiratory tract. Voice production. |
| Trachea | Flexible tube composed of C-shaped cartilaginous rings that are connected posteriorly to the trachealis muscle. Divides into the left and right main stem bronchi. | Cleans, warms, and moistens incoming air. |
| Bronchial tree | Right and left main stem bronchi subdivide within each lung into secondary bronchi, tertiary bronchi, and bronchioles, which contain smooth muscle. | Warms and moistens incoming air from trachea to alveoli. Smooth muscle constriction alters airflow. |
| Lungs | Paired organs located within pleural cavities of the thorax. The right lung has three lobes and the left has two lobes. | Contains air passageways distal to main stem bronchi, alveoli, and respiratory membranes. |
| Alveoli | Microscopic sacs at end of bronchial tree immediately adjacent to pulmonary capillaries. Functional unit of the lung. | Primary gas exchange site. Surfactant lines the alveoli to decrease surface tension and prevent complete closure during exhalation. |
| Pleurae | Double-layered, continuous serous membrane lining the inside of the thoracic cavity. Divided into parietal pleura (outer) and visceral pleura (inner). | Produces lubricating fluid that allows smooth gliding of lungs within the thorax. Potential space between parietal and visceral pleura. |

Sources: Adapted from E Marieb (ed). Human Anatomy and Physiology (3rd ed). Redwood City, CA: Benjamin-Cummings, 1995;743; and data from JR Moldover, J Stein, PG Krug. Cardiopulmonary Physiology. In EG Gonzalez, SJ Myers, JE Edelstein, et al. (eds), Downey & Darling's Physiological Basis of Rehabilitation Medicine (3rd ed). Boston: Butterworth–Heinemann, 2001;181–182.

**Table 2-2.** Primary and Accessory Respiratory Muscles with Associated Innervation

| Respiratory Muscles | Innervation |
| --- | --- |
| Primary inspiratory muscles | |
| Diaphragm | Phrenic nerve (C3–5) |
| External intercostals | Spinal segments T1–9 |
| Internal intercostals | Spinal segments T1–9 |
| Accessory inspiratory muscles | |
| Trapezius | Cervical nerve (C1–C4), spinal part of cranial nerve XI |
| Sternocleidomastoid | Spinal part of cranial nerve XI |
| Scalenes | Cervical/brachial plexus branches (C3–C8, T1) |
| Pectorals | Medial/lateral pectoral nerve (C5–8, T1) |
| Serratus anterior | Long thoracic nerve (C5–7) |
| Latissimus dorsi | Thoracodorsal nerve (C5–8) |
| Primary expiratory muscles | |
| Rectus abdominus | Spinal segments T5–12 |
| External obliques | Spinal segments T7–12 |
| Internal obliques | Spinal segments T8–12 |
| Accessory expiratory muscles | |
| Latissimus dorsi | Thoracodorsal nerve (C5–8) |

Sources: With data from FP Kendall, EK McCreary (eds). Muscles: Testing and Function (3rd ed). Baltimore: Williams & Wilkins, 1983;40,42–46,262; and JM Rothstein, SH Roy, SL Wolf. The Rehabilitation Specialist's Handbook (2nd ed). Philadelphia: FA Davis, 1998;123–144.

tions, stressors, pain, and visceral reflexes from lung tissue and other organ systems can also influence respiratory rate and depth.

### Respiratory Mechanics

After the respiratory muscles receive signals from the respiratory centers, two motions (bucket and pump handle) occur simultaneously with thoracic stabilization to create pressure changes within the thorax. Pressure changes result in the bulk flow of air (ventilation) in and out of the lungs. When alveolar pressure is less than atmospheric pressure, inspiration occurs; when alveolar pressure is greater than atmospheric pressure, expiration occurs. Changes in shape of the tho-

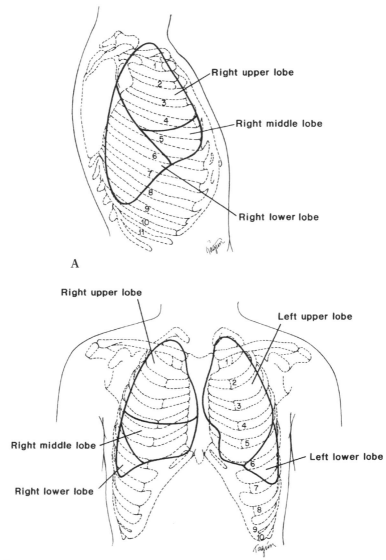

**Figure 2-1.** *A. Right lung positioned in the thorax. Bony landmarks assist in identifying normal right lung configuration. B. Anterior view of the lungs in the thorax in conjunction with bony landmarks. Left upper lobe is divided into apical and left lingula, which matches the general position of the right upper and middle lobes.*

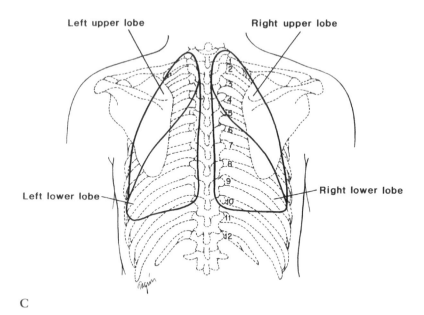

Figure 2-1. *Continued. C. Posterior view of the lungs in conjunction with bony landmarks. (With permission from E Ellis, J Alison [eds]. Key Issues in Cardiorespiratory Physiotherapy. Oxford, UK: Butterworth–Heinemann, 1992;12.)*

rax during inspiration and expiration result in these pressure changes between the atmosphere and the alveolar spaces. During inspiration, the diaphragm lowers, and the rib cage elevates and expands in anterior (pump handle) and lateral (bucket handle) directions to decrease the intrathoracic pressure. During expiration, the diaphragm relaxes passively and elevates, whereas the rib cage lowers to its resting position to increase the intrathoracic pressure. These motions are schematically outlined in Figure 2-2.[4,5]

*Gas Exchange*

Once air has reached the alveolar spaces, gas exchange can occur at the alveolar-capillary membrane. Diffusion of gases through the membrane is affected by the following:

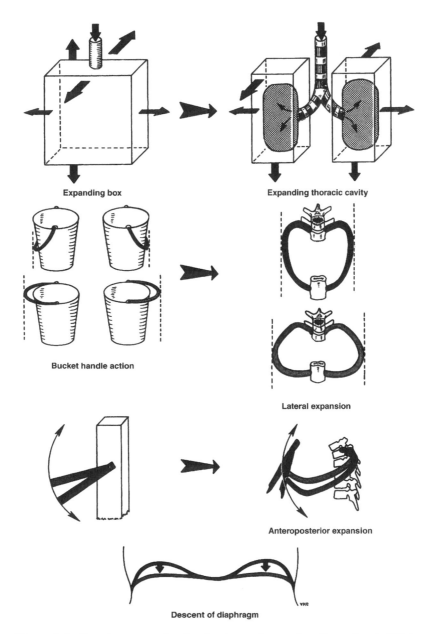

**Figure 2-2.** *Respiratory mechanics (bucket and pump handle motions). (With permission from RS Snell [ed]. Clinical Anatomy for Medical Students [5th ed]. Boston: Little, Brown, 1995;89.)*

1.    A concentration gradient in which gases will diffuse from areas of high concentration to areas of low concentration (e.g., alveolar $O_2$ = 100 mm Hg → capillary $O_2$ = 40 mm Hg)

2.    Surface area, or the total amount of alveolar-capillary interface available for gas exchange (e.g., the breakdown of alveolar membranes that occurs in emphysema will reduce the amount of surface area available for gas exchange)

3.    The thickness of the barrier (membrane) between the two areas involved (e.g., retained secretions in the alveolar spaces will impede gas exchange through the membrane)

### Ventilation and Perfusion Ratio

Gas exchange is optimized when the ratio of air flow (ventilation [$\dot{V}$]) to blood flow (perfusion [$\dot{Q}$]) approaches a 1:1 relationship. However, the actual $\dot{V}/\dot{Q}$ ratio is 0.8, as alveolar ventilation is approximately equal to 4 liters per minute and pulmonary blood flow is approximately equal to 5 liters per minute.[6]

Gravity, body position, and cardiopulmonary dysfunction can influence this ratio. Ventilation is optimized in areas of least resistance. For example, when a person is in a sitting position, the upper lobes initially receive more ventilation than the lower lobes; however, the lower lobes will have the largest net change in ventilation.

Perfusion is greatest in gravity-dependent areas. For example, when a person is in a sitting position, perfusion is the greatest at the base of the lungs; when a person is in a left side–lying position, the left lung receives the most blood.

A $\dot{V}/\dot{Q}$ mismatch (inequality in the relationship between ventilation and perfusion) can occur in certain situations. Two terms that are associated with $\dot{V}/\dot{Q}$ mismatch are dead space and shunt. Dead space occurs when ventilation is in excess of perfusion, as with a pulmonary embolus. A shunt occurs when perfusion is in excess of ventilation, as in alveolar collapse from secretion retention. These conditions are shown in Figure 2-3.

### Gas Transport

$O_2$ is transported away from the lungs to the tissues in two forms: (1) dissolved in plasma ($Po_2$) or (2) chemically bound to hemoglobin

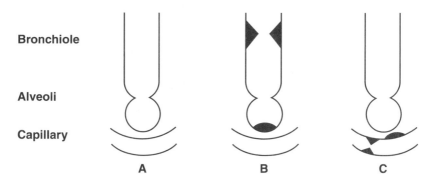

**Figure 2-3.** *Ventilation and perfusion mismatch. A. Normal alveolar ventilation. B. Capillary shunt. C. Alveolar dead space. (Artwork by Michele West.)*

on a red blood cell (oxyhemoglobin). As a by-product of cellular metabolism, $CO_2$ is transported away from the tissues to the lungs in three forms: (1) dissolved in plasma ($P_{CO_2}$), (2) chemically bound to hemoglobin (carboxyhemoglobin), and (3) as bicarbonate.

Approximately 97% of $O_2$ and $CO_2$ transport occurs in the combined forms of oxyhemoglobin, carboxyhemoglobin, and bicarbonate.[7] A smaller percentage, 3%, of $O_2$ and $CO_2$ is transported in dissolved forms. Dissolved $O_2$ and $CO_2$ exert a partial pressure within the plasma and can be measured by sampling arterial, venous, or mixed venous blood.[8] See the section Arterial Blood Gas Analysis for further description of this process.

## Evaluation

Respiratory evaluation is composed of patient history, physical examination, and interpretation of diagnostic test results.

### Patient History

In addition to the general chart review presented in Appendix I-A, other relevant information regarding respiratory dysfunction that should be ascertained from the chart review or patient interview is listed below[8-10]:

- History of smoking, including packs per day or pack years (packs per day × number of years smoked) and the amount of time that smoking has been discontinued (if applicable).

- Presence, history, and amount of $O_2$ therapy at rest, with activity, or both.

- Exposure to environmental or occupational toxins (e.g., asbestos).

- History of pneumonia, thoracic procedures, or surgery.

- History of assisted ventilation or intubation with mechanical ventilation.

- History or current reports of dyspnea either at rest or with exertion. Dyspnea is the subjective complaint of difficulty with respiration, also known as *shortness of breath*. Note: The abbreviation *DOE* represents "dyspnea on exertion."

- Level of activity before admittance.

- History of baseline sputum production.

- Sleeping position.

### Physical Examination

The physical examination of the respiratory system consists of inspection, auscultation, palpation, mediate percussion, and cough examination. Suggested guidelines for physical therapy intervention(s) that are based on examination findings and diagnostic test results are found at the end of this chapter.

### Inspection

A wealth of information can be gathered by simple observation of the patient at rest and with activity. Physical observation should proceed in a systematic fashion and include the following:

- General appearance and level of alertness.

- Ease of phonation.

- Skin color.

- Posture and chest shape.

• Respiratory pattern (including assessment of rate [12–20 breaths per minute is normal], depth, ratio of inspiration to expiration [1 to 2 is normal], sequence of chest wall movement during inspiration and expiration, comfort, presence of accessory muscle use, and symmetry). Respiratory patterns vary among individuals and may be influenced by (1) pain, (2) emotion, (3) body temperature, (4) sleep, (5) body position, (6) activity level, and (7) the presence of pulmonary, cardiac, metabolic, or nervous system disease. Table 2-3 provides a description of breathing patterns.

• Presence of digital clubbing.

• Presence of supplemental $O_2$ and other medical equipment. (Refer to Appendix III-A.)

• Presence and location of surgical incisions.

---

### Clinical Tip

• The optimal time, clinically, to examine a patient's breathing pattern is when he or she is unaware of the inspection. Knowledge of the physical examination can influence the patient's respiratory pattern. Therefore, compare the patient's respiratory pattern while he or she is asleep with the patient's respiratory pattern while he or she is awake, or compare the patient's respiratory pattern during conversation at rest with his or her respiratory pattern during activity.
• Objective observations of respiratory rate may not always be consistent with a patient's subjective complaints of dyspnea. For example, a patient may complain of shortness of breath but have a respiratory rate within normal limits. Therefore, the patient's subjective complaints, rather than the objective observations, may be a more accurate measure of treatment intensity.

---

### Auscultation
*Auscultation* is the process of listening to the sounds of air passing through the tracheobronchial tree and alveolar spaces. The sounds of airflow normally dissipate from proximal to distal airways, making

Table 2-3. Description of Breathing Patterns and Their
Associated Conditions

| Breathing Pattern | Description | Associated with |
| --- | --- | --- |
| Apnea | Lack of airflow to the lungs for >15 secs. | Airway obstruction, cardiopulmonary arrest, alterations of the respiratory center, narcotic overdose |
| Biot's respirations | Constant increased rate and depth of respiration followed by periods of apnea of varying lengths. | Elevated intracranial pressure, meningitis |
| Bradypnea | Respiratory rate <12 breaths per min. | Use of sedatives, narcotics, or alcohol; neurologic or metabolic disorders, excessive fatigue |
| Cheyne-Stokes respirations | Increasing depth of respiration followed by a period of apnea. | Elevated intracranial pressure, CHF, narcotic overdose |
| Hyperpnea | Increased depth of respiration. | Activity, pulmonary infections, CHF |
| Hyperventilation | Increased rate and depth of respiration resulting in decreased $P_{CO_2}$. | Anxiety, nervousness, metabolic acidosis |
| Hypoventilation | Decreased rate and depth of respiration resulting in increased $P_{CO_2}$. | Sedation or somnolence, neurologic depression of respiratory centers, overmedication, metabolic alkalosis |
| Kussmaul's respirations | Increased regular rate and depth of respiration. | Diabetic ketoacidosis, renal failure |
| Orthopnea | Dyspnea that occurs in a flat supine position. Relief occurs with more upright sitting or standing. | Chronic lung disease, CHF |
| Paradoxical respirations | Inward abdominal or chest wall movement with inspiration and outward movement with expiration. | Diaphragm paralysis, respiratory muscle fatigue, chest wall trauma |

Table 2-3. *Continued*

| Breathing Pattern | Description | Associated with |
|---|---|---|
| Sighing res- pirations | The presence of a sigh >2–3 times per min. | Angina, anxiety, dyspnea |
| Tachypnea | Respiratory rate >20 breaths per min. | Acute respiratory distress, fever, pain, emotions, anemia |

CHF = congestive heart failure; $P_{CO_2}$ = partial pressure of carbon dioxide.
Sources: Adapted from LD Kersten (ed). Comprehensive Respiratory Nursing: A Decision-Making Approach. Philadelphia: Saunders, 1989;119; and T Des Jardins, GG Burton (eds). Clinical Manifestations and Assessment of Respiratory Disease (3rd ed). St. Louis: Mosby, 1995;18.

the sounds less audible in the periphery as compared with the central airways. Alterations in airflow and respiratory effort result in distinctive sounds within the thoracic cavity that may indicate pulmonary disease or dysfunction.

Auscultation proceeds in a systematic, cephalocaudal fashion. Breath sounds on the left and right sides are compared in the anterior, lateral, and posterior segments of the chest wall, as shown in Figure 2-4. The diaphragm (flat side) of the stethoscope should be used for auscultation. The patient should be seated or lying comfortably in a position that allows access to all lung fields. Full inspirations and expirations are performed by the patient through the mouth, as the

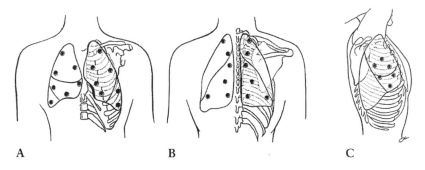

A    B    C

**Figure 2-4.** *Landmarks for lung auscultation on (A) anterior, (B) posterior, and (C) lateral aspects of the chest wall. (Artwork by Peter P. Wu.)*

clinician listens to the entire cycle of respiration before moving the stethoscope to another lung segment.

There are normal and abnormal (adventitious) breath sounds. Breath sounds should be documented according to the location and the phase of respiration (i.e., inspiration, expiration, or both) and in comparison with the opposite lung.

## Normal Breath Sounds

### Tracheal, Bronchial, or Bronchovesicular Sounds

Normal tracheal or bronchial breath sounds are loud, tubular sounds that are heard over the proximal airways, such as the trachea and main stem bronchi. A pause is heard between inspiration and expiration, with the expiratory phase being longer than the inspiratory phase. Normal bronchovesicular sounds are very similar to bronchial breath sounds; however, there is no pause between inspiration and expiration.[8,9]

### Vesicular Sounds

Vesicular sounds are soft, rustling sounds that are heard over the more distal airways and lung parenchyma. Inspiration is longer and more pronounced than expiration, as a decrease in airway lumen during expiration limits transmission of airflow sounds.[8,9]

Note: In most reference books, a distinction between normal bronchial and bronchovesicular sounds is made to help with standardization of terminology. This distinction, however, is often not used in the clinical setting.

---

### Clinical Tip

Clinically, tracheal or bronchial and vesicular breath sounds are generally documented as "normal" or "clear" breath sounds; however, the use of tracheal or vesicular breath sounds is more accurate. The abbreviation CTA is also frequently used and stands for "clear to auscultation."

---

## Abnormal Breath Sounds

Breath sounds are abnormal if they are heard outside their usual location in the chest or if they are qualitatively different from normal breath sounds.[11] Abnormal breath sounds with possible sources are outlined below:

| Sound | Possible Etiology |
|---|---|
| Bronchial (abnormal if heard in areas where vesicular sounds should be present) | Fluid or secretion consolidation (airlessness) that could occur with pneumonia |
| Decreased or diminished (less audible) | Hypoventilation, severe congestion, or emphysema |
| Absent | Pneumothorax or lung collapse |

## Adventitious Breath Sounds

Adventitious breath sounds occur from alterations or turbulence in airflow through the tracheobronchial tree and lung parenchyma. These sounds can be divided into continuous (wheezes and rhonchi) or discontinuous (crackles) sounds.[9,11]

### Continuous Sounds

*Wheeze.* Wheezes occur most commonly with airway obstruction from bronchoconstriction or retained secretions and are commonly heard on expiration. Wheezes may also be present during inspiration if the obstruction is significant enough. Wheezes can be high pitched (usually from bronchospasm or constriction, as in asthma) or low pitched (usually from secretions, as in pneumonia).

*Rhonchi.* Low-pitched or "snoring" sounds that are continuous characterize rhonchi. These sounds are generally associated with large airway obstruction, generally from secretions lining the airways.

*Stridor.* Stridor is an extremely high-pitched wheeze that occurs with significant upper airway obstruction and is present during both inspiration and expiration. The presence of stridor indicates a medical emergency. Stridor is also audible without a stethoscope.

---

### Clinical Tip

Acute onset of stridor during an intervention session warrants immediate notification of the nursing and medical staff.

---

### Discontinuous Sounds: Crackles

Crackles are bubbling or popping sounds that represent the presence of fluid or secretions, or the sudden opening of closed airways. Crackles that result from fluid (pulmonary edema) or secretions (pneumonia) are described as "wet" or "coarse," whereas crackles that occur from the sudden opening or closed airways (atelectasis) are referred to as "dry" or "fine."

Note: Wet crackles can also be referred to as *rales*, but the American Thoracic Society-American College of Chest Physicians has moved to eliminate this terminology for purposes of standardization.[12]

---

### Clinical Tip

Despite efforts to make the terminology of breath sounds more consistent, terminology may still vary from clinician to clinician and facility to facility. Always clarify the intended meaning of the breath sound description if your findings differ significantly from what has been documented or reported.

---

*Extrapulmonary Sounds*
These sounds are generated from dysfunction outside of the lung tissue. The most common sound is the *pleural friction rub*. This sound is heard as a loud grating sound, generally throughout both phases of respiration, and is almost always associated with pleuritis (inflamed pleurae rubbing on one another).[9,11]

*Voice Sounds*
Normal phonation is audible during auscultation, with the intensity and clarity of speech also dissipating from proximal to distal airways. Voice sounds that are more or less pronounced in distal lung regions, where vesicular breath sounds should occur, may indicate areas of consolidation or hyperinflation, respectively. The same areas of auscultation should be used when assessing voice sounds. The following three types of voice sound tests can be used to help confirm breath sound findings:

1.   Whispered pectoriloquy. The patient whispers "one, two, three." The test is positive for consolidation if phrases are clearly audible in distal lung fields. This test is positive for hyperinflation if the phrases are less audible in distal lung fields.

2.   Bronchophony. The patient repeats the phrase "ninety-nine." The results are similar to whispered pectoriloquy.

3.   Egophony. The patient repeats the letter "e." If the auscultation in the distal lung fields sound like "a," then fluid in the air
spaces or lung parenchyma is suspected.

---

Clinical Tip

To ensure accurate auscultation, do the following:
• Make sure stethoscope earpieces are pointing up and
inward before placing in the ears.
• Long stethoscope tubing may dampen sound transmission. Length of tubing should be approximately 30 cm (12
in.) to 55 cm (21–22 in.).[9]
• Always check proper function of the stethoscope before
auscultating by listening to finger tapping on the diaphragm while the earpieces are in place.
• Apply the stethoscope diaphragm firmly against the
skin so that it lays flat.
• Observe chest wall expansion and breathing pattern
while auscultating to help confirm palpatory findings of
breathing pattern (e.g., sequence and symmetry). For
example, decreased chest wall motion that was palpated
earlier in the left lower lung field may present with
decreased breath sounds in that same area.
    To minimize false-positive adventitious breath sound
findings, do the following:
• Ensure full, deep inspirations (decreased effort can be
misinterpreted as decreased breath sounds).
• Be aware of the stethoscope tubing's touching other
objects (especially ventilator tubing) or chest hair.
• Periodically lift the stethoscope off the chest wall to
help differentiate extraneous sounds (e.g., chest or nasogastric tubes, patient snoring) that may appear to originate
from the thorax.
• To maximize patient comfort, allow periodic rest periods between deep respirations to prevent hyperventilation
and dizziness.

---

Palpation

The third component of the physical examination is palpation of the
chest wall, which is performed in a cephalocaudal direction. Figure 2-5

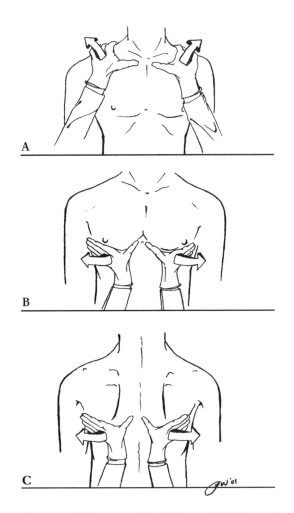

**Figure 2-5.** *Palpation of (A) upper, (B) middle, and (C) lower chest wall motion. (Artwork by Peter P. Wu.)*

demonstrates hand placement for chest wall palpation of the upper, middle, and lower lung fields. Palpation is performed to examine the following:

- Presence of fremitus (a vibration, caused by the presence of secretions or voice production, that is felt through the chest wall) during respirations.[8]

- Presence, location, and reproducibility of pain, tenderness, or both.

- Skin temperature.

- Presence of bony abnormalities, rib fractures, or both.

- Chest expansion and symmetry.

- Presence of *subcutaneous emphysema* (palpated as bubbles popping under the skin from the presence of air in the subcutaneous tissue; this finding is abnormal, as it represents air that has escaped or is escaping from the lungs. Subcutaneous emphysema can occur from a pneumothorax [PTX], a complication from central line placement, or after thoracic surgery).[1]

---

Clinical Tip

To decrease patient fatigue while palpating each of the chest wall segments for motion, all of the other items listed above can also be examined simultaneously.

---

**Mediate Percussion**

Mediate percussion can evaluate tissue densities within the thoracic cage, as well as indirectly measure diaphragmatic excursion during respirations. Mediate percussion can also be used to confirm other findings in the physical examination. The procedure is shown in Figure 2-6 and is performed by placing the palmar surface of the index finger, middle finger, or both of one hand flatly against the surface of the chest wall within the intercostal spaces. The tips of the other index finger, middle finger, or both then strike the distal third of the fingers that are resting against the chest wall. The clinician proceeds from side to side in a cephalocaudal fashion, within the intercostal spaces, for both anterior and posterior aspects of the chest wall. Sounds produced from mediate percussion can be characterized as one of the following:

- Resonant (over normal lung tissue)

- Hyperresonant (over emphysematous lungs or PTX)

- Tympanic (over gas bubbles in abdomen)

- Dull (from increased tissue density or lungs with decreased air)

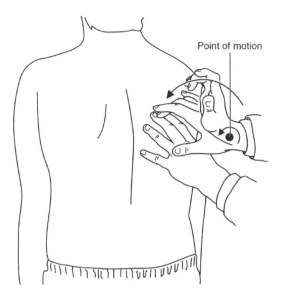

Point of motion

**Figure 2-6.** *Demonstration of mediate percussion technique. (With permission from EA Hillegass, HS Sadowsky [eds]. Essentials of Cardiopulmonary Physical Therapy. Philadelphia: Saunders, 1994;581.)*

- Flat (extreme dullness over very dense tissues, such as the thigh muscles)[9]

To evaluate diaphragmatic excursion with mediate percussion, the clinician first delineates the resting position of the diaphragm by percussing down the posterior aspect of one side of the chest wall until a change from resonant to dull (flat) sounds occurs. The clinician then asks the patient to inspire deeply and repeats the process, noting the difference in landmarks when sound changes occur. The difference is the amount of diaphragmatic excursion. The other side is also examined, and a comparison can then be made of the hemidiaphragms.

Note: Mediate percussion is a difficult skill and is performed most proficiently by experienced therapists or physicians. Mediate percussion can also be performed over the abdominal cavity to assess tissue densities, which is described further in Chapter 8. Also, do not confuse this examination technique with the intervention technique of *percussion,* which is used to help mobilize bronchopulmonary secretions in patients.

## Cough Examination

An essential component of bronchopulmonary hygiene is cough effectiveness. The cough mechanism can be divided into four phases: (1) full inspiration, (2) closure of the glottis with an increase of intrathoracic pressure, (3) abdominal contraction, and (4) rapid expulsion of air. The inability to perform one or more portions of the cough mechanism can lead to decreased pulmonary secretion clearance.

Cough examination includes the following components[9]:

- Effectiveness (ability to clear secretions)

- Control (ability to start and stop coughs)

- Quality (wet, dry, bronchospastic)

- Frequency (how often during the day and night cough occurs)

- Sputum production (color, quantity, odor, and consistency)

The effectiveness of a patient's cough can be examined directly by simply asking the patient to cough or indirectly by observing the above components when the patient coughs spontaneously.

---

### Clinical Tip

Hemoptysis, the expectoration of blood during coughing, may occur for many reasons. Hemoptysis is usually benign postoperatively if it is not sustained with successive coughs. The therapist should note whether the blood is dark red or brownish in color (old blood) or bright red (new or *frank* blood). The presence of new blood in sputum should be documented and the nurse or physician notified.

---

## Diagnostic Testing

### Oximetry

Pulse oximetry ($Spo_2$) is a noninvasive method of determining arterial oxyhemoglobin saturation ($Sao_2$). It also indirectly examines the partial pressure of $O_2$. Finger or ear sensors are generally applied to a patient on a continuous or intermittent basis. Oxyhemoglobin saturation is an indication of pulmonary reserve and is dependent on the

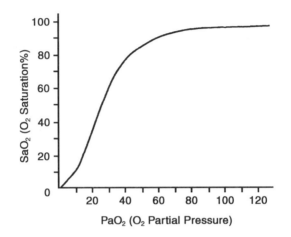

**Figure 2-7.** *The oxyhemoglobin dissociation curve. (Artwork by Marybeth Cuaycong.)*

$Po_2$ level in the blood. Figure 2-7 demonstrates the direct relationship of oxyhemoglobin saturation and partial pressures of $O_2$. As shown on the steep portion of the curve, small changes in $Po_2$ levels below 60 mm Hg will result in large changes in an oxygen saturation, which is considered moderately hypoxic.[8] The relationship between oxygen saturation and $Po_2$ levels is further summarized in Table 2-4. The affinity or binding of $O_2$ to hemoglobin is affected by changes in pH, $Pco_2$, temperature, and 2,3-diphosphoglycerate (a by-product of red blood cell metabolism) levels. Note that pulse oximetry can only measure changes in oxygenation ($Po_2$) indirectly and cannot measure changes in ventilation ($Pco_2$). Changes in ventilation need to be measured by arterial blood gas (ABG) analysis.[13]

---

### Clinical Tip

- To ensure accurate $O_2$ saturation readings, do the following: (1) check for proper waveform or pulsations, which indicate proper signal reception, and (2) compare pulse readings on $O_2$ saturation monitor with the patient's peripheral pulses or electrocardiograph readings (if available).
- $O_2$ saturation readings can be affected by poor circulation (cool digits), movement of sensor cord, cleanliness of

Table 2-4. Relationship between Oxygen Saturation, the Partial Pressure of Oxygen, and the Signs and Symptoms of Hypoxemia

| Oxyhemoglobin Saturation ($Sao_2$) (%) | Oxygen Partial Pressure ($Pao_2$) (mm Hg) | Signs and Symptoms of Hypoxemia |
|---|---|---|
| 97–99 | 90–100 | None |
| 95 | 80 | Tachypnea |
| | | Tachycardia |
| 90 | 60 | As above |
| | | Restlessness |
| | | Malaise |
| | | Impaired judgment |
| | | Incoordination |
| | | Vertigo |
| | | Nausea |
| 85 | 50 | As above |
| | | Labored respiration |
| | | Cardiac dysrhythmia |
| | | Confusion |
| 80 | 45 | As above |
| 75 | 40 | As above |

Source: Adapted from DL Frownfelter, E Dean (eds). Principles and Practice of Cardiopulmonary Physical Therapy (3rd ed). St. Louis: Mosby, 1996;237.

the sensors, nail polish, intense light, increased levels of carboxyhemoglobin ($Hbco_2$), jaundice, skin pigmentation, shock states, and severe hypoxia.[14,15]

## Arterial Blood Gas Analysis

ABG analysis examines acid-base balance (pH), ventilation ($CO_2$ levels), and oxygenation ($O_2$ levels), as well as guiding respiratory interventions, such as mechanical ventilation settings.[8] For proper cellular metabolism to occur, acid-base balance must be maintained. Disturbances in acid-base balance can be caused by respiratory or metabolic dysfunction. Normally, the respiratory and metabolic systems work in synergy to help maintain acid-base balance.

The ability to interpret ABGs provides the physical therapist with valuable information regarding the current medical status of the patient, the appropriateness for bronchopulmonary hygiene or exercise treatments, and the outcomes of medical and physical therapy intervention.

ABG measurements are usually performed on a routine basis, which is specified according to need in the critical care setting. For the critically ill patient, ABG sampling may occur every 1–3 hours. In contrast, ABGs may be sampled one or two times a day in a patient whose pulmonary or metabolic status has stabilized. Unless specified, arterial blood is sampled from an indwelling arterial line. Other sites of sampling include venous blood from a peripheral venous puncture or catheter and mixed venous blood from a pulmonary artery catheter. Appendix III-A describes vascular monitoring lines in more detail.

*Terminology*
The following terms are frequently used in ABG analysis:

| | |
|---|---|
| $Pao_2$ ($Po_2$) | The partial pressure of dissolved $O_2$ in plasma |
| $Paco_2$ ($Pco_2$) | The partial pressure of dissolved $CO_2$ in plasma |
| pH | The degree of acidity or alkalinity in blood |
| $HCO_3$ level | The level of bicarbonate in the blood |
| Percentage of $Sao_2$ ($O_2$ saturation) | A percentage of the amount of hemoglobin sites filled (saturated) with $O_2$ molecules ($Pao_2$ and $Sao_2$ are intimately related but are not synonymous) |

*Normal Values*
The normal values for ABGs are as follows[16]:
$Pao_2$     Greater than 80 mm Hg
$Paco_2$    35–45 mm Hg
pH     7.35–7.45
$HCO_3$    22–28 mEq/liter
ABGs are generally reported in the following format: $Pao_2$/$Paco_2$/ pH/ $HCO_3$ (e.g., 96/42/7.38/26).

*Arterial Blood Gas Interpretation*
Interpretation of ABGs includes the ability to determine any deviation from normal values and hypothesize a cause (or causes) for the acid-base disturbance in relation to the patient's clinical history.

The following terms are associated with ABG interpretation[17]:

- *Acidemia* occurs when the pH is less than 7.4.

- *Acidosis* is the process that causes acidemia.

- *Alkalemia* occurs when the pH is greater than 7.4.

- *Alkalosis* is the process that causes alkalemia.
- *Hypoxia* occurs when $Po_2$ is less than 80 mm Hg.
- *Hypercarbia* occurs when $Pco_2$ is greater than 50 mm Hg.

The following are the primary concepts of ABG interpretation:

1.   Respiratory or metabolic disorders can cause states of acidemia or alkalemia.

2.   If respiratory or metabolic disorders cause acid-base imbalances, then they are called the *primary process*.

3.   Acid-base imbalances can be *compensated* (pH is close to 7.35–7.45) for by the nonprimary system. For example, a primary respiratory acidosis can be compensated for by the metabolic system.

4.   If the nonprimary system fails to compensate for the primary system, the disorder is referred to as *uncompensated* (pH is higher or lower than 7.35–7.45).

5.   Acid-base imbalances can be also be *corrected* by addressing the primary process involved. For example, a primary metabolic alkalosis from renal system dysfunction can be corrected by administering medical therapy to the renal system.

Knowledge of uncompensated, compensated, or corrected acid-base disturbances provides insight into the patient's current medical status. The following outline provides basic guidelines for ABG interpretation:

1.   Examine the patient's pH level to determine acid-base balance.

   a.   If the patient's pH = 7.4, acid-base balance is normal.

   b.   If the patient's pH <7.4, the patient is acidotic.

   c.   If the patient's pH >7.4, the patient is alkalotic.

2.   To determine if the patient's pH change is due to a primary respiratory process, examine the $Pco_2$. For every 10-point change in $Pco_2$, there is a 0.08-change in pH in the opposite direction.

   a.   A low pH and a high $Pco_2$ indicate uncompensated respiratory acidosis.

    b.    A high pH and a low $P_{CO_2}$ indicate uncompensated respiratory alkalosis.

3.    To determine if the patient's pH change is due to a primary metabolic process, examine the $HCO_3$. For every 10-point change in $HCO_3$, there is a 0.15-change in pH in the same direction.

    a.    A low pH and a low $HCO_3$ indicate uncompensated metabolic acidosis.

    b.    A high pH and a high $HCO_3$ indicate uncompensated metabolic alkalosis.

4.    To determine if the patient's primary respiratory process has been compensated for by the renal system, examine $HCO_3$.

    a.    A high $HCO_3$ in respiratory acidosis indicates compensated respiratory acidosis.

    b.    A low $HCO_3$ in respiratory alkalosis indicates compensated respiratory alkalosis.

5.    To determine if the patient's primary metabolic process has been compensated for by the respiratory system, examine the $P_{CO_2}$.

    a.    A low $P_{CO_2}$ in metabolic acidosis indicates compensated metabolic acidosis.

    b.    A high $P_{CO_2}$ in metabolic alkalosis indicates compensated metabolic alkalosis.

The possible causes for these disorders are summarized in Table 2-5. Decreased levels of alertness may result from retained $CO_2$. A list of signs and symptoms of $CO_2$ retention is shown in Table 2-6.

---

### Clinical Tip

• Acid-base balance or pH is the most important ABG value to be within normal limits. It is important to relate ABG values with medical history and clinical course. ABG values and vital signs are generally documented on a daily flow sheet, an invaluable source of information. Changes in ABG values over time are more informative than a single ABG reading. Single ABG readings should be correlated with previous ABG readings, medical status, supplemental $O_2$ or ventilator changes, and medical procedures.

Table 2-5.  Common Causes of Acid-Base Imbalances

Causes of respiratory acidosis (low pH, high $CO_2$, normal bicarbonate)
  Obstructive lung disorder (acute or chronic)
  Central nervous system depression with or without neuromuscular disorders
  Hypoventilation from pain, oversedation, chest wall deformities, secretion
    retention
  Cardiopulmonary arrest
Causes of respiratory alkalosis (high pH, low $CO_2$, normal bicarbonate)
  Hyperventilation from nervousness and anxiety, fever, pain, or mechanical
    ventilation
  Hypoxia
  Pulmonary embolus, pulmonary fibrosis, asthma
  Pregnancy
  Brain injury
  Salicylates
  Congestive heart failure or hepatic insufficiency
Causes of metabolic alkalosis (high pH, high bicarbonate, normal $CO_2$)
  Fluid losses from upper gastrointestinal tract (e.g., vomiting or nasogastric
    tube aspiration of acid)
  Rapid correction of chronic hypercapnia (high $CO_2$)
  Diuretic or corticosteroid therapy
  Cushing's disease, hyperaldosteronism
  Severe potassium depletion
  Excessive ingestion of licorice
  Nonparathyroid hypercalcemia
Causes of metabolic acidosis (low pH, low bicarbonate, normal $CO_2$)
  Ketoacidosis from diabetes, starvation, or alcohol
  Poisonings from salicylates, ethylene glycol, methyl glycol, or paraldehyde
  Lactic acidosis
  Renal failure, renal tubular acidosis
  Diarrhea
  Drainage of pancreatic fluid
  Ureterosigmoidostomy
  Obstructed ileal loop
  Therapy with acetazolamide (Diamox) or with ammonium chloride
    ($NH_4Cl$)
  Intravenous hyperalimentation

Source: Adapted from CM Hudak, BM Gallo (eds). Critical Care Nursing, A Holistic
Approach (6th ed). Philadelphia: Lippincott, 1994.

**Table 2-6.** Clinical Presentation of Carbon Dioxide Retention and Narcosis

Altered mental status
  Lethargy
  Drowsiness
  Coma
Headache
Tachycardia
Hypertension
Diaphoresis
Tremor
Redness of skin, sclera, or conjuctiva

Source: Adapted from LD Kersten (ed). Comprehensive Respiratory Nursing: A Decision-Making Approach. Philadelphia: Saunders, 1989;351.

- Bicarbonate ($HCO_3$) levels are not routinely reported unless requested.
- Be sure to note if an ABG sample is drawn from mixed venous blood, as the normal $O_2$ value is lower. $P\bar{v}o_2$ of mixed venous blood is 35–40 mm Hg.

Note: Acid-base disturbances that occur clinically can arise from both respiratory and metabolic disorders; therefore, interpretation of the ABG results may not prove to be as straightforward as the example given above. Hence, the clinician must use this information as part of a complete examination process to gain full understanding of the patient's current medical status.

### Chest X-Rays

Radiographic information of the thoracic cavity in combination with a clinical history provides critical assistance in the differential diagnosis of pulmonary conditions. Figure 2-8 outlines the film markers of anatomic structures that are used for chest x-ray (CXR) interpretation.

Indications for CXRs are the following[18,19]:

- To assist in the clinical diagnosis and monitor the progression or regression of the following:

    Airspace consolidation (pulmonary edema, pneumonia, adult respiratory distress syndrome [ARDS], pulmonary hemorrhage, and infarctions)

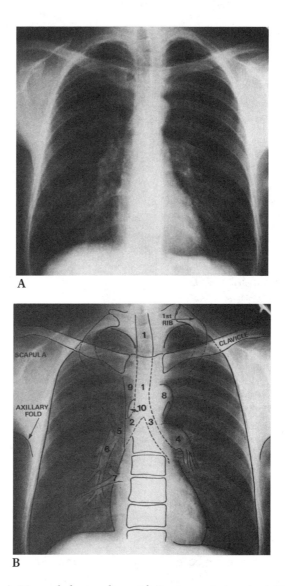

**Figure 2-8.** A. *Normal chest radiograph (posteroanterior view). B. Same radiograph as in A with normal anatomic structures labeled or numbered. (1 = trachea; 2 = right main stem bronchus; 3 = left main stem bronchus; 4 = left pulmonary artery; 5 = pulmonary vein to the right upper lobe; 6 = right interlobar artery; 7 = vein to right middle and lower lobes; 8 = aortic knob; 9 = superior vena cava; 10 = ascending aorta.) (With permission from RG Fraser, JA Peter Paré, PD Paré, et al. [eds]. Diagnosis of Diseases of the Chest, Vol. 1 [3rd ed]. Philadelphia: Saunders, 1988;287.)*

Large intrapulmonary air spaces and presence of mediastinal or subcutaneous air, as well as PTX

Lobar atelectasis

Other pulmonary lesions, such as lung nodules and abscesses

Rib fractures

• To determine proper placement of endotracheal tubes, central lines, chest tubes, or nasogastric tubes

• To evaluate structural features, such as cardiac or mediastinal size and diaphragmatic shape and position

CXRs are classified according to the direction of radiographic beam projection. The first word describes where the beam enters the body, and the second word describes the exit.

Common types of CXRs include the following:

| | |
|---|---|
| Posterior-anterior (P-A) | Taken while the patient is upright sitting or standing |
| Anterior-posterior (A-P) | Taken while the patient is upright sitting or standing, semireclined, or supine |
| Lateral | Taken while the patient is upright sitting or standing, or decubitus (lying on the side) |

Upright positions are preferred to allow full expansion of lungs without hindrance of the abdominal viscera and to visualize gravity-dependent fluid collections. Lateral films aid in three-dimensional, segmental localization of lesions and fluid collections not visible in P-A or A-P views.

### Clinical Tip

Diagnosis cannot be made by CXR alone. The therapist should use CXR reports as a guide for decision making and not as an absolute parameter for bronchopulmonary hygiene evaluation and treatment. CXRs sometimes lag behind significant clinical presentation (e.g., symptoms of pulmonary infection may resolve clinically, whereas CXR findings remain positive for infection).

## Sputum Analysis

Analysis of sputum includes culture and Gram's stain to isolate and identify organisms that may be present in the lower respiratory tract. Refer to Chapter 10 for more details on culture and Gram's stain. After the organisms are identified, appropriate antibiotic therapy can be instituted. Sputum specimens are collected when there is a rise in the patient's temperature or a change in the color or consistency of sputum occurs. They can also be used to evaluate the efficacy of antibiotic therapy. Sputum analysis can be inaccurate if a sterile technique is not maintained during sputum collection or if the specimen is contaminated with too much saliva, as noted microscopically by the presence of many squamous epithelial cells.

---

### Clinical Tip

• Therapists involved in bronchopulmonary hygiene and collecting sputum samples should have sterile sputum collection containers and equipment on hand before beginning the treatment session to ensure successful sputum collection.

• Patients who present with a sputum analysis that is negative for active infection may still have retained secretions which could hinder gas exchange and tolerance to activity; therefore, therapists will need to clinically evaluate the need for secretion clearance techniques.

---

## Flexible Bronchoscopy

A flexible, fiberoptic tube is used as a diagnostic and interventional tool to directly visualize and aspirate (suction) the bronchopulmonary tree. If a patient is mechanically ventilated, the bronchoscope is inserted through the endotracheal or tracheal tube. Please refer to Appendix III-B for more information on mechanical ventilation and endotracheal and tracheal tubes. If the patient is spontaneously breathing, a local anesthetic is applied, and the bronchoscope is inserted through one of the patient's nares. Table 2-7 summarizes the diagnostic and therapeutic indications of bronchoscopy.

Note: Bronchoscopy can also be performed with a rigid bronchoscope. This is primarily an operative procedure.[19–21,]

**Table 2-7.** Diagnostic and Therapeutic Indications for Flexible Bronchoscopy

Diagnostic indications
  Evaluation of neoplasms (benign or malignant) in air spaces and mediastinum, tissue biopsy
  Evaluation of the patient before and after lung transplantation
  Endotracheal intubation
  Infection, unexplained chronic cough, or hemoptysis
  Tracheobronchial stricture and stenosis
  Hoarseness or vocal cord paralysis
  Fistula or unexplained pleural effusion
  Localized wheezing or stridor
  Chest trauma or persistent pneumothorax
  Postoperative assessment of tracheal, tracheobronchial, bronchial, or stump anastomosis
Therapeutic indications
  Removal of retained secretions, foreign bodies, and/or obstructive endotracheal tissue
  Intubation or stent placement
  Bronchoalveolar lavage
  Aspiration of cysts or drainage of abscesses
  Pneumothorax or lobar collapse
  Thoracic trauma
  Airway maintenance (tamponade for bleeding)

Sources: Adapted from MR Hetzed (ed). Minimally Invasive Techniques in Thoracic Medicine and Surgery. London: Chapman & Hall, 1995;4; JM Rippe, RS Irwin, MP Fink, et al. (eds). Procedures and Techniques in Intensive Care Medicine. Boston: Little, Brown, 1994; and LM Malarkey, ME McMorrow (eds). Nurse's Manual of Laboratory Tests and Diagnostic Procedures (2nd ed). Philadelphia: Saunders, 2000;277–278.

## Ventilation-Perfusion Scan

The $(\dot{V}/\dot{Q})$ scan is used to rule out the presence of pulmonary embolism (PE) and other acute abnormalities of oxygenation and gas exchange and as pre- and postoperative evaluation of lung transplantation.

During a ventilation scan, inert radioactive gases or aerosols are inhaled, and three subsequent projections (i.e., after first breath, at equilibrium, and during washout) of airflow are recorded.

During a perfusion lung scan, a radioisotope is injected intravenously into a peripheral vessel, and six projections are taken (i.e., anterior, posterior, both laterals, and both posterior obliques). The scan is very sensitive to diminished or absent blood flow, and lesions of 2 cm or greater are detected.

Perfusion defects can occur with pulmonary embolus, asthma, emphysema and virtually all alveolar filling, destructive or space-occupying lesions in lung, and hypoventilation. A CXR a few hours after the perfusion scan helps the differential diagnosis.

Ventilation scans are performed first, followed by perfusion scan. The two scans are then compared to determine extent of $\dot{V}/\dot{Q}$ matching. As described earlier, in the Ventilation and Perfusion Ratio section, average reference $\dot{V}/\dot{Q}$ ratio is approximately equal to 0.8.[20,22]

**Pulmonary Function Tests**

Pulmonary function tests (PFTs) consist of measuring a patient's lung volumes and capacities, as well as inspiratory and expiratory flow rates. Lung capacities are comprised of two or more lung volumes. Quantification of these parameters helps in distinguishing obstructive from restrictive respiratory patterns, as well as determining how the respiratory system contributes to physical activity limitations. The respiratory system's volumes and capacities are shown in Figure 2-9. Alterations in volumes and capacities will occur with obstructive and restrictive diseases, and these changes are shown in Figure 2-10. Volume, flow, and gas dilution spirometers and body plethysmography are the measurement tools used for PFTs. A flow-volume loop is also included as part of the patient's PFTs and is shown in Figure 2-11. A comprehensive assessment of PFT results includes comparisons with normal values and prior test results. PFT results may be skewed according to a patient's effort. Table 2-8 outlines the measurements performed during PFTs.

The normal range of values for PFTs is variable and is based on a person's age, gender, height, ethnic origin, and weight (body surface area). Normal predicted values can be extrapolated from a nomogram or calculated from regression (prediction) equations obtained from statistical analysis.

For example, based on a nomogram, the following predicted values for forced vital capacity (FVC) and forced expiratory volume in 1 second ($FEV_1$) would be approximately[23]

- FVC = 4.1 liters, $FEV_1$ = 3 liters for a man who is 55 years old and 66 in. tall

- FVC = 2.95 liters, $FEV_1$ = 2.2 liters for a woman who is 55 years old and 62 in. tall

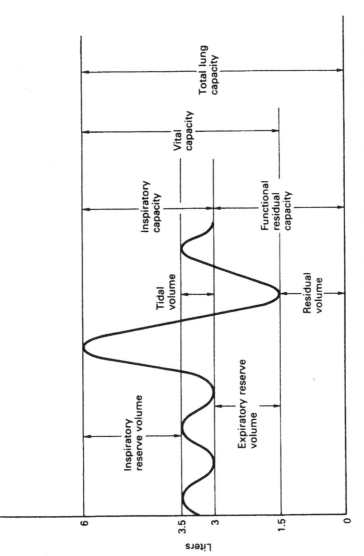
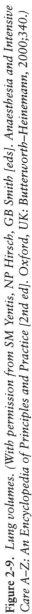

**Figure 2-9.** *Lung volumes. (With permission from SM Yentis, NP Hirsch, GB Smith [eds]. Anaesthesia and Intensive Care A–Z: An Encyclopedia of Principles and Practice [2nd ed]. Oxford, UK: Butterworth–Heinemann, 2000;340.)*

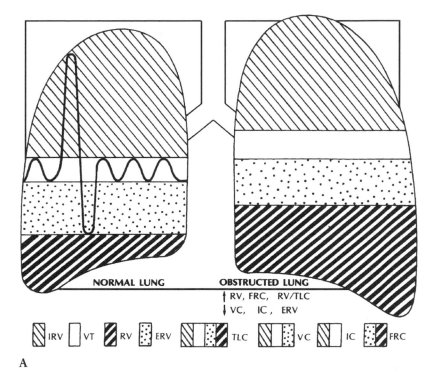

**Figure 2-10.** A. *How obstructive lung disorders alter lung volumes and capacities.*

Because there can be variability from person to person, it is most useful to compare a person's PFT results from his or her previous tests. Indications for PFTs are the following[23–25]:

- Detection and quantification of respiratory disease

- Evaluation of pulmonary involvement in systemic diseases

- Assessment of disease progression

- Evaluation of impairment, functional limitation, or disability

- Assessment for bronchodilator therapy or surgical intevention, or both, along with the subsequent response to the respective intervention

- Preoperative evaluation (high-risk patient identification)

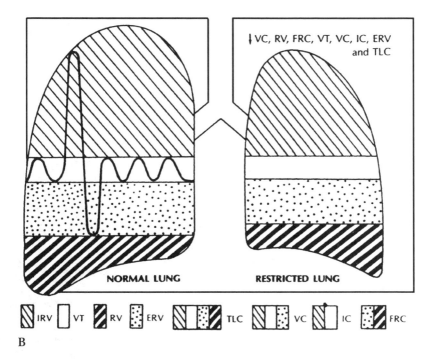

B

**Figure 2-10.** *Continued.* **B.** *How restrictive lung disorders alter lung volumes and capacities.* *(ERV = expiratory reserve volume; FRC = functional residual capacity; IC = inspiratory capacity; IRV = inspiratory reserve volume; RV = residual volume; TLC = total lung capacity; VC = tidal capacity; VT = tidal volume.)* *(With permission from T Des Jardins, GC Burton [eds]. Clinical Manifestations and Assessment of Respiratory Disease [3rd ed]. St. Louis: Mosby, 1995;40,49.)*

---

Clinical Tip

• $FEV_1$, FVC, and the $FEV_1$/FVC ratio are the most commonly interpreted PFT values. These measures represent the degree of airway patency during expiration, which affects airflow in and out of the lung.

• Predicted normal values for a person's given age, gender, and height will be provided in the PFT report for reference to the person's actual PFT result.

---

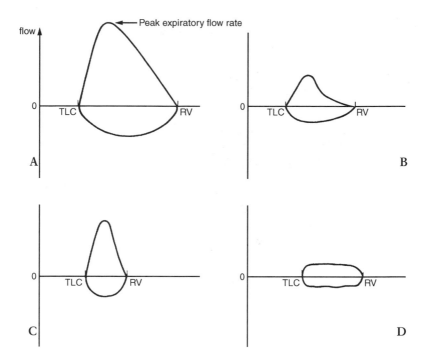

**Figure 2-11.** *Characteristic flow-volume loops: (A) normal, (B) obstructive lung disease, (C) restrictive lung disease, (D) tracheal/laryngeal obstruction. (RV = residual volume; TLC = total lung capacity.) (With permission from SM Yentis, NP Hirsch, GB Smith [eds]. Anaesthesia and Intensive Care A–Z: An Encyclopedia of Principles and Practice [2nd ed]. Oxford, UK: Butterworth–Heinemann, 2000;220.)*

## Pathophysiology

Respiratory disorders can be classified as obstructive or restrictive. A patient may present with single or multiple obstructive and restrictive processes, or with a combination of both as a result of environmental, traumatic, orthopedic, neuromuscular, nutritional, or drug-induced factors. These disorders may be infectious, neoplastic, or vascular in nature or involve the connective tissue of the thorax.[8]

**Table 2-8.** Description and Clinical Significance of Pulmonary Function Tests

| Test | Description | Significance |
| --- | --- | --- |
| Lung volume tests | | |
| Tidal volume (VT) | The volume of air inhaled or exhaled during a single breath in a resting state. | Decreased tidal volume could be indicative of atelectasis, fatigue, restrictive lung disorders, and tumors. |
| Inspiratory reserve volume (IRV) | The maximum amount of air that can be inspired following a normal inspiration. | Decreased IRV could be indicative of obstructive pulmonary disease. |
| Expiratory reserve volume (ERV) | The maximum amount of air that can be exhaled following a normal exhalation. | ERV is necessary to calculate residual volume and FRC. Decreased values could be indicative of ascites, pleural effusion, or pneumothorax. |
| Residual volume (RV) | The volume of air remaining in the lungs at the end of maximal expiration that cannot be forcibly expelled. | RV helps to differentiate between obstructive and restrictive disorders. An increased RV indicates an obstructive disorder, and a decreased RV indicates a restrictive disorder. |
| Total lung capacity (TLC) | The volume of air contained in the lung at the end of maximal inspiration. (TLC = VT + IRV + ERV + RV) | TLC helps to differentiate between obstructive and restrictive disorders. An increased TLC indicates an obstructive disorder; a decreased TLC indicates a restrictive disorder. |
| Vital capacity (VC) | The maximum amount of air that can be expired slowly and completely following a maximal inspiration. (VC = VT + IRV + ERV) | A decrease in VC can result from a decrease in lung tissue distensibility or depression of the respiratory centers in the brain. |
| Functional residual capacity (FRC) | The volume of air remaining in the lungs at the end of a normal expiration. | FRC values help differentiate between obstructive and restrictive respiratory patterns. |

| | Calculated from body plethysmography. (FRC = ERV + RV) | An increased FRC indicates an obstructive respiratory pattern, and a decreased FRC indicates a restrictive respiratory pattern. |
| Inspiratory capacity (IC) | The largest volume of air that can be inspired in one breath from the resting expiratory level. (IC = VT + IRV) | Changes in IC usually parallel changes in VC. Decreased values could be indicative of restrictive disorders. |
| Residual volume to total lung capacity ratio (RV:TLC ×100) | The percentage of air that cannot be expired in relation to the total amount of air that can be brought into the lungs. | Values >35% are indicative of obstructive disorders. |
| Ventilation tests | | |
| Minute volume (VE) or minute ventilation | The total volume of air inspired or expired in 1 min. (VE = VT × respiratory rate) | VE is most commonly used in exercise or stress testing. VE can increase with hypoxia, hypercapnia, acidosis, and exercise. |
| Respiratory dead space (VD) | The volume of air in the lungs that is ventilated but not perfused in conducting airways and nonfunctioning alveoli. | VD provides information about available surface area for gas exchange. Increased dead space = decreased gas exchange. |
| Alveolar ventilation (VA) | The volume of air that participates in gas exchange. Estimated by subtracting dead space from tidal volume. (VA = VT − VD) | VA measures the amount of oxygen available to tissue, but it should be confirmed by arterial blood gas measurements. |

**Table 2-8.** *Continued*

| Test | Description | Significance |
|---|---|---|
| Pulmonary spirometry tests | | |
| Forced vital capacity (FVC) | The volume of air that can be expired forcefully and rapidly after a maximal inspiration. | FVC is normally equal to VC, but FVC can be decreased in obstructive disorders. |
| Forced expiratory volume timed (FEVt) | The volume of air expired over a time interval during the performance of an FVC maneuver. | A decrease in $FEV_1$ can indicate either obstructive or restrictive airway disease. |
| | The interval is usually 1 sec ($FEV_1$). | With obstructive disease, a decreased $FEV_1$ results from increased resistance to exhalation. |
| | After 3 secs, FEV should equal FVC. | With restrictive disease, a subsequent decrease in $FEV_1$ results from a decreased ability to initially inhale an adequate volume of air. |
| FEV% (usually $FEV_1/FVC \times 100$) | The percent of FVC that can be expired over a given time interval, usually 1 sec. | FEV% is a better discriminator of obstructive and restrictive disorders than FEVt. |
| | | An increase in $FEV_1/FVC$ indicates a restrictive disorder, and a decrease in $FEV_1/FVC$ indicates an obstructive disorder. |
| Forced expiratory flow 25–75% ($FEF_{25-75\%}$) | The average flow of air during the middle 50% of a FEV maneuver. | A decrease in ($FEF_{25-75\%}$) generally indicates obstruction in the medium-sized airways. |
| | Used in comparison with VC. | |
| | Represents peripheral airway resistance. | |
| Peak expiratory flow rate (PEFR) | The maximum flow rate attainable at any time during an FEV. | PEFR can assist with diagnosing obstructive disorders such as asthma. |

| | | |
|---|---|---|
| Maximum voluntary ventilation (MVV) | The largest volume of air that can be breathed per minute by maximal voluntary effort. Test lasts 10–15 secs and is multiplied by six to four to determine the amount of air that can be breathed in a minute (liters/min). | MVV measures status of respiratory muscles, the resistance offered by airways and tissues, and the compliance of the lung and thorax. |
| Flow-volume loop (F-V loop) | A graphic analysis of the maximum forced expiratory flow volume followed by a maximum inspiratory flow volume | The distinctive curves of the F-V loop are created according to the presence or absence of disease. Restrictive disease demonstrates an equal reduction in flow and volume, resulting in a vertical oval-shaped loop. Obstructive disease demonstrates a greater reduction in flow compared with volume, resulting in a horizontal tear-shaped loop. |
| Gas exchange | | |
| Diffusing capacity of carbon monoxide (D$_{LCO}$) | A known mixture of carbon monoxide and helium gas is inhaled and then exhaled after 10 secs, and the amount of gases are remeasured. | D$_{LCO}$ assesses the amount of functioning pulmonary capillary bed in contact with functioning alveoli (gas exchange area). |

Sources: Adapted from JM Thompson, GK McFarland, JE Hirsch, et al (eds). Clinical Nursing Practice. St. Louis: Mosby, 1993;1410; and data from LM Malarkey, ME McMorrow (eds). Nurse's Manual of Laboratory Tests and Diagnostic Procedures (2nd ed). Philadelphia: Saunders, 2000;293–297.

Common terminology that is often used when describing respiratory dysfunction is listed below:

*Air trapping*: Retention of gas in the lung as a result of partial or complete airway obstruction

*Bronchospasm*: Smooth muscle contraction of the bronchi and bronchiole walls resulting in a narrowing of the airway lumen

*Consolidation*: Transudate, exudate, or tissue replacing alveolar air

*Hyperinflation*: Overinflation of the lungs at resting volume due to air trapping

*Hypoxemia*: A low level of oxygen in the blood, usually a $Pao_2$ less than 60–80 mm Hg

*Hypoxia*: A low level of oxygen in the tissues available for cell metabolism

*Respiratory distress*: The acute or insidious onset of dyspnea, respiratory muscle fatigue, abnormal respiratory pattern and rate, anxiety, and cyanosis related to inadequate gas exchange; the clinical presentation that usually precedes respiratory failure

*Respiratory failure*: The inability of the pulmonary system to maintain an adequate exchange of oxygen and carbon dioxide (see Appendix III-B)

### Obstructive Pulmonary Conditions

Obstructive lung diseases or conditions may be described by onset (acute versus chronic), severity (mild, moderate, or severe), and location (upper or lower airway). Obstructive pulmonary patterns are characterized by decreased air flow out of the lungs as a result of narrowing of the airway lumen. This causes increased dead space and decreased surface area for gas exchange. Table 2-9 outlines obstructive disorders, their general physical and diagnostic findings, and their general clinical management.

#### Asthma
Asthma is an immunologic response that can result from allergens (e.g., dust, pollen, smoke, pollutants), food additives, bacterial infection,

Table 2-9. Characteristics and General Management of Obstructive Disorders

| Disorder | Observation | Palpation | Auscultation | Cough | Chest X-Ray | Management |
|---|---|---|---|---|---|---|
| Asthma (exacerbation) | Tachypnea<br>Fatigue<br>Anxiety<br>Pursed lip breathing<br>Active expiration<br>Cyanosis, if severe | Tachycardia with weak pulse on inspiration<br>Increased A-P chest diameter<br>Decreased tactile and vocal fremitus<br>Hyperresonant percussion<br>Pulsus paradoxus (systolic blood pressure decreases on inspiration), if severe | Polyphonic wheezing on expiration > inspiration<br>Diminished breath sounds | Tight, usually nonproductive, then slightly productive of benign sputum | During exacerbation: translucent lung fields, flattened diaphragms, increased A-P diameter of chest, more horizontal ribs.<br>Chest x-ray is normal between asthma exacerbations. | Removal of causative agent<br>Bronchodilators<br>Corticosteroids<br>Supplemental $O_2$<br>IV fluid administration |

Table 2-9. *Continued*

| Disorder | Observation | Palpation | Auscultation | Cough | Chest X-Ray | Management |
|---|---|---|---|---|---|---|
| Chronic bronchitis | "Blue bloater" with stocky build and dependent edema<br><br>Tachypnea with prolonged expiratory phase<br><br>Pursed lip breathing<br><br>Accessory muscle use, often with fixed upper extremities<br><br>Elevated shoulders<br><br>Barrel chest<br><br>Fatigue<br><br>Anxiety | Tachycardia<br>Hypertension<br>Decreased tactile and vocal fremitus<br><br>Hyper-resonant percussion<br><br>Increased A-P chest diameter | Rhonchi<br>Diminished breath sounds<br>Crackles | Spasmodic cough<br>Sputum ranges from clear to purulent<br>Often most productive in the morning | Translucent lung fields.<br>Flattened diaphragms.<br>± Cardiomegaly with increased bronchovascular markings. | Smoking cessation<br>Bronchodilator<br>Steroids<br>Expectorants<br>Antibiotics if infection exists<br>Diuretics if cor pulmonale present<br>Supplemental $O_2$<br>Bronchopulmonary hygiene<br>Assisted or mechanical ventilation, if severe |

| | | | | | | |
|---|---|---|---|---|---|---|
| Emphysema | "Pink puffer" with cachexia<br>Otherwise, see Chronic bronchitis, above | See Chronic bronchitis, above | Very diminished breath sounds<br>Wheeze<br>Crackles | Usually absent and nonproductive | Translucent lung fields.<br>Flattened diaphragms.<br>Bullae.<br>± Small heart with decreased vascular markings. | Bronchodilators<br>Supplemental $O_2$<br>Nutritional support |
| Cystic fibrosis | Tachypnea<br>Fatigue<br>Accessory muscle use<br>Barrel chest<br>Cachexia<br>Clubbing | See Chronic bronchitis, above | Crackles<br>Diminished breath sounds<br>Rhonchi | Cough likely tight, either controlled or spasmodic<br>Usually very viscous, greenish sputum, ± blood streaks | Translucent lung fields.<br>Flattened diaphragms.<br>Fibrosis<br>Atelectasis<br>Enlarged right ventricle. | Antibiotics<br>Bronchodilators<br>Mucolytics<br>Supplemental $O_2$<br>Bronchopulmonary hygiene<br>Nutritional support<br>Psychosocial support<br>Lung transplantation |

Table 2-9. *Continued*

| Disorder | Observation | Palpation | Auscultation | Cough | Chest X-Ray | Management |
|---|---|---|---|---|---|---|
| Bronchiectasis | See Cystic fibrosis, above | See Chronic bronchitis, above | See Cystic fibrosis, above | Purulent, odorous sputum ± Hemoptysis | Patchy infiltrates. ± Atelectasis. + Honeycombing, if advanced. Increased vascular markings. Crowded bronchial markings. | Antibiotics Bronchodilators Corticosteroids Supplemental $O_2$ IV fluid administration Nutritional support Bronchopulmonary hygiene ± Pain control for pleuritic pain Lung transplantation |

± = with or without; A-P = anterior-posterior.

gastroesophageal reflux, stress, cold air, and exercise.[6] The asthmatic exacerbation may be immediate or delayed, resulting in air entrapment and alveolar hyperinflation during the episode with symptoms disappearing between attacks. The primary characteristics of an asthma exacerbation are

- Bronchial smooth muscle constriction

- Mucus production (without infection) due to the increased presence of leukocytes, such as eosinophils

- Bronchial mucosa inflammation and thickening due to cellular and fluid infiltration[26]

Admission to a hospital occurs if signs and symptoms of an asthma exacerbation do not improve after several hours of medical therapy, especially if $FEV_1$ is less than 50% of normal.[27] *Status asthmaticus* is a severe, life-threatening airway obstruction with the potential for cardiopulmonary complications, such as arrhythmia, heart failure, and cardiac arrest. Status asthmaticus is not responsive to basic medical therapies and is characterized by severe hypoxemia and hypercarbia that require assisted or mechanical ventilation.[28]

**Chronic Bronchitis**
Chronic bronchitis is the presence of cough and pulmonary secretion expectoration for at least 3 months, 2 years in a row.[29] Chronic bronchitis is usually linked to cigarette smoking or, less likely, to air pollution or infection. It begins with the following[6]:

- Narrowing of large, then small, airways due to inflammation of bronchial mucosa

- Bronchial mucous gland hyperplasia and bronchial smooth muscle cell hypertrophy

- Decreased mucociliary function

These changes result in air trapping, hyperinflated alveoli, bronchospasm, and excess secretion retention.

The definition of an acute exacerbation of chronic bronchitis is vague.[30] The patient often describes (1) worsened dyspnea at rest or with activity, with a notable inability to ambulate, eat, or sleep; (2) fatigue; and (3) abnormal sputum production or inability to clear sputum. On clinical examination, the patient may have hypoxemia, hypercarbia, pneumonia, cor pulmonale, or worsening of comorbidities. Hospital admission is determined by the degree of respiratory failure, hemodynamic stability, the number of recent physician visits, home oxygen use, and doses of pulmonary medications.[30]

### Emphysema

Emphysema may be genetic ($\alpha$1-antitrypsin protein deficiency) in origin, in which the lack of proteolytic inhibitors allows the alveolar interstitium to be destroyed, or it may be caused by cigarette smoking, air pollutants, or infection. Two types of emphysema occur: centriacinar and panlobular. *Centriacinar emphysema* affects the respiratory bronchioles and the proximal acinus. *Panlobular emphysema* affects the respiratory bronchioles, alveolar ducts and sacs, and alveoli.

Both types of emphysema have progressive destruction of alveolar walls and adjacent capillaries secondary to the following[6]:

- Decreased pulmonary elasticity

- Premature airway collapse

- Bullae formation (A *bulla* is a pocket of air surrounded by walls of compressed lung parenchyma.)

These changes result in decreased lung elasticity, air trapping, and hyperinflation.[31] Reasons for hospital admission are similar to those of a patient with chronic bronchitis, except cor pulmonale does not develop until the late stages of emphysema. A spontaneous PTX is a sequela of emphysema in which a *bleb* (a pocket of air between the two layers of visceral pleura) ruptures to connect with the pleural space.

### Cystic Fibrosis

Cystic fibrosis (CF) is a lethal, autosomal-recessive trait (chromosome 7) that affects exocrine glands of the entire body, particularly of the respiratory, gastrointestinal, and reproductive systems. Soon after birth, an initial pulmonary infection occurs that leads to the following changes throughout life[6]:

- Bronchial and bronchiolar walls become inflamed.

- Bronchial gland and goblet cells hypertrophy to create tenacious pulmonary secretions.

- Mucociliary clearance is decreased.

These changes result in bronchospasm, atelectasis, $\dot{V}/\dot{Q}$ mismatch, increased airway resistance, hypoxemia, and recurrent pulmonary infections.[31] Hospitalization may be indicated if there is increased sputum production or cough for longer than 2 weeks, worsened dyspnea or pulmonary function, weight loss, or the development of hemoptysis, PTX, or cor pulmonale.[32]

### Bronchiectasis

*Bronchiectasis* is an obstructive, restrictive disorder characterized by the following[6]:

- Destruction of the elastic and muscular bronchiole walls

- Destruction of the mucociliary escalator (in which normal epithelium is replaced by nonciliated mucus-producing cells)

- Bronchial dilatation

- Bronchial artery enlargement

It is defined as the permanent dilatation of airways that have a normal diameter of greater than 2 mm.[33] Bronchiectasis results in fibrosis and ulceration of bronchioles, chronically retained pulmonary secretions, atelectasis, and infection. The etiology of bronchiectasis includes previous bacterial respiratory infection, CF, tuberculosis, and immobile cilia syndromes.[33] In order of frequency, bronchiectatic changes occur in the left lower lobe, right middle lobe, lingula, entire left lung, right lower lobe, and entire right lung.[33] Hospitalization usually occurs when complications of bronchiectasis arise, including hemoptysis, pneumonia, PTX, empyema, or cor pulmonale.

### Restrictive Pulmonary Conditions

Restrictive lung diseases or conditions may be described by onset (acute versus chronic) or location (i.e., pulmonary or extrapulmonary). Restrictive patterns are characterized by low lung volumes that result from decreased lung compliance and distensibility and increased lung recoil. The end result is increased work of breathing. Table 2-10 outlines restrictive disorders, their general physical and diagnostic findings, and their general clinical management.

Table 2-10. Characteristics and General Management of Restrictive Disorders

| Disorder | Observation | Palpation | Auscultation | Cough | Chest X-Ray | Management |
|---|---|---|---|---|---|---|
| Atelectasis | ± Tachypnea<br>± Fever<br>± Shallow respirations | ± Tachycardia<br>Decreased tactile fremitus and vocal resonance | Crackles at involved area<br>Diminished breath sounds<br>If lobar collapse exists, absent or bronchial breath sounds | Dry or wet. Sputum ranges in color, depending on reason for atelectasis. | Linear opacity of involved area<br>If lobar collapse exists, white triangular-shaped density<br>Fissure and diaphragmatic displacement | Incentive spirometry<br>Supplemental O$_2$<br>Functional mobilization<br>Broncho-pulmonary hygiene |
| Pneumonia | See Atelectasis, above<br>Fatigue<br>± Accessory muscle use | See Atelectasis, above<br>Decreased chest expansion at involved area<br>Dull percussion | Crackles<br>Rhonchi<br>Bronchial breath sounds over area of consolidation | Initially dry to more productive.<br>Sputum may be yellow, tan, green, or rusty. | Well-defined density at the involved lobe(s)<br>± Air bronchogram<br>± Pleural effusion | Antibiotics<br>Supplemental O$_2$<br>IV fluid administration<br>Functional mobilization<br>Bronchopulmonary hygiene |

| | | | | | | |
|---|---|---|---|---|---|---|
| Pulmonary edema | Tachypnea Orthopnea Anxiety Accessory muscle use | Increased tactile and vocal fremitus | Symmetric wet crackles, especially at bases ± Wheeze | Thin, frothy, clear, white, or pink sputum. | Increased hilar vascular markings Kerley's B lines (short, horizontal lines at lung field periphery) ± Pleural effusion Left ventricular hypertrophy Cardiac silhouette Fluffy opacities | Diuretics Other medications dependent on etiology Supplemental O$_2$ Monitor hemodynamic status |
| Adult respiratory distress syndrome (ARDS) | Labored breathing and altered mental status at onset Tachypnea Increased PA pressure | Hypotension Tachy- or bradycardia Decreased bilateral chest wall expansion Dull percussion | Diminished breath sounds Crackles Wheezes Rhonchi (rare) | Generally without sputum, although sputum may be present if infection exists or from the presence of an endotracheal tube. | Pulmonary edema with diffuse bilateral patchy opacities | Mechanical ventilation Hemodynamic monitoring IV fluid administration Prone positioning Nitrous oxide therapy |

Table 2-10. *Continued*

| Disorder | Observation | Palpation | Auscultation | Cough | Chest X-Ray | Management |
|---|---|---|---|---|---|---|
| Pulmonary embolism (PE) | Rapid onset of tachypnea ± Chest pain Anxiety Dysrhythmia Light-headedness | Hypotension Tachycardia Decreased chest expansion on involved side | Diminished or absent breath sounds distal to PE Wheeze Crackles | Usually absent. | Nondiagnostic for PE. May show density at infarct site with lucency distal to the infarct Decreased lung volume Dilated PA with increased vascular markings ± Atelectasis | Anticoagulation Hemodynamic stabilization Supplemental $O_2$ or mechanical ventilation Inferior vena cava filter placement Thrombolysis Embolectomy |
| Lung contusion | Tachypnea Chest wall ecchymosis Cyanosis, if severe | Hypotension Tachycardia Crepitus due to rib fracture | Wet crackles Diminished or absent breath sounds at site | Weak cough if pain present, dry or wet. Sputum may be clear, white, or blood tinged. | Patchy, irregular opacities localized to a segment or lobe ± Consolidation | Pain management Supplemental $O_2$ Mechanical ventilation IV fluid administration |

± = with or without, PA = pulmonary artery.

## Atelectasis

Atelectasis involves the partial or total collapse of alveoli, lung segments(s), or lobe(s). It most commonly results from hypoventilation or ineffective pulmonary secretion clearance. The following conditions may also contribute to atelectasis:

- Inactivity

- Upper abdominal or thoracic incisional pain

- Compression of lung parenchyma

- Diaphragmatic restriction from weakness or paralysis

- Postobstructive pneumonia

- Presence of a foreign body

The result is hypoxemia from $\dot{V}/\dot{Q}$ mismatch, transpulmonary shunting, and pulmonary vasoconstriction of variable severity depending on the amount of atelectasis.[6] General risks for the development of atelectasis include cigarette smoking or pulmonary disease, obesity, and increased age. Peri- or postoperative risk factors include altered surfactant function from anesthesia, emergent or extended operative time, altered consciousness or prolonged narcotic use, hypotension, and sepsis.

## Pneumonia

*Pneumonia* is the multistaged inflammatory reaction of the distal airways from the inhalation of bacteria, viruses, microorganisms, foreign substances, gastric contents, dusts, or chemicals, or as a complication of radiation therapy.[6] Pneumonia is often described as *community* or *hospital (nosocomial) acquired*. *Nosocomial pneumonia* is defined as pneumonia occurring after 48 hours within a hospital stay and is associated with ventilator use, contaminated equipment, or poor hand washing.[34] The consequences of pneumonia are $\dot{V}/\dot{Q}$ mismatch and hypoxemia. The phases of pneumonia are the following[33]:

1.   Alveolar edema with exudate formation (0–3 days)

2.   Alveolar infiltration with bacterial colonization, red and white blood cells, and macrophages (2–4 days)

3.   Alveolar infiltration and consolidation with dead bacteria, white blood cells, and fibrin (4–8 days)

4.   Resolution with expectoration or enzymatic digestion of infil-
trative cells (after 8 days)

Pneumonia may be located in a single or multiple lobes either unilat-
erally or bilaterally. The complete clearance of pneumonia can take
up to 6 weeks.[34] Resolution of pneumonia is slower with increased
age, previous pneumonia, positive smoking history, poor nutritional
status, or with coexisting illness.

## Pulmonary Edema

The etiology of pulmonary edema can be categorized as either cardiogenic or noncardiogenic. *Cardiogenic pulmonary edema* is an imbalance of hydrostatic and oncotic pressures within the pulmonary
vasculature that results from backflow of blood from the heart.[6] This
backflow increases the movement of fluid from the pulmonary capillaries to the alveolar spaces. Initially, the fluid fills the interstitium and
then progresses to the alveolar spaces, bronchioles, and, ultimately,
the bronchi. A simultaneous decrease in the lymphatic drainage of the
lung may occur, exacerbating the problem. Cardiogenic pulmonary
edema can occur rapidly (*flash pulmonary edema*) or insidiously in
association with left ventricular hypertrophy, mitral regurgitation, or
aortic stenosis. Cardiogenic pulmonary edema results in atelectasis,
$\dot{V}/\dot{Q}$ mismatch, and hypoxemia.[6]

*Noncardiogenic pulmonary edema* can result from alterations in
capillary permeability (as in ARDS or pneumonia), intrapleural pressure from airway obstruction(s), or lymph vessel obstruction. The
results are similar to those of cardiogenic pulmonary edema.

---

### Clinical Tip

Beware of a flat position in bed or other positions that
worsen dyspnea during physical therapy intervention in
patients with pulmonary edema.

---

## Adult Respiratory Distress Syndrome

ARDS is an acute inflammation of the lung that is generally associated with aspiration, drug toxicity, inhalation injury, pulmonary
trauma, shock, systemic infections, and multisystem organ failure.[35] It
is considered a critical illness and has a lengthy recovery and a high
mortality rate. Characteristics of ARDS include the following:

1.   An exudative phase (hours to days) characterized by increased capillary permeability, interstitial and alveolar edema, hemorrhage, and alveolar consolidation with leukocytes and macrophages

2.   A proliferative stage (days to weeks) characterized by hyaline formation on alveolar walls and intra-alveolar fibrosis resulting in atelectasis, $\dot{V}/\dot{Q}$ mismatch, severe hypoxemia, and pulmonary hypertension

Latent pulmonary sequelae of ARDS are variable and range from no impairments to mild exertional dyspnea to mixed obstructive-restrictive abnormalities.[36]

### Pulmonary Embolism

PE is the partial or full occlusion of the pulmonary vasculature by one large or multiple small emboli from one or more of the following possible sources: thromboembolism originating from the lower extremity (more than 90% of the time),[37] air entering the venous system through catheterization or needle placement, fat droplets from traumatic origin, or tumor fragments. A PE results in[38]

- Decreased blood flow to the lungs distal to the occlusion

- Atelectasis and focal edema

- Bronchospasm from the release of humeral agents

- Possible parenchymal infarction

Emboli size and location determine the extent of $\dot{V}/\dot{Q}$ mismatch, pulmonary shunt, and thus the degree of hypoxemia and hemodynamic instability.[37] The onset of PE is usually extremely acute and may be a life-threatening emergency, especially if a larger artery is obstructed.

---

### Clinical Tip

- PT intervention should be discontinued if the signs and symptoms of PE arise during treatment (see Table 2-10). Seat or lay the patient down and call for help immediately.
- If you are evaluating the patient for the first time since a PE, make sure the patient has received a therapeutic level of anticoagulation medicine or that other medical treat-

ment has been completed. Refer to Chapter 6 for more information on anticoagulation.

## Interstitial Lung Disease

*Interstitial lung disease* (ILD) is a general term for the destruction of the respiratory membranes in multiple lung regions that occurs after an inflammatory phase in which the alveoli become infiltrated with macrophages and mononuclear cells, followed by a fibrosis phase in which the alveoli become scarred with collagen.[33] Fibrotic changes may extend proximally toward the bronchioles. There are more than 100 suspected predisposing factors for ILD, such as infectious agents, environmental and occupational inhalants, and drugs; however, no definite etiology is known.[6] Clinically, the patient presents with exertional dyspnea and bilateral diffuse chest radiograph changes, and without pulmonary infection or neoplasm.[39] ILD has a wide variety of clinical features and patterns beyond the scope of this text; however, the general sequela of ILD is a restrictive pattern with $\dot{V}/\dot{Q}$ mismatch.

## Lung Contusion

Lung contusion is the result of a sudden compression and decompression of lung tissue against the chest wall from a direct blunt (e.g., fall) or blast (e.g., air explosion) trauma. The compressive force causes shearing of the alveolar-capillary membrane and results in microhemorrhage, whereas the decompressive force causes a rebound stretching of the parenchyma.[40] There is a diffuse accumulation of blood and fluid in the alveoli and interstitium that causes alveolar shunting, decreased lung compliance, and increased pulmonary vascular resistance.[41] The resultant degree of hypoxemia is dependent on the size of contused tissue. Lung contusion is usually located below rib fracture(s) and is associated with PTX and flail chest.

### Restrictive Extrapulmonary Conditions

Disorders or trauma occurring outside of the visceral pleura may also affect pulmonary function. Table 2-11 outlines restrictive extrapulmonary disorders, their general physical findings, and their general medical management.

**Table 2-11.** Characteristics and General Management of Extrapleural Disorders

| Disorder | Observation | Palpation | Auscultation | Cough | Chest X-Ray | Management |
|---|---|---|---|---|---|---|
| Pleural effusion | Tachypnea ± Discomfort from pleuritis Decreased chest expansion on involved side | ± Tachycardia Decreased tactile fremitus Dull percussion | Normal to decreased breath sounds or bronchial breath sounds at the level of the effusion | Usually absent | Homogenous density in dependent lung Fluid obscures diaphragm and fills costophrenic angle Fluid shifts with change in patient position Mediastinal shift to opposite side, if severe | If effusion is small and respiratory status is stable, monitor only Supplemental $O_2$ Chest tube placement for moderate or large effusion Thoracocentesis, if persistent Pleurodesis Diuretics Work-up to determine cause if unknown Pain management if pleuritic pain present |

Table 2-11. *Continued*

| Disorder | Observation | Palpation | Auscultation | Cough | Chest X-Ray | Management |
|---|---|---|---|---|---|---|
| Pneumothorax (PTX) | See Pleural effusion, above | See Pleural effusion, above | Diminished breath sounds near involved site<br><br>Absent if tension PTX | Usually absent | Translucent area usually at apex of lung<br><br>± Associated depressed diaphragm, atelectasis, lung collapse, mediastinal shift, if severe | If PTX is small and respiratory status is stable, monitor only<br><br>If PTX is moderate-size or large, chest tube placement<br><br>Supplemental O$_2$<br><br>Pain management if pleuritic pain present |
| Hemothorax | See Pneumothorax, above | See Pleural effusion, above | See Pneumothorax, above | Usually absent, unless associated with significant lung contusion in which hemoptysis may occur | See Pleural effusion, above | Supplemental O$_2$<br><br>Chest tube placement<br><br>Pain management if pleuritic pain present<br><br>Monitor and treat for shock<br><br>Blood transfusion, as needed |

| | | | | | | |
|---|---|---|---|---|---|---|
| Flail chest | Tachypnea<br>Bony thorax discontinuity<br>Ecchymosis at site<br>± Cyanosis | Tachycardia<br>Hypertension<br>Dull percussion<br>Point tenderness at site<br>Crepitus at fracture site | Diminished breath sounds<br>Crackles | See Hemothorax, above | Opacity at site of associated lung contusion in nonsegmental or nonlobar pattern<br>Appears immediately<br>Rib fractures at site | Stabilization of thorax with mechanical ventilation<br>Pain management<br>Fluid balance |
| Empyema | See Pleural effusion, above | See Pleural effusion, above | See Pleural effusion, above | Usually absent | Homogenous density at involved area | See Pleural effusion, above<br>Antibiotics |
| Chylothorax | See Pleural effusion, above<br>Often asymptomatic | See Pleural effusion, above<br>Often asymptomatic | Diminished breath sounds at site | Usually absent | Homogenous density at area involved | See Pleural effusion, above<br>Nutritional support<br>Pleuroperitoneal shunt<br>Thoracic duct ligation |

± = with or without.

## Pleural Effusion

A *pleural effusion* is the presence of transudative or exudative fluid in the pleural space. *Transudative* fluid results from a change in the hydrostatic/oncotic pressure gradient of the pleural capillaries, which is associated with congestive heart failure, cirrhosis, PE, and pericardial disease.[42] *Exudative* fluid (containing cellular debris) occurs with pleural or parenchymal inflammation or altered lymphatic drainage, which is associated with neoplasm, tuberculosis (TB), pneumonia, pancreatitis, rheumatoid arthritis, and systemic lupus erythematosus.[6,42] Pleural effusions may be unilateral or bilateral, depending on the cause of the effusion, and may result in compressive atelectasis.

## Pneumothorax

PTX is the presence of air in the pleural space that can occur from (1) visceral pleura perforation with movement of air from within the lung (*spontaneous pneumothorax*), (2) chest wall and parietal pleura perforation with movement of air from the atmosphere (*traumatic* or *iatrogenic pneumothorax*), or (3) formation of gas by microorganisms associated with empyema. Spontaneous PTX can be a complication of chronic obstructive pulmonary disease or TB, or it can occur idiopathically in tall persons secondary to elevated intrathoracic pressures in the upper lung zones.[6] Traumatic PTX results from rib fracture, chest wounds, or other penetrating chest trauma. Complications of mechanical ventilation and central line placement are two examples of iatrogenic PTX. Pneumothoraces may also be described as follows:

*Closed*: Without air movement into the pleural space during inspiration and expiration (chest wall intact)

*Open*: With air moving in and out of the pleural space during inspiration and expiration (pleural space in contact with the atmosphere)

*Tension*: With air moving into the pleural space only during inspiration

PTX is usually unilateral. Complications of PTX include atelectasis and $\dot{V}/\dot{Q}$ mismatch. If a large or tension PTX exists, there can be lung collapse, mediastinal shift (displacement of the mediastinum) to the contralateral side, and cardiac tamponade (altered cardiac function secondary to decreased venous return to the heart from compression).[6]

## Hemothorax

*Hemothorax* is characterized by the presence of blood in the pleural space from damage to the pleura and great or smaller vessels (e.g., interstitial arteries). Causes of hemothorax are penetrating or blunt chest wall injury, draining aortic aneurysms, pulmonary arteriovenous malformations, and extreme coagulation therapy. Blood and air together in the pleural space, common after trauma, is a *hemopneumothorax*.

## Flail Chest

Flail chest is caused by the double fracture of three or more adjacent ribs, resulting from a crushing chest injury or vigorous cardiopulmonary resuscitation. The sequelae of this injury are[6]

- A paradoxical breathing pattern, with the discontinuous ribs moving inward on inspiration and outward on expiration as a result of alterations in atmospheric and intrapleural pressure gradients

- Contused lung parenchyma under the flail portion

In severe cases, mediastinal shift to the contralateral side occurs as air from the involved side is shifted and rebreathed (pendelluft).

## Empyema

Empyema is the presence of anaerobic bacterial pus in the pleural space, resulting from underlying infection (e.g., pneumonia, lung abscess) that crosses the visceral pleura or chest wall and parietal pleura penetration from trauma, surgery, or chest tube placement. Empyema formation involves pleural swelling and exudate formation, continued bacterial accumulation, fibrin deposition on pleura, and chronic fibroblast formation.

## Chylothorax

Chylothorax is the presence of thoracic duct lymph (chyle) in the pleural space that results most commonly from lymphoma and from trauma to the thoracic duct during thoracic surgery,[43] or less commonly from congenital malformation, hyperextension injury of the spine, or thoracic duct obstruction.

### Chest Wall Restrictions

A restrictive respiratory pattern may be caused by abnormal chest wall movement not directly related to pulmonary pathology. Musculoskeletal changes of the thoracic cage can occur with diseases such as anky-losing spondylitis, rheumatoid arthritis, and kyphoscoliosis, or with conditions such as pregnancy and obesity. Kyphoscoliosis and obesity are discussed in further detail because of their frequency in the clinical setting. Kyphoscoliosis can result in atelectasis from decreased thoracic cage mobility, respiratory muscle insufficiency, and parenchymal compression. Other consequences of kyphoscoliosis are progressive alveolar hypoventilation, increased dead space, hypoxemia with eventual pulmonary artery hypertension, cor pulmonale, or mediastinal shift (in very severe cases) toward the direction of the lateral curve of the spine.[6]

Obesity (defined as body weight 20–30% above age- and gender-predicted weight) can cause an abnormally elevated diaphragm position secondary to the upward displacement of abdominal contents, inefficient respiratory muscle use, and a noncompliant chest wall. These factors result in early airway closure (especially in dependent lung areas), tachypnea, altered respiratory pattern, $\dot{V}/\dot{Q}$ mismatch, and secretion retention.

## Management

### Pharmacologic Agents

The pharmacologic agents commonly used for the management of respiratory dysfunction include antihistamines (Appendix Table IV.7), antitussives (Appendix Table IV.11), bronchodilators (Appendix Table IV.13), inhaled corticosteroids (Appendix Table IV.16), expectorants (Appendix Table IV.18), intranasal steroids (Appendix Table IV.21), and mucolytics (Appendix Table IV.23).

---

Clinical Tip

• Be aware of respiratory medication changes, especially the addition or removal of medications from the regimen.
• Generally, nebulized medications are optimally active 15–20 minutes after administration.
• If a patient has an inhaler, it may be beneficial for the patient to bring it to physical therapy sessions in case of activity-induced bronchospasm.

---

## Thoracic Procedures

The most common thoracic operative and nonoperative procedures for respiratory disorders are described below in alphabetical order.[44,45]

*Bronchoplasty*: Also called a *sleeve resection*. Resection and re-anastomosis (reconnection) of a bronchus, most commonly performed for bronchial carcinoma (a concurrent pulmonary resection may be performed as well).

*Laryngectomy*: The partial or total removal of one or more vocal cords, most commonly performed for laryngeal cancer.

*Laryngoscopy*: Direct visual examination of the larynx with a fiberoptic scope, most commonly performed to assist with differential diagnosis of thoracic pathology or to assess the vocal cords.

*Lung volume reduction*: The unilateral or bilateral removal of one or more portions of emphysematous lung parenchyma, resulting in increased alveolar surface area.

*Mediastinoscopy*: Endoscopic examination of the mediastinum, most commonly performed for precise localization and biopsy of a mediastinal mass or for the removal of lymph nodes.

*Pleurodesis*: The obliteration of the pleural space, most commonly performed for persistent pleural effusions or pneumothoraces. A chemical agent is introduced into the pleural space via thoracostomy (chest) tube or with a thoracoscope.

*Pneumonectomy*: Removal of an entire lung, most commonly performed as a result of bronchial carcinoma, emphysema, multiple lung abscesses, bronchiectasis, or TB.

*Rib resection*: Removal of a portion of one or more ribs for accessing underlying pulmonary structures as a treatment for thoracic outlet syndrome or for bone grafting.

*Segmentectomy*: Removal of a segment of a lung, most commonly performed for a peripheral bronchial or parenchymal lesion.

*Thoracocentesis*: Therapeutic or diagnostic removal of pleural fluid via percutaneous needle aspiration.

*Thoracoscopy* (video-assisted thoracoscopic surgery): Examination, through the chest wall with a *thoracoscope*, of the pleura or lung parenchyma for pleural fluid biopsy or pulmonary resection.

*Tracheal resection and reconstruction*: Resection and re-anastomosis (reconnection) of the trachea, main stem bronchi, or both; most commonly performed for tracheal carcinoma, trauma, stricture, or tracheomalacia.

*Tracheostomy*: Incision of the second or third tracheal rings or the creation of a stoma or opening for a tracheostomy tube, preferred for airway protection and prolonged ventilatory support or after laryngectomy, tracheal resection, or other head and neck surgery.

*Wedge resection*: Removal of lung parenchyma without regard to segment divisions (a portion of more than one segment but not a full lobe), most commonly performed for peripheral parenchymal carcinoma.

### Physical Therapy Intervention

#### Goals
The primary physical therapy goals in the treatment of patients with primary lung pathology include promoting independence in functional mobility, maximizing gas exchange (by improving ventilation and airway clearance), and increasing aerobic capacity, respiratory muscle endurance, and the patient's knowledge of his or her condition. General treatment techniques to accomplish these goals are breathing retraining exercises, secretion clearance techniques, positioning, functional activity and exercise with vital sign monitoring, and patient education.

#### Basic Concepts for the Treatment of Patients with Respiratory Impairments
*Bronchopulmonary Hygiene*
The following are basic concepts for implementing a bronchopulmonary hygiene program for patients with respiratory dysfunction:

- A basic understanding of respiratory pathophysiology is necessary, because bronchopulmonary hygiene is not indicated for certain conditions, such as a pleural effusion or pulmonary edema.

- To develop a proper plan of care, the physical therapist must also understand whether the respiratory pathology is acute or chronic, reversible or irreversible, or stable or progressive, as well as the potential for alterations in other body systems.

- The bronchopulmonary hygiene treatment plan will vary in direct correlation to the patient's respiratory or medical status. The physical therapist must be cognizant of the potential for rapid decline in patient status and modify treatment accordingly.

- Bronchopulmonary hygiene requires constant reassessment before, during, and after physical therapy intervention as well as on a daily basis.

- Bronchopulmonary hygiene may be enhanced by the use of supplemental $O_2$ and medication such as bronchodilators. Both $O_2$ and bronchodilators are medications that require a physician's order.

- Tolerance to bronchopulmonary hygiene can be monitored by pulse oximetry and can help determine the need for supplemental $O_2$ during therapy sessions.

- Cough effectiveness can be enhanced with pain medication before therapy, splinting (if there is an incision or a rib fracture), positioning, and proper hydration.

- Patients with chronic respiratory diseases, such as CF or bronchiectasis, usually have an established routine for their bronchopulmonary hygiene. Although this routine may require modification in the hospital, maintaining this routine as much as possible will optimize the continuity of care. Be aware of the usual order of postural drainage positions and whether certain positions are uncomfortable.

- Document baseline sputum production, including certain times of the day when the patient is most productive.

- Patients with an obstructive pulmonary disorder generally do well with slow, prolonged exhalations, such as in pursed lip breathing. A patient may do this maneuver naturally. Frequent rest breaks between coughs are also helpful to prevent airtrapping and improve secretion clearance.

- Patients with a restrictive pulmonary disorder generally do well with therapeutic activities to improve inspiration, such as diaphragmatic breathing and chest wall stretching.

**Table 2-12.** Respiratory Evaluation Findings and Suggested Physical Therapy Interventions

| Evaluation | Finding | Suggested PT Intervention |
|---|---|---|
| Inspection | Dyspnea or tachypnea at rest or with exertion | Reposition for comfort or more upright posture. |
| | Asymmetric respiratory pattern | Relaxation techniques. |
| | | Energy conservation techniques. |
| | Abnormal sitting or standing posture | Diaphragmatic or lateral costal expansion exercise. |
| | | Incentive spirometry. |
| | | Postural exercises. |
| | | Stretching of trunk and shoulder musculature. |
| | | Administer or request supplemental $O_2$. |
| Palpation | Asymmetric respiratory pattern | Diaphragmatic or lateral costal expansion exercise. |
| | Palpable fremitus as a result of retained pulmonary secretions | Incentive spirometry. |
| | | Coughing exercises. |
| | | Upper extremity exercise. |
| | | Functional activity. |
| | | Manual techniques. |
| | | Postural drainage positions (See Appendix VIII). |
| | | Flutter valve, if applicable. |
| Percussion | Increased dullness as a result of retained pulmonary secretions | See Palpation, above. |
| Auscultation | Diminished or adventitious breath sounds as a result of retained pulmonary secretions | See Palpation, above. |
| Cough effectiveness | Ineffective cough | Position for comfort or to maximize expiratory force. |
| | | Incisional splinting, if applicable. |
| | | Huffing and coughing techniques. |
| | | Functional activity or exercise. |
| | | External tracheal stimulation (tracheal tickle). |
| | | Naso/endotracheal suctioning. |
| | | Request bronchodilator or mucolytic treatment. |

*Activity Progression*
The following are basic concepts of activity progression for patients with respiratory dysfunction:

- Rating of perceived exertion (see Chapter 1 for Borg's scale) is a better indicator of exercise intensity than heart rate because a patient's respiratory limitations, such as dyspnea, generally supersede cardiac limitations. Monitoring $O_2$ saturation can also assist in determining the intensity of the activity.

- Shorter, more frequent sessions of activity are often better tolerated than are longer treatment sessions. Patient education regarding energy conservation and paced breathing contributes to increased activity tolerance.

- A treatment session may need to be scheduled according to the patient's other hospital activities to ensure that the patient is not overfatigued for therapy.

- Document the need and duration of seated or standing rest periods during a treatment session to help measure functional activity progression or regression.

- Although $O_2$ may not be needed at rest, supplemental $O_2$ with exercise may decrease dyspnea and prolong exercise duration and intensity.

- Bronchopulmonary hygiene before an exercise session may optimize activity tolerance.

Table 2-12 provides some suggested treatment interventions based on common respiratory assessment findings.

# References

1. Thomas CL (ed). Taber's Cyclopedic Medical Dictionary (17th ed). Philadelphia: FA Davis, 1989;701, 1635, 2121.
2. Ganong WF (ed). Review of Medical Physiology (18th ed). Norwalk, CT: Appleton & Lange, 1997;626–630.
3. Scanlon VC, Sanders T (eds). Essentials of Anatomy and Physiology (3rd ed). Philadelphia: FA Davis, 1999;342–343.
4. Vander AJ, Sherman JH, Luciano DS (eds). Human Physiology, the Mechanisms of Body Function (4th ed). New York: McGraw-Hill, 1985;379.

5. Kelsen SG, Borberly BR. The Muscles of Respiration. In Dantzker DR, Scharf SM (eds), Cardiopulmonary Critical Care (3rd ed). Philadelphia: Saunders, 1998;115–120.
6. Des Jardins T (ed). Clinical Manifestations of Respiratory Disease (3rd ed). St. Louis: Mosby, 1995.
7. Guyton AC, Hall JE (eds). Textbook of Medical Physiology (9th ed). Philadelphia: Saunders, 1996;516.
8. Hillegass EA, Sadowsky HS (eds). Essentials of Cardiopulmonary Physical Therapy. Philadelphia: Saunders, 1994.
9. Butler SM. Clinical Assessment of the Cardiopulmonary System. In DL Frownfelter, E Dean (eds). Principles and Practice of Cardiopulmonary Physical Therapy (3rd ed). St. Louis: Mosby, 1996;217–clin tip, 222–percussion notes, plus most of chapters 209–228.
10. Humberstone N, Tecklin JS. Respiratory Evaluation. In S Irwin, JS Tecklin (eds), Cardiopulmonary Physical Therapy (3rd ed). St Louis: Mosby, 1995;334–335.
11. Boyars MC. Chest auscultation: how to maximize its diagnostic value in lung disease. Consultant 1997;37(2):415–417.
12. American College of CP & ATS Joint Committee on Pulmonary Nomenclature. Pulmonary terms and symbols. Chest 1975;67:583.
13. Sole ML, Byers JF. Ventilatory Assistance. In JC Hartshorn, ML Sole, ML Lamborn (eds), Introduction to Critical Care Nursing (2nd ed). Philadelphia: Saunders, 1997;139.
14. Gutierrez G, Arfeen QV. Oxygen Transport and Utilization. In DR Dantzker, SM Scharf (eds), Cardiopulmonary Critical Care (3rd ed). Philadelphia: Saunders,1998;195–196.
15. Ciesla ND, Murdock KR. lines, tubes, catheters, and physiologic monitoring in the ICU. Cardiopulmonary Phys Ther J 2000;11(1):18–19.
16. Kersten LD (ed). Comprehensive Respiratory Nursing: A Decision-Making Approach. Philadelphia: Saunders, 1989.
17. Hudak CM, Gallo BM (eds). Critical Care Nursing, A Holistic Approach (6th ed). Philadelphia: Lippincott, 1994;413.
18. Forrest JV, Feigin DS (eds). Essentials of Chest Radiology. Philadelphia: Saunders, 1982.
19. George RB, Matthay MA, Light RW, Matthay RA (eds). Chest Medicine: Essentials of Pulmonary and Critical Care Medicine (3rd ed). Baltimore: Williams & Wilkins, 1995;110.
20. Hetzed MR (ed). Minimally Invasive Techniques in Thoracic Medicine and Surgery. London: Chapman & Hall Medical, 1995;4.
21. Rippe JM, Irwin RS, Fink MP, et al (eds). Procedures and Techniques in Intensive Care Medicine. Boston: Little, Brown, 1994.
22. Lilington GA (ed). A Diagnostic Approach to Chest Diseases (3rd ed). Baltimore: Williams & Wilkins, 1987;23.
23. Ruppel GL (ed). Manual of Pulmonary Function Testing (7th ed). St. Louis: Mosby, 1998;1–7.
24. Thompson JM, Hirsch JE, MacFarland GK, et al. (eds). Clinical Nursing Practice. St. Louis: Mosby, 1986;136.
25. Wilson AF (ed). Pulmonary Function Testing, Indications and Interpretations. Orlando, FL: Orvine & Stratton, 1985.

26. Drazen MJ. Bronchial Asthma. In GL Baum, JD Crapo, BR Celli, JB Karlinsky (eds), Textbook of Pulmonary Diseases (6th ed). Philadelphia: Lippincott–Raven, 1998;791–805.
27. Staton GW, Ingram RH. Asthma. In DC Dale, DD Federman (eds), Scientific American Medicine, Vol. 3. New York: Scientific American, 1998;579–594.
28. Corbridge T, Hall JB. Status Asthmaticus. In JB Hall, GA Schmidt (eds), Principles of Critical Care (2nd ed). New York: McGraw-Hill, 1998; 579–594.
29. Fraser KL, Chapman KR. Chronic obstructive pulmonary disease: prevention, early detection, and aggressive treatment can make a difference. Postgrad Med 2000;108:103.
30. Celli BR. Clinical Aspects of Chronic Obstructive Pulmonary Disease. In GL Baum, JD Crapo, BR Celli, JB Karlinsky (eds), Textbook of Pulmonary Diseases (6th ed). Philadelphia: Lippincott–Raven, 1998;843–863.
31. Frownfelter DL, Dean E (eds). Principles and Practice of Cardiopulmonary Physical Therapy (3rd ed). St. Louis: Mosby, 1996.
32. Wood RE, Schafer IA, Karlinsky JB. Genetic Diseases of the Lung. In GL Baum, JD Crapo, BR Celli, JB Karlinsky (eds), Textbook of Pulmonary Diseases (6th ed). Philadelphia: Lippincott–Raven, 1998;1451–1468.
33. O'Riordan T, Adam W. Bronchiectasis. In GL Baum, JD Crapo, BR Celli, JB Karlinsky (eds), Textbook of Pulmonary Diseases (6th ed). Philadelphia: Lippincott–Raven, 1998;807–822.
34. Chesnutt MS, Prendergast TJ, Stauffer JL. Lung. In LM Tierney, SJ McPhess, MA Papadakis (eds), Currents: Medical Diagnosis and Treatment 1999 (38th ed). Stamford, CT: Appleton & Lange, 1999;225–337.
35. Fraser RS, Muller NL, Colman N, Pare PD (eds). Pulmonary Hypertension and Edema. In Fraser and Pare's Diagnosis of Diseases of the Chest, Vol. 3 (4th ed). Philadelphia: Saunders, 1999;1978.
36. O'Connor MF, Hall JB, Schmidt GA, Wood LDH. Acute Hypoxemic Respiratory Failure. In JB Hall, GA Schmidt, LDH Wood (eds), Principles of Critical Care (2nd ed). New York: McGraw-Hill, 1998;537–564.
37. Palevsky HI, Kelley MA, Fishman AP. Pulmonary Thromboembolic Disease. In AP Fishman (ed), Fishman's Pulmonary Diseases and Disorders, Vol. 1 (3rd ed). New York: McGraw-Hill, 1998:1297–1329.
38. Lazzara D. Respiratory distress. Nursing 2001;31:58–63.
39. Ragho G. Interstitial Lung Disease: A Clinical Overview and General Approach. In AP Fishman (ed), Fishman's Pulmonary Diseases and Disorders, Vol. 1 (3rd ed). New York: McGraw-Hill, 1998;1037–1053.
40. Vukich DJ, Markovick V. Thoracic Trauma. In P Rosen (ed), Emergency Medicine: Concepts and Clinical Practice, Vol. 1. St. Louis: Mosby, 1998;514–527.
41. Ruth-Sahd LA. Pulmonary contusions: management and implications for trauma nurses. J Trauma Nurs 1997;4:90–98.
42. Hayes DD. Stemming the tide of pleural effusions. Nursing 2001;31:49–52.
43. Fraser RS, Muller NL, Colman N, Pare PD (eds). Pleural Disease. In Fraser and Pare's Diagnosis of Diseases of the Chest, Vol. 4 (4th ed). Philadelphia: Saunders, 1999;2768.

44. Baue AE, Geha AS. Glenn's Thoracic and Cardiovascular Surgery, Vol. 1 (6th ed). Stamford, CT: Appleton & Lange, 1996.
45. Sabiston DC, Spencer FC. Surgery of the Chest, Vols. 1 and 2 (6th ed). Philadelphia: Saunders, 1995.

# 3

# Musculoskeletal System
*Michele P. West and James J. Gaydos*

## Introduction

An understanding of musculoskeletal pathology and medical-surgical intervention is often the basis of physical therapy evaluation and treatment planning for patients with acute orthopedic impairments. The primary goal of the physical therapist working with a patient in the acute care setting is to initiate rehabilitative techniques that foster early restoration of maximum functional mobility and reduce the risk of secondary complications. The objectives for this chapter are to provide the following:

1. A brief description of the structure and function of the musculoskeletal system

2. An overview of musculoskeletal evaluation, including physical examination and diagnostic tests

3. A description of fractures, including etiology, medical-surgical management, clinical findings, and physical therapy intervention

4. A description of joint arthroplasty and common surgeries of the spine, including surgical management and physical therapy intervention

5.    An overview of common soft tissue injuries, including surgical management and physical therapy intervention

6.    A brief overview of equipment commonly used in the acute care setting, including casts, braces, external fixators, and traction devices

## Structure and Function of the Musculoskeletal System

The musculoskeletal system is made up of the bony skeleton and contractile and noncontractile soft tissues, including muscles, tendons, ligaments, joint capsules, articular cartilage, and nonarticular cartilage. This matrix of soft tissue and bone provides the dynamic ability of movement, giving individuals the agility to move through space, absorb shock, convert reactive forces, generate kinetic energy, and perform fine motor tasks. The musculoskeletal system also provides housing and protection for vital organs and the central nervous system. As a result of its location and function, the musculoskeletal system commonly sustains traumatic injuries and degenerative changes. The impairments that develop from injury or disease can significantly affect an individual's ability to remain functional without further pathologic compromise.

## Musculoskeletal Examination

The initial evaluation of a patient with orthopedic dysfunction is invaluable to clinical management in the acute care setting. Physical therapy intervention for the patient with orthopedic impairments typically occurs postoperatively or after an injury is managed by the medical-surgical team.

### Patient History

In addition to a standard medical review (see Appendix I-A), information pertaining to the patient's musculoskeletal history should include the following:

• Cause and mechanism of injury at present

• Previous musculoskeletal, rheumatologic, or neurologic disease, injury, or surgery

- Functional level before admission
- Previous use of assistive device(s)
- Recreation or exercise level and frequency
- Need for adaptive equipment or footwear on a regular basis (e.g., a shoe lift)
- History of falls
- History of chronic pain

An understanding of the current medical-surgical management of musculoskeletal disease or injury should include

- Physician-dictated precautions or contraindications to treatment, such as weight-bearing status or activity level, or for the positioning of extremities
- The need for a splint, brace, or other equipment at rest or with activity
- Most recent lab values (e.g., hematocrit)
- Type and last dose of pain medication
- Whether the patient has been out of bed since admission to the hospital

*Pain*

Musculoskeletal pain quality and location should be determined subjectively and objectively. Use a pain scale appropriate for the patient's age, mental status, and vision. Note if pain is constant or variable, and if movement or position increases or decreases the pain. Refer to Appendix VI for more detailed information on pain assessment and management.

*Observation*

A wealth of information can be gathered by simple observation of the patient. This includes

- General appearance
- Level of alertness, anxiety, or stress
- Willingness to move or muscle guarding
- Presence of external orthopedic devices or equipment
- Muscle substitutions on active movement

More specifically, the physical therapist should observe posture, limb position, and skin integrity.

### Posture
Observe the patient's resting posture in supine, sitting, and standing positions. This includes inspection of the head, trunk, and extremities for alignment, symmetry, deformity, or atrophy.

### Limb Position
Observe the resting limb position of the involved extremity. Compare to both normal anatomic position and to the contralateral side. Note if the limb is in position naturally or if it is supported with a pillow, roll, or wedge.

---

### Clinical Tip

- A limb in a dependent position is at risk for edema formation, even if it is dependent for only a short period of time.
- Maintain joints in a neutral resting position to preserve motion and maintain soft tissue length.

---

### Skin Integrity
The patient's skin integrity should be inspected in general for edema, discoloration, bruising, or scars. If there is traumatic injury, carefully inspect the skin at the level of and distal to the injury. Note any lacerations or abrasions. If the patient has recently had surgery, observe the location, direction, and quality of incision(s). Note any pressure sores or potential for such. Refer to Chapter 7 for further discussion of skin integrity evaluation.

Clinical Tip

Pressure sores from prolonged or increased bed rest after trauma or orthopedic surgery can develop in anyone, regardless of age or previous functional abilities. Inspect the uninvolved extremity for skin breakdown too.

*Palpation*

Palpate skin temperature to touch, capillary refill, and peripheral pulses at the level of or distal to injury or the surgical site. Refer to Chapter 6 for further discussion of vascular examination. A discussion of special tests is beyond the scope of this text; however, the therapist should perform special testing if results of the interview or screening process warrant further investigation.

*Upper- and Lower-Quarter Screens*

Upper- and lower-quarter screening is the brief evaluation of bilateral range of motion (ROM), muscle strength, sensation, and deep tendon reflexes. It is a very efficient examination of gross neuromuscular status that guides the therapist to perform more specific testing.[1] The therapist should perform both an upper- or lower-quarter screen, regardless of the extremity involved. For example, for a patient with lower-extremity involvement who will require the use of an assistive device for functional mobility, both functional range and strength of the upper extremities must also be assessed. Tables 3-1 and 3-2 describe a modified version of an upper- and lower-quarter screen. Table 3-3 outlines normal ROM. Peripheral nerve innervations for the upper and lower extremities are listed in Tables 4-7 and 4-8, respectively. Dermatomal innervation is shown in Figure 4-6.

The sequencing of the upper- and lower-quarter screen is as follows[2]:

1.    Observe active ROM and test myotomes progressing from proximal to distal and beginning at the spinal level and moving dis-

Table 3-1. Upper-Quarter Screen

| Nerve Root | Myotome | Dermatome | Deep Tendon Reflex |
|---|---|---|---|
| C1 | Cervical rotation | No innervation | None |
| C2 | Shoulder shrug | Posterior head | None |
| C3 | Shoulder shrug | Posterior neck | None |
| C4 | Shoulder shrug | Acromioclavicular joint | None |
| C5 | Shoulder abduction | Lateral arm | Biceps |
| C5,6 | Elbow flexion | — | None |
| C6 | Wrist extension | Lateral forearm and palmar tip of thumb | Brachioradialis |
| C7 | Elbow extension and wrist flexion | Palmar distal phalanx of middle finger | Triceps |
| C8 | Thumb extension and finger flexion | Palmar distal aspect of little finger | None |
| T1 | Finger abduction | Medial forearm | None |

Sources: Adapted from ML Palmer, ME Epler (eds). Clinical Assessment Procedures in Physical Therapy. Philadelphia: Lippincott, 1990;32; and data from S Hoppenfeld. Physical Examination of the Spine and Extremities. East Norwalk, CT: Appleton & Lange, 1976.

tally to the extremities. Remember that it is imperative to assess these below the level of injury, as neurologic impairments may exist.

2.   Screen the patient's sensation to light touch, proximally to distally, as above.

3.   If weakness is found, assess strength using manual muscle testing. Break testing may also be performed as a modified way to assess isometric capacity of motor performance. If altered sensation to light touch is found, assess deep touch or other types of sensation further. Assess deep tendon reflexes if appropriate. Refer to Table 4-15 for the reflex grading and interpretation system.

### Clinical Tip

• Start the examination or screening process with the uninvolved side to minimize patient anxiety and pain response.
• If manual muscle testing is not possible secondary to conditions such as altered mental status, describe strength

Table 3-2. Lower-Quarter Screen

| Nerve Root | Myotome | Dermatome | Deep Tendon Reflex |
|---|---|---|---|
| L1 | Hip flexion | Antero-superior thigh just below the inguinal ligament | None |
| L2 | Hip flexion | Anterior medial thigh 2.5 in. below the anterior superior iliac spine | None |
| L3 | Knee extension with L4 | Middle third of anterior thigh | None |
| L4 | Knee extension with L3 and L5 | Patella and medial malleolus | Patellar tendon |
| L4,5 | Ankle dorsiflexion | — | None |
| L5 | Great toe extension | Fibular head and dorsum of foot | Posterior tibialis |
| S1 | Ankle plantar flexion | Lateral malleolus and plantar surface of foot | Achilles tendon |

Sources: Adapted from ML Palmer, ME Epler (eds). Clinical Assessment Procedures in Physical Therapy. Philadelphia: Lippincott, 1990;33; and data from S Hoppenfeld. Physical Examination of the Spine and Extremities. Norwalk, CT: Appleton & Lange, 1976.

in terms of quality or movement through an ROM (e.g., active hip flexion is one-third range in supine).
• Sensory testing is especially important over moderately or severely edematous areas, especially the distal extremities. The patient may not be aware of subtle changes in sensation.
• Girth measurements may be taken if edema of an extremity subjectively appears to increase.

## Functional Mobility and Safety

Functional mobility, including bed mobility, transfers, and ambulation on level surfaces and stairs, should be evaluated according to activity level, medical-surgical stability, and prior functional level. Safety is a key component of function. Evaluate the patient's willing-

Table 3-3. Normal Range of Motion Values Most Applicable in the Acute Care Setting

| Joint | Normal Range of Motion (Degrees) |
|---|---|
| Shoulder | |
| Flexion/extension | 0–180/0–60 |
| Abduction | 0–180 |
| Internal/external rotation | 0–70/0–90 |
| Elbow | |
| Flexion | 0–150 |
| Forearm | |
| Pronation/supination | 0–80/0–80 |
| Wrist | |
| Flexion/extension | 0–80/0–70 |
| Hip | |
| Flexion/extension | 0–120/0–30 |
| Abduction | 0–45 |
| Internal/external rotation | 0–45/0–45 |
| Knee | |
| Flexion | 0–135 |
| Ankle | |
| Dorsiflexion/plantar flexion | 0–20/0–45 |

ness to follow precautions with consistency. Observe for the patient's ability to maintain weight bearing or comply with equipment use. Monitor the patient's self-awareness of risk for falls, speed of movement, onset of fatigue, and body mechanics.

---

### Clinical Tip

• Safety awareness, or lack thereof, can be difficult to document. Try to describe a patient's level of safety awareness as objectively as possible (e.g., patient leaned on rolling tray table, unaware it could move).

• Nearly all patients will fear movement out of bed for the first time to some degree, especially if a fall or traumatic event led to the hospital admission. This is particularly true with elders. Before mobilization, use strategies to decrease fear. This includes an explanation of the treatment before mobilizing the patient and of the sensations the patient may feel (e.g., "Your foot will throb a little when you lower it to the floor.").

Because orthopedic injuries can often be the final result of other medical problems (e.g., balance disorders or visual or sensory impairments), it is important that the therapist take a thorough history, perform a musculoskeletal screen, and critically observe the patient's functional mobility. Medical problems may be subtle in presentation but may dramatically influence the patient's capabilities, especially with new variables, such as pain or the presence of a cast. Collectively, these factors lead to a decreased functional level.

---

### Clinical Tip

It may be the physical therapist who first appreciates an additional fracture, neurologic deficit, or pertinent piece of medical or social history. Any and all abnormal findings should be reported to the nurse or physician.

---

### Diagnostic Tests

The most commonly used diagnostic tests for the musculoskeletal system are listed in the following sections. These tests may be repeated during or after a hospital stay to assess bone and soft tissue healing and disease progression, or whether there is a sudden change in vascular or neurological status postoperatively.

### Radiography

More commonly known as *x-rays* or *plain films*, radiographic photographs are the mainstay in the detection of fracture, dislocation, bone loss, or foreign bodies or air in tissue. Sequential x-rays are standard intra- or postoperatively to evaluate component position with joint arthroplasty, placement of orthopedic hardware, or fracture reduction. X-rays may also detect soft tissue injuries, such as joint effusion, tendon calcification, or the presence of ectopic bone.[2]

### Computed Tomography

Computed tomography (CT) is the diagnostic test of choice for the evaluation of cortical bone in certain circumstances. For fracture and dislocations, CT can provide three-dimensional views for the spatial relationship of fracture fragments or to further evaluate fracture in anatomically complex joints, such as the pelvis, sacrum, spine, or shoulder.[3] CT is commonly used to define and localize spinal stenosis, disc protrusion or herniation, nerve entrapment, bone tumor, and osseous or articular bone infection or abscess.[4]

### Magnetic Resonance Imaging

Magnetic resonance imaging (MRI) is superior to x-ray or CT for the evaluation of soft tissue. MRI detects partial or complete tendon, ligament, or meniscal tears. MRI has also been used to (1) detect patellar tracking abnormalities, rotator cuff tears, and arthritis; (2) detect and localize soft tissue masses, such as hematoma, cyst, abscess, or lipoma; and (3) evaluate bone marrow. Finally, the high resolution of MRI reveals stress fractures and bone bruises that could be unobserved on x-ray.[3]

### Bone Scan

A bone scan is the radiographic picture of the uptake in bone of a radionuclide tracer. Scans of a portion of or the whole body may be taken at the instant the tracer is injected or 5–10 minutes or 2–4 hours postinjection. Bone scan reflects the metabolic status of the skeleton at the time of the scan and is extremely helpful in detecting metabolic abnormalities of bone before the appearance of structural changes on x-ray.[5] It is therefore used to detect skeletal metastases, especially in the base of the skull, sternum, scapula, and anterior ribs.[5] Other uses of bone scan include the diagnosis of stress fractures and other nondisplaced fractures, early osteomyelitis, inflammatory or degenerative arthritis, avascular necrosis (AVN), and myositis ossificans.

### Arthrography

An arthrogram is a radiograph of a joint with air or dye contrast. Performed primarily on the knee, shoulder, and hip, arthrography allows examination for internal joint derangements or soft tissue disruption. Arthrograms may diagnose meniscal and cruciate ligament tears or articular cartilage abnormalities of the knee, adhesive capsulitis or rotator cuff tears of the shoulder, and arthritis or intra-articular neoplasm of the hip.[6]

### Myelography

A myelogram is a radiograph or CT of the spinal cord, nerve root, and dura mater with dye contrast. A myelogram can demonstrate spinal stenosis, cord compression, intervertebral disc rupture, or nerve root injury.[7]

---

### Clinical Tip

• X-rays may be ordered after any new event, such as an in-hospital fall, abnormal angulation of an extremity, possible loss of fixation or reduction, or for a dramatic increase in pain. Regardless of the situation, defer physical therapy intervention until results are reported or the situation is managed.

• Physical therapy intervention is typically deferred for the patient post myelography secondary to specific post-procedure positioning and bed rest restrictions. (Refer to Myelography in Chapter 4.)

• As with any test that includes contrast media, contrast-related reactions post arthrogram or myelogram may occur. Check with the nurse or physician before physical therapy intervention.

---

## Fracture Management

### Types of Fracture

The analysis and classification of fracture reveal the amount of energy impacted on bone and the potential for secondary injury, and direct fracture management. Fractures can be described according to the following[8]:

1.  The maintenance of skin integrity:

    a.  A *closed fracture* is a bony fracture without disruption of the skin.

    b.  An *open fracture* is a bony fracture with open laceration of the skin or protrusion of the bone through the skin.

2.  The site of the fracture:

    a.    At the proximal third, distal third, or at the shaft of long bones.

    b.    An *intra-articular fracture* involves the articular surface. Intra-articular fractures are further described as linear, comminuted, impacted, or with bone loss. An *extra-articular* fracture does not involve the articular surface.

    c.    An *epiphyseal fracture* involves the growth plate.

3.    The configuration of the fracture (Figure 3-1):

    a.    A *linear fracture* can be *transverse* (fracture is perpendicular to the long axis of the bone), *oblique* (fracture is on a diagonal to the long axis of the bone), or *spiral* (fracture is similar to oblique with a greater surface area of shaft involvement secondary to a circular pattern).

    b.    A *comminuted fracture* has two or more fragments. A butterfly (wedge-shaped) fragment may or may not be present.

    c.    A *segmental fracture* has two or more fracture lines at different levels of the bone.

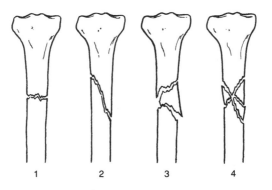

**Figure 3-1.** *Orientation of a fracture pattern. (1 = transverse; 2 = oblique; 3 = segmental; 4 = comminuted.) (With permission from A Unwin, K Jones [eds]. Emergency Orthopaedics and Trauma. Boston: Butterworth–Heinemann, 1995;22.)*

4.  The extent of the fracture:

   a.  An *incomplete fracture*, in which one portion of the cortex is interrupted.

   b.  A *complete fracture*, in which all cortices of bone are interrupted.

5.  The relative position of the fragments:

   a.  A *nondisplaced fracture* is characterized by anatomic alignment of fracture fragments.

   b.  A *displaced fracture* is characterized by abnormal anatomic alignment of fracture fragments.

## Clinical Goal of Fracture Management

The goal of fracture management is bony union of the fracture without further bone or soft tissue damage that enables early restoration of maximal function.[9] Early restoration of function minimizes cardiopulmonary compromise, muscle atrophy, and the loss of functional ROM. It also minimizes impairments associated with limited skeletal weight bearing (e.g., osteoporosis).

Fractures are managed either nonoperatively or operatively on an elective, urgent, or emergent basis depending on the location and type of fracture, presence of secondary injuries, and hemodynamic stability. *Elective* or *nonurgent* management (days to weeks) applies to stable fractures with an intact neurovascular system or fracture previously managed with conservative measures that have failed. *Urgent* management (24–72 hours) applies to closed, unstable fractures, dislocations, or long bone stabilization with an intact neurovascular system. *Emergent* management applies to open fractures, fractures/dislocations with an impaired neurovascular system or compartment syndrome, and spinal injuries with deteriorating neurologic deficits.[9]

*Fracture reduction* is the process of aligning and approximating fracture fragments. Reduction may be achieved by either closed or open methods. *Closed reduction* is noninvasive and is achieved by manual manipulation or traction. *Open reduction internal fixation* (ORIF) techniques require surgery and fixation devices (Figure 3-2), commonly referred to as *hardware*. ORIF is the treatment of choice

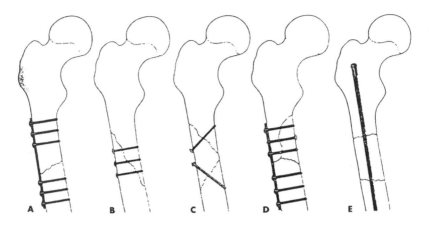

Figure 3-2. *Techniques of internal fixation. A. Plate and six screws for transverse or short oblique fracture. B. Screws for long oblique or spiral fracture. C. Screws for long butterfly fragment. D. Plate and screws for short butterfly fragment. E. Medullary nail for segmental fracture. (With permission from PG Beare, JL Myers [eds]. Adult Health Nursing [3rd ed]. St. Louis: Mosby, 1998;1243.)*

when closed methods cannot maintain adequate fixation throughout the healing phase. Immobilization of the fracture is required to maintain reduction and viability of the fracture site. Immobilization is accomplished through noninvasive (casts or splints) or invasive (screws, plates, rods, pins, and external fixators) techniques. Regardless of the method of immobilization, the goal is to promote bone healing.

Bone healing occurs in four stages: (1) hematoma formation within 72 hours, (2) fibrocartilage formation in 3 days to 2 weeks, (3) procallus formation in 3–10 days, and (4) remodeling or permanent callus formation in 3–10 weeks.[8,10] Table 3-4 lists the multitude of factors that contribute to the proper or improper healing of bone and affect the time frames for healing.

### Complications of Fracture

Complications of fracture may be immediate (within days), delayed (weeks to months), or late (months to years). The immediate or early

Table 3-4. Contributing Factors of Bone Healing

| Favorable | Unfavorable |
|---|---|
| Early mobilization<br>Early weight bearing<br>Maintenance of fracture reduction<br>Younger age<br>Good nutrition<br>Distal or proximal shaft fracture<br>Minimal soft tissue damage<br>Patient compliance<br>Presence of growth hormone | Presence of disease, such as diabetes, anemia, neuropathy, or malignancy<br>Vitamin deficiency<br>Osteoporosis<br>Infection<br>Irradiated bone<br>Severe soft tissue damage<br>Distraction of fracture fragments<br>Severe comminution<br>Bone loss<br>Multiple fracture fragments<br>Disruption of vascular supply to bone<br>Avascular necrosis<br>Corticosteroid use |

Sources: Adapted from CA Christian. General Principles of Fracture Treatment. In ST Canale (ed), Campbell's Operative Orthopaedics, Vol. 3 (9th ed). St. Louis: Mosby, 1998;1999; JM Black. Nursing Care of Clients with Musculoskeletal Trauma or Overuse. In JM Black, E Matassarian-Jacobs (eds), Medical-Surgical Nursing Clinical Management for Continuity of Care (5th ed). Philadelphia: Saunders, 1997;2134; and data from LN McKinnis. Fundamentals of Orthopedic Radiology. Philadelphia: FA Davis, 1997.

medical-surgical complications of special interest in the acute care setting include[10]

- Loss of fixation or reduction
- Deep vein thrombosis, pulmonary or fat emboli
- Nerve damage, such as paresthesia or paralysis
- Arterial damage, such as blood vessel laceration
- Compartment syndrome
- Incisional infection
- Shock

Delayed and late complications include[10]

- Loss of fixation or reduction

- *Delayed union* (fracture fails to unite in a normal time frame in the presence of unfavorable healing factors)

- *Nonunion* (failure of fracture to unite)

- *Malunion* (fracture healed with an angular or rotary deformity)

- *Pseudarthrosis* (formation of a false joint at the fracture site)

- Post-traumatic arthritis

- Osteomyelitis

- *Myositis ossificans* (heterotropic bone in muscle)

- AVN

### Fracture Management According to Body Region

#### Pelvis and Lower Extremity

*Pelvic Ring Fracture*
Pelvic fracture stability is defined by the degree of pelvic ring disruption. The pelvic ring is formed by the paired coxal bones, sacrum, sacroiliac joints, and symphysis pubis. *Unstable pelvic fractures* or dislocations occur in the anterior or posterior column of the pelvis owing to high-impact lateral or anteroposterior compression, or vertical shearing forces.[3] There is a disruption of the ring in two or more places, as shown in Figure 3-3.

*Stable pelvic fractures*, due to low-impact direct blows or falls, do not involve or minimally involve the displacement of the pelvic ring.[3] Stable pelvic fractures include localized iliac wing, pubic rami, or sacral fractures. Avulsion fractures of anterior superior iliac spine, anterior inferior iliac spine, or ischial tuberosity from strong contraction of muscle (typically seen in younger athletes) are considered stable pelvic fractures.[7] When a pelvic fracture is described as stable, it is inherent that further bony displacement will not occur on physiologic loading and that invasive procedures are not needed before mobilization.[11]

Chapter Appendix Table 3-A.1 describes the fracture classification and management of pelvic fractures. External fixation is used for stable

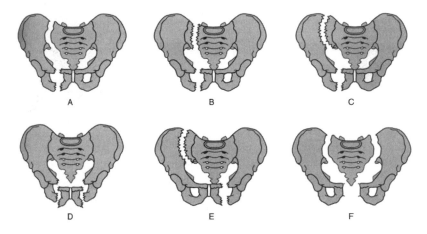

**Figure 3-3.** *Examples of unstable pelvic fractures include (A, B, and C) vertical shear (Malgaigne) fractures involving ischiopubic rami and disruption of an ipsilateral sacroiliac joint, be they (A) throughout the joint itself, (B) through a fracture of the sacral wing, or (C) through a fracture on the iliac bone. D. Straddle fractures, involving all four ischiopubic rami. E. Buckethandle fractures, involving an ischiopubic ramus and contralateral sacroiliac joint. F. Dislocations involving one or both sacroiliac joints and the symphysis pubis. (With permission from LN McKinnis [ed]. Fundamentals of Orthopedic Radiology. Philadelphia: FA Davis, 1997;225.)*

fractures only and can decrease post-traumatic hemorrhage. It is a good choice if abdominal injuries are present. External fixation will not stabilize vertical displacement.[11] ORIF techniques are the optimal choice of treatment for anterior and posterior pelvic displacement. Risks are high and should be taken only when benefits of anatomic reduction and rigid fixation outweigh problems of hemorrhage and infection.[11]

*Acetabular Fracture*
Acetabular fracture occurs when a high-impact blunt force is transmitted at one of four main points: the greater trochanter, a flexed knee, the foot (with the knee extended), or the posterior pelvis.[12] The exact location and severity of the fracture (Figure 3-4), with or without dislocation, can depend on the degree of hip flexion and extension, abduction and adduction, or internal and external rotation at the time of injury.[12] Acetabular fractures are highly associated with multiple injuries and shock. Common immediate and early complications associated with acetabular fracture include retroperitoneal

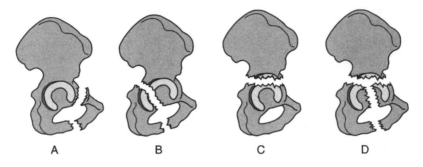

A    B    C    D

**Figure 3-4.** *Classification of acetabular fractures. A. Anterior column.*
*B. Posterior column. C. Transverse, involving both columns. D. Complex or*
*T shaped, involving both columns. (With permission from LN McKinnis [ed].*
*Fundamentals of Orthopedic Radiology. New York: Oxford University Press,*
*1997;227.)*

hematoma, gastrointestinal or urologic injury, degloving injury, deep venous thrombosis (DVT), pulmonary embolism, infection, and sciatic and superior gluteal nerve injury.[13] Common late complications include AVN of the femoral head or acetabular segment, hypertrophic ossification, and post-traumatic arthritis.[14] Chapter Appendix Table 3-A.2 describes the classification and management of acetabular fractures. Acetabular fractures are by nature intra-articular; hence, the management revolves around the restoration of a functional weight-bearing joint while avoiding osteoarthritis.[13] An acetabular fracture is a complex injury. Determinants of outcome include fracture pattern, degree of injury to the vascular status of the femoral head, the presence of neurologic injury, and the accuracy of reduction of the roof of the acetabulum.[15]

*Hip Dislocation*
Hip dislocation is the result of a high-velocity impact force and can occur in isolation or with a femoral or acetabular fracture. The majority of hip dislocations occur in a posterior direction, and anterior dislocations are rare.[16] A patient with a posteriorly dislocated hip has a limb that is shortened, internally rotated, and adducted in slight flexion.[17] An anteriorly dislocated hip appears adducted and externally rotated.[16]

Management of hip dislocation without fracture includes closed reduction under conscious sedation and muscle relaxation followed by traction or open reduction if closed reduction fails. Functional mobility (typically partial weight-bearing or weight-bearing as tolerated), exercise, and positioning are per physician order based on hip joint stability and associated neurovascular injury. Hip dislocation with fracture typically warrants surgical repair.

---

### Clinical Tip

* Posterior hip dislocation precautions typically exist after hip dislocation reduction. This limits hip flexion to 80–90 degrees, internal rotation to 0 degrees, and adduction to 0 degrees.
* Indirect restriction of hip movement after posterior dislocation during rest or functional activity can be achieved with the use of a knee immobilizer or hip abduction brace. This may be beneficial if the patient is confused or noncompliant.

---

### Femoral Head and Neck Fractures

Femoral head and neck fractures are often referred to as *hip fractures.* They can be classified as intracapsular or extracapsular. Femoral head and neck fractures occur from a direct blow to the greater trochanter, from a force with the hip externally rotated, or from a force along the femoral shaft.[18] In the elderly, a femoral neck fracture can occur with surprisingly little force owing to osteoporosis of the proximal femur. Femoral neck fractures in younger adults are almost always the result of high-impact forces, such as motor vehicle accidents (MVAs). *Intracapsular* fractures are located within the hip capsule and are also called *subcapital* fractures. The four-stage Garden Scale (Chapter Appendix Table 3-A.3) is used to classify femoral neck fractures and is based on the amount of displacement and the degrees of angulation (Figure 3-5). Clinically, Garden III and IV fractures are complicated by a disruption of the blood supply to the femoral head as a result of extensive capsular trauma. Poor blood supply from the circumflex femoral artery can lead to AVN of the femoral head, fracture nonunion, or both.[7]

*Extracapsular* fractures occur outside of the hip capsule. They can be further classified as intertrochanteric or subtrochanteric. *Intertrochanteric* fractures occur between the greater and lesser trochanters. *Subtrochanteric* fractures occur in the proximal one-third of the fem-

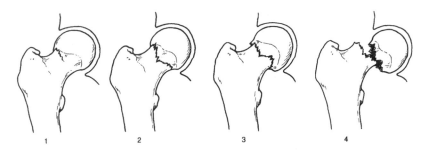

**Figure 3-5.** *Garden classification of subcapital fractures. 1, 2 = nondisplaced; 3, 4 = displaced. (With permission from A Unwin, K Jones [eds]. Emergency Orthopaedics and Trauma. Boston: Butterworth–Heinemann, 1995;193.)*

oral diaphysis and can occur with intertrochanteric or shaft fractures.[18] Inter- and subtrochanteric fractures are summarized in Chapter Appendix Table 3-A.4 and are shown in Figure 3-6.

*Femoral Shaft Fracture*
Femoral shaft fractures result from high-energy trauma and are often associated with major abdominal or pelvic injuries. Femoral shaft fractures can be accompanied by life-threatening systemic complications, such as hypovolemia, shock, or fat emboli. Often, there is significant bleeding into the thigh with hematoma formation. Hip dislocation and patellar fracture frequently accompany femoral shaft fractures.[19] Chapter Appendix Table 3-A.5 lists femoral shaft fracture management.

---

### Clinical Tip

• The uninvolved leg or a single crutch can be used to assist the involved lower leg in and out of bed.
• The patient should avoid rotation of and pivoting on the lower extremity after intramedullary rod placement, as microrotation of the intramedullary rod can occur and place stress on the fixation device.

---

*Distal Femoral Fractures*
Fractures of the distal femur are *supracondylar* (involving the distal femur shaft only), *unicondylar* (involving one femoral condyle), *inter-*

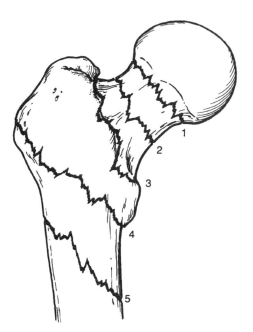

**Figure 3-6.** *Fractures of the proximal femur. (1 = subcapital; 2 = transcervical; 3 = basocervical; 4 = intertrochanteric; 5 = subtrochanteric.) (With permission from A Unwin, K Jones [eds]. Emergency Orthopaedics and Trauma. Boston: Butterworth–Heinemann, 1995;190.)*

*condylar* (involving both condyles), or a combination of these. Involvement of the articular surface of the knee joint complicates the fracture. Typically, this type of fracture is caused by high-energy trauma to the femur or a direct force that drives the tibia cranially into the intercondylar fossa. Distal femur fractures are often accompanied by injury to localized skin, muscle, and joint ligaments and cartilage with great potential for decreased knee joint mechanics.[20]

The management of distal femur fractures is summarized in Chapter Appendix Table 3-A.6. Complications of femur fracture include malunion, nonunion, infection, knee pain, and decreased knee ROM.[21]

*Patellar Fracture*
A patellar fracture results from direct trauma to the patella from a fall, blow, or MVA (e.g., dashboard injury). The knee is often flexed during injury, as the patella fractures against the femur. Patellar fracture may also occur from sudden forceful quadriceps contraction, as in sports or

from a stumbling fall.[7] Patellar fractures are associated with ipsilateral distal femoral or shaft fractures, proximal tibial condyle fractures, and posterior dislocation of the hip.[22] Late complications include patellofemoral or hardware pain, osteoarthritis, and decreased terminal extension from abnormal patellar mechanics, quadriceps weakness, or adhesions. Chapter Appendix Table 3-A.7 describes the management of patellar fractures. Most orthopedic surgeons perform partial or total patellectomy as a last resort because of the high incidence of an impaired quadriceps mechanism months later.[21]

*Tibial Plateau Fracture*
Tibial plateau fractures result from direct force on the proximal tibia (e.g., when a pedestrian is hit by an automobile), as shown by the Schatzker classification in Figure 3-7. This high-force injury often presents with open wounds, soft tissue injuries, ligamentous disruption, and dislocation. Contralateral collateral ligament injuries occur from varus or valgus force of injury.[7] Ligamentous injuries are most common in nondisplaced, compressed, and split compression fractures.[21]

The complexity of tibial plateau fractures cannot be overstated. Chapter Appendix Table 3-A.8 lists the management of tibial plateau fractures. Immediate or early complications of tibial plateau fractures include popliteal or peroneal nerve compression, compartment syndrome, infection, and DVT. Late complications include abnormal patellofemoral mechanics, lack of ROM or stability, and post-traumatic arthritis of the articular surface.

*Tibial Shaft and Fibula Fractures*
Tibial shaft and fibula fractures result from high-energy trauma (e.g., MVAs, crush injuries, skiing accidents) via direct blow, twisting of the ankle, or varus stress on the knee.[7] The higher the energy on impact, the more soft tissue and bone damage occurs. Tibial shaft fracture management (Chapter Appendix Table 3-A.9) is very complicated because of associated injuries similar to those of tibial plateau fractures. Immediate or early complications include anterior tibial artery damage, interosseous membrane rupture, peroneal nerve injury, or degloving injuries. Delayed or late complications include malunion, nonunion, osteomyelitis, secondary amputation, or reflex sympathetic dystrophy. The distal lower extremity must be thoroughly evaluated for concomitant ankle trauma (e.g., trimalleolar fracture, syndesmotic disruption, or talar dome fracture).

*Distal Tibial and Ankle Fractures*
Fractures of the distal tibia, distal fibula, and talus are described together because of their frequent simultaneous injury. Distal tibial

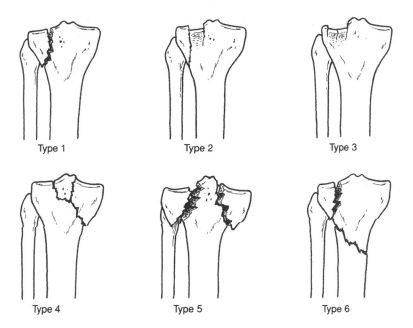

**Figure 3-7.** *Classification of tibial plateau fractures (Schatzker). Type 1 wedge fracture of the lateral tibial plateau. Type 2 wedge fracture of the lateral plateau with depression of the adjacent plateau. Type 3 central depression of the articular surface of the lateral plateau without a wedge fragment. Type 4 fracture of the medial tibial plateau. Type 5 bicondylar fracture. Type 6 tibial plateau fracture with separation of metaphysis from diaphysis. (With permission from A Unwin, K Jones [eds]. Emergency Orthopaedics and Trauma. Boston: Butterworth–Heinemann, 1995;226.)*

fractures (i.e., pilon fractures) are the result of high vertical loading forces, such as with parachuting accidents, falls from heights, sporting injuries, and MVAs.[23] Often, long axis compression throughout the proximal lower extremity can cause associated tibial plateau fracture, hip dislocation, or acetabular fracture.

Ankle fractures commonly result from torque caused by abnormal loading of the talocrural joint with body weight. Fractures may be simple, involving avulsion of a portion of the distal fibula, or complex, involving the entire mortise (trimalleolar fracture) with disruption of the syndesmosis. Fracture severity depends on the degree of foot inversion or eversion in relation to the subtalar joint at the time of injury.[23] Stability of the ankle depends on joint congruity and ligamentous integrity. Complications associated with ankle fractures are malunion, delayed union, traumatic arthritis, and osteomyelitis.[23] Chapter Appendix Table 3-A.10 lists distal tibial and ankle fracture management.

### Calcaneal and Forefoot Fractures

The most commonly fractured bone of the foot is the calcaneus, with fractures caused by a direct blow, such as a fall from a height or as an avulsion injury from a strong contraction of the triceps surae. Calcaneal fractures, usually bilateral, are associated with additional proximal leg injury or spinal fracture (e.g., burst fracture).[24] Latent complications of complex calcaneal fracture include joint pain, peroneal tendonitis, and heel spur from malunion.[24]

Forefoot fracture or metatarsal fracture occurs as a crush injury when a heavy object lands on the foot, as a twisting injury, as a stress fracture, or as an avulsion fracture at the base of the fifth metatarsal from forceful peroneus brevis contraction.[7] Chapter Appendix Table 3-A.11 lists the general types and management of calcaneal and forefoot fractures.

### Spine

In order of frequency, fractures of the spine are caused by automobile or motorcycle accidents, falls, sports accidents, and violence as a result of flexion, extension, rotation, and vertical compression forces.[25] Spinal fracture at any level is discussed in terms of location (anterior or posterior column) or stability (mechanical or neurologic). Anatomically, the anterior column refers to the vertebral bodies and intervertebral discs including the anterior and posterior longitudinal ligaments.[25] The posterior column refers to the transverse and spinous processes, pedicles, laminae, and facets, including the interspinous, infraspinous, supraspinous, and nuchal ligaments.[25]

A fracture may be considered stable if there is disruption of either the anterior or posterior column or an injury without neurologic compromise. An unstable fracture occurs if both the anterior and posterior columns are disrupted or if there is a potential for neurologic compromise. Potential neurologic injury can occur from progressive swelling at the site of the injury, hematoma formation, and associated intervertebral disc herniation or dislocation. Spinal fracture may occur with or without spinal cord injury (refer to Spinal Cord Injury in Chapter 4). Figures 3-8 and 3-9 are examples of high cervical (odontoid) and lumbar burst fractures.

Basic cervical and thoracolumbar fracture description and management are described in Chapter Appendix Tables 3-A.12 and 3-A.13,

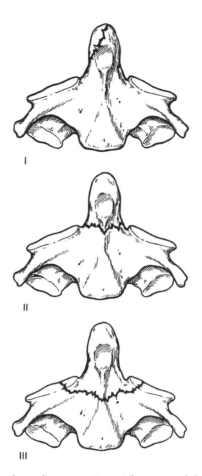

**Figure 3-8.** *Odontoid peg fractures. Type I fractures of the upper third of the peg. Type II fractures at the junction of the peg with the body of C2. Type III fractures essentially of the body of C2 at the base of the peg. (With permission from A Unwin, K Jones [eds]. Emergency Orthopaedics and Trauma. Boston: Butterworth–Heinemann, 1995;85.)*

respectively. If surgical management is required, it is performed as soon as the patient is medically stable. Secondary management of spinal fracture may also include the following:

- Examination and treatment of associated extremity fracture or head or internal injuries

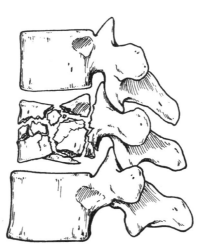

**Figure 3-9.** *Burst fracture. (With permission from A Unwin, K Jones [eds]. Emergency Orthopaedics and Trauma. Boston: Butterworth–Heinemann, 1995;85.)*

- Very frequent (every 15–30 minutes) neurovascular assessment by nursing
- Close monitoring of airway and breathing with cervical spine fractures

---

**Clinical Tip**

- Until the cervical, thoracic, and lumbar spines have been ruled out or "cleared" for fracture, do not remove temporary immobilization devices (e.g., cervical collar) until ordered to do so by the physician.
- Logroll precautions may exist before spine fracture clearance. This typically includes bed rest (with the head of the bed at a 30 degree angle or less) and turning the patient via *logroll* (with the head and torso as a unit).
- Refer to Physical Therapy Intervention after Spinal Surgery for additional tips on mobilizing a patient with back pain or after spinal stabilization.

---

## Upper Extremity

### Shoulder Girdle Fractures

Fracture of the scapula is rare and often requires little treatment (other than pain management), because the surrounding musculature serves to protect and immobilize the fracture. Scapular fractures occur most commonly in 35- to 45-year-olds as a result of axial loading on an outstretched arm or a direct blow or force from a fall onto the back or top of the shoulder.[26] Injuries associated with scapular fracture include rib fracture, pulmonary contusion, pneumothorax, and spinal fracture.

Fractures of the distal, middle, or medial third of the clavicle result from direct impact, such as falls or blows on the point of the shoulder. Management is conservative (sling immobilization for comfort) for nondisplaced fractures without ligamentous injury. ORIF is required acutely if the clavicle fracture is associated with neurovascular compromise, coracoclavicular ligament tear, floating shoulder (fracture of both the clavicle and surgical neck of the scapula), or for separation of fracture fragments by the deltoid or trapezius muscle.[27] Short-term immobilization is typical after ORIF.

Fractures involving the articulation of the glenohumeral joint or coracoid process are more complicated than scapular body and clavicular fractures. Intra-articular glenoid fractures may involve the spine of the scapula and are associated with shoulder dislocation or acromioclavicular injury.[28] Coracoid fractures occur at either the tip or base and may also involve the spine of the scapula.[28] Management for stable nondisplaced fractures is conservative (sling immobilization) or ORIF for displaced fractures.

The vast majority of glenohumeral dislocation occurs anteriorly as a result of forceful external rotation and extension while the arm is abducted.[7] Glenohumeral dislocation should be treated with immediate closed reduction to minimize injury to the neurovascular structures surrounding the joint. The need for strict dislocation precautions for the patient without risk factors for further dislocation is unlikely.[29]

### Proximal Humeral and Humeral Shaft Fractures

Proximal humeral fractures occur when the humerus is subjected to direct or indirect trauma and can be associated with glenohumeral dislocation, rotator cuff injuries, and brachial plexus or peripheral nerve damage. Fracture of the humeral head, anatomic neck, and lesser tuberosity are rare; however, fracture of the greater tuberosity is common.[7] The majority of these fractures are nondisplaced or minimally displaced.[30] Complications of proximal humeral fractures include nonunion, AVN of the humeral head, abnormal posture, and abnormal scapulothoracic rhythm.

Humeral shaft fractures are also the result of direct or indirect trauma, usually a fall on an outstretched hand, MVA, or direct load on the arm.[31] Humeral shaft fractures may be associated with radial nerve or brachial plexus injury. Chapter Appendix Table 3-A.14 summarizes proximal humerus and humeral shaft fracture management.

---

Clinical Tip

- When the patient is lying supine, placing a thin pillow or folded sheet under the upper arm will help maintain neutral alignment and reduce pain.
- Getting in and out of bed on the opposite side of an upper arm fracture is usually more comfortable for the patient.

---

*Distal Humeral, Olecranon, and Radial Head Fractures*
Distal humeral fractures are rare but complex fractures to manage because of the bony configuration of the elbow joint, adjacent neurovascular structures (Figure 3-10), and minimal soft tissue surrounding the joint.[32] The most common distal humerus fracture in the elderly is transcondylar (across the condyles of the olecranon fossa) as the result of a fall.[7] An intercondylar fracture (i.e., T- or Y-shaped condylar fracture) is the most common distal humeral fracture in adults. A direct impact of the ulna against the trochlea forces the condyles apart.[32] This is common after an MVA or high-impact fall. Treatment consists of (1) immobilization, followed by early ROM for a stable fracture; or (2) ORIF or total elbow arthroplasty (TEA) for severely comminuted intra-articular fractures. Late complications include hypomobility, nonunion, malunion, ulnar neuropathy, and heterotrophic ossification.

Olecranon fractures (Figure 3-11) result from direct trauma to a flexed elbow or a fall on an outstretched hand. Severe comminution of the olecranon is associated with humeral fracture and elbow dislocation. Late complications include loss of terminal elbow extension, painful hardware, and post-traumatic arthritis.[32]

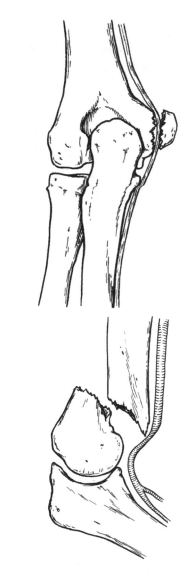

A

B

**Figure 3-10.** **A.** *Fracture of the medial epicondyle. Note the ulnar nerve runs immediately posterior to the fracture.* **B.** *The brachial artery is at risk in supracondylar fractures. (With permission from A Unwin, K Jones [eds]. Emergency Orthopaedics and Trauma. Boston: Butterworth–Heinemann, 1995;126, 128.)*

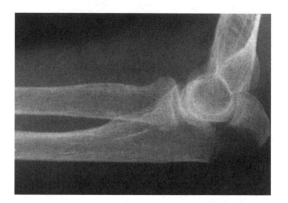

**Figure 3-11.** *Fracture of the olecranon. (With permission from A Unwin, K Jones [eds]. Emergency Orthopaedics and Trauma. Boston: Butterworth–Heinemann, 1995;130.)*

A fall onto an outstretched hand with a pronated forearm can cause a radial head or neck fracture (Figure 3-12). Associated injuries include elbow dislocation and disruption of the interosseous membrane, medial collateral ligament, or wrist fibrocartilage.[32] Complications of stable radial head fracture include residual pain and

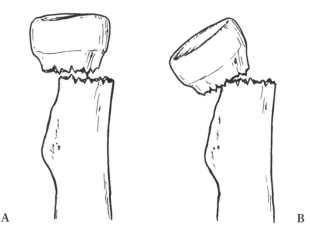

**Figure 3-12.** *Fractures of the radial neck. A. Displaced. B. Displaced and angulated. (With permission from A Unwin, K Jones [eds]. Emergency Orthopaedics and Trauma. Boston: Butterworth–Heinemann, 1995;130.)*

hypomobility, whereas unstable radial head fractures are associated with loss of fixation, nonunion, and painful hardware.[32] Olecranon and radial head fracture management is presented in Chapter Appendix Table 3-A.15.

*Forearm Fractures*
Fractures of the shaft or distal portion of the radius or ulna occur from a wide variety of direct trauma including falls, sports injuries, or MVAs. Owing to the high-energy impact, the fracture is usually displaced, affects an adjacent articulation, and involves a wrist or distal humeral fracture.[7] Management for forearm fracture is summarized in Chapter Appendix Table 3-A.16. Complications of forearm fracture include compartment syndrome, reflex sympathetic dystrophy, nonunion, malunion, radial nerve injury, post-traumatic arthritis, and hypomobility of the elbow, forearm, and wrist.[7,29]

*Carpal Fractures*
Carpal fractures and associated ligamentous injury or dislocation are typically due to compressive or hyperextension mechanisms of injury.[33] Management for the fracture of any carpal bone is similar. Nondisplaced fractures are treated with short arm cast immobilization with the wrist positioned in neutral flexion-extension with slight ulnar deviation.[33] Displaced fractures are treated with closed reduction and casting or ORIF with a postoperative splint or cast. Patients with isolated carpal fracture are usually treated in the ambulatory care setting.

---

### Clinical Tip

For patients who have concurrent lower- and upper-extremity injuries and require the use of a walker or crutches, a platform attachment placed on the assistive device will allow weight bearing to occur through the upper extremity proximal to the wrist.

---

*Metacarpal and Phalangeal Fractures*
Metacarpal fractures result from direct trauma, such as a crush injury, or by long-axis loading, as with punching injuries. The fracture may be accompanied by severe soft tissue injuries that can result in a treatment delay of 3–5 days to allow for a decrease in edema. Definitive treatment depends on the location of the fracture—either the articular surface

(ORIF), neck (closed reduction, percutaneous pinning, immobilization, or a combination of these), shaft (ORIF, percutaneous pinning, immobilization, or a combination of these), or base (percutaneous pinning and immobilization) of the metacarpal.

Phalangeal fractures result from crush forces and consequently are usually compounded by skin, tendon, and ligament damage. Management of nondisplaced phalangeal fracture is reduction and splinting. Management of displaced or intra-articular fracture is ORIF with splinting. Patients with isolated metacarpal and phalangeal fracture are usually treated in the ambulatory care setting.

## Joint Arthroplasty

Joint arthroplasty, the surgical reconstruction of articular surfaces with prosthetic components, is indicated to restore function and motion to a joint that is affected by degenerative arthritic changes.[34] Total joint arthroplasty is reserved for the individual with pain that is no longer responsive to conservative measures, such as anti-inflammatory medication, restriction or modification of activity, exercise, weight loss, or the use of an assistive device. This surgery is elective in nature and can be unilateral or bilateral. The incidence of bilateral total joint arthroplasties, simultaneous or staged, being performed in the acute care setting has increased in recent years. Bilateral joint arthroplasty has been established to be a safe procedure that reduces total rehabilitation time and hospital length of stay, thus decreasing medical costs and length of debilitation of the patient.[35]

Joint arthroplasty provides patients and caregivers with a predictable postoperative course in the acute orthopedic care setting. For this reason, there are high expectations for these patients to achieve specific short- and long-term functional outcomes. The following sections provide basic surgical information and clinical techniques and suggestions for the acute care physical therapist.

### Hip Arthroplasty

Hip arthroplasty involves the replacement of the femoral head, the acetabulum, or both with prosthetic components. A hip arthroplasty is most commonly performed on patients with severe hip arthritis (degenerative or rheumatoid), AVN, hip infection, or congenital dis-

**Table 3-5.**  Hip Disorders That May Require Total Hip Arthroplasty

Degenerative arthritis (hypertrophic or osteoarthritis)
Rheumatoid arthritis
Atraumatic avascular necrosis
Intrapelvic protrusio acetabuli*
Congenital subluxation or dislocation
Post-traumatic disorders (femoral neck, trochanteric, or acetabular
    fractures)
Failed reconstructive procedures (femoral osteotomy, arthrodesis, or
    resurfacing)
Metabolic disorders (Paget's disease, Gaucher's disease, or sickle cell
    anemia)
Fused hip or ankylosing spondylitis
Infectious disorders (tuberculosis and pyogenic arthritis)
Bone tumors
Neurologic disorders (cerebral palsy and Parkinson's disease)

*Chronic progression of the femoral head into the acetabulum and pelvis.
Source: Adapted from JW Harkess. Arthroplasty of Hip. In ST Canale (ed), Campbell's
Operative Orthopaedics, Vol. 1 (9th ed). St. Louis: Mosby, 1998.

orders. Refer to Table 3-5 for a complete list of hip disorders that may
require hip arthroplasty.

The most common type of hip arthroplasty, a *total hip arthroplasty*
(THA), is the replacement of both the femoral head and the acetabulum with a combination of metal (titanium or cobalt alloys) and polyethylene components (Figure 3-13). Technology and research have
introduced new materials for the weight-bearing components, such as
ultra-high-molecular-weight polyethylene and ceramic-on-ceramic and
metal-on-metal implants; however, long-term survival of such components is not yet known.[36]

The acetabular and femoral components may be *uncemented* or
*cemented*. Uncemented components are commonly used in the
younger, active patient, as well as in a patient with a revision THA
involving a failed cemented prosthesis. The uncemented components
have areas of porous coated metal on the surface that may be treated
with a biochemical agent, hydroxyapatite, to promote bony ingrowth
for improved fixation.[37] Press-fit prostheses are also being used and
have heavily textured surfaces that achieve fixation through interfer-
ence or interlocking of bone and metal surfaces.[34] Use of uncemented

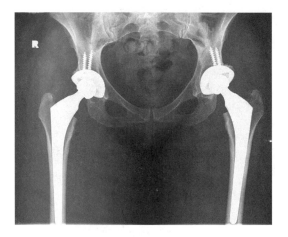

**Figure 3-13.** *Bilateral total hip arthroplasty.*

components has the advantage of biological fixation, reducing the incidence of *aseptic loosening* (the loosening caused by wear debris from the components). With uncemented components, weight bearing can be limited by surgeon protocol, but weight bearing should not be discouraged.[38] Weight bearing promotes bony ingrowth with the uncemented prosthetic components by allowing physiologic strain in the bone, thus increasing the activity of remodeling. With uncemented THA, the emphasis for the patient should be the prevention of torque or twisting on the operated leg while weight bearing.

The use of a cemented prosthesis (usually the femoral component) is reserved for an individual with a decreased ability to regenerate bone, such as a patient with osteopenia or osteoporosis.[39] A cemented prosthesis allows for full weight bearing early in the recovery phase.

A *bipolar* prosthesis consists of a metallic acetabular cup and polyethylene liner with a snap-fit socket placed over a femoral prosthesis, as shown in Figure 3-14.[40] A bipolar prosthesis is a type of hip arthroplasty used for revision when there is instability caused by osseous or muscular insufficiency that makes a patient's hip more likely to dislocate.

Surgical approaches and movement precautions for THA are presented in Table 3-6.[41,42] A good understanding of the surgical approach taken to expose the hip joint is necessary to determine movement precautions that prevent dislocation postoperatively. In the acute care setting, the risk of dislocation is significant because of the

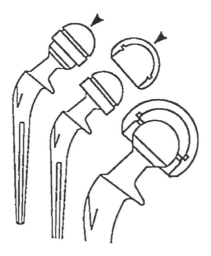

**Figure 3-14.** *Modified bipolar cup. Polyethylene cup is placed over head, and then the metal cup is pressed over it, polyethylene liner is locked in metallic cup, and head is locked in socket of polyethylene liner. Entire cup moves with femoral head as one unit, so cup cannot assume valgus or varus fixed position. Metal head can rotate in plastic socket in axis of neck. Cup must be used with the femoral prosthesis designed to fit properly into plastic liner. (With permission from JW Harkess. Arthroplasty of Hip. In AH Crenshaw [ed], Campbell's Operative Orthopaedics, Vol. 1 [8th ed]. St. Louis: Mosby, 1998.)*

**Table 3-6.** Surgical Approaches and Precautions for Total Hip Arthroplasty*

| Surgical Approach | Precautions |
| --- | --- |
| Posterolateral (most common) | No hip flexion beyond 90 degrees |
| | No excessive internal rotation |
| | No hip adduction past neutral |
| Lateral | No combined hip flexion beyond 90 degrees with adduction, internal rotation, or both |
| Anterolateral | Hip extension and external rotation are to be avoided |

*Hip surgery performed in conjunction with a trochanteric osteotomy (removal and reattachment of the greater trochanter) will require an additional movement restriction of no active abduction or passive adduction. Weight bearing of the surgical limb may be limited further.

incision made in the muscle mass and joint capsule for exposure of the hip during surgery. Consequently, the hip remains at risk for dislocation until these structures are well healed, edema is reduced, and the surrounding musculature is strengthened. Signs of dislocation include excessive pain with motion, abnormal internal or external rotation of the hip with limited active and passive motion, and shortening of the limb.[40]

Medical complications that may occur after THA include nerve injury, vascular damage and thromboembolism that can cause pulmonary embolism, myocardial infarction, and cerebral vascular accident. Complications pertaining to the implant can include fracture, aseptic loosening, osteolysis, heterotopic ossification, and infection.[43]

### Physical Therapy Intervention after Hip Arthroplasty

Early physical therapy intervention is focused on functional mobility, patient education about movement precautions during activities of daily living (ADLs), ROM, and strengthening of hip musculature. Physical therapy may assist in preventing complications, such as atelectasis, blockage of the intestines because of decreased peristalsis secondary to anesthesia (postoperative ileus), and DVT. Early mobilization improves respiration, digestion, and venous return from the lower extremities. Patients should be educated about these risks to assist in prevention of secondary complications.

- The priority of treatment is to achieve safe functional mobility (i.e., bed mobility, transfers, and ambulation with assistive devices) to maximize independence and functional outcome. Patient education is an important aspect of physical therapy. The physical therapist should educate the patient about movement precautions while encouraging use of the operated limb with functional activities. Verbal and tactile cueing may assist a patient in precaution maintenance; failure to do so may result in hip dislocation. The therapist should educate the patient that movement of the operated hip can decrease postoperative pain and stiffness.

- ROM (passive and active assisted) should be maintained within the parameters of the hip movement precautions. An overhead frame with a sling can promote active-assisted exercise.

- Isometric exercises for the quadriceps and gluteal muscles can be initiated immediately postoperatively, progressing to active-assisted exercises as tolerated. Muscle spasm often occurs in the musculature surrounding the hip postoperatively. Instructing the patient in exercises to gain control of the musculature involved in the surgery can help to reduce muscle spasms. Patients should be encouraged to perform all exercises independently.

• To assist in the prevention of DVT and reduce postoperative edema, the patient should be instructed to perform ankle-pumping exercises. This can be combined with external compression devices and antiembolic stockings to reduce the risk of a thromboembolic event. Before use of these modalities, ensure that the patient does not have cardiovascular insufficiency that may be exacerbated by their use.

• Before establishing an advanced strengthening program consisting of progressive resistive exercises or weight training, consult the surgeon, because excessive strain can hinder healing of surgically involved structures.

---

### Clinical Tip

• All peripheral innervations, dermatomal and myotomal, should be assessed on initial examination, with emphasis on the femoral nerve that innervates the quadriceps and the sciatic nerve that innervates the peroneals.[43] Neuropraxia of the femoral nerve can occur secondary to compression from surgical instrumentation and edema. A knee immobilizer may be necessary to provide stability if the quadriceps lacks adequate strength and stability for ambulation. If the peroneals are affected, resulting in a footdrop on the affected side, a custom-fit ankle-foot orthosis may be indicated for the patient to optimize gait.
• The use of a knee immobilizer reduces hip flexion by maintaining knee extension. This can be helpful in preventing dislocation in patients who are unable to maintain posterior hip precautions independently.
• Instruct the patient to avoid pivoting on the operated extremity when ambulating. Instead, the patient should turn by taking small steps and flexing the knee of the operated leg to clear the toes. To maintain movement precautions, the patient is encouraged to turn away from the operated limb.

- Emphasize to the patient that combining any of the restricted movements will increase the likelihood of dislocation. Provide the patient and family with written and illustrated education materials on all movement precautions.
- Elevation of the height of the bed can facilitate sit-to-stand transfers by reducing the degree of hip flexion and the work of the hip abductors and extensors. This is especially helpful for patients with bilateral THA. Also, instruct the patient to place the operated leg forward when performing a stand-to-sit transfer to decrease hip flexion.
- If available, a hip chair (or other elevated seating surface) and commode chair should be used to facilitate transfers while maintaining hip precautions. Pre- and postoperative education in the use of furniture of the appropriate height in the home should be initiated by the physical therapist.

### Knee Arthroplasty

Knee arthroplasty is indicated for patients with end-stage osteoarthritis, rheumatoid arthritis, traumatic arthritis, or nonseptic arthropathy. Pain reduction, gaining intrinsic joint stability, and restoration of function are the primary goals associated with knee arthroplasty and should only be considered when conservative measures have failed. The extent of damage within the joint determines the type of prosthesis implanted: unicompartmental or tricompartmental.

A *unicompartmental* (*unicondylar*) or *partial* knee arthroplasty is the replacement of the worn femoral and tibial articulating surfaces in either the medial or lateral compartment of the joint (Figure 3-15). This surgery is indicated for individuals who have osteoarthritis or osteonecrosis confined to one compartment. Proponents of the unicompartmental knee arthroplasty believe that it is a conservative measure to promote a more functional knee.[44] In unicompartmental knee arthroplasty, the goal is to maximize the preservation of the articular cartilage of the healthier compartment and spare bone that may in turn delay a total knee arthroplasty. More of the joint is preserved, including the cruciate ligaments, the opposite tibiofemoral compartment, and the patellofemoral joint. The rehabilitation is quicker, and

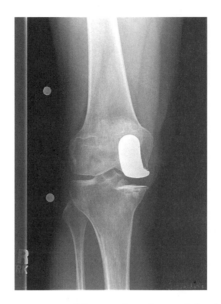

**Figure 3-15.** *Unicompartmental knee arthroplasty of the right medial compartment.*

an increased ROM is obtained because of more normal kinematics of the knee joint. Revision from a unicompartmental to a tricompartmental knee arthroplasty is often warranted at a later time because of continued degeneration; however, newer unicompartmental prosthetic designs may show improved results.[45] Associated valgus deformities may also be corrected by a tibial osteotomy and release of soft tissue during the partial knee replacement.

The *tricompartmental* or *total knee arthroplasty* (TKA) is the replacement of the femoral condyles, the tibial articulating surface, and the dorsal surface of the patella. This type of knee arthroplasty involves replacing the medial and lateral compartments of the joint, as well as resurfacing the patellofemoral articulation with prosthetic components (Figure 3-16A). These components are made of materials similar to those of the THA. The femoral condyles are replaced with a metal bearing surface that articulates with a polyethylene tray implanted on the proximal tibia. The dorsal aspect of the patella is often resurfaced if excessive erosion of the cartilage has occurred; however, some surgeons refrain from the patellar implant if the articular cartilage of the patella seems reasonably intact, as shown in Figure 3-16B.[46]

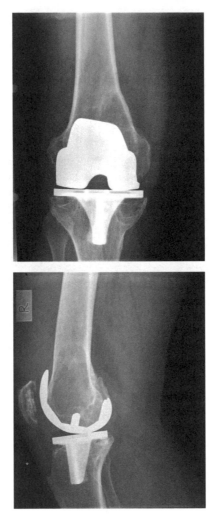

**Figure 3-16.** *A. Anterior view of a right total knee arthroplasty. B. Lateral view of a right total knee arthroplasty.*

The methods of fixation in TKA are similar to those of hip replacement. Cementing techniques can be used to fix the components, or the prosthetic design can allow for either porous ingrowth or press-fit. A press-fit prosthesis has surface modifications or grooves and bioactive hydroxyapatite to provide macrointerlock with the bone.[40] Many surgeons tend to use a hybrid technique by using a cemented tibial component with porous coated femoral and patellar prostheses. Partial weight bearing or weight bearing as tolerated often is allowed after TKA and is encouraged to promote use of the limb and promote bone remodeling.[46]

Patients who undergo either type of knee arthroplasty may have associated preoperative soft tissue contractures. A lateral retinacular release can be performed to centralize patellar tracking. If performed, there may be an increased risk of patellar subluxation with flexion. Special procedures that are performed in either type of knee arthroplasty should be taken into consideration by the physical therapist, because the surgeon may impose restrictions to ROM and weight bearing. Any additional procedure may prolong healing time secondary to increased edema and pain, which limits the patient's functional mobility and tolerance to exercise.

General medical complications after TKA are similar to those described with THA. Table 3-7 lists common complications specific to TKA.

### Physical Therapy Intervention after Knee Arthroplasty

Physical therapy intervention after knee arthroplasty is focused on increasing functional independence. The patients must also perform ROM and strengthening exercises and be educated in positioning techniques to help reduce swelling. Restrictions on weight bearing and precautions are also taught to the patient.

**Table 3-7.** Complications after Total Knee Arthroplasty

Thrombosis and thromboembolism
Poor wound healing
Infection
Joint instability
Fractures
Patellar tendon rupture
Patellofemoral instability, component failure, or loosening
Peroneal nerve injury
Component loosening or breakage
Wear and deformation

Source: Adapted from JL Guyton. Arthroplasty of Ankle and Knee. In ST Canale (ed), Campbell's Operative Orthopaedics, Vol. 1 (9th ed). St. Louis: Mosby, 1998.

• Evaluation and treatment of functional mobility to promote independence should begin immediately postoperatively. Bed mobility, transfer training, and gait training on level surfaces and stairs with appropriate assistive devices should be instructed to the patient to maximize functional outcomes and safety.

• Strengthening exercises may begin immediately postoperatively, emphasizing quadriceps exercises. Quadriceps retraining may be accomplished with overflow from the uninvolved limb or distal limb. Active-assisted quadriceps exercises should be performed to increase stability around the operated knee. The patient should be encouraged to perform exercises independently, within the limits of comfort.

• Knee immobilizers are often prescribed to protect the knee from twisting and buckling secondary to decreased quadriceps strength. With a lateral release, there may be increased pain and edema that may hinder quadriceps functioning; therefore, a knee immobilizer or brace may be required for a longer period of time.

• ROM exercises should begin immediately after TKA. ROM must be gained early in the rehabilitation of a TKA and is accomplished by passive or active-assisted exercises. If available, a continuous passive motion (CPM) machine may be used immediately postoperatively. The limitations to ROM are often attributed to pain, swelling, muscle guarding, and apprehension, all of which can be addressed through physical therapy interventions and patient education.

• Positioning and edema control should be initiated immediately to help reduce pain and increase ROM. The patient should be educated to elevate the operated extremity with pillows or towel rolls under the calf to promote edema reduction *and* promote knee extension. Ice should be applied after exercise or whenever needed for patient comfort.

---

### Clinical Tip

• Educate the patient to elevate the operated limb without putting pillows or towel rolls under the knee. This type of positioning keeps the knee flexed and will increase the risk of flexion contractures and edema.

- The therapist may place a towel roll or blanket along the lateral aspect of the femur, near the greater trochanter, to maintain the operated extremity in a neutral position. Any external rotation at the hip can result in slight flexion at the knee.
- The therapist should place a pillow or towel roll under the knee in the degree of available ROM while performing isometric exercises. This will produce a stronger quadriceps contraction by reducing passive stretch on joint receptors and pain receptors. This will also provide posterior support to the knee, providing increased tactile feedback for the patient.
- ROM for the majority of TKA is at least 90 degrees in the operating room. Consult the surgeon for the maximum amount of flexion obtained. This will provide the therapist with an idea of how much pain, muscle guarding, and edema are limiting patient performance.
- When performing active-assistive ROM, the use of hold/relax techniques to the hamstrings assists to decrease muscle guarding and increases knee flexion through reciprocal inhibition of the quadriceps muscle. This technique also provides a dorsal glide to the tibia, preparing the posterior capsule for flexion. Gentle massage of the quadriceps mechanism over the muscle belly or throughout the peripatellar region will improve ROM and reduce muscle guarding.
- With patients who have excessive edema with exercise, therapy sessions should be limited in duration and should concentrate on functional mobility. The use of a CPM in submaximal ranges in conjunction with ice will maintain knee ROM while assisting in edema reduction.
- If a brace or knee immobilizer is being used, the therapist should always check that it is applied properly. If the brace is not appropriately fitted to the patient or applied properly, it may keep the knee flexed. The therapist should adjust the brace or immobilizer to be certain that knee extension is maintained when worn by the patient. Nursing staff may need to be educated to different types of braces and the proper donning and doffing of the brace.
- Treatment sessions should be coordinated with administration of pain medication to increase patient comfort and compliance with ROM exercises.

## Shoulder Arthroplasty

Total shoulder arthroplasty (TSA) is indicated for patients with severe pain and limited ROM caused by osteoarthritis, rheumatoid arthritis, fracture, AVN, or traumatic arthritis. Conservative treatment should attempt to alleviate pain while increasing function. Only when these measures have failed should TSA be considered. If only the humeral head shows significant degeneration, a shoulder hemiarthroplasty may be considered. Prosthetic wear after TSA or shoulder hemiarthroplasty is of less concern than after THA or TKA, because the shoulder is not a weight-bearing structure.[47] The goal of surgery is to relieve pain and regain lost function.

TSA involves the replacement of the glenoid articulating surface and the humeral head with prosthetic components. A polyethylene glenoid unit with metal backing and keel articulates with a humeral prosthesis. Fixation of these components is either cemented or press-fit, processes similar to those in the other joint replacement surgeries.[48]

There are three types of TSA prostheses available: unconstrained, semiconstrained, and constrained. The most commonly used prosthesis is the unconstrained type that relies on soft tissue integrity of the rotator cuff and deltoid muscles. If these structures are insufficient or damaged, repair may take place during shoulder arthroplasty surgery and may prolong rehabilitation. The success of all TSA involves accurate surgical placement of the prosthesis and the ability of the surgeon to reconstruct the anatomic congruency of the joint. Proper orientation of the prosthetic components and preservation of structural length and muscular integrity are key aspects of the surgery that predispose favorable outcomes. The technical skill of the surgeon and advances in prosthetic components have improved outcomes with TSA. With appropriate patient selection and a properly functioning rotator cuff, a patient with a TSA can be rehabilitated to improve ROM and strength equal to that of the unaffected side.[47]

A proximal humeral hemiarthroplasty (Figure 3-17) can be performed when arthritic changes have affected only the humeral head. The humeral head is replaced with a prosthetic component through a similar technique as in TSA. Results are dependent on the integrity of the rotator cuff and deltoid, the precision of the surgeon, and the willingness of the patient to commit to a continual rehabilitation program. Rehabilitation of the shoulder hemiarthroplasty is similar to that of a TSA.

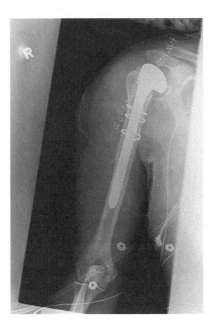

**Figure 3-17.** *Proximal hemiarthroplasty of the right shoulder.*

## Physical Therapy Intervention after Shoulder Arthroplasty

The rehabilitation after TSA or shoulder hemiarthroplasty should emphasize functional independence and patient education on therapeutic exercise. The physical therapist should confirm the presence of any precautions with the surgeon and educate the patient in passive and active-assisted ROM exercises to prevent the formation of adhesions. The stability of the shoulder is dependent on the rotator cuff and deltoid muscles, and the rehabilitation program may be dictated by their integrity. Maximum results from a TSA occur approximately 18–24 months after the surgery and a dedicated program of physical therapy.[47]

• Edema can be controlled with wrist and elbow ROM exercises and ice packs used in conjunction with elevation.

• A sling may be used for patient comfort but should be discontinued as soon as possible, following surgeon protocol, to increase ROM and strength. If there was extensive repair to the rotator cuff or deltoid, an abduction brace may be prescribed.

- The patient should be taught wand and pendulum exercises to promote shoulder flexion and abduction. With most TSAs, active external rotation should be performed in a pain-free ROM, but active abduction and flexion should be limited according to surgeon protocol. Outpatient physical therapy should begin shortly after the follow-up visit with the surgeon.

---

Clinical Tip

- A shoulder CPM can be ordered by the surgeon and applied postoperatively or for home use to assist with ROM and to prevent formation of adhesions.
- The physical therapist should initiate a consult for occupational therapy to instruct the patient on ADLs, especially if the patient's dominant arm is affected.

---

*Total Elbow Arthroplasty*

The reliability of TEA has progressed to outcomes comparable to those of other types of joint arthroplasty.[49] Indications for TEA are pain, instability, and elbow ankylosis. The patient population that demonstrates optimal results after TEA is those severely affected by rheumatoid arthritis.[50] Post-traumatic arthritis is also an indication for elbow arthroplasty; however, patient satisfaction and outcomes are inferior compared to those with rheumatoid arthritis.[51] The goal of TEA is the restoration of function through decreasing pain and increasing joint ROM and stability.

Early results of TEA with a fully constrained prosthesis have shown aseptic loosening. Conversely, an unlinked or less-constrained prosthesis demonstrates a decreased rate of loosening but has showed increased rates of failure secondary to weak collateral ligaments, anterior capsule, and reduced bone stock. Therefore, a semiconstrained prosthesis (Figure 3-18) is now favored for TEA to dissipate stress to the muscular and ligamentous structures surrounding the elbow, thus decreasing the rate of prosthetic loosening.[52] Unconstrained or resurfacing arthroplasties attempt to duplicate the anatomic surfaces within the joint and depend on intact ligaments and the anterior capsule for stability. A semiconstrained prosthesis may have a metal-to-polyethy-

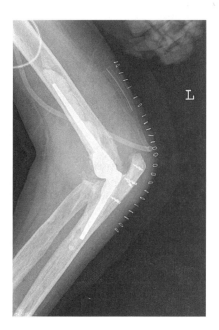

**Figure 3-18.** *Left total elbow arthroplasty shown in flexion.*

lene articulation that connects with a locking pin or snap-fit device[51] and is indicated for use if there is injury to the musculature and ligamentous structures of the elbow. Implants are constructed of materials similar to those of other total joint arthroplasties, and fixation techniques vary with cemented, uncemented, and hybrid (a combination of cemented and uncemented) fixation designs. Patient selection, surgical proficiency, and improved prosthetic design have improved outcomes and reduced complications after TEA.

Complications after a TEA include component loosening (usually the humeral component); joint instability, including dislocation or subluxation; ulnar nerve palsy; triceps weakness; delayed wound healing; and infection.[50]

Immediate rehabilitation of the patient with a TEA includes functional mobility training, ADL training, edema control, and ROM exercises per surgeon protocol. If available, an elbow CPM may be used. Passive elbow flexion and extension ROM may be allowed as tolerated according to patient pain levels while strengthening exercises are avoided.

## Total Ankle Arthroplasty

Total ankle arthroplasty has had difficulty gaining popularity due to increased failure rate with early prosthetic designs. There has been increased incidence of complications involving superficial and deep wound infections, loosening of the prosthesis, and associated subtalar and midtarsal degenerative joint disease. Debilitating arthritic pain is the primary indication for total ankle arthroplasty. Currently, the total ankle arthroplasty is optimal for an elderly patient with low physical demands, normal vascular status, good bone stock, and no immunosuppression.[53] Progress has been made with newer prosthetic designs and improved surgical techniques involving limited periosteal stripping, meticulous attention to positioning, and limited rigid internal fixation.

There are two types of prosthetic designs that have been developed to create a semiconstrained articulation. A two-component design with syndesmosis of the tibia and fibula consists of a tibial articular surface that is wider than the talar component. Fibular motion is eliminated, and a greater surface for fixation of the tibial component is created.[53] The second prosthetic design involves three components: a flat metal tibial plate, a metal talar component, and a mobile polyethylene bearing.[53] This system allows for multiplanar motion while maintaining congruency of the articulating surfaces. Both types of design consist of metal alloy and polyethylene components and rely on bony ingrowth for fixation. Technical skill and experience in component alignment and advanced instrumentation for component fixation are important aspects to be considered to improve postoperative outcomes. Current short-term results have shown reasonable increases in function, with little or no pain in appropriately selected patients.[53]

During the early postoperative period, care is taken to prevent wound complications. A short leg splint is used until sutures are removed, and the patient remains non weight bearing until bony ingrowth is satisfactory (approximately 3 weeks with hydroxyapatite-coated implants).[53] Early postoperative physical therapy treatment focuses on functional mobility and the patient's ability to maintain non weight bearing. The patient should be educated in edema reduction and early non-weight-bearing exercises, including ankle ROM and hip and knee strengthening if prescribed by the surgeon.

## Total Joint Arthroplasty Infection and Resection

The percentage of total joint arthroplasties that become infected (septic) is relatively small. However, a patient may present at any time after a joint arthroplasty with fever, wound drainage, persistent pain, and increased white blood cell count, erythrocyte sedimentation rate or C-reactive protein.[54] Infection is often diagnosed by aspirating the joint, culturing joint fluid specimens, and examining laboratory results from the aspirate. Once the type of organism is identified, there are several different avenues to follow for treatment of the infection. Treatment choices include antibiotic treatment and suppression, debridement with prosthesis retention or removal, primary exchange arthroplasty, two-stage reimplantation, or, in life-threatening instances, amputation.[55]

Within the early postoperative period, an infection in soft tissue with well-fixed implants can be treated with an irrigation and debridement procedure, exchange of polyethylene components, and antibiotic treatment. With an infection penetrating the joint space to the cement-bone interface, it is necessary to perform a *total joint arthroplasty resection*, consisting of the removal of prosthetic components, cement, and foreign material with debridement of surrounding tissue. A 6-week course of intravenous antibiotics should be followed before reimplantation of joint components.[45] The most successful results of deep periprosthetic infection have been obtained with the two-stage reimplantation and antibiotic treatment.[45] With reimplantation of prosthetic components, fixation depends on the quality of the bone, need for bone grafting, and use of antibiotic-impregnated bone cement.[43]

Resection arthroplasty of the hip or knee is commonly seen in the acute care orthopedic setting. A two-staged reimplantation is commonly performed. First, the hip or knee prosthetic is resected, and a cement spacer impregnated with antibiotics is placed in the joint to maintain tissue length and allow for increased weight bearing. Then, the prosthesis is re-implanted when the infection has cleared.[45,55] If the extent of the infection does not allow for reimplantation of prosthetic components, a knee resection arthroplasty or hip *Girdlestone* (removal of the femoral head, as in Figure 3-19),[55] may be the only option for the patient. Often, instability can be associated with these surgeries, leading to decreased function, and the patient often requires an assistive device for ambulation. Unlike a hip resection, a patient with a knee resection may undergo a knee arthrodesis or fusion with an intermedullary nail to provide a stable and painless limb.

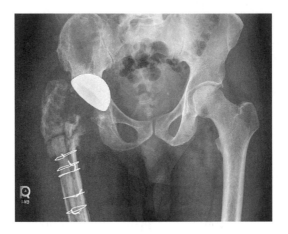

**Figure 3-19.** *Total hip arthroplasty resection (Girdlestone).*

## Physical Therapy Intervention after Resection Arthroplasty

Physical therapy after a resection arthroplasty without reimplantation or a two-staged reimplantation is dependent on the extent of joint or bone destruction caused by the infection and the removal of the prosthetic components, cement, and debridement of soft tissue. Weight-bearing restrictions may depend on use of cement spacers and vary from non weight bearing to weight bearing as tolerated, as established by the surgeon. Physical therapy sessions focus on functional mobility, safety, assistive device evaluation, and maintenance of muscle strength and endurance in anticipation for reimplantation of the joint.

- Patients who have an infection and joint resection arthroplasty may be compromised by general malaise and decreased endurance secondary to the infection, and, possibly, from increased blood loss during surgery. This may lead to decreased pain tolerance. The physical therapist should take these factors into account when mobilizing the patient. Functional mobility training should begin when the patient is stable, and physical therapy sessions should be modified for patient tolerance.

- THA precautions often do not pertain after removal of the prosthesis. The physical therapist should verify any other precautions, such as trochanteric precautions (see Table 3-6) and weight-bearing status, with the surgeon. Without movement precautions, most isometric, active, and active-assisted exercise may be appropriate. Progress the patient as tolerated to maximize function, strength, and endurance in preparation for eventual reimplantation of the prosthesis.

• For knee resection surgery, strengthening exercises for the quadriceps muscle can be initiated as long as the extensor mechanism is intact. Isometrics, active-assisted, and active-straight leg raises can be initiated according to patient comfort.

• Edema should be controlled with ice and elevation. Positioning of the limb is important to decrease discomfort from muscle spasm and the potential for deformities caused by muscle contractures around the hip and knee.

---

### Clinical Tip

• A hip Girdlestone procedure may leave a patient with a significant leg-length discrepancy. A patient's shoes should be adapted with a lift to correct gait and increase weight bearing on the affected extremity.
• With decreased leg length, the musculature surrounding the hip shortens. External (e.g., Buck) traction can be used to maintain muscle length and may be used while the patient is in bed. Shortened muscles may spasm. Isometric exercises should be encouraged to gain control of these muscles to reduce spasm.
• ROM should be minimal with knee resection so as to maintain integrity of bone surfaces if reimplantation is planned. A brace or knee immobilizer should be worn during functional activities to maintain knee extension but can be removed in bed. The unaffected limb can assist with lifting the affected limb with transfers out of bed.
• With a patient that is non weight bearing, a shoe on the unaffected side and a slipper sock on the affected side can assist with toe clearance when advancing the affected leg during the swing phase of gait. Conversely, with a patient who has a significant leg-length discrepancy, a slipper sock on the unaffected side and a shoe on the affected side can assist with ambulation until a shoe lift is obtained.

---

## Surgeries of the Spine

The vertebral column forms the central axial support of the body and consists of bony segments and fibrocartilaginous discs connected by ligamentous structures and supportive musculature. Degenerative, traumatic, or congenital changes can cause compensation in the vertebral bodies, intervertebral discs, facets, and intervertebral foramen. Any changes in these structures can result in dysfunction that, in turn, causes pain. Some common dysfunctions of the spine and associated structures are ligamentous sprain, muscle strain, herniated nucleus pulposus, rupture of the intervertebral disc, spinal stenosis with nerve root compression, spondylolisthesis, and degenerative disease of the disc, vertebral body, or facet joints. Any dysfunction can present itself in the cervical, thoracic, and lumbar spine.

Back pain is the major indication for spinal surgery. Pain can be disabling to a patient, limiting the ability to work or complete ADLs. Any acute injury, such as muscle spasm, herniated nucleus pulposus, and chronic low back pain exacerbations, should be managed conservatively before surgical treatment is recommended. Many injuries will heal with treatments, such as bed rest, anti-inflammatory medication, lifestyle modification, education in proper body mechanics, and outpatient physical therapy.[56] Surgery may be indicated when these measures fail to relieve a patient's symptoms or if there is a decline in the neurologic status of the patient.

Advances have been made in all areas of spinal surgery; however, there is still no cure for low back pain. Low back pain and leg pain can arise from degenerative disc disease and herniation or rupture of the intervertebral disc. Surgical procedures can be performed to relieve the symptoms associated with degenerative disc disease when conservative measures have failed. Open disc surgery and microdiscectomy remove disc fragments and herniated disc material that compress the adjacent nerve root. *Microdiscectomy* is a minimally invasive procedure that uses a microscope to view the surgical area, allowing for decreased surgical exposure.[56] Most microdiscectomy surgery can be done on an outpatient basis, and early return to activity can be accomplished. Symptom relief is high both initially postoperatively and on a long-term basis.[57] If additional exposure of the nerve root is needed, associated procedures, such as a laminectomy or foraminotomy, may be performed in conjunction with discectomy or spinal fusion. Refer to Table 3-8 for descriptions and indications for these procedures.

**Table 3-8.** Common Spinal Surgeries and Their Indications*

| Surgery | Indication | Procedure |
|---|---|---|
| Discectomy or microdiscectomy | Herniated nucleus pulposus (HNP) | Removal of the herniation or entire intervertebral disc. |
| Laminectomy | Spinal stenosis or nerve root compression | Removal of bone at the interlaminar space. |
| Foraminotomy | Spinal stenosis, HNP, or multiple nerve root compression | Removal of the spinous process and the entire laminae to the level of the pedicle. Usually done in conjunction with a fusion to maintain spinal stability. |
| Corpectomy | Multilevel stenosis, spondylolisthesis with nerve root compression | Removal of the vertebral body. The disc above and below the segment is removed, and a strut graft with instrumentation is used to fuse the anterior column. |
| Spinal fusion | Segmental instability, fractures, facet joint arthritis | Fusion of the facet joints using hardware and bone graft. May use fusion cages or pedicle screws and rods to achieve fixation. Approaches can vary, and a fusion can be done in conjunction with other spinal procedures to decompress nerve roots. |

*These procedures may be performed in any area of the spine when indicated. The approach may be anterior, posterior, or posterolateral.
Sources: Adapted from GW Wood. Lower Back Pain and Disorders of Intervertebral Disc. In ST Canale (ed), Campbell's Operative Orthopaedics, Vol. 1 (9th ed). St. Louis: Mosby, 1998; and JJ Regan. Endoscopic Spinal Surgery Anterior Approaches. In JW Frymoyer (ed), The Adult Spine Principles and Practice (2nd ed). New York: Lippincott–Raven, 1997.

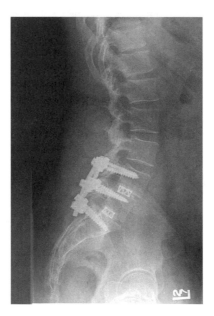

**Figure 3-20.** *Lateral view of a posterior interbody fusion with pedicle screws.*

Pain that arises from spinal instability caused by degenerative disc disease or degenerative joint disease may be treated surgically with a spinal fusion. Anterior or posterolateral spinal fusion with decompression attempts to fuse unstable spinal segments. This is achieved through implantation of various types of instrumentation with bone grafting to create a single motion segment and eliminate the source of pain, the disc.[58] The spinal segments are fixed using different types of rods, plates, and pedicle screws. The use of interbody fusion cages with instrumentation has become common practice for spinal fusion. An anterior lumbar interbody fusion, posterior lumbar interbody fusion (Figure 3-20), or combination can be performed.[56] Titanium alloy fusion cages are placed within the vertebral spaces, replacing the degenerated disc. These cages are then packed with bone graft harvested from the iliac crest (autograft) or from a bone bank (allograft). This bone graft can be supplemented with osteoinductive growth factors to facilitate fusion.[59] A combination of an anterior and posterior fusion can be successful when a single approach fails.

Experimental designs of the total disc replacement have been developed to reconstruct the disc, maintain disc height, and preserve segmental motion of the spine.[60] Developers of the artificial disc replacement believe that restoring mobility will decrease degeneration of spinal segments above and below the affected segment.[61] Artificial disc implantation has been occurring in Europe, and clinical trials are beginning in the United States. Many generations of the total disc design have shown promise, and if clinical trials are favorable, the total disc replacement may become a tool to combat back pain.[61]

Complications that can occur postoperatively from spinal surgery are neurologic injury, infection, cauda equina syndrome, dural tear with cerebrospinal fluid leak, and nonunion, as well as general surgical complications noted in previous sections.

## Physical Therapy Intervention after Spinal Surgery

In the acute care setting, physical therapy should emphasize early functional mobilization, education on proper body mechanics, gait training, and assessment of assistive devices to increase patient safety. Patients should be educated on movement precautions to minimize bending and twisting with activity, lifting restrictions per the surgeon, and use of braces or corsets if prescribed.

• Patients should be taught to logroll to get out of bed. The body rolls as a unit, minimizing trunk rotation. Functional mobility training should begin the first postoperative day. Ambulation should be stressed as the only formal exercise postoperatively for spinal surgery to promote healing of all tissues.

• Symptoms, such as radiating pain and sensory changes present before surgery, may persist for a significant period postoperatively secondary to edema surrounding the surgical site. Patients should be educated to this fact and told if any significant increase in pain or change in bladder and bowel function occurs, the patient should notify the nurse, surgeon, or both, immediately.

---

### Clinical Tip

• For surgical procedures with an anterior approach, the patient should be given a splinting pillow and educated in its use to promote deep breathing and coughing. A corset can be use to aid patient comfort with activity.

- Rolling walkers are useful to promote a step-through gait pattern and decrease stress on the spine caused by lifting a standard walker. Patients should progress to a cane or no assistive device to promote upright posture.
- If an iliac crest bone graft is harvested through a second incision, a patient may complain of increased pain at the surgical site. Ice can decrease swelling at the donor site. With this type of graft, a patient will likely need an assistive device to increase safety with ambulation and decrease pain.
- If interbody fusion cages are used, the patient should be encouraged to sit in a chair as soon as possible to increase compression on the cage and promote bone ingrowth. Sitting time can be unlimited according to patient comfort.[56]
- Patients who have undergone spinal fusion should be educated about the adverse effect that cigarette smoking has on the success of fusion.[62] The health-care team should emphasize smoking cessation, or the patient should be given the appropriate resources to assist with this task.
- The physical therapist should always check orders for braces used by the surgeon and any other restrictions on activity. Braces are usually worn when the patient is out of bed. If necessary, a surgeon may limit raising the head of the bed. Reverse Trendelenburg (putting the whole bed at a 45-degree angle, with head up) can assist with patient ADLs.
- Treatment should be coordinated with the administration of pain medication. Patients should be educated in relaxation techniques or breathing exercises to help manage their pain. The physical therapist should also be aware of any psychosocial factors that can interfere with patient recovery. If necessary, consult the psychiatric or chaplain services to assist with a patient's coping skills.

## Soft Tissue Surgeries

There is a wide variety of soft tissue surgeries encountered in the acute care orthopedic setting. The majority of these surgeries are aimed at improving joint stability by repairing the functional length of muscles, tendons, and ligaments. Common soft tissue surgeries include tendon transfers, muscle repairs, fasciotomies, cartilage resections or repairs, and ligament reconstructions. Many of these surgeries have progressed to be ambulatory surgery, but discharge may be delayed until the day after surgery secondary to inadequate pain control or adverse reactions to anesthesia.

Arthroscopic surgery has become common practice in the repair of joint structures in the acute care setting. *Arthroscopy* is indicated for a variety of joint problems not only as a diagnostic tool, but also, with advances in instrumentation, to repair joint structures injured by trauma or degeneration. The benefits of arthroscopic surgery are a reduced postoperative morbidity; decreased size of incision; decreased local inflammation; improved diagnosis; absence of secondary effects, such as neuroma, scarring, and functional imbalance; decreased hospital costs; and reduced complication rates.[63] However, complications after arthroscopy can still occur (Table 3-9).

### Knee Arthroscopy

In the acute care setting, a patient may be admitted after an arthroscopic procedure, such as an anterior cruciate ligament (ACL) repair. An ACL repair performed arthroscopically involves the replacement of the ACL with an autograft or allograft from the extensor mechanism, hamstring tendons, or Achilles tendon. Fixation of grafts involves the use of inter-

Table 3-9. Complications of Arthroscopy

---

Intraoperative
  Damage to intra-articular structures leading to chondromalacic changes
    and degenerative arthritis
  Damage to extra-articular structures, such as blood vessels, nerves, ligaments, and tendons
  Surgical instrument failure
  Fracture
Postoperative
  Hemarthrosis
  Thrombophlebitis
  Infection
  Reflex sympathetic dystrophy

---

Source: Data from BB Phillips. General Principles of Arthroscopy. In ST Canale (ed), Campbell's Operative Orthopaedics, Vol. 2 (9th ed). Boston: Mosby, 1998.

ference screws and washers, nonabsorbable sutures secured with staples, or bone plugs attached with screws or wires into tibial and femoral tunnels (Figure 3-21). Associated meniscal and ligamentous repairs, such as meniscal repairs or *meniscectomy*, may be performed with an ACL reconstruction or independently. Refer to Table 3-10 for a description of these procedures and physical therapy interventions.

### Shoulder Arthroscopy

Shoulder surgeries for soft tissue dysfunctions are common in the acute care setting and include subacromial decompression, acromioplasty, anterior capsular shift, and rotator cuff repair. These surgeries can be performed arthroscopically depending on the extent of damage. Rota-

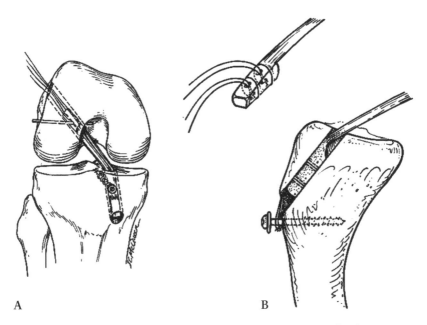

A                                    B

**Figure 3-21.** *Fixation of graphs with bone fragments. A. Patellar bone piece fixed in femoral tunnel by Kirschner wire; tibial bone piece fixed in tibial tunnel by small fragment AO screw. B. Heavy, nonabsorbable sutures are placed through two holes in bone and tied around screw. (With permission from RH Miller III. Knee Injuries. In ST Canale [ed], Campbell's Operative Orthopaedics, Vol. 2 [9th ed]. Boston: Mosby, 1998.)*

tor cuff repairs may require increased exposure so an open repair or mini-open repair may be performed with associated procedures, such as subacromial decompression.[64] Refer to Table 3-11 for a description of these procedures and associated physical therapy interventions. Functional training may be necessary for the older patient or for the patient with an existing functional limitation prior to admission.

**Table 3-10.** Soft Tissue Repair and Reconstruction Surgeries of the Knee and Physical Therapy Intervention

| Type of Repair and Reconstruction | Procedure | Physical Therapy Intervention |
| --- | --- | --- |
| Meniscectomy | Removal of all or part of the medial or lateral meniscus secondary to an irreparable tear | Edema management. Proximal and distal ROM exercises. Quadriceps and hamstring strengthening, as permitted by surgeon protocol. Functional training per weight-bearing precautions. |
| Meniscal repair | Repair of a torn meniscus in the vascular portion of the meniscus, where the likelihood of healing is greatest | As above. Restrictions on ROM and weight bearing may be imposed by the surgeon. Hinged brace, if prescribed. |
| Lateral retinacular release | Release of the synovium, capsular and retinacular structures lateral to the patella, and proximal muscle fibers of the vastus lateralis | Gentle ROM exercises per surgeon protocol. Edema management. Isometric exercises and quadriceps strengthening consisting of straight-leg raises (SLRs). Short-arc quadriceps strengthening should be avoided. Functional training per weight-bearing precautions. |

Table 3-10. *Continued*

| Type of Repair and Reconstruction | Procedure | Physical Therapy Intervention |
|---|---|---|
| Anterior cruciate ligament (ACL) reconstruction | Reconstruction of the insufficient ligament using autograft or allograft of the patellar tendon or hamstring tendon | Edema management. Use of a brace per surgeon (education to don/doff brace). Active and passive knee ROM exercises. (A CPM may be prescribed for home use.) Isometric exercises (quadriceps and hamstring) and quadriceps strengthening consisting of SLR per surgeon protocol. Functional training per weight-bearing precautions. |
| Posterior cruciate ligament (PCL) reconstruction | Reconstruction of the insufficient ligament with autograft or allograft using the central third of the patellar tendon or Achilles tendon | See anterior cruciate ligament, above. |
| Quadricepsplasty | Separation of the quadriceps mechanism, lengthening of the quadriceps mechanism, or both | Limitation of ROM to less-than-full flexion using a hinged brace. Gentle ROM exercise and CPM to maximum of 90 degrees. Passive knee extension. Active and active-assisted exercises for quadriceps and hamstrings. Functional training per weight-bearing precautions. |

CPM = continuous passive motion; ROM = range of motion.
Source: Data from BB Phillips. Arthroscopy of Lower Extremity. In ST Canale (ed), Campbell's Operative Orthopaedics, Vol. 2 (9th ed). St. Louis: Mosby, 1998.

Table 3-11. Soft Tissue Repair and Reconstruction Surgeries
of the Shoulder and Physical Therapy Intervention

| Type of Repair and Reconstruction | Procedure | Physical Therapy Intervention |
|---|---|---|
| Subacromial decompression or acromioplasty | Resection of the undersurface of the acromion | Use of a sling as indicated. Edema management. Hand, wrist, and elbow ROM. Pendulum exercises. Active and active-assisted shoulder ROM exercises. |
| Rotator cuff repair (arthroscopic, open, or mini-open procedure) | Can include repair of the biceps tendon, supraspinatus tendon, or avulsed rotator cuff | See Subacromial decompression or acromioplasty, above. Self-assisted ROM exercises per surgeon protocol (can be limited by the extent of repair). |
| Anterior reconstruction (Bankart repair) | Indicated for recurrent anterior instability Includes an anterior capsular shift, labral repair, or both | Immobilization using a sling, as indicated. Hand, wrist, and elbow ROM Edema management. Passive ROM within parameters, if indicated by the surgeon. |

ROM = range of motion.
Source: Data from BB Phillips. Arthroscopy of Upper Extremity. In ST Canale (ed), Campbell's Operative Orthopaedics, Vol. 2 (9th ed). St. Louis: Mosby, 1998.

## Experimental Soft Tissue Surgery

The advent of *autologous cartilage transplantation* is a recent advance in technology aimed at the repair of chondral defects in the knee. The clinical outcomes will, it is hoped, slow the progression of arthritic changes that may lead to more extensive surgery. Short-term results have shown promising results for repairing osteochondritis dissecans lesions on the femoral condyles.[65] Articular cartilage is harvested by arthroscopy from a non-weight-bearing surface in the affected knee, and growth of these cartilage cells then takes place in a laboratory. After the cells are cultured, another surgical procedure is performed in which the cartilage cells are injected onto a patch of periosteum covering the articular defect in the involved joint, as demonstrated in Figure 3-22.[66] Weight bearing is limited to approximately 40 pounds of the involved extremity, and ROM with a CPM is encouraged to promote nutrition in the articular cartilage.[65] Exercise and weight bearing are dependent on the location of the defect, and all precautions should be verified with the surgeon.

## Equipment for Fracture and Soft Tissue Injury Management

### Casts

A cast is a circumferential rigid dressing used to provide the immobilization of joints proximal and distal to fracture fragments necessary for bone healing. Casts can be made of plaster, fiberglass, or synthetic material and can be used on almost any body part. The rigidity of the cast allows for fracture stabilization, prevention of deformity, pain management, and protection.[10] Specific joint positioning is determined by the physician. Table 3-12 lists the common types of casts. Some casts may be split into two pieces (*bivalved cast*) to allow periodic visualization of the involved area or to relieve pressure. A small piece of cast may be cut out (i.e., window) to allow access for pulse monitoring, wound or drain care, or to relieve intra-abdominal pressure in a body cast.[67] Casts can also be used to provide low-load, prolonged, passive stretch to soft tissue to improve ROM. This is known as *serial casting*. A *cast brace* is the combination of casting material with orthotic components (e.g., hinge joints). It is commonly used in the treatment of nondisplaced fractures of the elbow or knee or as an adjunct to internal fixation.[68]

Complications associated with casts include

- *Compartment syndrome* is neurovascular compromise caused by microvascular and venous congestion within a muscle compartment that can lead to tissue hypoxia.[69] This may be caused by excessive swelling or the improper fit of a cast. The pressure increases within a facial compartment(s) of an extremity and, left untreated, can

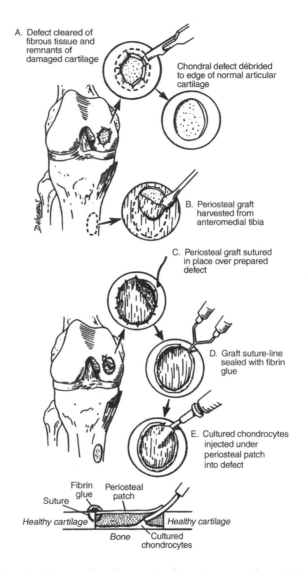

**Figure 3-22.** *Autologous chondrocyte implantation procedure. (With permission from the Orthopaedic and Sports Sections of the American Physical Therapy Association. SD Gillogly, M Voight, T Blackburn, Treatment of the Articular Cartilage Defects of the Knee with Autologous Chondrocyte Implantation. J Orthop Sports Phys Ther 1998;28:245.)*

**Table 3-12.** Common Types of Casts

| Type of Cast | Description |
| --- | --- |
| Short leg cast (SLC) | Extends from metatarsal heads to tibial tubercle. For distal tibia/fibula, ankle, and foot fractures. Immobilizes foot and ankle, usually 90 degrees neutral or slight dorsiflexion. Plantar flexion immobilization for Achilles tendon rupture. |
| Patellar tendon-bearing cast | Extends from metatarsal heads to mid- or suprapatella. For midshaft tibia fractures. Used for weight bearing activity. A patellar tendon bar dissipates some limb loading force to the external cast shell. Knee position is 90 degrees flexion, neutral ankle, or slight dorsiflexion. |
| Long leg cast (LLC), cylinder cast | Extends from metatarsal heads to the proximal/mid femur (to stabilize the tibia) or to the greater trochanter (to stabilize the distal femur). For proximal tibia and distal femur fractures. Knee immobilized in full extension or 5-degree flexion. A cylinder cast is essentially an LLC that does not enclose the foot. |
| Hip spica | Extends from lower trunk/pelvis to the involved distal thigh (single hip spica) or to the involved entire lower extremity and thigh of the uninvolved side (1 1/2 hip spica). For proximal femur and hip joint fractures or hip dislocation. Hip is immobilized approximately 30 degrees of hip flexion and abduction with 30 degrees knee flexion. Used rarely in adults. |
| Short arm cast (SAC) | Extends from MCP joint to proximal forearm. For radius and ulna fractures. Wrist immobilized in best position for fracture reduction or slight extension. Allows elbow flexion/extension and thumb/finger movement. |

| Type of Cast | Description |
| --- | --- |
| Long arm cast (LAC) | Extends from MCP joint to proximal upper arm, or to the axilla/shoulder to limit abduction and external rotation. |
| | For distal humerus, elbow, and forearm fractures. |
| | Elbow flexion typically immobilized at 90 degrees. |
| Thumb spica | Extends from tip of thumb to any point on the forearm. |
| | For distal radius, wrist, or thumb fractures. |
| | Wrist immobilized in neutral to slight extension with thumb under second and third fingers. |
| Shoulder spica | Essentially a two-piece cast composed of a long arm cast and modified body cast connected by stabilizing bars. |
| | The cast does not cover either shoulder. |
| | For complex humerus fractures or shoulder dislocation. |
| | Shoulder immobilized in best position for reduction, usually 30 degrees flexion, abduction, and external rotation. |
| Body cast | Extends from above the nipple line to the pubis, enclosing the chest and abdomen. |
| | For stable spine injuries, such as burst fractures. |
| | Immobilizes the thoracic and lumbar spine. |

MCP = metacarpophalangeal.
Source: Data from ML Stills, K Christensen. Management of Extremity Fractures: Principles of Casting and Orthotics. In MM Lusardi, CC Nielsen, Orthotics and Prosthetics in Rehabilitation. Boston: Butterworth–Heinemann, 2000.

progress to tissue necrosis. The most reliable signs and symptoms of compartment syndrome are pain (out of proportion to the injury, unrelieved by pain medicine, and increased by passive ROM or touch) and paresthesia.[69] Other signs and symptoms include pallor, weakness, decreased peripheral pulses, and dense tissues.

• Nerve compression is compression of a peripheral nerve over a bony prominence (e.g., peroneal nerve on the fibular head) by the cast. This form of nerve entrapment can result in transient or permanent nerve damage depending on the duration of compression.

• Skin breakdown can occur secondary to increased pressure, moisture development in the cast (causing blister formation), open skin lesions, or any combination of these.

Clinical Tip

• Notify the nurse, physician, or both immediately for any signs and symptoms of compartment syndrome, nerve compression, suspected skin breakdown, or new drainage from within the cast.
• The therapist should elevate all distal extremities 4–5 in. above the heart to allow gravity to assist venous return. Elevation of more than 5 in. can increase venous pressure, causing increased cardiovascular work load, and may be contraindicated for patients with congestive heart failure.
• Casts, especially plaster casts, should not get wet. The therapist should instruct the patient to wrap the cast in a waterproof bag during bathing or showering. Exposing casting materials to water weakens the structure and traps moisture against the skin.
• The therapist should instruct the patient to contact the physician if the following develop: symptoms of burning or warmth, numbness, or tingling; movement of the limb within the cast; increased edema; a discolored and cool hand or foot; or a strong odor from within the cast.
• The therapist should discourage patients from sliding objects in the cast to scratch itchy skin. Such objects can be lost in the cast or displace the stockinet beneath the cast and cause a wound or increase the risk of pressure sore formation. Because the cast provides a moist and warm environment, bacterial growth can develop at an accelerated rate and progress into a gangrenous lesion. To relieve itching below the cast, gently tap the cast or blow cool air into it.[68]
• Most casts are not rigid enough to withstand the forces of weight bearing. Weight-bearing parameters must be clarified by the physician.
• A nonslip cast boot should be provided for patients who have casts encompassing the foot and are allowed to weight bear with transfers and ambulation.
• It is important to reinforce that the patient move all joints proximal and distal to the cast to maintain functional ROM.

*Braces and Splints*

Braces and splints are used in conjunction with medical and surgical intervention techniques for management of musculoskeletal dysfunctions. Functional bracing is based on the concept that continued function during healing promotes osteogenesis (bone growth) and enhances soft tissue healing while preventing joint hypomobility and disuse atrophy. Bracing and splinting can be used to maintain fracture alignment during healing, joint stabilization, and anatomic joint alignment, and to minimize weight-bearing forces. Braces can be applied immediately at the time of injury or used as part of a progressive treatment course after conventional casting or traction. They may be prefabricated or custom made. Table 3-13 lists some of the most commonly used braces and splints, including spinal orthoses. Complications with braces and splints include improper fit, skin breakdown, and improper use or poor compliance.

**Table 3-13.** Braces, Splints, and Orthoses Commonly Used in the Acute Care Setting

| Type of Orthosis | Description |
| --- | --- |
| Spine/trunk | |
| Soft cervical collar | Foam cylinder with a cloth cover that secures posteriorly (more extended spine) or anteriorly (more flexed spine). |
| | For injuries that do not require rigid cervical fixation (e.g., whiplash injury). |
| | Serves primarily as a kinesthetic reminder to limit neck movement. |
| Reinforced cervical collar (Philadelphia, Miami J, Aspen) | Bivalved total-contact padding reinforced within a semirigid plastic frame that secures with Velcro. |
| | Enclosing the neck, the chin is supported anteriorly, the occiput posteriorly, and it rests on the superior trunk. |
| | An anterior opening can accommodate a tracheostomy tube. |
| | For situations that require moderate limitations of neck movement (e.g., s/p fusion). |

Table 3-13. *Continued*

| Type of Orthosis | Description |
| --- | --- |
| Sterno-occipito-mandibular (SOMI) immobilizer | T-shaped yoke worn over the shoulders and anterior chest connects to an occipital support via a U-shaped metal rod. The distal yoke is anchored by a strap around the midtrunk, and a mandibular support attaches to the yoke by a single metal post and to the occipital support by straps. For instability at or above C4. Strictly controls flexion. Metal supports can be adjusted to position the neck in neutral or slight flexion/extension. |
| Halo vest | Percutaneous pins to the skull connect at the level of the forehead to a circumferential frame, which is attached via vertical rods to a vest lined with sheepskin. Used for strict immobilization of the cervical or high thoracic spine (e.g., s/p unstable fracture). |
| Abdominal binder | Wide elastic fabric secured by Velcro. Placed around the abdomen, pelvis, or both. Provides external abdominal support (e.g., used after abdominal surgery to support a large incision) and a kinesthetic reminder to minimize lower thoracic or lumbar movement. |
| Jewitt brace | Anterolateral aluminum frame with pads at the sternum, lateral midline of the trunk, pubis, and lumbar spine. Used to limit flexion and encourage hyperextension (e.g., lower thoracic or lumbar compression fracture). |
| Molded thoracolumbosacral orthosis (TLSO) | Custom-fabricated, total-contact thermoplastic shell (single unit or bivalved) secured with Velcro. Used to limit trunk flexion/extension, sidebending, and rotation (e.g., fracture or deformity of the thoracic or upper lumbar spine). |
| Lower extremity Post-op shoe | Sandal-type shoe with open areas at the toe and dorsum of the foot. Velcro connects the medial and lateral sides. |

| Type of Orthosis | Description |
|---|---|
| | Used for an edematous foot, to accommodate a bulky dressing on the foot, or for painful toe/foot conditions (e.g., s/p open-toe amputation, patient with congestive heart failure). |
| Ankle stirrup (Air-cast) | Stirrup shaped, molded, and plastic-lined with an air-filled compartment. |
| | Medial and lateral sides connect with Velcro. |
| | Worn in a shoe. |
| | Permits plantar- and dorsiflexion but limits inversion/eversion. |
| | For moderate–severe ankle sprains. |
| Short leg walking boot | Prefabricated, bivalved, hard, plastic outer shell with foam-filled air cells that encloses the foot and lower leg below the knee. |
| | The plantar aspect has a nonslip rubber grip. |
| | Used for conditions that allow weight bearing but require intermittent immobilization (stable ankle fracture) or cushioning (e.g., bruised calcaneus). |
| Solid ankle–foot orthosis (AFO) | Thermoplastic posterior shell extends from just below the knee to the plantar aspect of the foot. |
| | Secured proximally by Velcro and worn inside a shoe. |
| | For mediolateral ankle stability, footdrop prevention, control of knee hyperextension or flexion (e.g., hypertonicity, peroneal nerve palsy). |
| Knee immobilizer | Cylinder-shaped foam secured with Velcro with either posterior or medial/lateral aluminum stays. |
| | Extends from the upper thigh to the calf. |
| | Promotes knee extension. |
| | For knee injuries not requiring rigid immobilization (e.g., ligamentous injury). |
| Drop-lock brace (Bledsoe) | Lateral and medial metal struts at the thigh and lower leg connect to a hinge mechanism at the knee. |
| | The hinge has a dial to select the desired degree of flexion or extension at the knee. |
| | The metal struts, which secure with Velcro, adhere to foam at the thigh and calf. |
| | For knee injuries requiring intermittent rigid immobilization (e.g., s/p anterior cruciate ligament repair or patellar fracture). |

**Table 3-13.** *Continued*

| Type of Orthosis | Description |
|---|---|
| Hip abduction orthosis | A padded pelvic band with a lateral extension toward the greater trochanter connects to a thigh cuff by a metal upright, including an adjustable hip joint. |
| | The thigh cuff extends medially across the knee joint. |
| | May be used with a spine orthosis or AFO. |
| | For injuries or conditions that require limitation of hip flexion/extension (e.g., s/p total hip revision, hip dislocation, or spine and pelvis trauma). |
| Upper extremity | |
| Simple arm sling | Fabric sling with a strap around the neck positions the elbow in approximately 90-degree flexion across the chest with the shoulder internally rotated. |
| | Used for comfort and gentle support of the shoulder and upper extremity (e.g., s/p stable clavicle or humeral fracture). |
| Rowe sling | As above, a simple arm sling with a second strap around the trunk to limit shoulder abduction and external rotation. |
| | For conditions requiring stricter intermittent immobilization (e.g., s/p open rotator cuff repair). |
| Resting hand splint | Thermoplastic splint placed on the dorsal aspect of the hand, wrist, and forearm. |
| | Positions the distal upper extremity at mid pronation/supination, 20–30-degree wrist extension, proximal interphalangeal flexion, distal interphalangeal extension, and partial thumb opposition. |
| | Used to support, protect, or maintain a functional position of the wrist and hand (e.g., neuromuscular disorders). |

s/p = status post.
Source: Data from MM Lusardi, CC Nielsen (eds). Orthotics and Prosthetics in Rehabilitation. Boston: Butterworth–Heinemann, 2000.

**Clinical Tip**

• Patient education is vital for any patient receiving a brace, splint, or orthosis. The patient or caregiver should have a good working knowledge of the function and purpose of the device, as well as the ability to don and doff the device.

• Often, a manufacturer's brand name is used to identify its most popular brace or splint. Therefore, it is important to clarify and understand the specific *function* of the brace or splint, not just the style or popular name.

## *External Fixators*

An *external fixator* is a device consisting of aluminum or titanium percutaneous pins inserted at oblique or right angles to the long axis of a bone that connect externally to a frame. The frame provides the alignment forces to fracture fragments and maintains reduction while healing occurs.[67] In pin fixation, the frame is rod shaped. In ring fixation, the frame is circular and is placed around the extremity. External fixation devices are often the treatment of choice for severely comminuted or open fractures; fractures with severe soft tissue, vascular, or burn injures; or when infection is present.[70] An additional use of external fixation is to compress or lengthen a long bone.[9] An advantage of external fixation is the ability to manage associated injuries, such as skin grafts and areas of debridement. It also allows for early functional mobilization. External fixators can be placed on the upper extremity, lower extremity, and pelvis. Complications of external fixation devices include[9]

• Pin site infection

• Nerve, blood vessel, muscle, or tendon impingement or impalement damage secondary to pin placement

• Loss of fracture reduction or refracture

• Nonunion or malunion

• Compartment syndrome

---

**Clinical Tip**

• It is important to maintain full ROM of all joints proximal and distal to the external fixator. A footplate can be attached to the lower leg fixator to maintain neutral ankle dorsiflexion.

• The external fixator is very sturdy and can be used to assist in moving the involved limb, if permitted by the physician.

• Take extra care in the prevention of inadvertent tapping or banging of the external fixator against objects, such as a walker or footstool, as the force (vibration) is transferred to the bone and is painful.

• Clear drainage, as well as slight bleeding, redness, and swelling, at the pin sites, is normal.

---

### Traction

Traction involves the use of a distractive force on an extremity to reduce fracture, immobilize a joint, or decrease muscle spasm.[71] A system of weights and pulleys restores the alignment of bone and muscle. The traction apparatus connects to the patient (positioned in supine) by either direct (skeletal traction) or indirect (skin traction) means.[10] *Skeletal traction* uses pins or wires placed through the bone to provide a prolonged distractive force. It is maintained continuously; therefore, the patient is on strict bed rest. Skeletal traction is more effective as a distraction tool than skin traction. *Skin traction* uses boots, slings, or belts applied directly to the skin that can be removed for intermittent use of the involved extremity per physician's orders. Table 3-14 lists the different types of traction.

Complications associated with traction include[67]

• Hypomobility of the involved joint and hypermobility at the joint closest to the skeletal pin site

• Generalized muscle atrophy of the immobilized limb

• Deconditioning of the cardiovascular system and the general side effects of prolonged bed rest (see Appendix 1-B)

Table 3-14. Common Types of Traction

| Type | Description |
|------|-------------|
| Buck | Prefabricated boot on lower leg exerts a straight pull to distract lower extremity. The hip may be positioned in neutral or slight abduction. Typically used for femoral head or shaft fractures, hip dislocations, hip arthritis, post Girdlestone procedure, sciatica, or to decrease hip muscle spasm. |
| Russell | Essentially Buck traction with a sling below the knee. Used for femoral head or tibial plateau fractures, or various knee injuries. |
| Pelvic | A belt is applied to the lumbar spine and pelvis, and the HOB is elevated 20–30 degrees with the foot of the bed elevated 45 degrees, or a sling suspends the buttocks just off the bed. Used for back pain or pubic symphysis fracture, respectively. |
| Overhead 90-90 | An L-shaped frame over the entire arm and a sling at the forearm suspend the upper extremity at 90 degrees each of shoulder and elbow flexion with the arm across the chest (0-degree abduction). Used for fracture and dislocation of the shoulder and upper arm. |
| Side arm | Traction set-up and indications similar to Overhead 90-90, except arm position is 90 degrees of abduction, 90 degrees of elbow flexion, with palm facing foot of bed. |
| Cervical | Cervical halter with a chin strap exerts a straight pull on the cervical spine. The HOB may be flat or slightly elevated. Used for cervical spine fracture, ruptured disc, or severe ligamentous strain and sprain. |

HOB = head of bed.
Sources: With permission from Zimmer Traction Handbook. Zimmer, Inc., 1996; and WC Dubuisson. Nursing Management of Adults with Musculoskeletal Trauma. In PG Beare, JL Meyers. Adult Health Nursing (3rd ed). St. Louis: Mosby, 1998.

- Skin breakdown or decubitus ulcer formation of the immobilized limb over high-pressure areas (See Pathophysiology of Wounds in Chapter 7)
- Infection of traction pin sites or osteomyelitis
- Compartment syndrome

**Clinical Tip**

• Do not adjust, remove, or reapply traction unless there is a good working knowledge of the traction apparatus. Physician orders must be received to remove or adjust the traction unit.

• The patient's body alignment or the position of the bed is specifically selected for proper countertraction; therefore, the therapist must not change the positioning of the head or foot of the bed or the placement of blanket rolls or sandbags.

• Keep weights hanging free when the patient is in traction. Be careful not to lower the height of the bed so as to let the weight inadvertently rest on the floor.

• Never hang a weight over a patient.

• Notify the nurse of any frayed traction rope, loose knots, or any other alteration of the traction apparatus.

• It is important to monitor the patient's skin integrity, pain report, and lower-extremity position when in traction, because abnormal traction or extremity position can cause discomfort or nerve palsy (e.g., external hip rotation can compress the peroneal nerve against a suspension device).

• Include isometric or active exercise of both the involved and uninvolved extremities as appropriate to minimize strength loss, joint stiffness, and restlessness associated with prolonged bed rest, as well as to promote a positive body image.

# References

1. Palmer ML, Epler M (eds). Gross Evaluations. Clinical Assessment Procedures in Physical Therapy. Philadelphia: Lippincott, 1990;2–6.
2. Magee DJ (ed). Principles and Concepts. Orthopedic Physical Assessment (3rd ed). Philadelphia: Saunders, 1997;1–52.
3. Sonin AH, Rogers LF. Skeletal Trauma. In RG Grainger, D Allison (eds), Grainger and Allison's Diagnostic Radiology: A Textbook of Medical Imaging, Vol. 3 (3rd ed). New York: Churchill Livingstone, 1997;1573–1627.

4. Golding SJ, Genant HJ. Computed Tomography of the Musculoskeletal System. In RG Grainger, D Allison (eds), Grainger and Allison's Diagnostic Radiology: A Textbook of Medical Imaging, Vol. 3 (3rd ed). New York: Churchill Livingstone, 1997;1879–1891.

5. Greyson ND. Radionuclide Bone Scanning. In RG Grainger, D Allison (eds), Grainger and Allison's Diagnostic Radiology: A Textbook of Medical Imaging, Vol. 3 (3rd ed). New York: Churchill Livingstone, 1997;1915–1929.

6. Murphy WA. Joint Disease. In RG Grainger, D Allison (eds), Grainger and Allison's Diagnostic Radiology: A Textbook of Medical Imaging, Vol. 3 (3rd ed). New York: Churchill Livingstone, 1997;1804–1807.

7. McKinnis LN (ed). Fundamentals of Orthopedic Radiology. Philadelphia: FA Davis, 1997.

8. Lundon K (ed). Injury, Regeneration, and Repair in Bone. In Orthopedic Rehabilitation Science: Principles for Clinical Management of Bone. Boston: Butterworth–Heinemann, 2000;93–113.

9. Christian CA. General Principles of Fracture Management. In ST Canale (ed), Campbell's Operative Orthopaedics, Vol. 3 (9th ed). St. Louis: Mosby, 1998;1939–2041.

10. Black JM. Nursing Care of Clients with Musculoskeletal Trauma or Overuse. In JM Black, E Matassarin-Jacobs (eds), Medical-Surgical Nursing Clinical Management for Continuity of Care (5th ed). Philadelphia: Saunders, 1997;2129–2170.

11. Cryer HG, Johnson E. Pelvic Fractures. In DV Feliciano, EE Moore, KL Mattox (eds), Trauma (3rd ed). Stamford CT: Appleton & Lange, 1996;635–660.

12. DiPasquale TG, Nowinski RJ. The Acute Care and Evaluation of Acetabular Fractures. In M Bosse, JF Kellam, TJ Fisher, P Tornetta (eds), Orthopaedic Knowledge Update: Trauma (2nd ed). Rosemont, IL: American Academy of Orthopaedic Surgeons, 2000;239–253.

13. Perry DC, DeLong W. Acetabular fractures. Orthop Clin North Am 1997;28:405–417.

14. Tile M. Fractures of the Acetabulum. In CA Rockwood, DP Green, RW Bucholz, JD Heckman (eds). Rockwood and Green's Fractures in Adults (4th ed). Philadelphia: Lippincott–Raven Publishers, 1996;1617–1658.

15. Tornetta P. Displaced acetabular fractures: indications for operative and nonoperative management. J Am Acad Orthop Surg 2001;9:18–28.

16. Leighton RK, Lammens P. Hip Dislocations and Fractures of the Femoral Head. In M Bosse, JF Kellam, TJ Fisher, P Tornetta (eds), Orthopaedic Knowledge Update: Trauma (2nd ed). Rosemont, IL: American Academy of Orthopaedic Surgeons, 2000;311–316.

17. JL Guyton. Fractures of the Hip, Acetabulum, and Pelvis. In ST Canale (ed), Campbell's Operative Orthopaedics, Vol. 3 (3rd ed). St. Louis: Mosby, 1998;2181–2262.

18. DeLee JC. Fractures and Dislocations of the Hip. In CA Rockwood, DP Green, RW Bucholz, JD Heckman (eds). Rockwood and Green's Fractures in Adults (4th ed). Philadelphia: Lippincott–Raven Publishers, 1996;1659–1744.

19. Unwin A, Jones K (eds). The Femur. Emergency Orthopaedics and Trauma. Oxford, U.K.: Butterworth–Heinemann, 1995;203–207.
20. Geel CW. Extra-Articular and Intra-Articular Fractures of the Distal End Segment of the Femur. In M Bosse, JF Kellam, TJ Fisher, P Tornetta (eds), Orthopaedic Knowledge Update: Trauma (2nd ed). Rosemont, IL: American Academy of Orthopaedic Surgeons, 2000;147–155.
21. Whittle AP. Fractures of the Lower Extremity. In ST Canale (ed), Campbell's Operative Orthopaedics, Vol. 3 (3rd ed). St. Louis: Mosby, 1998;2042–2164.
22. Johnson EE. Fractures of the Patella. In CA Rockwood, DP Green, RW Bucholz, JD Heckman (eds), Rockwood and Green's Fractures in Adults, Vol. 2 (4th ed). Philadelphia: Lippincott–Raven, 1996;1956–1972.
23. Geissler WB, Tsao AK, Hughes JL. Fractures and Injuries of the Ankle. In CA Rockwood, DP Green, RW Bucholz, JD Heckman (eds), Rockwood and Green's Fractures in Adults, Vol. 2 (4th ed). Philadelphia: Lippincott–Raven, 1996;2201–2266.
24. Heckman JD. Fractures and Dislocations of the Foot. Fractures and Injuries of the Ankle. In CA Rockwood, DP Green, RW Bucholz, JD Heckman (eds), Rockwood and Green's Fractures in Adults, Vol. 2 (4th ed). Philadelphia: Lippincott–Raven, 1996;2267–2405.
25. Hockberger RS, Kirshenbaum KJ, Doris PE. Spinal Injuries. In P Rosen (ed), Emergency Medicine Concepts and Clinical Practice, Vol. 1 (4th ed). St. Louis: Mosby, 1998;462–475.
26. KP Butters. Fractures and Dislocations of the Scapula. In CA Rockwood, DP Green, RW Bucholz, JD Heckman (eds), Rockwood and Green's Fractures in Adults, Vol. 2 (4th ed). Philadelphia: Lippincott–Raven, 1996;1163–1192.
27. Crenshaw AH. Fractures of the Shoulder Girdle, Arm, and Forearm. In ST Canale (ed), Campbell's Operative Orthopaedics, Vol. 3 (3rd ed). St. Louis: Mosby, 1998;2281–2362.
28. Blachut PA, Broekhuyse HM. Fractures of the Scapula and Clavicle and Injuries of the Acromioclavicular and Sternoclavicular Joints. In Orthopaedic Knowledge Update: Trauma (2nd ed). Rosemont, IL: American Academy of Orthopaedic Surgeons, 2000;3–12.
29. Schmidt AH. Fractures of the Proximal Humerus and Dislocation of the Glenohumeral Joint. In Orthopaedic Knowledge Update: Trauma (2nd ed). Rosemont, IL: American Academy of Orthopaedic Surgeons, 2000;13–22.
30. Williams GR, Wong KL. Two-part and three-part fractures: open reduction and internal fixation versus closed reduction and percutaneous pinning. Orthop Clin North Am 2000;31:1–21.
31. Zuckman JD, Koval KJ. Fractures of the Shaft of the Humerus. In CA Rockwood, DP Green, RW Bucholz, JD Heckman (eds), Rockwood and Green's Fractures in Adults, Vol. 2 (4th ed). Philadelphia: Lippincott–Raven, 1996;1025–1053.
32. Kuntz DG, Baratz ME. Fractures of the Elbow. Elbow Trauma and Reconstruction. Orthop Clin North Am 1999;30:37–61.
33. Kellam JF. Carpal Fractures and Dislocations. In M Bosse, JF Kellam, TJ Fisher, P Tornetta (eds), Orthopaedic Knowledge Update: Trauma (2nd

ed). Rosemont, IL: American Academy of Orthopaedic Surgeons, 2000;85–89.

34. Daniels AU, Tooms RE, Harkess JW. Arthroplasty: Introduction and Overview. In Canale ST (ed), Campbell's Operative Orthopaedics, Vol. 1 (9th ed). St. Louis: Mosby, 1998;211–231.

35. Reuben JD, Meyers SJ, Cox DD, et al. Cost comparison between bilateral simultaneous, staged, and unilateral total joint arthroplasty. J Arthroplasty 1998;13(2):172–179.

36. Roberson JR. Bearing surfaces and wear in total hip replacement: current developments. Semin Arthroplasty 2000;11(3):161–166.

37. Callaghan JJ. Options for fixation in total hip replacement. Semin Arthroplasty 2000;11(3):151–160.

38. Rao RR, Sharkey PF, Hozack WJ, et al. Immediate weightbearing after uncemented total hip arthroplasty. Clin Orthop 1998;349:156–162.

39. Tate D, Sculco TP. Advances in total hip arthroplasty. Am J Orthop 1998;24(4):274–282.

40. Harkess JW. Arthroplasty of Hip. In AH Crenshaw (ed). Campbell's Operative Orthopaedics, Vol. 1 (8th ed). St. Louis: Mosby, 1992;441–626.

41. Roberson JR. Primary total hip replacement: the case for the posterolateral approach. Semin Arthroplasty 2000;11(3):143–150.

42. Kavanagh, BF. Anterolateral exposure to the hip for total hip replacement. Seminars Arthroplasty 2000;11(3):137–142.

43. Harkess JW. Arthroplasty of Hip. In ST Canale (ed), Campbell's Operative Orthopaedics, Vol 1. (9th ed). St. Louis: Mosby, 1998;296–471.

44. Buly RL, Sculco TP. Recent advances in total knee replacement surgery. Curr Opin Rheumatol 1995;7:107–113.

45. Guyton JL. Arthroplasty of Ankle and Knee. In ST Canale (ed), Campbell's Operative Orthopaedics, Vol. 1 (9th ed). St. Louis: Mosby, 1998;232–295.

46. Tooms RE. Arthroplasty of Ankle and Knee. In AH Crenshaw (ed), Campbell's Operative Orthopaedics, Vol. 1 (9th ed). St. Louis: Mosby, 1992;389–439.

47. Sisk TD, Wright PE. Arthroplasty of Shoulder and Elbow. In AH Crenshaw (ed), Campbell's Operative Orthopaedics, Vol. 1 (8th ed). St. Louis: Mosby, 1992;627–673.

48. Torchia ME, Cofield RH, Settergren CR. Total shoulder arthroplasty with the Neer prosthesis: long-term results. J Shoulder Elbow Surg 1997;6(6):495–505.

49. Hargreaves D, Emery, R. Total elbow replacement in the treatment of rheumatoid disease. Clin Orthop 1999;366:61–71.

50. Kudo H, Iwano K, and Nishino J. Total elbow arthroplasty with use of a nonconstrained humeral component inserted without cement in patients who have rheumatoid arthritis. J Bone Joint Surg Am 1999; 81(9):1268–1280.

51. Azar FM, Wright PE. Arthroplasty of Shoulder and Elbow. In ST Canale (ed), Campbell's Operative Orthopaedics, Vol. 1 (9th ed). St. Louis: Mosby, 1998;473–518.

52. O'Driscoll SW. Elbow arthritis: treatment options. J Am Acad Orthop Surg 1993;1(2):106–116.

53. Saltzman CL, McIff TE, Buckwalter JA, Brown TD. Total ankle replacement revisited. J Orthop Sports Phys Ther 2000;30(2):56–67.
54. Tattevin P, Cremieux AC, Pottier P, et al. Prosthetic joint infection: When can prosthesis salvage be considered? Clin Infect Dis 1999;29 (2):292–295.
55. Westrich GH, Salvati EA, Brause B. Postoperative Infection. In JV Bono, JC McCarthy, TS Thornhill, et al. (eds), Revision Total Hip Arthroplasty. New York: Springer-Verlag, 1999;371–390.
56. Wood GW. Lower Back Pain and Disorders of Intervertebral Disc. In ST Canale (ed), Campbell's Operative Orthopaedics, Vol. 3 (9th ed). Boston: Mosby, 1998;3014–3092.
57. Findlay GF, Hall BI, Musa BS, et al. A 10-year follow-up of the outcome of lumbar microdiscectomy. Spine 1998;23(10):1168–1171.
58. Miyakoshi N, Abe E, Shimada Y, et al. Outcome of one-level posterior lumbar interbody fusion for spondylolisthesis and postoperative intervertebral disc degeneration adjacent to the fusion. Spine 2000;25(14): 1837–1842.
59. Sandhu HS. Anterior lumbar interbody fusion with osteoinductive growth factors. Clin Orthop 2000;371:56–60.
60. Zeegers WS, Bohnen LMLJ, Laaper M, Verhaegen MJA. Artificial disc replacement with the modular type SB Charité III: 2-year results in 50 prospectively studied patients. Eur Spine J 1999;8:210–217.
61. Cinotti G, David T, Postacchini F. Results of disc prosthesis after a minimum follow-up period of 2 years. Spine 1996;21(8):995–1000.
62. Glassman SD, Anagnost SC, Parker A, et al. The effect of cigarette smoking and smoking cessation on spinal fusion. Spine 2000;25(20): 2608–2615.
63. Philips BB. General Principles of Arthroscopy. In ST Canale (ed), Campbell's Operative Orthopaedics, Vol. 2 (9th ed). St. Louis: Mosby, 1998;1453–1469.
64. Norberg FB, Field LD, Savoie FH. Repair of the rotator cuff, mini-open and arthroscopic repairs. Clin Sports Med 2000;19(1):77–97.
65. Minas T, Peterson L. Chondrocyte transplantation. Operative Techniques Orthop 1997;7(4):323–333.
66. Bentley G, Minas T. Treating joint damage in young people. BMJ 2000;320(7249):1585–1588.
67. Bryant GG. Modalities for Immobilization. In: AH Maher, SW Salmond, TA Pellino (eds), Orthopaedic Nursing (2nd ed). Philadelphia: Saunders, 1998;296–322.
68. Stills ML, Christensen K. Management of Extremity Fractures: Principles of Casting and Orthotics. In MM Lusardi, CC Nielsen (eds), Orthotics and Prosthetics in Rehabilitation. Boston: Butterworth–Heinemann, 2000;291–306.
69. Tumbarello C. Acute Extremity Compartment Syndrome. J Trauma Nurs 2000;7:30–36.
70. Dubuisson WC. Nursing Management of Adults with Musculoskeletal Trauma. In PG Beare, JL Myers (eds), Adult Health Nursing (3rd ed). St. Louis: Mosby, 1998;1228–1231.
71. Zimmer Traction Handbook: A Complete Reference Guide to the Basics of Traction. Zimmer, Inc., 1996.

# Appendix 3-A: Management and Physical Therapy Interventions for Fractures

*Michele P. West*

Note: This appendix was created as a guide for the physical therapist—these tables are not all-inclusive. Specific fracture classification systems are used only if they are universal or very commonly used; otherwise, fractures are listed by general type such as nondisplaced or displaced, closed or open, or stable or unstable. The authors encourage the therapist to consult other resources for specific fracture patterns or eponyms not described here. The weight-bearing status is provided as an estimate in the setting of a localized fracture; therefore, be sure to follow physician mandated orders for weight-bearing, ROM, and exercise, especially if there is a secondary fracture or associated soft tissue injury. Finally, it is inherent that patient/ family education is a part of each treatment session; thus it is not specifically listed in this appendix.

"Gentle ROM" as it appears in this appendix, is defined as active-assisted range of motion techniques that are within the patient's tolerance. Tolerance is determined in part by the subjective report of pain as well as objective limitations of muscle guarding and pattern of motion.

**Table 3-A.1.** Young Classification, Management, and Physical Therapy Intervention for Pelvic Ring Fractures

| Fracture Type | Management Options | Physical Therapy Intervention |
|---|---|---|
| APC, type I—disruption of the pubic symphysis with <2.5 cm of diastasis; no significant posterior pelvic injury | Symptomatic pain management | Functional mobility PWB or WBAT as tolerated Hip and distal joint A/AAROM |
| APC, type II—disruption of the pubic symphysis of >2.5 cm with tearing of the anterior sacroiliac, sacrospinous, and sacrotuberous ligaments | External fixation Anterior ORIF | Functional mobility NWB, TDWB, or PWB Hip and distal joint AA/AROM Lower-extremity exercise |
| APC, type III—complete disruption of the pubic symphysis and posterior ligament complexes, with hemipelvic displacement | External fixation Posterior percutaneous pinning Anterior and posterior ORIF | Functional mobility NWB or TDWB (usually limited to transfer out of bed only) on the least-involved side Distal lower-extremity A/AAROM |
| LC, type I—posterior compression of the SIJ without ligament disruption; oblique pubic ramus fracture | Symptomatic pain management | See APC, type I, above |
| LC, type II—rupture of the posterior sacroiliac ligament; pivotal internal rotation of the hemipelvis on the SIJ with a crush injury of the sacrum and an oblique pubic ramus fracture | External fixation Anterior and posterior ORIF | See APC, type III, above |

| | | |
|---|---|---|
| LC, type III—findings in type II with evidence of an APC injury to the contralateral pelvis | Anterior and posterior ORIF | See APC, type III, above |
| Vertical shear—complete ligament or bony disruption of a hemipelvis associated with hemipelvic displacement | Traction if not medically cleared for surgery<br>Percutaneous fixation (SIJ)<br>External fixation<br>Anterior and posterior ORIF | See APC, type III, above<br>Positioning, breathing exercise, and uninvolved extremity exercise if on bed rest |

A/AAROM = active/active-assistive range of motion; APC = anteroposterior compression; LC = lateral compression; PWB = partial weight bearing; NWB = non weight bearing; ORIF = open-reduction internal fixation; SIJ = sacroiliac joint; TDWB = touch-down weight bearing; WBAT = weight bearing as tolerated.

Sources: Adapted from HG Cryer, E Johnson. Pelvic Fractures. In DV Feliciano, EE Moore, KL Mattox (eds), Trauma (3rd ed). Stamford, CT: Appleton & Lange, 1996;640; and data from AR Burgess, AL Jones. Fractures of the Pelvic Ring. In CA Rockwood, DP Green, RW Bucholz, JD Heckman (eds), Rockwood and Green's Fractures in Adults (4th ed). Philadelphia: Lippincott–Raven, 1996.

Table 3-A.2. Management and Physical Therapy Intervention for Acetabular Fractures*

| Fracture Type | Management Options | Physical Therapy Intervention |
|---|---|---|
| Stable (displacement of <2–5 mm in the dome with an intact weight bearing surface) (e.g., distal anterior column, distal transverse, or both-column fracture without major posterior column displacement) | Traction with bed rest<br><br>Closed reduction | Functional mobility TDWB or PWB<br><br>Gentle ROM exercise<br><br>Positioning, breathing exercise, and uninvolved extremity exercise if on bed rest<br><br>Continuous passive motion at knee for indirect hip ROM |
| Unstable (any fracture with a nonintact weight-bearing dome) (e.g., large anterior, large posterior, superior transverse, or T-shaped fracture) | Percutaneous pinning<br><br>Open reduction internal fixation (may involve trochanteric osteotomy if posterior wall fracture)<br><br>Total hip arthroplasty | Functional mobility PWB or weight bearing as tolerated<br><br>Gentle hip ROM<br><br>Hip precautions per physician for total hip arthroplasty |

PWB = partial weight bearing; ROM = range of motion; TDWB = touch-down weight bearing.

*The patient may have hip dislocation precautions if the acetabular fracture is associated with hip dislocation.

Sources: Data from TG DiPasquale, RJ Nowinski. The Acute Care and Evaluation of Acetabular Fractures. In M Bosse, JF Kellam, TJ Fisher, P Tornetta (eds), Orthopaedic Knowledge Update: Trauma (2nd ed). Rosemont, IL: American Academy of Orthopaedic Surgeons, 2000; and M Tile. Fractures of the Acetabulum. In CA Rockwood, DP Green, RW Bucholz, JD Heckman (eds), Rockwood and Green's Fractures in Adults (4th ed). Philadelphia: Lippincott–Raven, 1996.

**Table 3-A.3.** Garden Classification, Management, and Physical Therapy
Intervention for Intracapsular Hip Fractures

| Fracture Type | Management Options | Physical Therapy Intervention |
|---|---|---|
| Garden I (impacted, incomplete fracture) | Closed reduction and percutaneous pinning<br>Closed reduction and spica cast[a] | Functional mobility PWB or NWB (spica)<br>A/AAROM exercises (limited by pain)<br>Lower-extremity strengthening |
| Garden II (complete fracture without displacement)[b] | Closed reduction, internal pin fixation<br>ORIF | Functional mobility PWB<br>A/AAROM exercises (limited by pain)<br>Lower-extremity strengthening |
| Garden III (complete fracture with partial displacement, capsule partially intact) | ORIF | See Garden II, above |
| Garden IV (complete fracture with full displacement and capsule disruption) | ORIF<br>Unipolar or bipolar arthroplasty | Functional mobility PWB or WBAT, A/AAROM exercises and strengthening, usually with posterior hip precautions |

A/AAROM = active/active-assisted range of motion; NWB = non weight bearing; ORIF
= open-reduction internal fixation; PWB = partial weight bearing, WBAT = weight bearing as tolerated.
[a]Rarely used secondary to risk of disimpaction of the fracture. Considered if the patient is agile and extremely compliant with NWB.
[b]Garden II is considered unstable despite nondisplacement because of a lack of bone impaction of the femoral head.
Source: Data from JL Guyton. Fractures of Hip, Acetabulum, and Pelvis. In ST Canale (ed), Campbell's Operative Orthopaedics, Vol. 3 (9th ed). St. Louis: Mosby, 1998.

**Table 3-A.4.** Evans and Russell-Taylor Classification, Management, and Physical Therapy Intervention for Intertrochanteric and Subtrochanteric Fractures

| Fracture Type | Management Options | Physical Therapy Intervention |
|---|---|---|
| Intertrochanteric, Evans type I (fracture line extends upward and outward from the lesser trochanter) | Closed reduction internal fixation (CRIF) ORIF | Functional mobility PWB Gentle hip ROM exercise Distal LE strengthening exercises |
| Intertrochanteric, Evans type II (fracture line extends down and outward from lesser trochanter) | ORIF ± osteotomy and bone grafting Bipolar arthroplasty | Functional mobility TDWB Gentle hip ROM exercise Distal LE strengthening exercise |
| Subtrochanteric, Russell-Taylor type IA (single fracture line extends from below lesser trochanter to the distal greater trochanter) | ORIF IM rod | See Intertrochanteric, Evans type I, above |
| Subtrochanteric, Russell-Taylor type IB (as in type IA with a second fracture line to the superior aspect of the lesser trochanter) | ORIF IM rod | See Intertrochanteric, Evans type I, above |
| Subtrochanteric, Russell-Taylor type IIA (single fracture line extends from below the lesser trochanter into the greater trochanter) | ORIF/DHS IM rod | See Intertrochanteric, Evans type I, above |
| Subtrochanteric, Russell-Taylor type IIB (as in type IIA, with a second fracture line to the superior aspect of the lesser trochanter) | ORIF/DHS Bone grafting | Functional mobility NWB or TDWB Gentle hip ROM exercise Distal LE strengthening exercise |

± = with or without; DHS = dynamic hip screw; IM = intramedullary; LE = lower extremity; NWB = non weight bearing; ORIF = open-reduction internal fixation; PWB = partial weight bearing; ROM = range of motion; TDWB, touch-down weight bearing.
Source: Data from JL Guyton. Fractures of Hip, Acetabulum, and Pelvis. In ST Canale (ed), Campbell's Operative Orthopaedics, Vol. 3 (9th ed). St. Louis: Mosby, 1998.

**Table 3-A.5.** Management and Physical Therapy Intervention for Femoral Shaft Fractures

| Fracture Type | Management Options | Physical Therapy Intervention |
|---|---|---|
| Closed; simple or non-displaced | IM rod<br>ORIF | Functional mobility NWB, TDWB, or WBAT<br>Gentle ROM exercise |
| Closed; comminuted, impacted, or both | Traction on bed rest<br>IM rod<br>ORIF | Functional mobility NWB or TDWB<br>Lower extremity ROM exercise per physician order<br>Positioning, breathing exercise, and uninvolved extremity exercise if on bed rest |
| Open; comminuted and displaced | Irrigation and debridement with immediate or delayed wound closure<br>Short-term skeletal traction on bed rest<br>External fixation<br>IM rod | See Closed; comminuted, impacted, or both, above |

IM = intramedullary; NWB = non weight bearing; ORIF = open-reduction internal fixation; ROM = range of motion; TDWB = touch-down weight bearing; WBAT = weight bearing as tolerated.
Source: Data from JL Guyton. Fractures of Hip, Acetabulum, and Pelvis. In ST Canale (ed), Campbell's Operative Orthopaedics, Vol. 3 (9th ed). St. Louis: Mosby, 1998.

**Table 3-A.6.** Management and Physical Therapy Intervention for Distal Femur Fractures

| Fracture Type | Management Options | Physical Therapy Intervention |
|---|---|---|
| Supracondylar; extra-articular, simple, nondisplaced | Long leg cast | Functional mobility NWB<br>Distal and proximal A/AAROM exercise |
| Supracondylar; extra-articular, displaced, or comminuted | Traction on bed rest<br>Closed reduction with percutaneous plate fixation<br>Intramedullary nail<br>ORIF<br>Knee immobilizer or hinged knee brace (stable fixation) or cast (less-stable fixation)<br>Continuous passive motion | Functional mobility light PWB<br>Distal and proximal A/AAROM exercise<br>Positioning, breathing exercise, and uninvolved extremity exercise if on bed rest |
| Unicondylar; intra-articular, nondisplaced | Long leg cast with close monitoring for loss of reduction | Functional mobility NWB or TDWB<br>Distal and proximal A/AAROM exercise |
| Unicondylar; intra-articular, displaced | Traction on bed rest<br>Closed-reduction and percutaneous fixation<br>ORIF<br>Long leg splint or cast | Functional mobility TDWB<br>Gentle ROM exercise<br>Continuous passive motion per physician order or type of immobilization device |

| Fracture Type | Management Options | Physical Therapy Intervention |
|---|---|---|
| Intercondylar; intra-articular | Long-term traction ORIF Cast brace if less-stable fixation achieved | Functional mobility TDWB or light PWB Delayed gentle ROM and quadriceps exercise Maintenance of functional ROM of hip and ankle |

A/AAROM = active/active-assisted range of motion; NWB = non weight bearing; ORIF = open-reduction internal fixation; PWB = partial weight bearing; ROM = range of motion; TDWB = touch-down weight bearing.
Source: Data from AP Whittle. Fractures of the Lower Extremity. In ST Canale (ed), Campbell's Operative Orthopaedics, Vol. 3 (3rd ed). St. Louis: Mosby, 1998.

**Table 3-A.7.** Management and Physical Therapy Intervention for Patellar Fractures

| Fracture Type | Management Options | Physical Therapy Intervention |
|---|---|---|
| Nondisplaced | Closed reduction Long leg cast (or other immobilization brace) with full knee extension | Functional mobility PWB or WBAT Avoid strong straight leg raise and strong quadriceps contraction because it can stress the fracture site |
| Displaced (simple vertical or transverse fracture) | ORIF with immobilization of the knee at full extension Continuous passive motion | See Nondisplaced, above AAROM (per physician) after few days of immobilization |
| Comminuted | ORIF (with fragment removal, if applicable) | Functional mobility NWB, PWB, or WBAT |

Table 3-A.7. *Continued*

| Fracture Type | Management Options | Physical Therapy Intervention |
|---|---|---|
| | Partial patellectomy (when one large fragment remains) or total patellectomy (if no large fragments remain) and quadriceps tendon repair | See Nondisplaced, above, in regard to quadriceps |
| | Immobilization with long leg cast, long leg brace, or posterior splint at full knee extension or slight flexion | |

AAROM = active-assisted range of motion; ORIF = open-reduction internal fixation; NWB = non weight bearing; PWB = partial weight bearing; WBAT = weight bearing as tolerated.
Source: Data from AP Whittle. Fractures of Lower Extremity. In ST Canale (ed.) Campbell's Operative Orthopaedics, Vol. 3 (9th ed). St. Louis: Mosby, 1998.

Table 3-A.8. Management and Physical Therapy Intervention for Tibial Plateau Fractures

| Fracture Type | Management Options | Physical Therapy Intervention |
|---|---|---|
| Nondisplaced | Closed reduction | Functional mobility |
| | Cast-brace immobilization or postoperative knee brace | TDWB or PWB |
| | | AAROM exercise, continuous passive motion to knee joint, or both |
| | Ligament repair (if applicable) | |

| Fracture Type | Management Options | Physical Therapy Intervention |
|---|---|---|
| Displaced; single condylar or split compression fracture | External fixation<br><br>ORIF<br><br>Cast-brace application or postoperative knee brace | Functional mobility NWB, TDWB, or PWB<br><br>AAROM exercise, continuous passive motion to knee joint, or both |
| Displaced; impacted, or severely comminuted bicondylar fracture | Skeletal traction and bed rest (≤1 wk) to allow for soft tissue healing<br><br>ORIF ± bone graft<br><br>Simultaneous ligament or meniscal repair, if applicable<br><br>Immobilization brace | Functional mobility NWB, TDWB, or PWB<br><br>Delayed knee A/AAROM<br><br>Positioning, breathing exercise, and uninvolved extremity exercise if on bed rest |

A/AAROM = active/active-assisted range of motion; AAROM = active-assisted range of motion; NWB = non weight bearing; ORIF = open-reduction internal fixation; PWB = partial weight bearing; TDWB = touch-down weight bearing.

Source: Data from AP Whittle. Fractures of Lower Extremity. In ST Canale (ed), Campbell's Operative Orthopaedics, Vol. 3 (9th ed). St. Louis: Mosby, 1998.

**Table 3-A.9.** Medical-Surgical Management and Physical Therapy Intervention for Tibial Shaft Fractures

| Fracture Type | Management Options | Physical Therapy Intervention |
|---|---|---|
| Closed; minimally displaced | Closed reduction<br>Long leg cast | Functional mobility TDWB, PWB, or WBAT<br>Quadriceps strengthening<br>Edema management |
| Closed; moderately displaced | Open-reduction internal fixation (ORIF)<br>Short leg cast | Functional mobility NWB, TDWB<br>Knee ROM exercise<br>Quadriceps strengthening<br>Edema management |
| Closed; severely displaced, comminuted, or both | External fixation<br>Temporary calcaneal traction to allow for soft tissue healing<br>ORIF | Functional mobility NWB<br>Ankle ± knee ROM exercises<br>Quadriceps strengthening<br>Edema management |
| Open | External fixation | See Closed; severely displaced, comminuted, or both, above |

± = with or without; NWB = non weight bearing; PWB = partial weight bearing; ROM = range of motion; TDWB = touch-down weight bearing; WBAT = weight bearing as tolerated.

**Table 3-A.10.** Medical-Surgical Management and Physical Therapy Intervention for Distal Tibial and Ankle Fractures

| Fracture Type | Medical-Surgical Options | Physical Therapy Intervention |
|---|---|---|
| Distal tibial; closed, minimally displaced | Closed reduction<br>Short leg cast | Functional mobility NWB<br>Knee ROM exercises<br>Proximal joint strengthening<br>Edema management |
| Distal tibial; closed, moderately displaced | ORIF<br>Short leg cast | See Distal tibial; closed, minimally displaced, above |

| Fracture Type | Medical-Surgical Options | Physical Therapy Intervention |
|---|---|---|
| Distal tibial; closed, severely displaced | Temporary calcaneal traction<br>External fixation<br>ORIF | Functional mobility NWB<br>Lower-extremity isometrics<br>Neutral ankle positioning<br>Proximal joint strengthening<br>Edema management |
| Distal tibial; open | External fixation | Functional mobility NWB<br>Ankle ROM exercise<br>Neutral ankle positioning<br>Proximal joint strengthening<br>Edema management |
| Ankle; closed, nondisplaced | Closed reduction<br>Short leg cast or walking cast | Functional mobility NWB or PWB<br>Edema management<br>Proximal lower-extremity strengthening exercise |
| Ankle; closed, displaced, multi-fracture, or both | Closed reduction<br>ORIF<br>Cast application or other immobilization method dependent on degree of edema | Functional mobility NWB<br>Edema management<br>Proximal lower-extremity strengthening exercise<br>Foot and ankle exercise as per physician and type of immobilization device |
| Ankle; open | Irrigation and debridement with immediate or delayed wound closure<br>Traction<br>External fixation<br>ORIF | See Ankle; closed, displaced, multifracture, or both, above |

NWB = non weight bearing; ORIF = open-reduction internal fixation; PWB = partial weight bearing; ROM = range of motion.
Source: Data from WB Geissler, AK Tsao, JL Hughes. Fractures and Injuries of the Ankle. In CA Rockwood, DP Green, RW Bucholz, JD Heckman (eds), Rockwood and Green's Fractures in Adults (4th ed). Philadelphia: Lippincott–Raven, 1996.

**Table 3-A.11.** Management and Physical Therapy Intervention for Calcaneal and Forefoot Fractures*

| Fracture Type | Management Options | Physical Therapy Intervention |
|---|---|---|
| Calcaneal; extra-articular, minimally displaced | Closed reduction<br>SLC | Functional mobility<br>NWB<br>Proximal lower-extremity strengthening and ROM exercise<br>Edema management<br>Ankle/forefoot exercise as per physician and type of immobilization device |
| Calcaneal; avulsion | Closed reduction<br>ORIF<br>SLC | See Calcaneal; extra-articular, minimally displaced, above |
| Calcaneal; intra-articular fracture involving the subtalar joint | Skeletal traction<br>Immediate or delayed SLC<br>Closed reduction and percutaneous pinning<br>ORIF<br>Arthrodesis if fracture is very severe | See Calcaneal; extra-articular, minimally displaced, above |
| Calcaneal; open | Irrigation and debridement with immediate or delayed wound closure<br>Skeletal traction<br>External fixation | See Calcaneal; extra-articular, minimally displaced, above |

| Fracture Type | Management Options | Physical Therapy Intervention |
|---|---|---|
| Forefoot; minimally displaced | Closed reduction<br>Percutaneous pinning<br>SLC or walking cast | Functional mobility NWB, PWB, or WBAT, dependent on exact location and severity of fracture<br>Proximal lower-extremity strengthening and ROM exercise<br>Edema management |
| Forefoot; moderate or severe displacement, with fragmentation or angulation | ORIF<br>Percutaneous pinning<br>SLC | See Forefoot; minimally displaced, above |
| Forefoot; open | See Calcaneal; open, above<br>ORIF | See Forefoot; minimally displaced, above |

NWB = non weight bearing; ORIF = open-reduction internal fixation; PWB = partial weight bearing; ROM = range of motion; SLC = short leg cast; WBAT = weight bearing as tolerated.
*For calcaneal fractures, cast application may not be in the neutral ankle position to protect the fracture site from strong ankle muscle contractions.
Source: Data from JD Heckman. Fractures and Dislocations of the Foot. In CA Rockwood, DP Green, RW Bucholz, JD Heckman (eds). Rockwood and Green's Fractures in Adults (4th ed). Philadelphia: Lippincott–Raven, 1996.

**Table 3-A.12.** Management and Physical Therapy Intervention for Common Cervical Spine Fractures

| Fracture Type | Management Options | Physical Therapy Intervention |
|---|---|---|
| Hangman's fracture, or bilateral pedicle fracture of axis (C1)<br><br>Type I—no angulation and <3 mm displacement of C2 on C3<br><br>Type II—>3 mm displacement of C2 on C3<br><br>Type IIA—minimal displacement and significant angulation of C2<br><br>Type III—full uni- or bilateral facet dislocation | Cervical collar immobilization for type I<br><br>Cervical traction/ reduction followed by halo vest for type II and IIA (cervical collar for type II possible)<br><br>Posterior open reduction and halo vest or C1-3 fusion for type III | Functional mobility with logroll precautions<br><br>Posture and body mechanics training<br><br>Therapeutic exercise and active–assisted/passive range of motion dependent on neurologic injury<br><br>Balance and scapular exercises for the patient in a halo vest |
| Odontoid process fracture<br><br>Type I—oblique avulsion fracture of the tip of the odontoid<br><br>Type II—fracture of the neck of the odontoid<br><br>Type III—fracture extending to the C2 vertebral body | Cervical collar immobilization for type I<br><br>Closed reduction or ORIF with halo vest, anterior or posterior C1-2 fusion ± bone grafting with cervical collar for type II<br><br>Closed reduction or open-reduction internal fixation with halo vest for type III | See Hangman's fracture, or bilateral pedicle fracture of axis (C1), above |

| Fracture Type | Management Options | Physical Therapy Intervention |
|---|---|---|
| Vertebral body (stable wedge) fracture—bony impaction and concavity of the vertebral body | Cervical collar | Functional mobility<br>Posture and body mechanics training |
| Spinous process (stable, isolated) or laminal fracture | Cervical collar | See Vertebral body (stable wedge) fracture, above |

± = with or without; ORIF = open-reduction internal fixation.
Sources: Data from RC Sasso, TM Reilly. Odontoid and Hangman's Fractures. Orthopaedic Knowledge Update: Trauma (2nd ed). Rosemont, IL: American Academy of Orthopaedic Surgeons, 2000; and RS Hockberger, KJ Kirshenbaum, PE Doris. Spinal Injuries. In P Rosen (ed), Emergency Medicine Concepts and Clinical Practice (4th ed). St. Louis: Mosby, 1998.

**Table 3-A.13.** Management and Physical Therapy for Common Thoracolumbar Spine Fractures

| Fracture Type | Management Options | Physical Therapy Intervention |
|---|---|---|
| Spinous process, transverse process, laminar, or facet fracture (stable, isolated) | Cervicothoracic or thoracolumbar orthosis | Functional mobility with logroll precautions<br>Posture and body mechanics training<br>Therapeutic exercise and active-assisted/passive range of motion dependent on neurologic injury |
| Vertebral body compression (impacted anterior wedge) fracture—stable | Short-term bed rest<br>Vertebroplasty<br>Thoracolumbar or thoracolumbosacral orthosis or hyperextension brace<br>Fusion (if severe) | See Spinous process, transverse process, laminar, or facet fracture (stable, isolated), above |

**Table 3-A.13.** *Continued*

| Fracture Type | Management Options | Physical Therapy Intervention |
|---|---|---|
| Vertebral body burst (axial compression) fracture—unstable | Short-term bed rest<br>Thoracolumbosacral orthosis<br>Anterior/posterior decompression and reconstruction ± bone grafting | See Spinous process, transverse process, laminar, or facet fracture (stable, isolated), above |
| Multidirectional fracture with disc involvement and facet dislocation—unstable | Anterior/posterior decompression and fusion<br>Thoracolumbosacral orthosis | See Spinous process, transverse process, laminar, or facet fracture (stable, isolated), above |

± = with or without.
Source: Data from AR Vaccaro, K Singh. Thoracolumbar Injuries: Nonsurgical Treatment. DC Kwok. Thoracolumbar Injuries: The Posterior Approach. In Orthopaedic Knowledge Update: Trauma (2nd ed). Rosemont, IL: American Academy of Orthopaedic Surgeons, 2000.

**Table 3-A.14.** Management and Physical Therapy Intervention of Proximal Humeral* and Humeral Shaft Fractures

| Fracture Type | Management Options | Physical Therapy Intervention |
|---|---|---|
| Proximal humeral; displaced, one-part | Closed reduction<br>Sling immobilization | Functional mobility NWB<br>Pendulum exercises and passive range of motion per physician<br>Elbow, wrist, and hand range-of-motion exercises<br>Edema management |

| Fracture Type | Management Options | Physical Therapy Intervention |
| --- | --- | --- |
| Proximal humeral; displaced, two-part | Closed reduction with percutaneous pinning<br>ORIF<br>Intramedullary rod<br>Sling immobilization | See Proximal humeral; displaced, one-part, above |
| Proximal humeral; displaced, three-part | ORIF<br>Hemiarthroplasty | See Proximal humeral; displaced, one-part, above<br>See section Physical Therapy Intervention after Shoulder Arthroplasty in Chapter 3 |
| Proximal humeral; displaced, four-part | Transcutaneous reduction with fluoroscopy<br>Percutaneous pinning<br>ORIF | See Proximal humeral; displaced, three-part, above |
| Comminution of humeral head | Hemiarthroplasty<br>Sling immobilization | See Proximal humeral; displaced, one-part, above |
| Humeral shaft; closed, minimal displacement | Closed reduction<br>Sling, hanging arm cast, or functional brace | Functional mobility NWB<br>Shoulder and elbow active/active-assisted range-of-motion exercise per physician and type of immobilization<br>Isometric scapulothoracic exercise<br>Wrist and hand exercise<br>Edema management |

**Table 3-A.14.** *Continued*

| Fracture Type | Management Options | Physical Therapy Intervention |
|---|---|---|
| Humeral shaft; closed, displaced with angulation | ORIF<br>Intramedullary nails<br>Long arm splint | See Humeral shaft; closed, minimal displacement, above |
| Humeral shaft; open | Irrigation and debridement with immediate or delayed wound closure<br>External fixation<br>ORIF | See Humeral shaft; closed, minimal displacement, above |

NWB = non weight bearing; ORIF = open-reduction internal fixation.
*Proximal humeral fractures according to the Neer classification.
Sources: Data from GR Williams, KL Wong. Two-Part and Three-Part Fractures: Open Reduction and Internal Fixation Versus Closed Reduction and Percutaneous Pinning. Orthop Clin North Am 2000;31:1–21; and JD Zuckman, KJ Koval. Fractures of the Shaft of the Humerus. In CA Rockwood, DP Green, RW Bucholz, JD Heckman (eds), Rockwood and Green's Fractures in Adults (4th ed). Philadelphia: Lippincott–Raven, 1996.

**Table 3-A.15.** Management and Physical Therapy Intervention for
Olecranon and Radial Head Fractures

| Fracture Type | Management Options | Physical Therapy Intervention |
|---|---|---|
| Olecranon; closed, nondisplaced | Long arm cast with elbow in midflexion | Functional mobility NWB |
| | | Initiation of elbow active-assisted range of motion in pain-free range per physician |
| | | Distal and proximal joint active range of motion |
| | | Edema management |
| Olecranon; closed, displaced | ORIF | See Olecranon; closed, nondisplaced, above |
| Olecranon; closed, comminuted | ORIF Immobilization | See Olecranon; closed, nondisplaced, above |
| Radial head; closed, non-, or minimally displaced | Closed reduction with early immobilization | See Olecranon; closed, nondisplaced, above |
| | Hematoma aspiration | |
| | Sling or short-term splint | |
| Radial head; closed, displaced | Closed reduction and short-term splinting if range of motion (ROM) adequate or ORIF if ROM inadequate | See Olecranon; closed, nondisplaced, above |
| | Partial or total radial head excision | |
| Radial head; closed, comminuted | ORIF with immobilization | See Olecranon; closed, nondisplaced, above |
| | Radial head excision ± radial head prosthesis, ± bone grafting | |

± = with or without; NWB = non weight bearing; ORIF = open-reduction internal fixation.
Source: Data from RN Hotchkiss. Fractures and Dislocations of the Elbow. In CA
Rockwood, DP Green, RW Bucholz, JD Heckman (eds), Rockwood and Green's Fractures in Adults (4th ed). Philadelphia: Lippincott–Raven, 1996.

**Table 3-A.16.** Management and Physical Therapy Intervention for
Forearm Fractures

| Fracture Type | Management Options | Physical Therapy Intervention |
|---|---|---|
| Shaft fracture of radius or ulna | Closed reduction with casting, or casting alone if nondisplaced<br><br>ORIF (if displaced) with functional brace | Functional mobility NWB<br><br>Distal and proximal range-of-motion exercises<br><br>Edema management |
| Distal radius; extra-articular | Closed reduction and percutaneous pinning<br><br>Sugar-tong splint or cast<br><br>ORIF ± functional brace | See Shaft fracture, above |
| Distal radius; intra-articular | ORIF<br><br>Closed reduction with external fixation ± percutaneous pinning<br><br>Arthroscopic controlled internal fixation | See Shaft fracture, above<br><br>Active and passive finger movement if patient has an external fixator |
| Distal radius; intra-articular, comminuted | Closed reduction with external fixation<br><br>ORIF<br><br>Bone grafting<br><br>Splint | See Distal radius; intra-articular, above |

± = with or without; NWB = non weight bearing; ORIF = open-reduction internal fixation.
Source: Adapted from DL Fernandez, AK Palmer. Fracture of the Distal Radius. In DP Green, RN Hotchkiss, WL Pederson (eds), Green's Operative Hand Surgery, Vol. 1 (4th ed). New York: Churchill Livingstone, 1998;950.

# 4

# Nervous System
*Michele P. West*

## Introduction

The nervous system is linked to every system of the body and is responsible for the integration and regulation of homeostasis. It is also involved in the action, communication, and higher cortical function of the body. A neurologic insult and its manifestations therefore have the potential to affect multiple body systems. To safely and effectively prevent or improve the neuromuscular, systemic, and functional sequelae of altered neurologic status in the acute care setting, the physical therapist requires an understanding of the neurologic system and the principles of neuropathology. The objectives of this chapter are to provide the following:

1.   A brief review of the structure and function of the nervous system

2.   An overview of neurologic evaluation, including the physical examination and diagnostic tests

3.   A description of common neurologic diseases and disorders, including clinical findings, medical and surgical management, and physical therapy interventions

## Structure and Function of the Nervous System

The nervous system is divided as follows:

1. The central nervous system (CNS), consisting of the brain and spinal cord

2. The peripheral (voluntary) nervous system, consisting of efferent and afferent somatic nerves outside the CNS

3. The autonomic (involuntary) nervous system, consisting of the sympathetic and parasympathetic systems

### Central Nervous System

#### Brain

The brain is anatomically divided into the cerebral hemispheres, diencephalon, brain stem, and cerebellum. A midsagittal view of the brain is shown in Figure 4-1A. Although each portion of the brain has its own function, it is linked to other portions via tracts and rarely works in isolation. When lesions occur, disruption of these functions can be predicted. Figure 4-1B shows the basal ganglia and the internal capsule. Tables 4-1 and 4-2 describe the basic structure, function, and dysfunction of the cerebral hemispheres, diencephalon, brain stem, and cerebellum.

*Protective Mechanisms*
The brain is protected by the cranium, meninges, ventricular system, and blood-brain barrier.

#### Cranium
The cranium encloses the brain. It is composed of eight cranial and 14 facial bones connected by sutures and contains approximately 85 foramen for the passage of the spinal cord, cranial nerves (CNs), and blood vessels.[1] The cranium is divided into the cranial vault, or calvaria (the superolateral and posterior aspects), and the cranial floor, which is composed of fossae (the anterior fossa supports the frontal lobes; the middle fossa supports the temporal lobes; and the posterior fossa supports the cerebellum, pons, and medulla).[2]

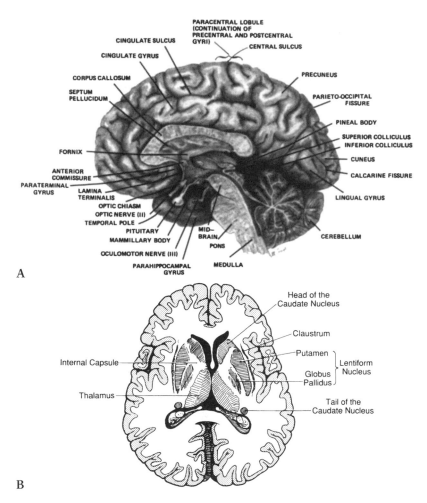

**Figure 4-1. A.** *Medial (midsagittal) view of a hemisected brain. (With permission from S Gilman, SW Newman [eds]. Manter and Gatz's Essentials of Neuroanatomy and Neurophysiology [7th ed]. New York: Oxford University Press, 1987;9.)* **B.** *Horizontal section of the cerebrum showing the basal ganglia. (With permission from RJ Love, WG Webb [eds]. Neurology for the Speech-Language Pathologist [4th ed]. Boston: Butterworth–Heinemann, 2001;38.)*

**Table 4-1.** Structure, Function, and Dysfunction of the Cerebral Hemispheres

| Lobe of Cerebrum | Structure | Function | Dysfunction |
|---|---|---|---|
| Frontal lobe | Precentral gyrus | Voluntary motor cortex of contralateral face, arm, trunk, and leg | Contralateral mono- or hemiparesis or hemiplegia |
| | Supplementary motor area | Advanced motor planning Contralateral head and eye turning (connections to cranial nerves III, IV, VI, IX, X, and XII nuclei) | Contralateral head and eye paralysis |
| | Prefrontal pole | Personality center, including abstract ideas, concern for others, conscience, initiative, judgment, persistence, and planning | Loss of inhibition and demonstration of antisocial behaviors Ataxia, primitive reflexes, and hypertonicity |
| | Paracentral lobule | Bladder and bowel inhibition | Urinary and bowel incontinence |
| | Broca's area | D: Motor speech center ND: Appreciation of intonation and gestures with vocalization | Broca's (expressive) aphasia |
| Parietal lobe | Postcentral gyrus | Somatosensory cortex of contralateral pain, posture, proprioception, and touch of arm, trunk, and leg | Contralateral sensation loss |
| | Parietal pole | D: Ability to perform calculations | D: Acalculia, agraphia, finger agnosia |

| | | | |
|---|---|---|---|
| Temporal lobe | Wernicke's area | ND: Ability to construct shapes, awareness of external environment, and body image<br>D: Sensory speech (auditory and written) comprehension center<br>ND: Appreciation of content of emotional language (e.g., tone of voice) | ND: Constructional apraxia, geographic agnosia, dressing apraxia, anosognosia<br>Wernicke's (receptive) aphasia |
| | Optic radiation | Visual tract | Lower homonymous quadrantanopia |
| | Gustatory cortex | Perception of taste | Dysfunction is very uncommon |
| | Superior temporal gyrus (auditory cortex) | D: Appreciation of language<br>ND: Appreciation of music, rhythm, and sound | D: Decreased ability to hear<br>ND: Decreased ability to appreciate music |
| | Middle and inferior temporal gyri | Learning and memory centers | Learning and memory deficits |
| | Limbic lobe and olfactory cortex | Affective and emotion center, including mood, primitive behavior, self-preservation, short-term memory, visceral emotion processes, and interpretation of smell | Aggressive or antisocial behaviors<br>Inability to establish new memories |
| | Wernicke's area | See Parietal lobe, above | Wernicke's (receptive) aphasia |

**Table 4-1.** *Continued*

| Lobe of Cerebrum | Structure | Function | Dysfunction |
|---|---|---|---|
| | Optic radiation | Visual tract | Upper homonymous quadrantanopia |
| Occipital lobe | Striate and parastriate cortices | Perception of vision (visual cortex) | Homonymous hemianopsia with or without macular involvement |

D = dominant, ND = nondominant.

Sources: Data from KW Lindsay, I Bone, R Callander (eds). Neurology and Neurosurgery Illustrated (2nd ed). Edinburgh, UK: Churchill Livingstone, 1991; S Gilman, SW Newman (eds). Manter and Gatz's Essentials of Clinical Neuroanatomy and Neurophysiology (7th ed). Philadelphia: FA Davis, 1989; JA Kiernan (ed). Introduction to Human Neuroscience. Philadelphia: Lippincott, 1987; EN Marieb (ed). Human Anatomy and Physiology (5th ed). San Francisco: Benjamin-Cummings, 2001; and L Thelan, J Davie, M Lough (eds). Critical Care Nursing: Diagnosis and Management (2nd ed). St. Louis: Mosby, 1994.

**Table 4-2.** Structure, Function, and Dysfunction of the Diencephalon, Brain Stem, and Cerebellum

| Brain Structure | Substructure | Function | Dysfunction |
|---|---|---|---|
| **Diencephalon** | | | |
| Thalamus | Specific and association nuclei | Cortical arousal | Altered consciousness |
| | | Integrative relay station for all ascending and descending motor stimuli and all ascending sensory stimuli except smell | Signs and symptoms of increased ICP |
| | | | Contralateral hemiplegia, hemiparesis, or hemianesthesia |
| | | Memory | Altered eye movement |
| Hypothalamus | Mamillary bodies | Autonomic center for sympathetic and parasympathetic responses | Altered autonomic function and vital signs |
| | Optic chiasm | | Headache |
| | Infundibulum (stalk) connects to the pituitary gland | Visceral center for regulation of body temperature, food intake, thirst, sleep and wake cycle, water balance | Visual deficits |
| | Forms inferolateral wall of third ventricle | Produces ADH and oxytocin | Vomiting with signs and symptoms of increased ICP |
| | | Regulates anterior pituitary gland | See Chapter 11 for more information on hormones and endocrine disorders |
| | | Association with limbic system | |

**Table 4-2.** *Continued*

| Brain Structure | Substructure | Function | Dysfunction |
|---|---|---|---|
| Epithalamus | Pineal body<br>Posterior commissure, striae medullares, habenular nuclei and commissure | Association with limbic system | Dysfunction unknown |
| Subthalamus | Substantia nigra<br>Red nuclei | Association with thalamus for motor control | Dyskinesia and decreased motor control |
| Pituitary | Anterior and posterior lobes | Production, storage, and secretion of reproductive hormones<br>Secretion of ADH and oxytocin | See Chapter 11 for more information on hormones and endocrine disorders |
| Internal capsule | Fiber tracts connecting thalamus to the cortex | Conduction pathway between the cortex and spinal cord | Contralateral hemiparesis or hemiplegia and hemianesthesia |
| Brain stem<br>Midbrain | Superior cerebellar peduncles<br>Superior and inferior colliculi<br>Medial and lateral lemniscus<br>CNs III and IV nuclei<br>Reticular formation<br>Cerebral aqueduct in its center | Conduction pathway between higher and lower brain centers<br>Visual reflex<br>Auditory reflex | Contralateral hemiparesis or hemiplegia and hemianesthesia, altered consciousness and respiratory pattern, cranial nerve palsy |

| | | | |
|---|---|---|---|
| Pons | Middle cerebellar peduncles<br>Respiratory center<br>CNs V–VIII nuclei<br>Forms anterior wall of fourth ventricle | Conduction pathway between higher and lower brain centers | See Midbrain, above |
| Medulla | Decussation of pyramidal tracts<br>Inferior cerebellar peduncles<br>Inferior olivary nuclei<br>Nucleus cuneatus and gracilis<br>CNs IX–XII nuclei | Homeostatic center for cardiac, respiratory, vasomotor functions | See Midbrain, above |
| Cerebellum<br>Anterior lobe | Medial portion<br>Lateral portion | Sensory and motor input of trunk<br>Sensory and motor input of extremities for coordination of gait | Ipsilateral ataxia and discoordination or tremor of extremities |
| Posterior lobe | Medial and lateral portions | Sensory and motor input for coordination of motor skills and postural tone | Ipsilateral ataxia and discoordination of the trunk |

**Table 4-2.** *Continued*

| Brain Structure | Substructure | Function | Dysfunction |
|---|---|---|---|
| Flocculonodular | Flocculus nodule | Sensory input from ears | Ipsilateral facial sensory loss and Horner's syndrome, nystagmus, visual overshooting |
| | | Sensory and motor input from eyes and head for coordination of balance and eye and head movement | Loss of balance |

ADH = antidiuretic hormone; CN = cranial nerve; ICP = intracranial pressure.

Sources: Data from KW Lindsay, I Bone, R Callander (eds). Neurology and Neurosurgery Illustrated (2nd ed). Edinburgh, UK: Churchill Livingstone, 1991; S Gilman, SW Newman (eds). Manter and Gatz's Essentials of Clinical Neuroanatomy and Neurophysiology (7th ed). Philadelphia: FA Davis, 1989; JA Kiernan (ed). Introduction to Human Neuroscience. Philadelphia: Lippincott, 1987; EN Marieb (ed). Human Anatomy and Physiology (5th ed). San Francisco: Benjamin-Cummings, 2001; and L Thelan, J Davie, M Lough (eds). Critical Care Nursing: Diagnosis and Management (2nd ed). St. Louis: Mosby, 1994.

## Meninges

The meninges are three layers of connective tissue that cover the brain and spinal cord. The dura mater, the outermost layer, lines the skull (periosteum) and has four major folds (Table 4-3). The arachnoid, the middle layer, loosely encloses the brain. The pia mater, the inner layer, covers the convolutions of the brain and forms a portion of the choroid plexus in the ventricular system. The three layers create very important anatomic and potential spaces in the brain, as shown in Figure 4-2 and described in Table 4-4.

## Ventricular System

The ventricular system nourishes the brain and acts as a cushion by increasing the buoyancy of the brain. It consists of four ventricles and a series of foramen, through which cerebrospinal fluid (CSF) passes to surround the CNS. CSF is a colorless, odorless solution produced by the choroid plexus of all ventricles. CSF circulates in a pulse-like fashion through the ventricles and around the spinal cord with the beating of ependymal cilia that line the ventricles and intracranial blood volume changes that occur with breathing and cardiac systole.[3] The flow of CSF under normal conditions, as shown in Figure 4-3, is as follows[4]:

**Table 4-3.**  Dural Folds

| | |
|---|---|
| Falx cerebri | Vertical fold that separates the two cerebral hemispheres to prevent horizontal displacement of these structures |
| Falx cerebelli | Vertical fold that separates the two cerebellar hemispheres to prevent horizontal displacement of these structures |
| Tentorium cerebelli | Horizontal fold that separates occipital lobes from the cerebellum to prevent vertical displacement of these structures |
| Diaphragm sellae | Horizontal fold that separates that subarachnoid space from the sella turcica and is perforated by the stalk of the pituitary gland |

Source: Data from JL Wilkinson (ed). Neuroanatomy for Medical Students (3rd ed). Oxford, UK: Butterworth–Heinemann, 1998.

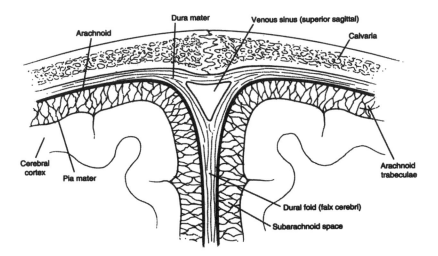

Figure 4-2. *Coronal section of cranial meninges showing a venous sinus and dural fold. (With permission from PA Young, PH Young. Basic Clinical Neuroanatomy. Philadelphia: Williams & Wilkins, 1997;8.)*

- From the lateral ventricles via the interventricular foramen to the third ventricle

- From the third ventricle to the fourth ventricle via the cerebral aqueduct

- From the fourth ventricle to the cisterns, subarachnoid space, and spinal cord via the median and lateral apertures

Table 4-4. Dural Spaces

| | |
|---|---|
| Epidural (extradural) space | Potential space between the skull and outer dura mater. |
| Subdural space | Potential space between the dura and the arachnoid mater; a split in the dura contains the venous sinus. |
| Subarachnoid space | Anatomic space between the arachnoid and pia mater containing cerebrospinal fluid and the vascular supply of the cortex. |

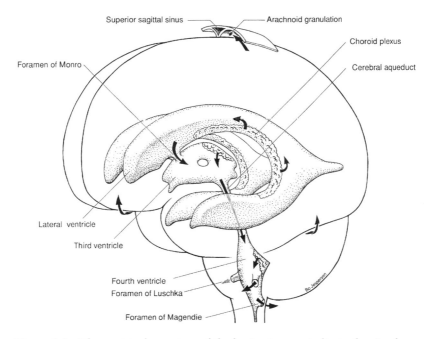

**Figure 4-3.** *The ventricular system of the brain. Arrows indicate the circulation of cerebrospinal fluid from the site of formation in the choroid plexus to the site of absorption in the villi of the sagittal sinus. (With permission from J Bogousslavsky, M Fisher [eds]. Textbook of Neurology. Boston: Butterworth–Heinemann, 1998;656.)*

When ventricular pressure is greater than venous pressure, CSF is absorbed into the venous system via the arachnoid villi, capillary walls of the pia mater, and lymphatics of the subarachnoid space near the optic nerve.[2]

### Blood-Brain Barrier

The blood-brain barrier is the physiologic mechanism responsible for keeping toxins, such as amino acids, hormones, ions, and urea, from altering neuronal firing of the brain. It readily allows water, oxygen, carbon dioxide, glucose, some amino acids, and substances that are highly soluble in fat (e.g., alcohol, nicotine, and anesthetic agents) to pass across the barrier.[5,6] The barrier consists of fused endothelial cells on a basement membrane that is surrounded by astrocytic foot extensions.[6] Substances must therefore pass through, rather than

around, these cells. The blood-brain barrier is absent near the hypothalamus, pineal region, anterior third ventricle, and floor of the
fourth ventricle.[3]

### Central Brain Systems

The central brain systems are the reticular activating system and the
limbic system. The reticular activating system is responsible for
human consciousness level and integrates the functions of the brain
stem with cortical, cerebellar, thalamic, hypothalamic, and sensory
receptor functions.[5]

The limbic system is a complex interactive system, with primary
connections between the cortex, hypothalamus, and sensory receptors.[5] The limbic system is the emotional system, mediating cortical
autonomic function of internal and external stimuli.

### Circulation

The brain receives blood from the internal carotid and vertebral arteries, which are linked together by the circle of Willis, as shown in Figure 4-4. Each vessel supplies blood to a certain part of the brain
(Table 4-5). The circulation of the brain is discussed in terms of a sin-

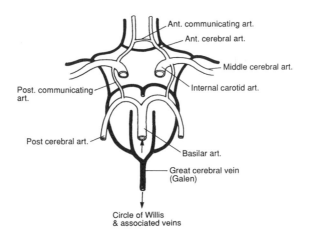

**Figure 4-4.** *Schematic representation of the arterial circle of Willis and
accompanying veins. (Ant. = anterior; art. = artery; Post. = posterior.) (With
permission from EG Gonzalez, SJ Meyers [eds]. Downey and Darling's Physiological Basis of Rehabilitation Medicine [3rd ed]. Boston: Butterworth–
Heinemann, 2001;22.)*

**Table 4-5.** Blood Supply of the Major Areas of the Brain

| Artery | Area of Perfusion |
| --- | --- |
| Anterior circulation | |
| Internal carotid artery (ICA) | The dura, optic tract, basal ganglia, midbrain, uncus, lateral geniculate body, and tympanic cavity. Ophthalmic branch supplies the eyes and orbits. |
| External carotid artery (ECA) | All structures external to the skull, the larynx, and the thyroid. |
| Anterior cerebral artery (ACA) | Medial and superior surface of frontal and parietal lobes. Medial striate branch supplies anterior portion of the internal capsule, optic chiasm and nerve, portions of the hypothalamus, and basal ganglia. |
| Middle cerebral artery (MCA) | Lateral surface of the frontal, parietal, and occipital lobes, including the superior and lateral surfaces of temporal lobes. |
| Posterior circulation | |
| Vertebral artery | Medulla, dura of the posterior fossa, including the falx cerebri and tentorium cerebelli. |
| Basilar artery | Pons and midbrain. |
| Posterior inferior cerebellar artery (PICA) | Posterior and inferior surface of cerebellum. |
| Anterior inferior cerebellar artery (AICA) | Anterior surface of the cerebellum, flocculus, and inferior vermis. |
| Superior cerebellar artery (SCA) | Superior surface of cerebellum and vermis. |
| Posterior cerebellar artery (PCA) | Occipital lobe and medial and lateral surfaces of the temporal lobes, thalamus, lateral geniculate bodies, hippocampus, and choroid plexus of the third and lateral ventricles. |

Sources: Data from CL Rumbaugh, A Wang, FY Tsai (eds). Cerebrovascular Disease Imaging and Interventional Treatment Options. New York: Igaku-Shoin Medical Publishers, 1995; and KL Moore (ed). Clinically Oriented Anatomy (2nd ed). Baltimore: Williams & Wilkins, 1985.

gle vessel or by region (usually as the anterior or posterior circulation). There are several anastomotic systems of the cerebral vasculature that provide essential blood flow to the brain. Blood is drained from the brain through a series of venous sinuses. The superior sagittal sinus, with its associated lacunae and villi, is the primary drainage site. The superior sagittal sinus and sinuses located in the dura and scalp then drain blood into the internal jugular vein for return to the heart.

### Spinal Cord

The spinal cord lies within the spinal column and extends from the foramen magnum to the first lumbar vertebra, where it forms the conus medullaris and the cauda equina and attaches to the coccyx via the filum terminale. Divided into the cervical, thoracic, and lumbar portions, it is protected by mechanisms similar to those supporting the brain. The spinal cord is composed of gray and white matter and provides the pathway for the ascending and descending tracts, as shown in cross section in Figure 4-5 and outlined in Table 4-6.

### Peripheral Nervous System

The peripheral nervous system consists of the cranial and spinal nerves and the reflex system. The primary structures include peripheral nerves, associated ganglia, and sensory receptors. There are 12 pairs of CNs, each with a unique pathway and function (sensory, motor, mixed, or autonomic). Thirty-one pairs of spinal nerves (all mixed) exit the spinal cord to form distinct plexuses (except T2 through T12). The peripheral nerves of the upper and lower extremities and thorax are listed in Tables 4-7 through 4-9, and the dermatomal system is shown in Figure 4-6. The reflex system includes spinal, deep tendon, stretch, and superficial reflexes and protective responses.

### Autonomic Nervous System

The portion of the peripheral nervous system that innervates glands and cardiac and smooth muscle is the autonomic nervous system. The parasympathetic division is activated in time of rest, whereas the sympathetic division is activated in times of work or "fight or flight" situations. The two divisions work closely together, with dual innervation of most organs, to ensure homeostasis.

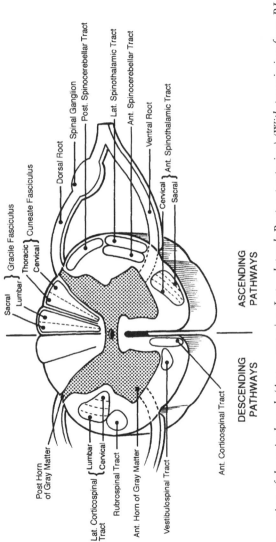

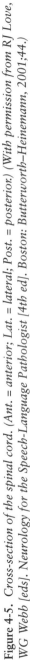

**Figure 4-5.** *Cross-section of the spinal cord. (Ant. = anterior; Lat. = lateral; Post. = posterior.) (With permission from RJ Love, WG Webb [eds]. Neurology for the Speech-Language Pathologist [4th ed]. Boston: Butterworth–Heinemann, 2001;44.)*

**Table 4-6.** Major Ascending and Descending White Matter Tracts*

| Tract | Function |
| --- | --- |
| Fasciculus gracilis | Sensory pathway for lower-extremity and lower-trunk joint proprioception, vibration, two-point discrimination, graphesthesia, and double simultaneous stimulation |
| Fasciculus cuneatus | Sensory pathway for upper-extremity, upper-trunk, and neck joint proprioception, vibration, two-point discrimination, graphesthesia, and double simultaneous stimulation |
| Lateral spinothalamic | Sensory pathway for pain, temperature, and light touch |
| Ventral spinocerebellar | Sensory pathway for ipsilateral subconscious proprioception |
| Dorsal spinocerebellar | Sensory pathway for ipsilateral and contralateral subconscious proprioception |
| Lateral corticospinal (pyramidal) | Motor pathway for contralateral voluntary fine muscle movement |
| Anterior corticospinal (pyramidal) | Motor pathway for ipsilateral voluntary movement |
| Rubrospinal (extra-pyramidal) | Motor pathway for gross postural tone |
| Tectospinal (extra-pyramidal) | Motor pathway for contralateral gross postural muscle tone associated with auditory and visual stimuli |
| Vestibulospinal (extra-pyramidal) | Motor pathway for ipsilateral gross postural adjustments associated with head movements |

*Sensory tracts ascend from the spinal cord; motor tracts descend from the brain to the spinal cord.
Sources: Data from S Gilman, SW Newman (eds). Manter and Gatz's Essentials of Clinical Neuroanatomy and Neurophysiology (7th ed). Philadelphia: FA Davis, 1989; and EN Marieb (ed). Human Anatomy and Physiology (5th ed). San Francisco: Benjamin-Cummings, 2001.

**Table 4-7.** Major Peripheral Nerves of the Upper Extremity

| Nerve | Spinal Root | Innervation |
|---|---|---|
| Dorsal scapular | C5 | Levator scapulae, rhomboid major and minor |
| Suprascapular | C5 and C6 | Supraspinatus, infraspinatus |
| Lower subscapular | C5 and C6 | Teres major |
| Axillary | C5 and C6 | Teres minor, deltoid |
| Radial | C5, C6, C7, and C8 | Triceps, brachioradialis, anconeus, extensor carpi radialis longus and brevis, supinator, extensor carpi ulnaris, extensor digitorum, extensor digiti minimi, extensor indicis, extensor pollicis longus and brevis, abductor pollicis brevis |
| Ulnar | C8 and T1 | Flexor digitorum profundus, flexor carpi ulnaris, palmaris brevis, abductor digiti minimi, flexor digiti minimi brevis, opponens digiti minimi, palmar and dorsal interossei, third and fourth lumbricals |
| Median | C6, C7, C8, and T1 | Pronator teres, flexor carpi radialis, palmaris longus, flexor digitorum superficialis and profundus, flexor pollicis longus, pronator quadratus, abductor pollicis brevis, opponens pollicis, flexor pollicis brevis, first and second lumbricals |
| Musculo-cutaneous | C5, C6, and C7 | Coracobrachialis, brachialis, biceps |

Source: Data from FH Netter (ed). Atlas of Human Anatomy. Summit City, NJ: CIBA-GEIGY Corporation, 1989.

# Neurologic Examination

The neurologic examination is initiated on hospital admission or in the field and is reassessed continuously, hourly or daily, as necessary. The neurologic examination consists of patient history; mental status examination; vital sign measurement; vision, motor, sensory, and coordination testing; and diagnostic testing.

**Table 4-8.** Major Peripheral Nerves of the Lower Extremity

| Nerve | Spinal Root | Innervation |
|---|---|---|
| Femoral | L2, L3, and L4 | Iliacus<br>Psoas major<br>Sartorius<br>Pectinous<br>Rectus femoris<br>Vastus lateralis, intermedius, and medialis<br>Articularis genu |
| Obturator | L2, L3, and L4 | Obturator externus<br>Adductor brevis, longus, and magnus<br>Gracilis |
| Sciatic | L4, L5, S1, S2, and S3 | Biceps femoris<br>Adductor magnus<br>Semitendinosus<br>Semimembranosus |
| Tibial | L4, L5, S1, S2, and S3 | Gastrocnemius<br>Soleus<br>Flexor digitorum longus<br>Tibialis posterior<br>Flexor hallucis longus |
| Common peroneal | L4, L5, S1, and S2 | Peroneus longus and brevis<br>Tibialis anterior<br>Extensor digitorum longus<br>Extensor hallucis longus<br>Extensor hallucis brevis<br>Extensor digitorum brevis |

Source: Data from FH Netter (ed). Atlas of Human Anatomy. Summit City, NJ: CIBA-GEIGY Corporation, 1989.

*Patient History*

A detailed history, initially taken by the physician, is often the most helpful information used to delineate whether a patient presents with a true neurologic event or another process (usually cardiac or metabolic in nature). The history may be presented by the patient or, more commonly, by a family member or person witnessing the acute or progressive event(s) responsible for hospital admission. One common

Table 4-9. Major Peripheral Nerves of the Trunk

| Nerve | Spinal Root | Innervation |
|---|---|---|
| Spinal accessory | C3 and C4 | Trapezius |
| Phrenic | C3, C4, and C5 | Diaphragm |
| Long thoracic | C5, C6, and C7 | Serratus anterior |
| Medial pectoral | C6, C7, and C8 | Pectoralis minor and major |
| Lateral pectoral | C7, C8, and T1 | Pectoralis major |
| Thoracodorsal | C7 and C8 | Latissimus dorsi |
| Intercostal | Corresponds to nerve root level | External intercostals Internal intercostals Levatores costarum longi and brevis |
| Iliohypogastric and ilioinguinal | L1 | Transversus abdominus Internal abdominal oblique |
| Inferior gluteal | L4, L5, S1, and S2 | Gluteus maximus |
| Superior gluteal | L4, L5, and S1 | Gluteus medius and minimus Tensor fascia latae |

Source: Data from FH Netter (ed). Atlas of Human Anatomy. Summit City, NJ: CIBA-GEIGY Corporation, 1989.

framework for organizing questions regarding *each* neurologic complaint, sign, or symptom is presented here[7,8]:

- What is the patient feeling?
- When did the problem initially occur and has it progressed?
- What relieves or exacerbates the problem?
- What is the onset, frequency, and duration of signs or symptoms?

In addition to the general medical record review (see Appendix I-A), questions relevant to a complete neurologic history include the following:

- Does the problem involve loss of consciousness?
- Did a fall precede or follow the problem?

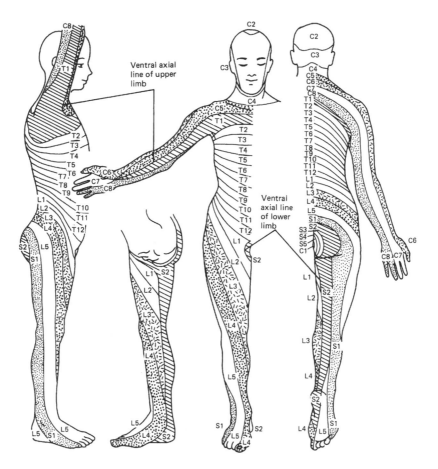

**Figure 4-6.** *Dermatome chart based on embryologic segments. (With permission from GD Maitland [ed]. Vertebral Manipulation [5th ed]. Oxford, UK: Butterworth–Heinemann, 1986;46.)*

- Is there headache, dizziness, or visual disturbance?
- What are the functional deficits associated with the problem?
- Is there an alteration of speech?
- Does the patient demonstrate memory loss or altered cognition?

- Does the patient have an altered sleep pattern?

- What is the handedness of the patient? (Handedness is a predictor of brain [language] dominance.)

*Observation*

Data that can be gathered from close or distant observation of the patient include the following:

- Level of alertness, arousal, distress, or the need for restraint

- Body position

- Head, trunk, and extremity posture, including movement patterns

- Amount and quality of active movement

- Amount and quality of interaction with the environment or family members

- Degree of ease or difficulty with activities of daily living

- Presence of involuntary movements, such as tremor

- Eye movement(s)

- Presence of hemibody or hemispace neglect

- Presence of muscle atrophy

- Respiratory rate and pattern

---

Clinical Tip

The therapist should correlate these observations with other information from the chart review and other health care team members to determine (1) if the diagnosis is consistent with the physical presentation, (2) what types of commands or tone of voice to use, (3) how much assistance is needed, and (4) how to prioritize the portions of the physical therapy evaluation.

---

## Mental Status Examination

The mental status examination includes assessment of level of consciousness, cognition, emotional state, and speech and language ability.

### Level of Consciousness

*Consciousness* consists of arousal and the awareness of self and environment, including the ability to interact appropriately in response to any normal stimulus.[9] Coma is often considered the opposite of consciousness. Table 4-10 describes the different states of consciousness. Evaluating a patient's level of consciousness is important because it serves as a baseline to monitor stability,

**Table 4-10.** Normal and Abnormal States of Consciousness

| | |
|---|---|
| Alert | Completely awake. |
| | Aware of all stimuli. |
| | Able to interact meaningfully with clinician. |
| Lethargic or somnolent | Arousal with stimuli. |
| | Falls to sleep when not stimulated. |
| | Decreased awareness. |
| | Loss of train of thought. |
| Obtundent | Difficult to arouse. |
| | Requires constant stimulation for all activities. |
| | Confused. |
| Stuporous | Arousal only with vigorous stimulation. |
| | Unable to complete mental status examination because responses are usually incomprehensible words. |
| Coma | Unarousable. |
| | Nonverbal. |
| Delirium | State of disorientation marked by irritability or agitation, suspicion and fear, and misperception of stimuli. |
| | Patient demonstrates offensive, loud, and talkative behaviors. |
| Dementia | Alteration in mental processes secondary to organic disease that is not accompanied by a change in arousal. |

Sources: Data from RL Strub, FW Black (eds). Mental Status Examination in Neurology (2nd ed). Philadelphia: FA Davis, 1985; and F Plum, J Posner (eds). The Diagnosis of Stupor and Coma (3rd ed). Philadelphia: FA Davis, 1980.

improvement, or decline in the patient's condition. It also helps determine the severity and prognosis of neurologic insult or disease state, thus directing the medical plan of care.

---

### Clinical Tip

- Level of consciousness is often vaguely described in medical charts; therefore, be specific when documenting a patient's mental status. Describe the intensity of stimulus needed to arouse the patient, the patient's best response, and the patient's response to the removal of the stimulus.[9]
- Changes in body position, especially the transition from a recumbent position to sitting upright, often stimulate increased alertness. Other stimuli to increase alertness include daylight, radio or television sound, or a cold cloth on the forehead.
- Use a progressive intensity of stimuli to arouse a patient with decreased alertness or level of consciousness. For example, call the patient's name in a normal tone of voice before using a loud tone of voice, or tap the patient's shoulder before rubbing the shoulder.
- Time of day, fatigue, and side effects of medication are factors that can cause variable levels of alertness or participation in physical therapy. The documentation of these factors is important for communication among the health care team and for the rehabilitation screening process.
- A & O × 3 is a common abbreviation for *a*lert and *o*riented to person, place, and time. The number may be modified to reflect the patient's orientation (e.g., A & O × 1 [self]).

---

### Glasgow Coma Scale

The Glasgow Coma Scale (GCS) is a widely accepted measure of level of consciousness and responsiveness and is described in Table 4-11. The GCS evaluates best eye opening (E), motor response (M), and verbal response (V). To determine a patient's overall GCS, add each

Table 4-11.   The Glasgow Coma Scale

| Response | Score |
|---|---|
| Eye opening (E) | |
| Spontaneous: eyes open without stimulation | 4 |
| To speech: eyes open to voice | 3 |
| To pain: eyes open to noxious stimulus | 2 |
| Nil: eyes do not open despite variety of stimuli | 1 |
| Motor response (M) | |
| Obeys: follows commands | 6 |
| Localizes: purposeful attempts to move limb to stimulus | 5 |
| Withdraws: flexor withdrawal without localizing | 4 |
| Abnormal flexion: decorticate posturing to stimulus | 3 |
| Extensor response: decerebrate posturing to stimulus | 2 |
| Nil: no motor movement | 1 |
| Verbal response (V) | |
| Oriented: normal conversation | 5 |
| Confused conversation: vocalizes in sentences, incorrect context | 4 |
| Inappropriate words: vocalizes with comprehensible words | 3 |
| Incomprehensible words: vocalizes with sounds | 2 |
| Nil: no vocalization | 1 |

Source: Data from B Jennett, G Teasdale (eds). Management of Head Injuries. Philadelphia: FA Davis, 1981.

score (i.e., E + M + V). Scores range from 3 to 15. A score of 8 or less signifies coma.[10]

---

### Clinical Tip

Calculation of the GCS usually occurs at regular intervals. The GCS should be used to confirm the type and amount of cueing needed to communicate with a patient, determine what time of day a patient is most capable of participating in physical therapy, and delineate physical therapy goals.

---

## Cognition

Cognitive testing includes the assessment of attention, orientation, memory, abstract thought, and the ability to perform calculations or construct figures. General intelligence and vocabulary are estimated with questions regarding history, geography, or current events. Table 4-12 lists typical methods of testing the components of cognition.

**Table 4-12.** Tests of Cognitive Function

| Cognitive Function | Definition | Task |
|---|---|---|
| Attention | Ability to attend to a specific stimulus or task | Repetition of a series of numbers or letters |
| | | Spelling words forward and backward |
| Orientation | Ability to orient to person, place, and time | Identify name, age, current date and season, birth date, present location, town, etc. |
| Memory | Immediate recall | Recount three words after a few seconds |
| | Short-term memory | Recount words (after a few minutes) or recent events |
| | Long-term memory | Recount past events |
| Calculation | Ability to perform verbal or written mathematical problems | Add, subtract, multiply, or divide whole numbers |
| Construction | Ability to construct a two- or three-dimensional figure or shape | Draw a figure after a verbal command or reproduce a figure from a picture |
| Abstraction | Ability to reason in an abstract rather than a literal or concrete fashion | Interpret proverbs. Discuss how two objects are similar or different |
| Judgment | Ability to reason (according to age and lifestyle) | Demonstrate common sense and safety |

Source: Data from LS Bickley, RA Hoekelman (eds). Bate's Guide to Physical Examination and History Taking (7th ed). Philadelphia: Lippincott, 1999.

## Emotional State

Emotional state assessment entails observation and direct questioning to ascertain a patient's mood, affect, perception, and thought process, as well as to evaluate for behavioral changes. Evaluation of emotion is not meant to be a full psychiatric examination; however, it provides insight as to how a patient may complete the cognitive portions of the mental status examination.[11]

---

### Clinical Tip

It is important to note that a patient's culture may affect particular emotional responses.

---

## Speech and Language Ability

The physician should perform a speech and language assessment as soon as possible according to the patient's level of consciousness. The main goals of this assessment are to evaluate the patient's ability to articulate and produce voice and the presence, extent, and severity of aphasia.[12] These goals are achieved by testing comprehension and repetition of spoken speech, naming, quality and quantity of conversational speech, and reading and writing abilities.[12]

A speech-language pathologist is often consulted to perform a longer, more in-depth examination of cognition, speech, and swallow using standardized tests and skilled evaluation of articulation, phonation, hearing, and orofacial muscle strength testing.

---

### Clinical Tip

• The physical therapist should be aware of and use, as appropriate, the speech-language pathologist's suggestions for types of commands, activity modification, and positioning as related to risk of aspiration.

• The physical therapist is often the first clinician to notice the presence or extent of speech or language dysfunction during activity, especially during higher-level tasks or those activities that cause fatigue. The physical therapist should report these findings to other members of the health care team.

---

*Vital Signs*

The brain is the homeostatic center of the body; therefore, vital signs are an indirect measure of neurologic status and the body's ability to perform basic functions, such as respiration and temperature control.

Blood pressure, heart rate, respiratory rate and pattern (see Table 2-3), temperature, and other vital signs from invasive monitoring (see Appendix III-A) are assessed continuously or hourly to determine neurologic and hemodynamic stability.

---

Clinical Tip

The therapist should be aware of blood pressure parameters determined by the physician for the patient with neurologic dysfunction. These parameters may be set greater than normal to maintain adequate perfusion to the brain or lower than normal to prevent further injury to the brain.

---

*Cranial Nerves*

CN testing provides information about the general neurologic status of the patient and the function of the special senses. The results assist in the differential diagnosis of neurologic dysfunction and may help in determining the location of a lesion. CNs I through XII are tested on admission, daily in the hospital, or when there is a suspected change in neurologic function (Table 4-13).

*Vision*

Vision testing is an important portion of the neurologic examination, because alterations in vision can indicate neurologic lesions, as illustrated in Figure 4-7. In addition to the visual field, acuity, reflexive, and ophthalmoscopic testing performed by the physician during CN assessment, the pupils are further examined for the following:

- Size and equality. Pupil size is normally 2–4 mm or 4–8 mm in diameter in the light and dark, respectively.[13] The pupils should be

**Table 4-13.** Origin, Purpose, and Testing of the Cranial Nerves

| Nerve/*Origin* | Purpose | How to Test | Signs/Symptoms of Impairment |
|---|---|---|---|
| Olfactory (CN I)/ *cerebral cortex* | Sense of smell | Have the patient close one nostril, and ask the patient to sniff a mild-smelling substance and identify it. | Anosmia |
| Optic (CN II)/*thalamus* | Central and peripheral vision | Acuity: Have the patient cover one eye, and ask patient to read a visual chart. | Blindness |
| | | Fields: Have the patient cover one eye, and hold an object (e.g., pen cap) at arm's length from the patient in his or her peripheral field. Hold the patient's head steady. Slowly move the object centrally, and ask the patient to state when he or she first sees the object. Repeat the process in all quadrants. | |

| Cranial nerve/location | Function | Test | Signs |
| --- | --- | --- | --- |
| Oculomotor (CN III)/*midbrain* | Upward, inward, and inferomedial eye movement | CNs III, IV, and VI are tested together. | Ophthalmoplegia with eye deviation downward and outward |
| | Eyelid elevation | Pupil reaction to light: Shine a flashlight into one eye and observe bilateral pupil reaction. | Ptosis |
| | Pupil constriction / Visual focusing | Gaze: Hold object (e.g., pen) at arm's length from the patient, and hold the patient's head steady. Ask the patient to follow the object with a full horizontal, vertical, and diagonal gaze. | Loss of ipsilateral pupillary light and accommodation reflexes |
| Trochlear (CN IV)/*midbrain* | Inferolateral eye movement and proprioception | See Oculomotor (CN III), above. | Diplopia / Head tilt to unaffected side / Weakness in depression of ipsilateral adducted eye |
| Trigeminal (CN V)/*pons* | Sensation of face | Conduct touch, pain, and temperature sensory testing over the patient's face. | Loss of facial sensation |
| | Mastication | Observe for deviation of jaw. | Ipsilateral deviation of opened jaw |

**Table 4-13.** *Continued*

| Nerve/*Origin* | Purpose | How to Test | Signs/Symptoms of Impairment |
|---|---|---|---|
| | Corneal reflex | Wisp of cotton on the patient's cornea. | Loss of ipsilateral corneal reflex |
| | Jaw jerk* | Palpate masseter as the patient clamps his or her jaw. | |
| Abducens (CN VI)/*pons* | Lateral eye movement and proprioception | See Oculomotor (CN III), above. | Diplopia Convergent strabismus Ipsilateral abductor paralysis |
| Facial (CN VII)/*pons* | Taste (anterior two-thirds of tongue) | Ask the patient to smile, wrinkle brow, purse lips, and close eyes tightly. | Paralysis of ipsilateral upper and lower facial muscles, loss of lacrimation, dry mouth, loss of taste on ipsilateral two-thirds of tongue. |
| | Facial expression | Inspect closely for symmetry. | |
| | Autonomic innervation of lacrimal and salivary glands | — | — |
| Vestibulocochlear (CN VIII)/ *pons* | Vestibular branch: sense of equilibrium | Oculocephalic reflex (Doll's eyes): Rotate the patient's head and watch for eye movement. | Vertigo, nystagmus, disequilibrium, neural deafness |

| | | | |
|---|---|---|---|
| | Cochlear branch: sense of hearing | Cochlear: Vibrate a tuning fork, place it on the mid forehead, and ask the patient if sound is heard louder in one ear. | (Normal oculocephalic reflex is that the eyes will move in the opposite direction of the head prior to return to midline) |
| Glossopharyngeal (CN IX)/ *medulla* | Gag reflex Motor and proprioception of superior pharyngeal muscle Autonomic innervation of salivary gland Taste (posterior one-third of tongue) Blood pressure regulation | Test CNs IX and X together. Induce gag with tongue depressor (one side at a time). Patient phonates a prolonged vowel sound or talks for an extended period of time. Listen for voice quality and pitch. | Loss of gag reflex, dysphagia, dry mouth, loss of taste ipsilateral one-third of tongue |
| Vagus (CN X)/*medulla* | Swallowing Proprioception of pharynx and larynx Parasympathetic innervation of heart, lungs, and abdominal viscera | See Glossopharyngeal (CN IX), above. | Dysphagia, soft palate paralysis, contralateral deviation of uvula, ipsilateral anesthesia of pharynx and larynx, hoarseness |

**Table 4-13.** *Continued*

| Nerve/*Origin* | Purpose | How to Test | Signs/Symptoms of Impairment |
|---|---|---|---|
| Spinal accessory (CN XI)/ *medulla* | Motor control and proprioception of head rotation, shoulder elevation | Ask patient to rotate the head or shrug the shoulders. Offer gentle resistance to movement. | Weakness with head turning to the opposite side and ipsilateral shoulder shrug |
| | Motor control of pharynx and larynx | — | — |
| Hypoglossal (CN XII)/ *medulla* | Movement and proprioception of tongue for chewing and speech | Ask the patient to stick out his or her tongue and observe for midline. Observe for other tongue movements. Listen for articulation problems. | Ipsilateral deviation of tongue during protrusion Consonant imprecision |

CN = cranial nerve.
*Rarely tested.
Sources: Data from KW Lindsay, I Bone, R Callander (eds). Neurology and Neurosurgery Illustrated (2nd ed). Edinburgh, UK: Churchill Livingstone, 1991; EN Marieb (ed). Human Anatomy and Physiology (5th ed). San Francisco: Benjamin-Cummings, 2001; RJ Love, WG Webb (eds). Neurology for the Speech-Language Pathologist (4th ed). Boston: Butterworth–Heinemann, 2001; and adapted from PA Young, PH Young (eds). Basic Clinical Neuroanatomy. Baltimore: Williams & Wilkins, 1997;295–297.

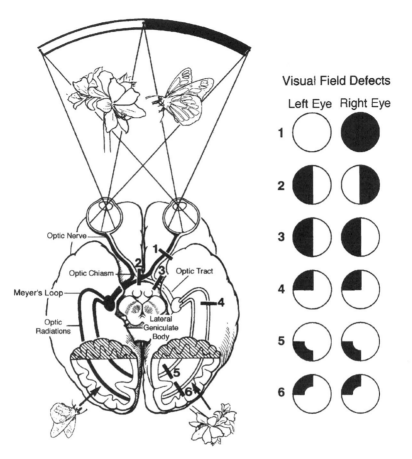

**Figure 4-7.** *Visual pathway with lesion sites and resulting visual field defects. The occipital lobe has been cut away to show the medial aspect and the calcarine sulci. (With permission from RJ Love, WG Webb [eds]. Neurology for the Speech-Language Pathologist [4th ed]. Boston: Butterworth–Heinemann, 2001;103.)*

of equal size, although up to a 1-mm difference in diameter can normally occur between the left and right pupils.[14]

• Shape. Pupils are normally round but may become oval or irregularly shaped with neurologic dysfunction.

• Reactivity. Pupils normally constrict in response to light, as a consensual response to light shown in the opposite eye or when fixed on a near object. Conversely, pupils normally dilate in the dark. Constriction and dilation occur briskly under normal circumstances. A variety of deviations of pupil characteristics can occur. Pupil reactivity can be tested by shining a light directly into the patient's eye. Dilated, nonreactive (fixed), malpositioned, or disconjugate pupils can signify very serious neurologic conditions (especially oculomotor compression, increased intracranial pressure [ICP], or brain herniation).[14]

---

Clinical Tip

• Note any baseline pupil changes, such as those associated with cataract repair (keyhole shape).
• If the patient's vision or pupil size or shape changes during physical therapy intervention, discontinue the treatment and notify the nurse or physician immediately.
• For a patient with diplopia (double vision), a cotton or gauze eye patch can be worn temporarily over one eye to improve participation during physical therapy sessions.
• PERRLA is an acronym that describes pupil function: *p*upils *e*qual, *r*ound, and *r*eactive to *l*ight and *a*ccommodation.

---

*Motor Function*

The evaluation of motor function consists of strength, tone, and reflex testing.

**Strength Testing**
*Strength* is the force output of a contracting muscle directly related to the amount of tension that it can produce.[15] Strength can be graded in the following ways in the acute care setting:

• Graded 0–5/0–N (normal) with manual muscle testing

• Graded as strong or weak with resisted isometrics

• Graded by the portion of a range of motion in which movement occurs (e.g., hip flexion through one-fourth of available range)

• Graded functionally

Clinical Tip

• The manner in which muscle strength is tested depends on the patient's ability to follow commands, arousal, cooperation, and activity tolerance, as well as on constraints on the patient, such as positioning, sedation, and medical equipment.

• If it is not possible to grade strength in any of the described ways, then only the presence, frequency, and location of spontaneous movements are noted instead.

**Muscle Tone**

Muscle tone has been described in a multitude of ways; however, neither a precise definition nor a quantitative measure has been determined.[16] It is beyond the scope of this chapter to discuss the various definitions of tone, including variants such as clonus and tremor. For simplicity, muscle tone is discussed in terms of hyper- or hypotonicity. *Hypertonicity*, an increase in muscle contractility, includes *spasticity* (velocity-dependent increase in resistance to passive stretch) and *rigidity* (increased agonist and antagonist muscle tension) secondary to a neurologic lesion of the CNS or upper motor neuron system. [17] *Hypotonicity*, a decrease in muscle contractility, includes *flaccidity* (diminished resistance to passive stretching and tendon reflexes)[17] from a neurologic lesion of the lower motor neuron system (or as in the early stage of spinal cord injury [SCI]). Regardless of the specific definition of muscle tone, clinicians agree that muscle tone may change according to a variety of factors, including stress, febrile state, pain, body position, medical status, medication, CNS arousal, and degree of volitional movement.[18]

Muscle tone can be evaluated in the following ways:

• Passively as mild (i.e., mild resistance to movement with quick stretch), moderate (i.e., moderate resistance to movement, even without quick stretch), or severe (i.e., resistance great enough to prevent movement of a joint)[19]

• Passively or actively as the ability or inability to achieve full joint range of motion

• Actively as the ability to complete functional mobility and volitional movement

• As abnormal decorticate (flexion) or decerebrate (extension) posturing. (*Decortication* is the result of a hemispheric or internal capsule lesion that results in a disruption of the corticospinal tract.[14] *Decerebration* is the result of a brain stem lesion and is thus considered a sign of deteriorating neurologic status.[14] A patient may demonstrate one or both of these postures.)

### Reflexes

A *reflex* is a motor response to a sensory stimulus and is used to assess the integrity of the motor system in the conscious or unconscious patient. The reflexes most commonly tested are deep tendon reflexes (DTRs). A DTR should elicit a muscle contraction of the tendon stimulated. Table 4-14 describes DTRs according to spinal level and expected response. DTR testing should proceed in the following manner:

1.　The patient should be sitting or supine and as relaxed as possible.

2.　The joint to be tested should be in midposition to stretch the tendon.

3.　The tendon is then directly tapped with a reflex hammer. Both sides should be compared. Reflexes are typically graded as present (normal, exaggerated, or depressed) or absent. Reflexes can also be graded on a scale of 0–4, as described in Table 4-15. Depressed reflexes signify lower motor neuron disease or neuropathy. Exaggerated reflexes signify upper motor neuron disease, or they may be due to hyperthyroidism, electrolyte imbalance, or other metabolic abnormalities.[20]

**Table 4-14.** Deep Tendon Reflexes of the Upper and Lower Extremities

| Reflex | Spinal Level | Normal Response |
|---|---|---|
| Biceps | C5 | Elbow flexion |
| Brachioradialis | C6 | Elbow flexion |
| Triceps | C7 | Elbow extension |
| Patellar | L4 | Knee extension |
| Posterior tibialis | L5 | Plantar flexion and inversion |
| Achilles | S1 | Plantar flexion |

Table 4-15. Deep Tendon Reflex Grades and Interpretation

| Grade | Response | Interpretation |
| --- | --- | --- |
| 0 | No response | Abnormal |
| 1+ | Diminished or sluggish response | Low normal |
| 2+ | Active response | Normal |
| 3+ | Brisk response | High normal |
| 4+ | Very brisk response, with or without clonus | Abnormal |

Source: Data from LS Bickley, RA Hoekelman. Bate's Guide to Physical Examination and History Taking (7th ed). Philadelphia: Lippincott, 1999.

Clinical Tip

The numeric results of DTR testing may appear in a stick figure drawing in the medical record. The DTR grades are placed next to each of the main DTR sites. An arrow may appear next to the stick figure as well. Arrows pointing upward signify hyper-reflexia; conversely, arrows pointing downward signify hyporeflexia.

A superficial reflex should elicit a muscle contraction from the cornea, mucous membrane, or area of the skin that is stimulated. The most frequently tested superficial reflexes are the corneal (which involve CNs V and VII), gag and swallowing (which involve CNs IX and X), and perianal (which involves S3–S5). These reflexes are evaluated by physicians and are graded as present or absent. Superficial reflexes may be abnormal cutaneous responses or recurrent primitive reflexes that are graded as present or absent. The most commonly tested cutaneous reflex is the *Babinski sign*. A positive (abnormal) Babinski sign is great-toe extension with splaying of the toes in response to stroking the lateral plantar surface of the foot with the opposite end of a reflex hammer. It indicates corticospinal tract damage.

## Sensation

Sensation testing evaluates the ability to sense light and deep touch, proprioception, temperature, vibration sense, and superficial and deep pain. For each modality, the neck, trunk, and extremities are tested bilaterally, proceeding in a dermatomal pattern. For more reliable sensation testing results, the patient should look away from the area being tested. Table 4-16 outlines the method of sensation testing by stimulus.

**Table 4-16.** Sensation Testing

| Sensation | Modality and Method |
| --- | --- |
| Superficial pain | Touch a pin or pen cap over the extremities or trunk. |
| Deep pain | Squeeze the patient's forearm or calf bulk. |
| Light touch | Apply light pressure with the finger, a cotton ball, or washcloth over the extremities or trunk. |
| Proprioception | Lightly grasp the distal interphalangeal joint of the patient's finger or great toe, and move the joint slowly up and down. Ask the patient to state in which direction the joint is moved. Test distal to proximal (e.g., toe to ankle to knee). |
| Vibration | Activate a tuning fork and place on a bony prominence. Ask the patient to state when the vibration slows and stops. Proceed distal to proximal. |
| Temperature | Place test tubes filled with warm or cold water on the area of the patient's body to be tested. Ask the patient to state the temperature. (Rarely done in the acute care setting.) |
| Stereognosis | Place a familiar object in the patient's hand and ask the patient to identify it. |
| Two-point discrimination | Place two-point caliper or drafting compass on area to be tested. Ask the patient to distinguish whether it has one or two points. |
| Graphesthesia | Trace a letter or number in the patient's open palm and ask the patient to state what was drawn. |
| Double simultaneous stimulation | Simultaneously touch two areas on the same side of the patient's body. Ask patient to locate and distinguish both points. |

Sources: Data from KW Lindsay, I Bone, R Callander (eds). Neurology and Neurosurgery Illustrated (2nd ed). Edinburgh, UK: Churchill Livingstone, 1991; S Gilman, SW Newman (eds). Manter and Gatz's Essentials of Clinical Neuroanatomy and Neurophysiology (7th ed). Philadelphia: FA Davis, 1989; and JV Hickey (ed). The Clinical Practice of Neurological and Neurosurgical Nursing (4th ed). Philadelphia: Lippincott, 1997.

Clinical Tip

Before completing the sensory examination, the physical therapist should be sure that the patient can correctly identify stimuli (e.g., that a pinprick feels like a pinprick).

## Coordination

Although each lobe of the cerebellum has its own function, coordination tests cannot truly differentiate among them. Coordination tests evaluate the presence of ataxia (general incoordination), dysmetria (overshooting), and dysdiadochokinesia (inability to perform rapid alternating movements) with arm, leg, and trunk movements, as well as with gait.[8] The results of each test (Table 4-17) are described in terms of the patient's ability to complete the test, accuracy, regularity of rhythm, and presence of tremor.[21]

Another test is the *pronator drift test*, which is used to qualify loss of position sense. While the patient is sitting or standing, he or she flexes both shoulders and extends the elbows with the palms upward. The patient is then asked to close his or her eyes. The forearm is observed for 10–20 seconds for (1) pronation or downward drift, which suggests a contralateral corticospinal lesion, or (2) an upward or sideward drift, which suggests loss of position sense.[22]

## Diagnostic Procedures

A multitude of diagnostic tests and procedures is used to evaluate, differentiate, and monitor neurologic dysfunction. Each has its own cost, accuracy, advantages, and disadvantages. For the purposes of this text, only the procedures most commonly used in the acute care setting are described.

### X-Ray

X-rays can provide anterior and lateral views of the skull that are used to assess the presence of calcification, bone erosion, or fracture, especially after head or facial trauma or if a tumor is suspected. Anterior, lateral, and posterior views of the cervical, thoracic, lumbar, and sacral spine are used to assess the presence of bone erosion, fracture,

**Table 4-17.** Coordination Tests

| Test | Method |
|------|--------|
| Upper extremity | |
| Finger to nose | Ask the patient to touch his or her nose. Then, ask patient to touch his or her nose and then touch your finger (which should be held an arm's length away). Ask the patient to repeat this rapidly. |
| Supination and pronation | Ask the patient to rapidly and alternately supinate and pronate his or her forearms. |
| Tapping | Ask the patient to rapidly tap his or her hands on a surface simultaneously, alternately, or both. |
| Arm bounce | Have the patient flex his or her shoulder to 90 degrees with elbow fully extended and wrist in the neutral position, then apply a brief downward pressure on the arm. (Excessive swinging of the arm indicates a positive test.) |
| Rebound phenomenon | Ask the patient to flex his or her elbow to approximately 45 degrees. Apply resistance to elbow flexion, then suddenly release the resistance. (Striking of the face indicates a positive test.) |
| Lower extremity | |
| Heel to shin | Ask the patient to move his or her heel down the opposite shin and repeat rapidly. |
| Tapping | Ask the patient to rapidly tap his or her feet on the floor simultaneously, alternately, or both. |
| Romberg test | Ask the patient to stand (heels together) with eyes open. Observe for swaying or loss of balance. Repeat with eyes closed. |
| Gait | Ask the patient to walk. Observe gait pattern, posture, and balance. Repeat with tandem walking to exaggerate deficits. |

Source: Data from KW Lindsay, I Bone, R Callander (eds). Neurology and Neurosurgery Illustrated (2nd ed). Edinburgh, UK: Churchill Livingstone, 1991.

dislocation, spondylosis, spur, or stenosis, especially after trauma or if there are motor or sensory deficits.[14,23]

### Computed Tomography

In computed tomography (CT), coronal or sagittal views of the head, with or without contrast media, are used to assess the density, displacement, or abnormality (location, size, and shape) of the cranial vault and fossae, cortical sulci and sylvian fissures, ventricular system, and gray and white matter. CT is also used to assess the presence of extraneous abscess, blood, calcification, contusion, cyst, hematoma, hydrocephalus, or tumor.[14,23] CT of spine or orbits is also available. Head CT is the preferred neuroimaging test for the evaluation of acute cerebrovascular accident (CVA), as it can readily distinguish a primary ischemic from a primary hemorrhagic process and thus determine the appropriate use of tissue plasminogen activator (tPa) (see Appendix IV).[24]

### Magnetic Resonance Imaging and Angiography

Views in any plane of the head, with or without contrast, taken with magnetic resonance imaging (MRI) are used to assess intracranial neoplasm, degenerative disease, cerebral and spinal cord edema, ischemia, hemorrhage, arteriovenous malformation (AVM), and congenital anomalies.[14,23] Magnetic resonance angiography (MRA) is used to assess the intracranial vasculature for CVA, transient ischemic attack (TIA), venous sinus thrombosis, AVM, and vascular tumors or extracranially for carotid bifurcation stenosis.[25]

### Doppler Flowmetry

*Doppler flowmetry* is the use of ultrasound to assess blood flow.

#### Transcranial Doppler Sonography

*Transcranial Doppler sonography* (TCD) involves the passage of low-frequency ultrasound waves over thin cranial bones (temporal) or over gaps in bones to determine the velocity and direction of blood flow in the anterior, middle, or posterior cerebral and basilar arteries. It is used to assess arteriosclerotic disease, collateral circulation, vasospasm, and brain death, and to identify AVMs and their supply arteries.[14,23]

### Carotid Noninvasives

Carotid noninvasives use the passage of high-frequency ultrasound waves over the common, internal, and external carotid arteries to determine the velocity of blood flow in these vessels. It is used to assess location, presence, and severity of carotid occlusion and stenosis.[14,23]

### Digital-Subtraction Angiography

Digital-subtraction angiography (DSA) is the computer-assisted radiographic visualization of the carotids and cerebral vessels with a minimal view of background tissues. An image is taken before and after the injection of a contrast medium. The first picture is "subtracted" from the second, a process that creates a highlight of the vessels. Digital-subtraction angiography is used to assess aneurysm, AVM, fistula, occlusion, or stenosis. It is also used in the operating room (i.e., television display) to examine the integrity of anastomoses or cerebrovascular repairs.[14,23]

### Cerebral Angiography

Cerebral angiography involves the radiographic visualization (angiogram) of the displacement, patency, stenosis, or vasospasm of intra- or extracranial arteries after the injection of a radiopaque contrast medium via a catheter (usually femoral). It is used to assess aneurysm, AVMs, or intracranial lesions as a single procedure or in the operating room to examine blood flow after surgical procedures (e.g., after an aneurysm clipping).[14]

---

### Clinical Tip

Patients are on bed rest with the involved hip and knee immobilized for approximately 8 hours after cerebral angiography to ensure proper healing of the catheter insertion site.

---

## Lumbar Puncture

A lumbar puncture (LP) is the collection of CSF from a needle placed into the subarachnoid space below the L1 vertebra, usually between L3 and L4. The patient is placed in a side-lying position with the neck and hips flexed as much as possible (to open the laminae for the best access to the subarachnoid space). Multiple vials of CSF are collected and tested for color, cytology, chlorine, glucose, protein, and pH. The opening and closing pressures are noted. LP is used to assist in the diagnosis of autoimmune and infectious processes, and, in certain circumstances, it is used to verify subarachnoid hemorrhage (SAH). LP provides access for the administration of spinal anesthesia, intrathecal antibiotics, or for therapeutic CSF removal.[14,23]

---

Clinical Tip

Headache is a common complaint after an LP secondary to meningeal irritation or CSF leakage. A patient may be placed on bed rest for several hours after an LP to minimize upright positioning, which increases headache. Other short-term complications of LP include backache, bleeding at the needle site, voiding difficulty, and fever.

---

## Positron Emission Tomography

Positron emission tomography (PET) produces three-dimensional cross-section images of brain tissue after the injection of nuclide positrons that produce gamma rays and are detected by a scanner. This physiological image measures cerebral glucose uptake, oxygen metabolism and blood flow.[14] A PET scan may be best used to assist in the diagnosis of cerebrovascular disease or trauma, epilepsy, dementia or psychiatric disorders.

## Electroencephalography

Electroencephalography is the recording of electrical brain activity, using electrodes affixed to the scalp at rest or sleep, after sleep deprivation, after hyperventilation, or after photic stimulation. Brain waves may show abnormalities of activity, amplitude, pattern, or speed. Electroencephalography is used in conjunction with other neurodiagnostic tests to assess seizure focus, sleep and metabolic disorders, dementia, and brain death.[14,23]

### Evoked Potentials

Evoked potentials are electrical responses generated by the stimulation of a sensory organ. A visual evoked potential is measured using electrodes that are placed over the occipital lobe to record occipital cortex activity after a patient is shown flashing lights or a checkerboard pattern. Visual evoked potentials are used to assess optic neuropathies and optic nerve lesions. A brain stem auditory evoked response is measured using electrodes that are placed over the vertex to record CN VIII, pons, and midbrain activity after a patient listens to a series of clicking noises through headphones. Brain stem auditory evoked responses are used to assess acoustic tumors, brain stem lesions in multiple sclerosis (MS), or brain stem function (in comatose patients). A somatosensory evoked potential is measured using electrodes over the contralateral sensory cortex after the median or posterior tibial nerve is electrically stimulated. Somatosensory evoked potentials are used to assess SCI, cervical disc disease, sensory dysfunction associated with MS, or parietal cortex tumor.[14,23]

### Electromyography and Nerve Conduction Velocity Studies

Electromyography (EMG) is the recording of muscle activity at rest, with voluntary movement, and with electrical stimulation with needle electrodes. Nerve conduction velocity studies are the measurement of the conduction time and amplitude of an electrical stimulus along a peripheral nerve(s). EMG and nerve conduction velocity studies are used to assess and differentiate myopathy and peripheral nerve injury, respectively.[14]

### Myelography

Myelography uses x-ray to show how a contrast medium flows through the subarachnoid space and around the vertebral column after the removal of a small amount of CSF and the injection of dye via LP. It is used to assess bone displacement, disc herniation, cord compression, or tumor.[14,23]

---

Clinical Tip

Depending on the type of dye used, a patient may have positioning restrictions after a myelogram. If water-based dye was used, the patient should remain on bed rest with the head of the bed at 30 degrees for approximately 8–24 hours, because the dye may cause a seizure if it reaches the cranium. If an oil-based dye was used, the patient may have to remain in bed with the bed flat for 6–24 hours. Additionally, the patient may experience headache, back spasm, fever, nausea, or vomiting, regardless of the type of dye used.[23]

---

## Pathophysiology

### Traumatic Brain Injury

The medical-surgical treatment of traumatic brain injury (TBI) is a complex and challenging task. Direct or indirect trauma to the skull, brain, or both typically results in altered consciousness and systemic homeostasis. TBI can be described by the following[26]:

1.    Location. TBI may involve damage to the cranium only, the cranium and brain structures, or brain structures only. Frequently, head trauma is categorized as (1) closed (protective mechanisms are maintained), (2) open (protective mechanisms are altered), (3) coup (the lesion is deep to the site of impact), (4) contrecoup (the lesion is opposite the site of impact), or (5) coup-contrecoup (a combination of coup and contrecoup).

2.    Extent. TBI may be classified as primary (in reference to the direct biomechanical changes in the brain) or secondary (in reference to the latent intracranial or systemic complications that exacer-

bate the original injury). The terms *focal* and *diffuse* are often used to describe a specific or gross lesion, respectively.

3.　Severity. In addition to diagnostic tests, TBI may be classified according to cognitive skill deficit and GCS as mild (13–15), moderate (9–12), or severe (3–8).

4.　Mechanism of injury. The two mechanisms responsible for primary TBI are acceleration-deceleration and rotation forces. These forces may be of low or high velocity and result in the compression, traction, or shearing of brain structures.

Secondary brain injury occurs within minutes to hours of the traumatic primary injury and is characterized by inflammatory, vascular, and biomolecular abnormalities. These changes include the release of cytokines and a disruption of the blood-brain barrier, which causes the development of vasogenic (extracellular) brain edema; impaired cerebral autoregulation and ischemia in the setting of hypoxia and hypotension; tissue acidosis and an influx of electrolytes, which causes cytotoxic (intracellular) brain edema; and the loss of neurons, glial cells, and presynaptic terminals from neurochemical and oxygen free radical reactions.[27,28]

Table 4-18 defines the most common types of TBI and describes the clinical findings. The management of these conditions is discussed later in General Management and in Table 4-21.

## Spinal Cord Injury

Spinal cord injury (SCI) and the resultant para- or quadriplegia are typically due to trauma or, less frequently, impingement of the spinal cord from abscess, ankylosing spondylitis, or tumor. *Primary* SCI, the direct trauma at the time of injury, can be described according to location or mechanism of injury[29]:

1.　Location. SCI may involve the cervical, thoracic, or lumbar spines.

2.　Mechanism of injury. SCI may result from blunt or penetrating injuries. Blunt forces include (1) forward hyperflexion, causing the discontinuity of the posterior spinal ligaments, disc herniation, and

**Table 4-18.** Clinical Findings and General Management of Traumatic Brain Injuries

| Injury | Definition | Clinical Findings |
| --- | --- | --- |
| Cerebral concussion | Shaking of the brain secondary to acceleration-deceleration forces, usually as a result of a fall or during sports activity. Can be classified as mild or classic. Signs and symptoms of cerebral concussion are reversible. | Brief loss of consciousness or "dazed" presentation, headache, dizziness, irritability, inappropriate laughter, decreased concentration and memory, retro- or antegrade amnesia, altered gait |
| Cerebral contusion | Bruise (small hemorrhage) secondary to acceleration-deceleration forces or beneath a depressed skull fracture, most commonly in the frontal or temporal areas. | See Cerebral concussion, above |
| Cerebral laceration | Tear of the cortical surface secondary to acceleration-deceleration forces, commonly in occurrence with cerebral contusion over the anterior and middle fossa where there are sharp bony surfaces. | S/S dependent on area involved, ICP, and degree of mass effect |
| Diffuse axonal injury (DAI) | Occurs with widespread white matter shearing secondary to high-speed acceleration-deceleration forces, usually as a result of a motor vehicle accident. Can be classified as mild (6–24 hrs of coma), moderate (greater than 24 hrs coma), or severe (days to weeks of coma). | Coma, abnormal posturing (if severe), other S/S dependent on area involved, ICP, and degree or mass effect |

**Table 4-18.** *Continued*

| Injury | Definition | Clinical Findings |
|---|---|---|
| Epidural hematoma (EDH) | Blood accumulation in the epidural space secondary to tearing of meningeal arteries that compresses deep brain structures. Associated with cranial fractures, particularly the thin temporal bone and frontal and middle meningeal tears. | Headache, altered consciousness, abnormal posture, contralateral hemiparesis, and other S/S dependent on specific location of the lesion, ICP, and degree of mass effect |
| Subdural hematoma (SDH) | Blood accumulation in the subdural space that compresses brain structures as a result of traumatic rupture or tear of cerebral veins, increased intracranial hemorrhage, or continued bleeding of a cerebral contusion. | See Epidural hematoma, above |
|  | The onset of symptoms may be acute (up to 24 hrs), subacute (2 days to 3 wks), or chronic (3 wks to 3–4 mos). | Can present with a "lucid" interval before loss of consciousness for a second time |
| Intracerebral hematoma (ICH) | Blood accumulation in the brain parenchyma secondary to acceleration-deceleration forces, the shearing of cortical blood vessels, or beneath a fracture. | See Epidural hematoma, above |

| Injury | Definition | Clinical Findings |
|--------|-----------|-------------------|
| | May also arise as a complication of hypertension or delayed bleeding with progression of blood into the dural, arachnoid, or ventricular spaces. | |

ICP = intracranial pressure, S/S = signs and symptoms.
Sources: Data from JV Hickey (ed). The Clinical Practice of Neurological and Neurosurgical Nursing (4th ed). Philadelphia: Lippincott, 1997; and SA Mayer, LP Rowland. Head Injury. In LP Rowland (ed). Merritt's Neurology (10th ed). Philadelphia: Lippincott, Williams & Wilkins, 2000.

vertebral dislocation or fracture; (2) hyperextension, causing discontinuity of the anterior spinal ligaments, disc herniation, and vertebral dislocation or fracture; and (3) axial compression, rotation, contusion, laceration, or transection. Penetrating forces, such as gunshot or stab wounds, may be (1) low velocity, in which the spinal cord and protective structures are injured directly, or (2) high velocity, in which a concussive force injures the spinal cord, and the protective structures remain intact.

*Secondary* SCI is a complex series of pathologic vascular and inflammatory responses to primary SCI, which further compound the original injury over the course of several days. A summary of secondary SCI includes (1) vasospasm of superficial spinal vessels, intraparenchymal hemmorhage and disruption of the blood-brain and spinal cord barrier, complicated by neurogenic shock and loss of autoregulation, and (2) increased calcium levels, which stimulate free radical production to cause further ischemia, the release of catecholamines and opioids, and the accumulation of activated microglia and macrophages.[29,30]

The severity of SCI is most commonly classified by the American Spinal Injury Association (ASIA) Impairment Scale.[31] This scale classifies SCI acccording to motor and sensory function[32]:

A = Complete—No sensory or motor function is preserved in S4-5.

B = Incomplete—The preservation of sensory function without motor function below the neurological level and includes S4-5.

C = Incomplete—The preservation of motor function below the neurological level. Muscle function of more than half of key muscles below this level is less than $3/5$.

D = Incomplete—The preservation of motor function below the neurological level. Muscle function of at least half of key muscles below this level is less than $3/5$.

E = Normal—Motor and sensory function are intact.

The most common types of incomplete SCI syndromes are described in Table 4-19. The immediate physiologic effect of SCI is spinal shock; the triad of hypotension, bradycardia, and hypothermia is secondary to altered sympathetic reflex activity.[31] It is beyond the scope of this book to discuss in detail the physiologic sequelae of SCI. However, other major physiologic effects of SCI include autonomic dysreflexia; orthostatic hypotension; impaired respiratory function; bladder, bowel, and sexual dysfunction; malnutrition; stress ulcer; diabetes insipidus; syndrome of inappropriate secretion of antidiuretic hormone; edema; and increased risk of deep venous thrombosis.

---

**Clinical Tip**

• If, during physical therapy intervention, a patient with SCI develops signs and symptoms associated with autonomic dysreflexia, return the patient to a reclined sitting position, and notify the nurse or physician immediately. Signs and symptoms of autonomic dysreflexia include headache, bradycardia, hypertension, and diaphoresis.[33]
• During the early mobilization of the patient with SCI into the sitting position, consider using compression stockings or Ace wraps on the legs and an abdominal binder to prevent or minimize orthostatic hypotension.

---

The management of SCI typically includes medical stabilization with ventilatory support (if indicated); immobilization of the spine with a collar, orthosis, traction, halo vest, or surgical repair; methylpredisolone or other pharmacologic therapies; treatment of secondary injures; pain management; and psychosocial support.

**Table 4-19.** Spinal Cord Injury Syndromes

| Syndrome | Mechanism of Injury | Description |
|---|---|---|
| Central cord | Hyperextension injury, or as a result of tumor, rheumatoid arthritis, or syringomyelia | Lesion of the central cord exerts pressure on anterior horn cells. Typically presents with bilateral motor paralysis of upper extremities greater than lower extremities, variable sensory deficits, and possible bowel/bladder dysfunction. |
| Anterior cord | Hyperflexion injury, acute large disc herniation, or as a result of anterior spinal artery injury | Lesion of the anterior cord damages the anterolateral spinothalamic tract, cortical spinal tract, and anterior horn (gray matter). Typically presents with bilateral loss of pain and temperature sensation and motor function with retained light touch, proprioception, and vibration sense. |
| Brown-Séquard | Penetrating spinal trauma (e.g., stab wound), epidural hematoma, spinal arteriovenous malformation, cervical spondylosis, or unilateral articular process fracture or dislocation | Lesion of one-half of the spinal cord; typically presents with contralateral loss of pain and temperature sensation; ipsilateral loss of touch, proprioception, and vibration sense; and ipsilateral motor paresis or paralysis. |

Sources: Data from DA Buckley, MM Guanci. Spinal cord trauma. Nurs Clin North Am 1999;34(3); and JV Hickey (ed). The Clinical Practice of Neurological and Neurosurgical Nursing (4th ed). Philadelphia: Lippincott, 1997.

## Cerebrovascular Disease and Disorders

A patent cerebral vasculature is imperative for the delivery of oxygen to the brain. Alterations of the vascular supply or vascular structures can cause neurologic dysfunction from cerebral ischemia or infarction.

### Transient Ischemic Attack

A TIA is characterized by the sudden onset of focal neurologic deficits, such as hemiparesis or altered speech secondary to cerebral, retinal, or cochlear ischemia, commonly from carotid or vertebrobasilar disease.[34] These deficits last less than 24 hours without residual effects. The management of TIAs involves observation, treatment of causative factor (if possible), anticoagulation, and carotid endarterectomy. TIA is often a strong prognostic indicator of stroke.

### Cerebrovascular Accident

A CVA, otherwise known as a *stroke* or *brain attack*, is characterized by the sudden onset of focal neurologic deficits of more than 24 hours' duration secondary to insufficient oxygen delivery to the brain.

The most prominent risk factors for CVA include older age, male gender, black race, hypertension, coronary artery disease, hyperlipidemia, atrial fibrillation, hypercoagulable state, diabetes mellitus, obesity, smoking, and alcohol abuse.[35]

*Ischemic* CVA is the result of cerebral hypoperfusion. An ischemic CVA has a slow onset and is due to thrombotic disease, such as carotid artery stenosis or arteriosclerotic intracranial arteries, or an embolus from the heart in the setting of atrial fibrillation, meningitis, prosthetic valves, patent foramen ovale, or endocarditis. The management of ischemic CVA involves blood pressure control (normal to elevated range), treatment of causative factors (if possible), anticoagulation, recombinant tPA,[36] cerebral edema control, prophylatic anticonvulsant therapy, and carotid endarterectomy (if indicated).

---

### Clinical Tip

A patient who has received tPA is at risk for intracranial hemmorhage or bleeding from other sites and requires strict blood pressure control during the first 24 hours of infusion.[37] Physical therapy is usually not initiated during this time frame.

---

Hemorrhagic CVA involves cerebral hypoperfusion, which is abrupt in onset and is secondary to intraparenchymal hemorrhage associated with hypertension, AVM, trauma, aneurysm, or SAH. The management of hemorrhagic CVA involves blood pressure control (low to normal range), treatment of causative factors (if possible), corticosteroids, anticoagulation (for reperfusion), prophylactic anticonvulsant therapy, and surgical hematoma evacuation (if appropriate).

Experimental treatment options for CVA include cytoprotective drugs and gene transfer therapy.[38] The signs and symptoms of CVA depend on the location (anterior vs. posterior and cortical vs. subcortical) and the extent of the cerebral ischemia or infarction. General signs and symptoms include contralateral motor and sensory loss, speech and perceptual deficits, altered vision, abnormal muscle tone, headache, nausea, vomiting, and altered effect.

Other terms commonly used to describe CVA include the following:

*Completed stroke.* A CVA in which the neurologic impairments have fully evolved

*Stroke-in-evolution.* A CVA in which the neurologic impairments continue to evolve or fluctuate over hours or days[38]

*Lacunar stroke.* A cerebral infarct of deep white matter (less than 1.5 cm in diameter) due to the thrombosis of very small penetrating cerebral vessels[39]

*Watershed stroke.* A cerebral infarct between the terminal areas of perfusion of two different arteries, typically between the anterior and middle cerebral arteries[14]

### Arteriovenous Malformation

AVM is a malformation in which blood from the arterial system is shunted to the venous system (thereby bypassing the capillaries) through abnormally thin and dilated vessels. An AVM can occur in a variety of locations, shapes, and sizes. The result of the bypass of blood is degeneration of brain parenchyma around the site of the AVM, which creates a chronic ischemic state. Signs and symptoms of AVM include headache, dizziness, fainting, seizure, aphasia, bruit, and motor and sensory deficits.[34] Management of AVM includes cerebral angiogram to evaluate the precise location of the

AVM, followed by surgical AVM repair, embolization, radiosurgery (stereotactic), or photon beam therapy.[14]

### Cerebral Aneurysm

Cerebral aneurysm is the dilation of a cerebral blood vessel wall owing to a smooth muscle defect through which the endothelial layer penetrates. Cerebral aneurysms most commonly occur at arterial bifurcations and in the larger vessels of the anterior circulation. Signs and symptoms of unruptured cerebral aneurysm are determined by size and location, such as[34]

Anterior communicating artery—Visual field deficits, endocrine dysfunction, frontal headache

Middle cerebral artery—Aphasia, focal arm weakness, paresthesias

Basilar bifurcation—Oculomotor paresis

Signs and symptoms of ruptured aneurysm include violent headache, stiff neck, photophobia, vomiting, hemiplegia, aphasia, seizure, and CN (III, IV, VI) palsy.[14] Management of cerebral aneurysm involves CT scan or angiogram to closely evaluate the aneurysm, followed by aneurysm clipping, embolization, or balloon occlusion.

### Subarachnoid Hemorrhage

Subarachnoid hemorrhage (SAH), the accumulation of blood in the subarachnoid space, is most commonly the result of aneurysm rupture, or less commonly a complication of AVM, tumor, infection, or trauma. It is graded from I to V according to the Hunt and Hess scale[14]:

I.    Asymptomatic

II.    Moderate to severe headache, nuchal rigidity, without neurologic deficit

III.    Drowsiness, confusion, with mild focal neurologic deficit

IV.    Stupor, moderate to severe focal deficits, such as hemiplegia

V.    Comatose, abnormal posturing

SAH is diagnosed by history, clinical examination, CT scan, LP, or angiogram. The management of SAH depends on its severity and may

include surgical aneurysm repair with blood evacuation; ventriculostomy; and supportive measures to maximize neurologic, cardiac, and respiratory status, rehydration, and fluid-electrolyte balance.
Complications of SAH include rebleeding, hydrocephalus, seizure, and vasospasm. *Vasospasm* is the spasm (constriction) of one or more cerebral arteries that occurs 4–12 days after SAH.[40] Diagnosed by either transcranial Doppler, cerebral angiography or CT, the exact etiology of vasospasm is unknown. Vasospasm results in cerebral ischemia distal to the area of spasm if untreated. The signs and symptoms of vasospasm are worsening level of consciousness, agitation, decreased strength, altered speech, pupil changes, headache, and vomiting, and they may wax and wane with the degree of vasospasm. Vasospasm is treated with induced hypertension, hypervolemia, and hemodilution.[40]

### Ventricular Dysfunction

### Hydrocephalus
Hydrocephalus is the acute or gradual accumulation of CSF, causing excessive ventricular dilation and increased ICP. CSF permeates through the ventricular walls into brain tissue secondary to a pressure gradient. There are two types of hydrocephalus:

1.   *Noncommunicating* (obstructive) hydrocephalus, in which there is an obstruction of CSF flow within the ventricular system. There may be thickening of the arachnoid villi or an increased amount or viscosity of CSF. This condition may be congenital or acquired, often as the result of aqueduct stenosis, tumor obstruction, abscess, or cyst, or as a complication of neurosurgery.[4]

2.   *Communicating* hydrocephalus, in which there is an obstruction in CSF flow as it interfaces with the subarachnoid space. This condition can occur with meningitis, after head injury, with SAH, or as a complication of neurosurgery.[2]

Hydrocephalus may be of acute onset characterized by headache, altered consciousness, decreased upward gaze, and papilledema.[8] Management includes treatment of the causative factor if possible, or ventriculoperitoneal (VP) or ventriculoatrial (VA) shunt.

*Normal-pressure hydrocephalus* (NPH) is a type of comminucating hydrocephalus without an associated rise in ICP and occurs primarily in the elderly.[34] It is diagnosed by history, head CT, and, possibly, LP. The hallmark triad of the signs of NPH is altered mental status (confusion), altered gait, and urinary incontinence. NPH is typically gradual and idiopathic but may be associated with previous meningitis, trauma, or SAH.[8] Management of NPH is typically with a VP shunt.

### Cerebrospinal Fluid Leak

A CSF leak is the abnormal discharge of CSF from a scalp wound, the nose (rhinorrhea), or the ear (otorrhea) as a result of a meningeal tear. A CSF leak can occur with anterior fossa or petrous skull fractures or, less commonly, as a complication of neurosurgery. With a CSF leak, the patient becomes at risk for meningitis with the altered integrity of the dura. A CSF leak, which usually resolves spontaneously in 7–10 days,[14] is diagnosed by clinical history, CT cisternography, and testing of fluid from the leak site. If the fluid is CSF (and not another fluid, e.g., mucus), it will test positive for glucose. The patient may also complain of a salty taste in the mouth. Management of CSF leak includes prophylactic antibiotics (controversial), lumbar drainage for leaks persisting more than 4 days, dural repair for leaks persisting more than 10 days, or VP or VA shunt.[34]

---

### Clinical Tip

If it is known that a patient has a CSF leak, the therapist should be aware of vital sign or position restrictions before physical therapy intervention. If a CSF leak increases or a new leak occurs during physical therapy intervention, the therapist should stop the treatment, loosely cover the leaking area, and notify the nurse immediately.

---

### Seizure

A *seizure* is a phenomenon of excessive cerebral cortex activity with or without loss of consciousness. The signs and symptoms of the seizure depend on the seizure locus on the cortex (e.g., visual hallucinations accompany an occipital cortex locus). Seizures can occur as a complication of CVA, head trauma, meningitis, or surgery. Febrile state, hypoxia, hyper- or hypoglycemia, hyponatremia, severe uremia or hepatic encephalopathy, drug overdose, and drug or alcohol withdrawal are also associated with seizure.[41] Seizures are classified as *partial* (originating in a focal region of one hemisphere) or *generalized* (originating in both hemispheres or from a deep midline focus). Types of partial seizures include the following[41]:

• *Simple partial seizures* are partial seizures without loss of consciousness.

• *Complex partial seizures* involve a brief loss of consciousness marked by motionless staring.

• *Partial seizures with secondary generalization* involve a progression to seizure activity in both hemispheres.

Types of generalized seizures include the following[41]:

• *Tonic seizures* are characterized by sudden flexor or extensor rigidity.

• *Tonic-clonic seizures* are characterized by sudden extensor rigidity followed by flexor jerking. (This type of seizure may be accompanied by incontinence or a crying noise owing to rigidity of the truncal muscles.)

• *Clonic seizures* are characterized by rhythmic jerking muscle movements without an initial tonic phase.

• *Atonic seizures* are characterized by a loss of muscle tone.

• *Absence seizures* are characterized by a very brief period (seconds) of unresponsiveness with blank staring and the inability to complete any activity at the time of the seizure.

• *Myoclonic seizures* are characterized by local or gross rapid, nonrhythmic jerking movements.

Seizures are of acute onset, with or without any of the following: aura, tremor, paresthesia, sensation of fear, gustatory hallucinations, lightheadedness, and visual changes. Medical management of seizures involves the treatment of causative factor (if possible) and antiepilep-

tic drugs. Surgical management for seizure refractory to medical management may consist of the resection of the seizure focus or the implantation of a vagal nerve stimulator.[42]
Terms related to seizure include the following[14,41]:

*Epilepsy* or *seizure disorder.* Refers to recurrent seizures.

*Status epilepticus.* More than 30 minutes of continuous seizure activity or two or more seizures without full recovery of consciousness between seizures. Generalized tonic-clonic status epilepticus is a medical emergency marked by the inability to sustain spontaneous ventilation with the potential for hypoxia requiring pharmacologic and life support.

*Prodrome.* The signs and symptoms (e.g., smells, auditory hallucinations, a sense of déjà vu) that precede a seizure by hours.

*Aura.* The signs and symptoms (as above) that precede a seizure by seconds or minutes.

*Postictal state.* The period of time immediately after a seizure.

---

### Clinical Tip

Establish the seizure history, including prodrome or aura (if any), for the patient with a recent seizure or epilepsy by either chart review or interview to be as prepared as possible to assist the patient if seizure activity should occur.

---

### Syncope

Syncope is the transient loss of consciousness and postural tone secondary to cerebral hypoperfusion, usually accompanied by bradycardia and hypotension.[42] Syncope can be any of the following[43]:

- Cardiogenic syncope, resulting from drug toxicity; dysrhythmias, such as atrioventricular block or supraventricular tachycardia; cardiac tamponade; atrial stenosis; aortic aneurysm; pulmonary hypertension; or pulmonary embolism

- Neurologic syncope, resulting from benign positional vertigo, cerebral atherosclerosis, seizure, spinal cord lesions, or peripheral neuropathy associated with diabetes mellitus or with degenerative diseases, such as PD

- Reflexive syncope, resulting from carotid sinus syndrome, pain, emotions, or a vasovagal response after eating, coughing, or defecation

- Orthostatic syncope, resulting from the side effects of drugs, volume depletion, or prolonged bed rest

Syncope is diagnosed by clinical history, ECG, Holter or continuous-loop event recorder, or tilt-table testing. CT and MRI are only performed if new neurologic deficits are found.[43] The management of syncope, dependent on the etiology and frequency of the syncopal episode(s), may include treatment of the causative factor; pharmacologic agents, such as beta-adrenergic blockers; or cardiac pacemaker placement.

## Neuroinfectious Diseases

See Chapter 10 for a description of encephalitis, meningitis, and poliomyelitis.

## Common Degenerative Central Nervous System Diseases

### Amyotrophic Lateral Sclerosis

Amyotrophic lateral sclerosis (ALS), or Lou Gehrig disease, is the progressive degeneration of upper and lower motor neurons, primarily the motor cells of the anterior horn and the corticospinal tract. The etiology of ALS is unknown except for familial cases. Signs and symptoms of ALS depend on the predominance of upper or lower motor neuron involvement and may include hyper-reflexia, muscle atrophy, fasciculation, and weakness, which result in dysarthria, dysphagia, respiratory weakness, and immobility.[44] ALS is diagnosed by clinical presentation and EMG.[8] Owing to the progressive nature of ALS, management is typically supportive or palliative, depending on the disease state, and may include pharmacologic therapy Relutek (Riluzole) spasticity control, bronchopulmonary hygiene, and nutritional and psychosocial support.[34]

## Guillain-Barré Syndrome

Guillain-Barré syndrome (GBS), or acute inflammatory demyelinating polyradiculopathy, is caused by the breakdown of Schwann cells by antibodies.[34] There is an onset of paresthesia, pain (especially of the lumbar spine), symmetric weakness (commonly proximal followed by distal, including the facial and respiratory musculature), and autonomic dysfunction approximately 1–3 weeks after a viral infection. GBS is diagnosed by history, clinical presentation, CSF sampling (increased protein level), and EMG studies (which show decreased motor and sensory velocities).[8] Once diagnosed, the patient with GBS is hospitalized because of the potential for rapid respiratory muscle paralysis.[45] Functional recovery varies from full independence to residual weakness that takes 12–24 months to resolve.[34] GBS is fatal in 5% of cases.[45] The management of GBS may consist of pharmacologic therapy (immunosuppressive agents), plasma exchange, intravenous immunoglobulin, respiratory support, physical therapy, and the supportive treatment of associated symptoms (e.g., pain management).

## Multiple Sclerosis

MS is the demyelination of the white matter of the CNS and of the optic nerve, presumably an autoimmune reaction. MS is categorized by onset and progression as relapsing-remitting (clearly defined relapses with full recovery or with residual deficit), primary progressive (occasional plateaus in disease progression and only temporary improvements), secondary progressive (initial relapsing-remitting followed by disease progression with or without relapses or plateaus), or progressive relapsing (progressive from onset with acute relapses, with or without full recovery).[34]

MS typically occurs in 20- to 40-year-olds and in women more than men. It is diagnosed by history (the onset of symptoms must occur and resolve more than once), clinical presentation, CSF sampling (increased myelin protein and immunoglobulin G levels), and by MRI (which shows the presence of two or more plaques of the CNS).[8] These plaques are located at areas of demyelination where lymphocytic and plasma infiltration and gliosis have occurred. Signs and symptoms of the early stages of MS may include focal weakness, fatigue, diplopia, blurred vision, equilibrium loss (vertigo), and urinary incontinence. Additional signs and symptoms of the latter stages of MS may include ataxia, paresthesias, spasticity, sensory deficits, hyper-reflexia, tremor, and nystagmus.[44] The management of MS may include pharmacologic therapy (corticosteroids), skeletal muscle relaxants, physical therapy, and the treatment of associated disease manifestations (e.g., bladder dysfunction).

### Parkinson's Disease

*Parkinson's disease* (PD) is the idiopathic progressive onset of bradykinesia, altered posture and postural reflexes, resting tremor, and cogwheel rigidity. Other signs and symptoms may include shuffling gait characterized by the inability to start or stop, blank facial expression, drooling, decreased speech volume, an inability to perform fine motor tasks, and dementia.[44] PD is diagnosed by history, clinical presentation, and MRI (which shows a light rather than dark substantia nigra).[8] The management of PD mainly includes pharmacologic therapy with antiparkinsonian agents and physical therapy. Stereotactic thalamotomy and the placement of a high-frequency thalamic stimulator are surgical options for symptoms refractory to medical therapy.[34]

## General Management

### Intracranial and Cerebral Perfusion Pressure

The maintenance of normal ICP or the prompt recognition of elevated ICP is one of the primary goals of the team caring for the postcraniosurgical patient or the patient with cerebral trauma, neoplasm, or infection.

*ICP* is the pressure CSF exerts within the ventricles. This pressure (normally 4–15 mm Hg) fluctuates with any systemic condition, body position, or activity that increases cerebral blood flow, blood pressure, or intrathoracic or abdominal pressure or that decreases venous return or increases cerebral metabolism.

The three dynamic variables within the fixed skull are blood, CSF, and brain tissue. As ICP rises, these variables change in an attempt to lower ICP via the following mechanisms: cerebral vasoconstriction, compression of venous sinuses, decreased CSF production, or shift of CSF to the subarachnoid space. When these compensations fail, compression of brain structures occurs, and fatal brain herniation will develop if untreated (Figure 4-8). The signs and symptoms of increased ICP are listed in Table 4-20. The methods of controlling ICP, based on clinical neurologic examination and diagnostic tests, are

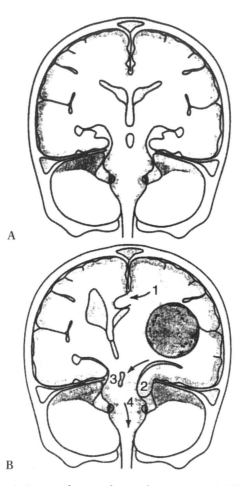

**Figure 4-8.** *Herniation syndromes depicted. Intracranial shifts from supratentorial lesions. A. Normal location of structures. B. Various herniation syndromes are demonstrated. 1. Cingulate gyrus is herniating under falx cerebri. 2. Temporal lobe is herniating downward through the tentorial notch. 3. Compression of contralateral cerebral peduncle is seen. 4. Downward displacement of brain stem through tentorial notch is a central herniation syndrome. (With permission from PG Beare, JL Myers [eds]. Adult Health Nursing [3rd ed]. Philadelphia: Saunders, 1998;919.)*

**Table 4-20.** Early and Late Signs of Increased Intracranial Pressure

| Observation | Early | Late |
| --- | --- | --- |
| Level of consciousness | Confusion, restlessness, lethargy | Coma |
| Pupil appearance | Ipsilateral pupil sluggish to light, ovoid in shape, with gradual dilatation | Papilledema, ipsilateral pupil dilated and fixed or bilateral pupils dilated and fixed (if brain herniation has occurred) |
| Vision | Blurred vision, diplopia, and decreased visual acuity | Same as early signs but more exaggerated |
| Motor | Contralateral paresis | Abnormal posturing Bilateral flaccidity if herniation has occurred |
| Vital signs | Stable blood pressure and heart rate | Hypertension and bradycardia (Cushing's response), altered respiratory pattern, increased temperature |
| Additional findings | Headache, seizure, cranial nerve palsy | Headache, vomiting, altered brain stem reflexes |

Source: Data from JV Hickey. The Clinical Practice of Neurological and Neurosurgical Nursing (4th ed). Philadelphia: Lippincott, 1997.

outlined in Table 4-21. Appendix Table III-A.5 describes the different types of ICP monitoring systems.

Cerebral perfusion pressure (CPP), or cerebral blood pressure, is mean arterial pressure minus ICP. It indicates oxygen delivery to the brain. Normal CPP is 70–100 mm Hg. CPPs at or less than 60 mm Hg for a prolonged length of time correlate with ischemia and anoxic brain injury.[46]

Following are terms related to ICP:

*Brain herniation.* The displacement of brain parenchyma through an anatomic opening; named according to the location of the displaced structure (e.g., *transtentorial herniation* is the herniation of the cerebral hemispheres, diencephalon, or midbrain beneath the tentorium cerebelli)

*Mass effect.* The combination of midline shift, third ventricle compression, and hydrocephalus[8]

**Table 4-21.** Treatment Options to Decrease Intracranial Pressure (ICP)

| Variable | Treatment |
|---|---|
| Blood pressure | Inotropic drugs to maintain mean arterial pressure >90 mm Hg to aid in cerebral perfusion, or antihypertensives |
| Osmotherapy | Osmotic diuretic to minimize cerebral edema |
| Mechanical ventilation | Normocapnia* to maximize cerebral oxygen delivery by limiting cerebral ischemia from the vasoconstrictive effects of decreased $Paco_2$ |
| Cerebrospinal fluid drainage | Ventriculostomy to remove cerebrospinal fluid |
| Sedation/paralysis | Barbiturates to decrease cerebral blood flow or other medication to decrease the stress of noxious activities |
| Positioning | Head of the bed at 30–45 degrees to increase cerebral venous drainage |
| | Promote neutral cervical spine and head position |
| Environment | Dim lights, decreased noise, frequent rest periods to decrease external stimulation |
| Seizure control | Prophylactic anticonvulsant medication |
| Temperature control | Normothermia or induced hypothermia to 32–35°C (e.g., cooling blanket or decreased room temperature) to decrease cerebral metabolism |

*Routine aggressive hyperventilation is no longer used for the control of elevated ICP. Hyperventilation can contribute to secondary brain injury because of a rebound increase in cerebral blood flow and volume in response to a decreased cerebrospinal fluid pH.
Source: Data from F Wong. Prevention of secondary brain injury. Crit Care Nurs 2000;20:18–27.

*Midline shift.* The lateral displacement of the falx cerebri secondary to a space-occupying lesion

*Space-occupying lesion.* A mass lesion, such as a tumor or hematoma, that displaces brain parenchyma and may result in the elevation of ICP and shifting of the brain

Another primary goal of the team is to prevent further neurologic impairment. The main components of management of the patient with neurologic dysfunction in the acute care setting include pharmacologic therapy, surgical procedures, and physical therapy intervention.

## Pharmacologic Therapy

A multitude of pharmacologic agents can be prescribed for the patient with neurologic dysfunction. These include anticonvulsant agents (see Appendix Table IV.5), osmotic diuretics (see Appendix Table IV.26), adrenocorticosteroids (see Appendix Table IV.1), skeletal muscle relaxants (see Appendix Table IV.28), and antiparkinsonian agents (see Appendix Table IV.9). Additional pharmacologic agents for medical needs include antibiotics (e.g., for infection or after neurosurgery), antihypertensives, thrombolytics, anticoagulants, chemotherapy and radiation for CNS neoplasm, stress ulcer prophylaxis (e.g., after SCI), pain control, and neuromuscular blockade.

## Neurosurgical Procedures

The most common surgical and nonsurgical neurologic procedures are described below (see Table 3-8 for a description of surgical spine procedures and Appendix III-A for a description of ICP monitoring devices).

*Aneurysm clipping.* The obliteration of an aneurysm with a surgical clip placed at the stem of the aneurysm.

*Burr hole.* A small hole made in the skull with a drill for access to the brain for the placement of ICP monitoring systems, hematoma evacuation, or stereotactic procedures; a series of burr holes is made before a craniotomy.

*Craniectomy.* The removal of incised bone, usually for brain (bone flap) tissue decompression; the bone may be permanently removed or placed in the bone bank or temporarily placed in the subcutaneous tissue of the abdomen (to maintain blood supply).

*Cranioplasty.* The reconstruction of the skull with a bone graft or acrylic material to restore the protective properties of the scalp and for cosmesis.

*Craniotomy.* An incision through the skull for access to the brain for extensive intracranial neurosurgery, such as aneurysm or AVM repair or tumor removal; craniotomy is named according to the area of the bone affected (e.g., frontal, bifrontal, frontotemporal [pterional], temporal, occipital).

*Embolization.* The use of arterial catheterization (entrance usually at the femoral artery) to place a material, such as a detachable coil, balloon, or sponge, to clot off an AVM or aneurysm.

*Evacuation.* The removal of an epidural, subdural, or intraparenchymal hematoma via burr hole or craniotomy.

*Shunt placement.* The insertion of a shunt system that connects the ventricular system with the right atrium (VA shunt) or peritoneal cavity (VP shunt) to allow the drainage of CSF when ICP rises.

*Stereotaxis.* The use of a stereotactic frame (a frame that temporarily attaches to the patient's head) in conjunction with head CT results to specifically localize a pretargeted site, as in tumor biopsy; a burr hole is then made for access to the brain.

---

### Clinical Tip

• The physical therapist should be aware of the location of a craniectomy, because the patient should not have direct pressure applied to that area. Look for signs posted at the patient's bedside that communicate positioning restrictions.
• Pay close attention to head of bed positioning restrictions for the patient who has recently had neurosurgery. Often, the head of bed is at 30 degrees, or it may be flat for an initial 24 hours and then gradually elevated 15–30 degrees per day depending on the location of surgery (supratentorial or infratentorial, respectively).[14]

---

### Physical Therapy Intervention

#### Goals

The primary physical therapy goals in treating patients with primary neurologic pathology in the acute care setting include maximizing independence and promoting safety with gross functional activity. Another main goal is to assist in the prevention of the secondary manifestations of neurologic dysfunction and immobility, such as pressure sores, joint contracture, and the deleterious effects of bed rest (see Appendix I-B).

## Basic Concepts for the Treatment of Patients with Neurologic Dysfunction

• A basic understanding of neurologic pathophysiology is necessary to create appropriate functional goals for the patient. The therapist must appreciate the difference between reversible and irreversible and between nonprogressive and progressive disease states.

• There are a number of natural changes of the nervous system with aging, such as decreased coordination, reflexes, balance, and visual acuity. Be sure to accommodate for these normal changes in the examination of and interaction with the elderly patient.

• Take extra time to observe and assess the patient with neurologic dysfunction, as changes in neurologic status are often very subtle.

• A basic knowledge of the factors that affect ICP and the ability to modify treatment techniques or conditions during physical therapy intervention for the patient with head trauma, after intracranial surgery, or other pathology interfering with intracranial dynamics is necessary for patient safety.

• Patient and family or caregiver education is an important component of physical therapy. Incorporate information about risk factor reduction (e.g., stroke prevention) and reinforce health care team recommendations (e.g., swallowing strategies per the speech-language pathologist).

• There are a variety of therapeutic techniques and motor control theories for the treatment of the patient with neurologic dysfunction. Do not hesitate to experiment with or combine techniques from different schools of thought.

• Be persistent with patients who do not readily respond to typical treatment techniques, because these patients most likely present with perceptual impairments superimposed on motor and sensory deficits.

• Recognize that it is rarely possible to address all of the patient's impairments at once; therefore, prioritize the plan of care according to present physiologic status and future functional outcome.

## References

1. Marieb EN (ed). Human Anatomy and Physiology. Redwood City, CA: Benjamin-Cummings, 1989;172.
2. Moore KL. The Head. In KL Moore (ed), Clinically Oriented Anatomy (2nd ed). Baltimore: Williams & Wilkins, 1985;794.
3. Westmoreland BF, Benarroch EE, Daube JR, et al. (eds). Medical Neurosciences: An Approach to Anatomy, Pathology, and Physiology by Systems and Levels (3rd ed). New York: Little, Brown, 1986;107.
4. Young PA, Young PH (eds). Basic Clinical Neuroanatomy. Baltimore: Williams & Wilkins, 1997;251–258.
5. Marieb EN (ed). Human Anatomy and Physiology. Redwood City, CA: Benjamin-Cummings, 1989;375.
6. Wilkinson JL (ed). Neuroanatomy for Medical Students (3rd ed). Oxford, UK: Butterworth–Heinemann, 1998;189–200.
7. Goldberg S (ed). The Four-Minute Neurological Exam. Miami: Med-Master, 1992;20.
8. Lindsay KW, Bone I, Callander R (ed). Neurology and Neurosurgery Illustrated (2nd ed). Edinburgh, UK: Churchill Livingstone, 1991.
9. Plum F, Posner J (eds). The Diagnosis of Stupor and Coma (3rd ed). Philadelphia: FA Davis, 1980;1.
10. Jennett B, Teasdale G (eds). Management of Head Injuries. Philadelphia: FA Davis, 1981;77.
11. Strub RL, Black FW (eds). Mental Status Examination in Neurology (2nd ed). Philadelphia: FA Davis, 1985;9.
12. Love RJ, Webb WG (eds). Neurology for the Speech-Language Pathologist (4th ed). Boston: Butterworth–Heinemann, 2001;205.
13. Specter RM. The Pupils. In HK Walker, WD Hall, JW Hurst (eds), Clinical Methods: The History, Physical, and Laboratory Examinations (3rd ed). Boston: Butterworth, 1990;300.
14. Hickey JV. The Clinical Practice of Neurological and Neurosurgical Nursing (4th ed). Philadelphia: Lippincott–Raven Publishers, 1997.
15. Kisner C, Colby LA. Therapeutic Exercise Foundations and Techniques (3rd ed). Philadelphia: FA Davis, 1996;57.
16. Katz RT, Dewald J, Schmit BD. Spasticity. In RL Braddon (ed). Physical Medicine and Rehabilitation (2nd ed). Philadelphia: Saunders, 2000;592.
17. Victor M, Ropper AH. Motor Paralysis. In M Victor, AH Ropper (eds), Adam and Victor's Principles of Neurology. New York: McGraw-Hill, 2001;50–58.
18. O'Sullivan SB. Motor Control Assessment. In SB O'Sullivan, TJ Schmitz (eds). Physical Rehabilitation: Assessment and Treatment (3rd ed). Philadelphia: FA Davis, 1998;115.
19. Charness A. Gathering the Pieces: Evaluation. In A Charness (ed), Stroke/Head Injury: A Guide to Functional Outcomes in Physical Therapy Management. Rockville, MD: Aspen, 1986;1.
20. Swartz MH. The Nervous System. In MH Swartz, W Schmitt (eds), Textbook of Physical Diagnosis History and Examination (3rd ed). Philadelphia: Saunders, 1998;529.

21. Gelb DJ. The Neurologic Examination. In DJ Gelb (ed), Introduction to Clinical Neurology (2nd ed). Boston: Butterworth–Heinemann, 2000; 43–90.
22. Bickley LS, Hoekelman RA. The Nervous System. In LS Bickley, B Bates, RA Hoekelman (eds), Bate's Guide to Physical Examination and History Taking (7th ed). Philadelphia: Lippincott, 1999;585.
23. Shpritz DW. Neurodiagnostic studies. Nurs Clin North Am 1999;34: 593.
24. Kelley RE, Gregory T. CT versus MRI: Which is better for diagnosing stroke? Patient Care. 1999;33:175–178, 181–182.
25. Delapaz R, Chan S. Computed Tomography and Magnetic Resonance Imaging. In LP Rowland (ed), Merritt's Neurology (10th ed). Philadelphia: Lippincott, Williams & Wilkins, 2000;55–63.
26. McNair ND. Traumatic brain injury. Nurs Clin North Am 1999;34:637–659.
27. Wong F. Prevention of secondary brain injury. Crit Care Nurs 2000;20:18–27.
28. Zink BJ. Traumatic brain injury outcome: concepts for emergency care. Ann Emerg Med 2001;37:318–332.
29. Dubendorf P. Spinal cord injury pathophysiology. Crit Care Nurs Q 1999;22:31–35.
30. Mautes A, Weinzierl MR, Donovan F, Noble LJ. Vascular events after spinal cord injury: contribution to secondary pathogenesis. Phys Ther 2000;80:673–687.
31. Mitcho K, Yanko JR. Acute care management of spinal cord injuries. Crit Care Nurs Q 1999;22:60–79.
32. Selzer ME, Tessler AR. Plasticity and Regeneration in the Injured Spinal Cord. In EG Gonzalez, SJ Myers (eds), Downey and Darling's Physiological Basis of Rehabilitation Medicine (3rd ed). Boston: Butterworth–Heinemann, 2001;629–632.
33. Buckley DA, Guanci MM. Spinal cord trauma. Nurs Clin North Am 1999;34:661–687.
34. Bradley WG, Daroff RB, Fenichel GM, Marsden CD (eds). Pocket Companion to Neurology in Clinical Practice (3rd ed). Boston: Butterworth–Heinemann, 2000.
35. Ingall TJ. Preventing ischemic stroke. Postgrad Med 2000;107:34–50.
36. Meschia JF. Management of acute ischemic stroke. Postgrad Med 2000;107:85–93.
37. Blank F, Keyes M. Thrombolytic therapy for patients with acute stroke in the ED setting. J Emerg Nurs 2000;26:24–30.
38. Hock NH. Brain attack: the stroke continuum. Nurs Clin North Am 1999;34:689–724.
39. Flemming KD, Brown RD. Cerebral infarction and transient ischemic attacks. Postgrad Med 2000;107:55–83.
40. Mower-Wade D, Cavanaugh MC, Bush D. Protecting a patient with ruptured cerebral aneurysm. Nursing 2001;31:52–57.
41. Drury IJ, Gelb DJ. Seizures. In DJ Gelb (ed), Introduction to Clinical Neurology (2nd ed). Boston: Butterworth–Heinemann, 2000;129–151.

42. Aminoff MJ. Nervous System. In LM Tierney, SJ McPhee, MA Papadakis (eds), Current Medical Diagnosis and Treatment 2001 (40th ed). New York: Lange Medical Books/McGraw-Hill, 2001;979–980, 983–986.
43. Cox MM, Kaplan D. Uncovering the Cause of Syncope. Patient Care 2000;34:39–48, 59.
44. Fuller KS. Degenerative Diseases of the Central Nervous System. In CC Goodman, WG Boissonnault (eds). Pathology: Implications for the Physical Therapist. Philadelphia: Saunders, 1998;723.
45. Worsham TL. Easing the course of Guillain-Barré syndrome. RN 2000;63:46–50.
46. King BS, Gupta R, Narayan RJ. The early assessment and intensive care unit management of patients with severe traumatic brain and spinal cord injuries. Surg Clin North Am 2000;80:855–870.

# 5

# Oncology

*Susan Polich*

## Introduction

*Cancer* is a term that applies to a group of diseases characterized by the abnormal growth of cells. The physical therapist requires an understanding of underlying cancer pathology, as well as the side effects, considerations, and precautions related to cancer care to enhance clinical decision making to safely and effectively treat the patient with cancer. This knowledge will also assist the physical therapist with the early detection of previously undiagnosed cancer. The objectives for this chapter are to provide the following:

1.  An understanding of the medical assessment and diagnosis of a patient with cancer, including staging and classification

2.  An understanding of the various medical and surgical methods of cancer management

3.  A better understanding of a variety of the different body system cancers

4.  Examination, evaluation, and intervention considerations for the physical therapist

## Definitions

The terms *neoplasm, tumor,* and *cancer* are currently used interchangeably. *Neoplasm* means "new growth" and applies to any abnormal mass of tissue which exceeds the growth of normal tissue, grows at the expense of its host, and persists even after the stimulus to grow is removed. The term *tumor* originally applied to the swelling caused by inflammation but now refers only to a new growth. *Cancer* is the layperson's term for all malignant neoplasms.[1–4]

Normal cells change in size, shape, and type, known collectively as *dysplasia,* if the proper stimulus is provided. *Hyperplasia* refers to an increase in cell number. *Metaplasia* is the change of one cell type to another. Hyperplasia and metaplasia can be reversible and normal— or persistent and abnormal.[1,2,4]

Neoplasms, or persistent, abnormal dysplastic cell growth, are classified by cell type, growth pattern, anatomic location, degree of dysplasia, tissue of origin, and their ability to spread or remain in the original location. Two general classifications for neoplasm are benign and malignant. *Benign* tumors are usually considered harmless and slow growing and have cells that closely resemble normal cells of adjacent tissue. However, these benign tumors may occasionally become large enough to encroach on surrounding tissues and impair their function. *Malignant* neoplasms, or *malignant tumors,* grow uncontrollably, invading normal tissues and causing destruction to surrounding tissues and organs. Malignant neoplasms may spread, or *metastasize,* to other areas of the body through the cardiovascular or lymphatic system.[1–5]

Tumors may also be classified as primary or secondary. *Primary* tumors are the original tumors in the original location. *Secondary* tumors are those metastases that have moved from the primary site.[4]

## Nomenclature

Benign and malignant tumors are named by their cell of origin (Table 5-1). Benign tumors are customarily named by attaching *-oma* to the cell of origin. Malignant tumors are usually named by adding *carcinoma* to the cell of origin if they originate from epithelium and *sarcoma* if they originate in mesenchymal tissue.[1–3] Variations to this naming exist, such as *melanoma* and *leukemia.*

Table 5-1. Classification of Benign and Malignant Tumors

| Tissue of Origin | Benign | Malignant |
|---|---|---|
| Epithelium | | |
| Surface epithelium | Papilloma | Carcinoma |
| Epithelial lining of gland or ducts | Adenoma | Adenocarcinoma |
| Connective tissue and muscle | | |
| Fibrous tissue | Fibroma | Fibrosarcoma |
| Cartilage | Chondroma | Chondrosarcoma |
| Bone | Osteoma | Osteosarcoma |
| Smooth muscle | Leiomyoma | Leiomyosarcoma |
| Striated muscle | Rhabdomyoma | Rhabdomyosarcoma |
| Nerve tissue | | |
| Glial | — | Glioma |
| Meninges | Meningioma | Meningeal sarcoma |
| Retina | — | Retinoblastoma |
| Lymphoid tissue | — | Lymphoma/ lymphosarcoma |
| Bone marrow | | |
| White blood cells | — | Leukemias |
| Plasma cells | — | Multiple myeloma |

Source: With permission from S Baird (ed). A Cancer Source Book for Nurses (6th ed). Atlanta: American Cancer Society, 1991;28.

## Etiology and Risk Factors

The causes, or etiologies, of neoplasm are often divided into two categories, external or environmental and genetic. There are risk factors that are thought to predispose a person to cancer. Most cancers probably develop from a combination of factors. The most common etiologies can be found in Table 5-2. Risk factors can be found in Table 5-3.

## Signs and Symptoms

Signs and symptoms of cancer are most often due to the tumor's growth and invasion of surrounding tissues. The American Cancer Society has the acronym CAUTION for several common signs of cancer[6]:

Table 5-2. Cancer Etiologies

| |
| --- |
| Viruses |
|   Human papilloma virus |
|   Epstein-Barr virus |
| Chemical agents |
|   Tar |
|   Soot |
|   Dyes |
|   Polycyclic hydrocarbons |
|   Nickel |
|   Arsenic |
|   Excessive ethanol ingestion |
|   Vinyl chloride |
|   Benzene |
| Physical agents |
|   Ionizing radiation |
|   Ultraviolet light |
|   Asbestos |
|   Wood dust |
| Drugs |
|   Some chemotherapeutic agents |
| Hormones |
|   Estrogen |

Source: Adapted from LM Tierney, SJ McPhee, MA Papadakis (eds). Current Medical Diagnosis and Treatment. Stamford, CT: Appleton & Lange, 1999.

- C = Change in bowel or bladder habits

- A = A sore that does not heal

- U = Unusual bleeding or discharge

- T = Thickening or lump in the breast or elsewhere

- I = Indigestion or difficulty in swallowing

- O = Obvious change in a wart or mole

- N = Nagging cough or hoarseness

Additional signs and symptoms that may indicate cancer include fever, unexplained weight loss of more than 10 lb, undue fatigue, unexplained pain, anorexia, anemia, and weakness.[2]

**Table 5-3.** Risk Factors for Selected Cancer Sites

| Cancer Site | High-Risk Factors |
| --- | --- |
| Lung | Heavy smoker, older than age 40 yrs |
| | Smoked one pack per day for 20 yrs |
| | Started smoking at age 15 or before |
| | Smoker working with or near asbestos |
| Breast | Lump in breast |
| | Nipple discharge |
| | History of breast cancer |
| | Family history of breast cancer |
| | Benign breast disease |
| | High-fat diet |
| | Nulliparous or first child after age 30 yrs |
| | Early menarche or menopause |
| Colon/rectum | History of rectal polyps or colonic adenomatosis |
| | Family history of rectal polyps |
| | Ulcerative colitis or Crohn's disease |
| | Obesity |
| | Increasing age |
| Uterine | Unusual vaginal blood or discharge |
| | History of menstrual irregularity |
| | Late menopause |
| | Nulliparity |
| | Infertility through anovulation |
| | Diabetes, hypertension, and obesity |
| | Age 50–64 yrs |
| Skin | Excessive exposure to the sun |
| | Fair complexion that burns easily |
| | Presence of congenital moles or history of dysplastic nevi or cutaneous melanoma |
| | Family history of melanoma |
| Oral | Heavy smoker and alcohol drinker |
| | Poor oral hygiene |
| | Long-term exposure to the sun, particularly to the lips |
| Ovary | History of ovarian cancer among close relatives |
| | Nulliparity or delayed age at first pregnancy |
| | Age 50–59 yrs |

Table 5-3. *Continued*

| Cancer Site | High-Risk Factors |
| --- | --- |
| Prostate | Increasing age |
| | Occupations relating to the use of cadmium |
| | Family history |
| Stomach | History of stomach cancer among close relatives |
| | Diet heavy in smoked, pickled, or salted foods |

Source: With permission from S Baird (ed). A Cancer Source Book for Nurses (6th ed). Atlanta: American Cancer Society, 1991;32.

Paraneoplastic syndromes are symptoms that cannot be related directly to the cancer's growth and invasion of tissues. They are thought to be due to abnormal hormonal secretions by the tumor. The syndromes are present in approximately 15% of persons diagnosed with cancer and often are the first sign of malignancy. Clinical findings are similar to endocrinopathies (Cushing's syndrome, hypoglycemia), nerve and muscle syndromes (myasthenia), dermatologic disorders (dermatomyositis), vascular and hematologic disorders (venous thrombosis, anemia), and others.[1,7]

## Diagnosis

After obtaining a medical history and performing a physical examination, the physician uses specific medical tests to diagnose cancer. These tests may include medical imaging, blood tests for cancer markers, and several types of biopsy. *Biopsy*, or removal and examination of tissue, is the definitive test for cancer identification. Table 5-4 lists common medical tests used to diagnose cancer.

## Staging and Grading

After the diagnosis of cancer is established, staging is performed to describe the location and size of the primary site of the tumor, the extent of lymph node involvement, and the presence or absence of metastasis. Staging helps to determine treatment options, predict life expectancy, and determine prognosis for complete resolution.

**Table 5-4.** Diagnostic Tests for Cancer

| Test | Description |
|------|-------------|
| Biopsy | Tissue is taken via incision, needle, aspiration procedures. A pathologist examines the tissue to identify the presence or absence of cancer cells; if cancer is present, the tumor is determined to be benign or malignant. The cell or tissue of origin, staging, and grading are also performed. |
| Blood tests | Blood can be assessed for the presence or absence of tumor markers: |

| Marker | Cancer |
|--------|--------|
| Prostate surface antigen | Prostate disease |
| Carcinoembryonic antigen | Colon cancer |
| Prostatic-acid phosphatase | Prostate cancer |
| Alpha-fetoprotein | Liver cell cancer |
| CA125 | Ovarian cancer |
| CA19-9 | Colon cancer |
| CA15-3 | Stool guaiac |

| Test | Description |
|------|-------------|
| Stool guaiac | Detects small quantities of blood in stool. |
| Sigmoidoscopy | The sigmoid colon is examined with a sigmoidoscope. |
| Colonoscopy | The upper portion of the rectum is examined with a colonoscope. |
| Mammography | A radiographic method is used to look for a mass or calcification in breast tissue. |
| Radiography | X-ray is used to detect a mass. |
| Magnetic resonance imaging and computerized axial tomography | These noninvasive imaging techniques are used to assess lesions suspected of being cancerous. |
| Bone scan | Radionuclide imaging used to detect the presence, amount of metastatic disease, or both in bones. |
| Pap smear | A type of biopsy in which cells from the cervix are removed and examined. |
| Sputum cytology | A sputum specimen is inspected for cancerous cells. |
| Bronchoscopy | A tissue or sputum sample can be taken by rigid or flexible bronchoscopy. |

CA = carbohydrate antigen.

The mostly commonly used method to stage cancer is the TNM system. Tumors are classified according to the American Joint Committee on Cancer using this system based on the size of the primary tumor (T), presence or absence of tumor in local lymph nodes (N), and presence or absence of metastasis (M) (Table 5-5).[1]

Grading reports the degree of dysplasia, or differentiation, from the original cell type. The higher the grade, the greater the differentiation, or appearance, from the original cell. In some cases, tumor cells may look so unlike any normal cell that no cell of origin can be determined. Higher degree of differentiation is linked to aggressive, fatal tumors (Table 5-6).[1]

## Management

Not all cancers are curable. Physicians may therefore focus treatment on quality of life with palliative therapies rather than on curative therapies. Four major treatment options include:

- Surgical removal of the tumor

- Radiation to destroy or shrink the tumor

- Chemotherapy

- Biotherapy (including immunotherapy, hormonal therapy, bone marrow transplantation, and monoclonal antibodies)

**Table 5-5.** TNM System

| |
| --- |
| T: Primary tumor |
|    TX: Primary tumor cannot be assessed. |
|    T0: No evidence of primary tumor. |
|    Tis: Carcinoma in situ (site of origin). |
|    T1, T2, T3, T4: Progressive increase in tumor size and local involvement. |
| N: Regional lymph node involvement |
|    NX: Nodes cannot be assessed. |
|    N0: No metastasis to local lymph nodes. |
|    N1, N2, N3: Progressive involvement of local lymph nodes. |
| M: Distant metastasis |
|    MX: Presence of distant metastasis cannot be assessed. |
|    M0: No distant metastasis. |
|    M1: Presence of distant metastasis. |

**Table 5-6.** Grading of Neoplasms

| Grade I | Tumor cells closely resemble original tissue. |
|---|---|
| Grades II and III | Tumor cells are intermediate in appearance, moderately differentiated. |
| Grade IV | Tumor cells are so poorly differentiated (anaplastic) that the cell of origin is difficult or impossible to determine. |

Additional treatments may include physical therapy, nutritional support, acupuncture, chiropractic treatment, alternative medicine, and hospice care.

Treatment protocols differ from physician to physician and from cancer to cancer. Standard treatment includes some combination of surgery, radiation, and chemotherapy.

## Surgery

Surgical intervention is determined by the size, location, and type of cancer, as well as the patient's age, general health, and functional status. The following are the types of general surgical procedures for resecting or excising a neoplasm:

• *Exploratory surgery* is the removal of regions of the tumor to explore for staging or discover the extent or invasion of the tumor.

• *Excisional surgery* is the removal of cancerous cells and the surrounding margin of normal tissue. Tissue cells are sent to pathology to determine the type of cancer cell and to determine whether the entire growth was removed.

• *Debulking* is an incomplete resection used to reduce the size of a large tumor to make the patient more comfortable or prevent the tumor from impinging vital tissue. This surgery is usually used when the cancer is considered "incurable."

• *Mohs' surgery* is a microscopically controlled surgery in which layers of the tumor are removed and inspected microscopically until all layers have been removed.[8]

• *Lymph node dissection* involves the removal or resection of malignant lymph nodes to help control the spread of cancer.

• *Skin grafting* may be indicated in large resections of tumors to replace areas of skin removed during resection of a neoplasm with donor skin (see Chapter 7).

• *Reconstructive surgery* is the surgical repair of a region with a flap of skin, fascia, muscle, and vessels. It aids in a more cosmetic and functional result of surgical repair and protects the underlying resected area.

---

Clinical Tip

• Special care must be taken with skin grafts. Patients usually remain on bed rest to allow the graft to begin to adhere. (Length of bed rest is dependent on physician's protocol, ranging from 0 to 36 days.[9–11]) During bed rest, therapeutic exercise may be performed with extremities not involving the skin graft site.
• Muscle contraction in newly constructed muscle flaps should be minimized or avoided.

---

*Radiation*

High-ionizing radiation is used to destroy or prevent cancer cells from growing further, while minimizing the damage to surrounding healthy tissues. Radiation therapy reduces the size of a tumor to allow for resection surgically, to relieve compression on structures surrounding the tumor, and to relieve pain (by relieving compression on pain-sensitive structures). Reducing the size of a tumor with radiation therapy may also help to reduce the need for a large resection, amputation, or complete mastectomy.[7]

Radiation may be delivered via supervoltage radiotherapy (*teletherapy*) or by planting radioactive material near the tumor (*seeding* or *brachytherapy*). Radiation destroys cells in its path; therefore, special consideration is given to irradiating as little normal tissue as possible. Teletherapy uses various methods, such as linear acceleration and modifying-beam wedges, to permit greater localization.[7] Seeding may destroy all surrounding tissues, including healthy tissue. Radioactive seeds are implanted for several days, then removed.

Common side effects of radiation therapy include skin reactions, slow healing of wounds, limb edema, contractures, fibrosis, alopecia, neuropathy, headaches, cerebral edema, seizures, visual disturbances, bone marrow suppression, cough, pneumonitis, fibrosis, esophagitis, nausea, vomiting, diarrhea, cystitis, and urinary frequency.[6,7]

---

**Clinical Tip**

• Physical therapy should be deferred while the person has implanted radioactive seeds.
• Massage and heating modalities should be withheld for 1 year in an irradiated area.
• Persons undergoing irradiation by beam (teletherapy) will have blue markings where the radiation is being delivered. Caution should be taken with the skin and underlying tissues in that area, because it will be very fragile. Persons who have received the maximum allowable radiation in an area will have that area outlined in black. Special care should be taken with the skin and other tissues in that area, because it will be very fragile.
• A patient may be prescribed antiemetics (see Appendix IV, Table IV-6) after radiation treatment to control nausea and vomiting. Notify the physician if antiemetic therapy is insufficient to control the patient's nausea or vomiting during physical therapy sessions.

---

*Chemotherapy*

The overall purpose of chemotherapy is to treat or prevent metastatic disease and reduce the size of the tumor for surgical resection or palliative care. Patients may receive single agents or a combination of agents. Chemotherapy can be performed preoperatively and postoperatively. Chemotherapy is usually delivered systemically, via intravenous or central lines, but may be directly injected in or near a tumor. Patients may receive a single or multiple rounds of chemotherapy over time to treat their cancer and to possibly minimize side effects. Side effects of chemotherapy include nausea, vomiting, "cancer pain," and loss of hair and other fast-growing cells, including platelets and red and white blood cells.

Different types of chemotherapeutic agents have different mechanisms of action. Alkylating agents and nitrosoureas inhibit cell growth and division by reacting with DNA. Antimetabolites prevent cell growth by competing with metabolites in production of nucleic acid. Plant alkaloids prevent cellular reproduction by disrupting cell mitosis.[12]

Chemotherapeutic agents are listed in Appendix IV, Tables IV-15.A–H.

---

### Clinical Tip

- Some chemotherapeutic agents are so toxic to humans that patients may have to remain in their rooms while the agents are being delivered to avoid risk to other patients and health care workers. Physical therapists should check with the patient's physician if unsure.
- Nausea and vomiting after chemotherapy vary on a patient-to-patient basis. The severity of these side effects may be due to the disease stage, chemotherapeutic dose, or number of rounds. Some side effects may be so severe as to limit physical therapy, whereas others can tolerate activity. Rehabilitation should be delayed or modified until the side effects from chemotherapy are minimized or alleviated.
- Patients may be taking antiemetics, which help to control nausea and vomiting after chemotherapy. The physical therapist should alert the physician when nausea and vomiting limit the patient's ability to participate in physical therapy so that the antiemetic regimen may be modified or enhanced. Antiemetics are listed in Appendix IV, Table IV-6.
- Chemotherapy agents affect the patient's appetite and ability to consume and absorb nutrients. This decline in nutritional status can inhibit the patient's progression in strength and conditioning programs. Proper nutritional support should be provided and directed by a nutritionist. Consulting with the nutritionist may be beneficial when planning the appropriate activity level that is based on a patient's caloric intake.
- Patients should be aware of the possible side effects and understand the need for modification or delay of rehabilitation efforts. Patients should be given emotional

support and encouragement when they are unable to achieve the goals that they have initially set. Intervention may be coordinated around the patient's medication schedule.

• Vital signs should always be monitored, especially when patients are taking the more toxic chemotherapy agents that affect the heart, lungs, and central nervous system.

• Platelet and red and white blood cell counts should be monitored with a patient on chemotherapy. The Bone Marrow Transplant section in Chapter 12 suggests therapeutic activities with altered blood cell counts.

• Patients receiving chemotherapy can become neutropenic. They can be at risk for infections and sepsis.[7] (A *neutrophil* is a type of leukocyte or white blood cell that is often the first immunologic cell at the site of infection; *neutropenia* is an abnormally low neutrophil count. Refer to Bone Marrow Transplantation in Chapter 12 for reference value of neutropenia.) Therefore, patients undergoing chemotherapy may be on neutropenic precautions, such as being in isolation. Follow the institution's guidelines for precautions when treating these patients to help reduce the risk of infections. Examples of these guidelines can be found in the Bone Marrow Transplantation section of Chapter 12.

*Biotherapy*

Hormonal therapy and immunotherapy also play an important role in managing cancer. Hormonal therapy includes medically or surgically eliminating the hormonal source of cancer (e.g., orchiectomy, oophorectomy, or adrenalectomy) or pharmacologically changing hormone levels.[6,7] Immunotherapy includes enhancing the patient's immune system and changing the immune system's response to the cancer, most commonly with recombinant growth factors, such as interferon-alpha or interleukin.

Hormonal therapy is most commonly used to treat breast and prostate cancer. Some breast tumor cells contain estrogen in their cytoplasm (estrogen-receptor positive). Use of antiestrogens, such as tamoxifen, may keep the tumor from enlarging or metastasizing.

Elimination of the source of androgens in prostate cancer via orchiectomy may also reduce the cancer's spread.

Colony-stimulating factors may be used to sustain the patient with low blood counts during cancer treatment. Colony-stimulating factors, such as erythropoietin, may be given to reduce anemia.[7]

*Monoclonal antibodies* are antibodies of a single type produced by a single line of B lymphocytes. The antibodies are produced specifically to attach themselves to specific types of tumor cells. These antibodies can be used alone to attack cancer cells or may have radioactive material bound to them.

## Cancers in the Body Systems

Cancers can invade or affect any organ or tissue in the body. The following is a description of various cancers in each body system.

### Pulmonary Cancers

Cancer can affect any structure of the pulmonary system. The common types of lung cancer are *squamous cell carcinoma, adenocarcinoma, small cell carcinoma,* and *large cell carcinoma.*[6,7] Symptoms associated with these include chronic cough, dyspnea, adventitious breath sounds (e.g., wheezing, crackles), chest pain, and hemoptysis.[7]

Nonsurgical techniques, such as x-ray, computerized axial tomography, and positron emission tomography, can be used to stage lung cancer.[13] Table 5-7 describes pulmonary cancer sites and

**Table 5-7.** Surgical Interventions for Pulmonary Cancers

| Area Involved | Surgical Procedure | Excision of |
|---|---|---|
| Pleura | Pleurectomy | Portion of pleura |
| Rib | Rib resection | Portion of rib |
| Trachea and bronchi | Tracheal repair and reconstruction | Trachea |
| | Sleeve resection | Portion of main stem bronchus |
| Lung | Pneumonectomy | Entire single lung |
| | Lobectomy | Single or multiple lobes of the lung |
| | Wedge resection | Wedge-shaped segment of lung |

surgical procedures used in their management. Recent surgical advances include the use of video-assisted, non-rib spreading lobectomy to remove tumor and the use of an intraoperative ultrasound probe to aid in tumor localization.[14,15]

---

Clinical Tip

• Thoracic surgery may involve a large incision on the thoracic wall. Surgical incisions into the pleural space will cause deflation of the lung. Deep-breathing exercises, along with mucus clearance techniques with incisional splinting and range-of-motion exercises of the upper extremity on the side of the incision, are important to prevent postoperative pulmonary complications and restore shoulder and trunk mobility.
• Patients may have chest tubes in place immediately after surgery (see Appendix III-A).
• Oxygen supplementation may be required in post-thoracic surgical patients. Oxyhemoglobin saturation ($Sao_2$) should be monitored to ensure adequate oxygenation, especially when increasing activity levels.
• Caution must be taken when positioning patients after pneumonectomy. Placing patients with the existing lung in the dependent position may adversely affect ventilation, perfusion, and, ultimately, oxygenation. Positioning guidelines should be clarified with the surgeon, if not already stated.[16]

---

*Musculoskeletal Cancers*

Tumors of bone are most commonly discovered after an injury or fracture or during a medical work-up for pain. Some tumors in the bone or muscle may arise from other primary sites. Common primary tumors that metastasize to bone include breast, lung, prostate, kidney, and thyroid tumors.[17] Treatment of musculoskeletal tumors can include radiation, chemotherapy, amputation, arthroplasty (joint replacement), and reconstruction using an allograft (cadaver bone). Types of primary orthopedic cancers are described in Table 5-8.

Although not all metastases to bone cause pathologic fractures, surgical intervention can be used for a patient with a bone metastasis because of the risk of pathologic fracture. These procedures may

Table 5-8. Orthopedic Cancers

| Type of Tumor | Common Age Group | Common Site of Tumors |
|---|---|---|
| Osteosarcoma | Young children and young adults | Distal femur, proximal tibia Commonly metastasize to lung |
| Chondrosarcoma | Adults | Pelvis or femur |
| Fibrosarcoma | Adults | Femur or tibia |
| Rhabdomyosarcoma (Ewing's sarcoma) | Children and adolescents | Trunk, pelvis, and long bones |

include the use of intramedullary rods, plates, and prosthetic devices (e.g., total joint arthroplasty) and are described in Chapter 3 under Fracture Management, Appendix, and Total Joint Arthroplasty sections, respectively.

---

### Clinical Tip

• A patient with bone metastases must receive clearance from the physician before mobility, along with clarifying the patient's weight-bearing status.
• Patients commonly experience fractures owing to metastatic disease in the vertebrae, proximal humerus, and femur.[18] Therefore, patients should be instructed in safety management to avoid falls or trauma to involved areas.
• Check the weight-bearing status of patients after bone grafting, as weight bearing may be restricted.

---

### Breast Cancer

Breast cancer, although more prevalent in women, is also diagnosed in men to a lesser extent. It may be discovered during routine breast examinations or mammography. Common surgical procedures for the treatment of breast cancer are listed in Table 5-9.

**Table 5-9.** Surgical Interventions for Breast Cancer

| Surgical Intervention | Tissues Involved |
|---|---|
| Radical mastectomy | Removal of breast tissue, skin, pectoralis major and minor, rib, and lymph nodes |
| Modified radical mastectomy | Removal of breast, skin, and sampling axillary lymph nodes |
| Simple or total mastectomy | Removal of breast, then, in another procedure, a sampling of the axillary lymph nodes |
| Partial mastectomy | Removal of tumor and surrounding wedge of tissue |
| Lumpectomy or local wide excision | Removal of tumor and axillary lymph nodes resection in separate procedure |
| Reconstruction—implants | Saline implanted surgically beneath the skin or muscle |
| Reconstruction—muscle flap transfer | Muscle from stomach or back, including layers of skin fat and fascia, transferred to create a breast |

## Clinical Tip

• The physical therapist should check the physician's orders regarding upper-extremity range-of-motion restrictions, especially with muscle transfers. The therapist must know what muscles were resected or transferred during the procedure, the location of the incision, and whether there was any nerve involvement before mobilization. Once this information is clarified, the therapist should proceed to assess the range of motion of the shoulder and neck region, as it may be affected during surgical interventions for breast cancer.

• Patients may exhibit postoperative pain, lymphedema, or nerve injury due to trauma or traction during the operative procedure.

• Postoperative drains may be in place immediately after surgery, and the physical therapist should take care to avoid manipulating these drains. Range-of-motion exercises may cause the drain to be displaced.

- Incisions, resulting from muscle transfer flaps involving the rectus abdominis, pectoralis, or latissimus dorsi, should be supported when the patient coughs.
- The physical therapist should instruct the patient in the logroll technique, which is used to minimize contraction of the abdominal muscles while the patient is getting out of bed. The therapist should also instruct the patient to minimize contraction of the shoulder musculature during transfers.
- Lymphedema may need to be controlled with lymphedema massage, elevation, exercise while wearing nonelastic wraps, elastic garments, or compression pneumatic pumps, especially when surgery involves lymph nodes that are near the extremities. These techniques have been shown to be of value in decreasing lymphedema.[19-21] Circumferential or water displacement measurements of the involved upper extremity may be taken to record girth changes and to compare with the noninvolved extremity.
- The physical therapist should consider the impact of reconstructive breast surgery on the patient's sexuality, body image, and psychological state.[9]

## Gastrointestinal and Genitourinary Cancers

Gastrointestinal cancers can involve the esophagus, stomach, colon, and rectum. Cancers of the liver and pancreas, although considered gastrointestinal, will be discussed separately. Genitourinary cancers can involve the uterus, ovaries, testicles, prostate, bladder, and kidney. Surgical procedures used to treat genitourinary cancers are listed in Table 5-10; surgical procedures used to treat gastrointestinal cancers are described in Table 5-11.

### Clinical Tip

- Patients with genitourinary cancer may experience urinary incontinence. Bladder control training, pelvic floor exercises, and biofeedback or electrical stimulation may be necessary to restore control of urinary flow.[22-24]

**Table 5-10.**  Surgical Interventions for Genitourinary System Cancers

|  | Surgical Intervention | Excision |
|---|---|---|
| Uterus | Hysterectomy | Uterus through abdominal wall or vagina |
|  | Total abdominal hysterectomy | Body of uterus and cervix through abdominal wall |
|  | Subtotal abdominal hysterectomy | Uterus (cervix remains) |
| Ovary | Oophorectomy | One ovary |
| Ovaries and oviducts | Bilateral salpingo-oophorectomy | Both ovaries and oviducts |
| Prostate | Radical prostatectomy | Entire prostate |
| Testes | Orchiectomy | One or both testes |

• Patients with gastrointestinal cancer may experience bowel as well as urinary incontinence.

• Both bowel and bladder incontinence can lead to areas of dampened skin, which are prone to breakdown.[25] Therefore, physical therapists should be careful to minimize shearing forces in these areas during mobility.

**Table 5-11.**  Surgical Interventions for Gastrointestinal System Cancers

| Area Involved | Surgical Intervention | Excision |
|---|---|---|
| Stomach | Subtotal gastrectomy | Portion of the stomach |
|  | Near-total gastrectomy | Body of the stomach |
|  | Total gastrectomy | Entire stomach |
|  | Gastroduodenostomy | Portion of the stomach and duodenum |
|  | Gastrojejunostomy | Portion of the stomach and jejunum |
| Colon | Hemicolectomy | Portion of the colon |
| Rectum | Anterior or low-anterior resection | Upper-third of the rectum |
|  | Abdominal perineal resection | Middle- and lower-third of the rectum |

## Hepatobiliary Cancers

Primary liver tumors can arise from hepatic cells, connective tissue, blood vessels, or bile ducts. Primary malignant liver carcinomas are almost always associated with cirrhosis. Benign liver tumors are associated with women taking oral contraceptives. Most benign liver tumors are asymptomatic.

*Hepatic adenomas* (benign hepatic cell tumors) are highly vascular, and patients carry the risk of hepatic rupture. *Hepatomas*, or malignant hepatic parenchymal cell tumors, are closely associated with male gender, excessive ethanol use, hepatitis B, and hepatitis C. Treatment is usually with chemoembolization or tumor resection. Patients with a small, nonmetastasizing hepatoma may be treated with liver transplantation. Untreated hepatoma has a very poor prognosis. Five-year survival rates for treated tumors are 15–45%.[7]

Cancer of the biliary tract is usually found during surgery for another biliary disease or when metastasizing to other organs, particularly the liver. Treatment is by surgery, but prognosis is poor.

In both hepatic cancer and biliary cancer, laboratory values are used to diagnose, prognose, and monitor the course of treatment. Liver function tests may include bilirubin, aspartate aminotransferase (AST), alanine aminotransferase (ALT), lactate dehydrogenase (LDH), gamma-glutamyltransferase, alkaline phosphatase, coagulation factors, and serum proteins.

Surgical interventions for the hepatobiliary system are outlined in Table 5-12.

Table 5-12. Surgical Interventions for the Hepatobiliary System

| Area Involved | Surgical Intervention | Excision |
| --- | --- | --- |
| Pancreas | Whipple procedure | Duodenum and proximal pancreas |
| Liver | Segmental resection | Complete segment of liver |
| | Subsegmental resection | Portion of a segment of liver |

## Clinical Tip

Any patient with hepatic adenoma must be cautioned to avoid lifting heavy objects or performing maneuvers that increase intra-abdominal pressure.

## Pancreatic Cancer

The incidence of pancreatic cancer doubled in the late twentieth century.[26] Most pancreatic tumors arise from the pancreatic duct and are found in the head of the pancreas. Pain and jaundice are the most usual clinical manifestations; these symptoms occur as the tumor invades surrounding tissue, especially the liver and gallbladder. Treatment usually focuses on tumor resection, alleviation of pain, and prevention of gastric outlet obstruction. Surgery (Table 5-12), radiation, and chemotherapy are used as treatment. Recent treatments include supravoltage radiation plus chemotherapy.[27] Patients with nonresectable tumors have benefited from placement of a biliary stent or gastric operative bypass.[28] Even so, prognosis is poor because the disease has usually metastasized by the time it is diagnosed.[3]

## Hematologic Cancers

Hematologic cancers can arise from any blood-forming tissue. These malignancies include the leukemias, lymphomas, and multiple myeloma. The malignant cells can occur in the blood stream, bone marrow, spleen, lymph nodes, and thymus, and, in some cases, they can invade bone itself.

### Leukemia

The leukemias are malignancies of white blood cells, most commonly granulocytes (neutrophils or polymorphonuclear leukocytes) and lymphocytes. These malignant cells first occupy the bone marrow, replacing normal cells, then spill into the blood stream.

Because the malignant cells first occupy the bone marrow, they can occlude the space occupied by normal bone marrow cells. As a result, patients can have anemia, thrombocytopenia, and leukopenia. Often,

Table 5-13. Types of Leukemia

| Type | Cells Involved | Age Range (yrs) |
|------|---------------|-----------------|
| Acute lymphocytic leukemia | Lymphocytes | 3–7 |
| Acute nonlymphocytic leukemia | Stem cells | 15–40 |
| Chronic myelogenous leukemia | Granulocytes | 25–60 |
| Chronic lymphocytic leukemia | Lymphocytes | 50+ |

the clinical manifestations of leukemia are fatigue, easy bruising, and infections. (Refer to Chapter 6 for hematologic information.)

Leukemia is classified as acute or chronic, depending on the maturity of the malignant cell. Acute leukemia is from a more immature white blood cell; disease progression tends to be rapid. Chronic leukemias are from more mature cells; disease progression is usually slower. Acute leukemias tend to occur in children and young adults. Chronic leukemia tends to occur in older adults. Types of leukemia, cells affected, and common age ranges are listed in Table 5-13.

### Lymphomas

Lymphomas are malignancies of lymphocytic cells and lymph tissues. Unlike leukemic cells that occupy bone marrow and spill into the blood stream, lymphomas occupy lymph tissue (lymph nodes and spleen). Occupation of the lymph nodes usually causes painless enlargement, often the first sign of lymphoma.

The most common type of lymphoma is Hodgkin's lymphoma. The other most common types of lymphoma are non-Hodgkin's (malignant or lymphosarcoma) and Burkitt's lymphomas. Burkitt's lymphoma is a solid tumor of B-cell origin, endemic in Africa.[1,7] Characteristics of Hodgkin's and non-Hodgkin's lymphomas can be found in Table 5-14.

Table 5-14. Characteristics of Hodgkin's and Non-Hodgkin's Lymphomas

| | Hodgkin's Lymphoma | Non-Hodgkin's Lymphoma |
|---|---|---|
| Nodal involvement | Usually involves single node site | Usually involves more than one site |
| Spread | Usually orderly | Nonorderly |
| Extranodal involvement | Uncommon | Common |

Table 5-15.   Stages of Lymphoma, Ann Arbor Classification

| Stage | Distribution of Disease |
|-------|-------------------------|
| I | Single lymph node region or single extralymphatic organ or site involved |
| II | Two or more lymph node regions on the same side of the diaphragm involved or involvement of limited continuous extralymphatic organ |
| III | Lymph node regions on both sides of the diaphragm, limited contiguous extralymphatic organ involvement, or both |
| IV | Multiple, disseminated involvement of one or more extralymphatic organs, with or without lymphatic involvement |

Source: Adapted from Carbone PP, Kaplan HS, Musshoff K, et al. Report of the Committee on Hodgkin's Disease Staging Classification. Cancer Res 1971;31(11):1860–1861.

For lymphoma, the TNM system has generally been replaced by the Ann Arbor Classification. This classification is based on the number and location of lymph nodes involved. The Ann Arbor Classification can be found in Table 5-15.

*Prognosis*
If left untreated, all leukemias and lymphomas are fatal. Malignant cells can infiltrate all major blood vessels and organs, causing occlusion and infarction. Infiltration into the musculoskeletal structures can result in joint hemorrhage, rheumatologic-type symptoms, and synovitis. Infiltration of neurologic tissues can result in nerve palsies, encephalopathy, headache, vomiting, blurred vision, and auditory problems.[1] In addition, the decreased number of normal immunologic cells leaves the patient highly susceptible to infection.

*Treatment*
Leukemias are treated with chemotherapy, radiation, hormone therapy, and bone marrow transplantation. Lymphoma is treated with chemotherapy, irradiation, or both. Some of the slower-growing leukemias are left untreated, especially if the patient is elderly.[3] Bone marrow transplantation is discussed in Chapter 12.

Clinical Tip

Platelet counts and hematocrit should be assessed to determine a safe level of activity or exercise. See Bone Marrow Transplant in Chapter 12 for specific guidelines.

## Multiple Myeloma

*Multiple myeloma* is a malignancy of plasma cells, which are derived from B-lymphocytes (B-cells), and are responsible for creating antibodies. The disease is characterized by the tumor's arising in the bone marrow of flat bones and the infiltration of the myeloma cells into the bone and, eventually, other organs. These malignant cells produce a single type of antibody that may increase the viscosity of the blood. Classically, the disease produces bone pain and decreased number of normal hematologic cells (e.g., red blood cells, white blood cells, and platelets).

The disease has a slow progression. Most persons affected with multiple myeloma have an asymptomatic period that can last up to 20 years.[1] Bone pain, usually the first symptom, occurs when the myeloma cells have destroyed bone. Lesions created in the bone by the malignant cells can cause pathologic fractures, especially in the vertebral bodies. As further bone is destroyed, calcium and phosphorus are released, causing renal stones and renal failure.[1,2,7]

Amyloidosis may occur in patients with multiple myeloma. Deposition of this glycoprotein in tissues may cause them to become hard and waxy.

Myeloma is treated with chemotherapy, biotherapy, radiation, and bone marrow transplantation. No treatment is curative.

---

### Clinical Tip

- People with advanced stages of multiple myeloma may be dehydrated. Ensure proper hydration before any type of intervention.
- Activity clearance should be obtained from the physician before mobilizing anyone with bone lesions.

---

### Head, Neck, and Facial Tumors

Head, neck, and facial cancers involve the paranasal sinuses, nasal and oral cavities, salivary glands, pharynx, and larynx. Environmental factors and personal habits (e.g., tobacco use) are often closely associated with the development of cancer in this region.[29]

Physical therapy intervention may be indicated after the treatment of head, neck, and facial tumors. Surgical procedures include radical neck dissection, laryngectomy, and reconstructive surgery. Radical neck dissections may include removal or partial removal of the larynx, tonsils, lip, tongue, thyroid gland, parotid gland, cervical musculature (including the sternocleidomastoid, platysma, omohyoid, and floor of the mouth), internal and external jugular veins, and lymph nodes.[30] Reconstructive surgery may include a skin flap, muscle flap, or both to cover resected areas of the neck and face. The pectoralis or trapezius muscle is used during muscle flap reconstructive procedures. A facial prosthesis is sometimes used to help the patient attain adequate cosmesis and speech.

### Clinical Tip

• Postoperatively, impairment of the respiratory system should be considered in patients with head, neck, and facial tumors because of possible obstruction of the airway or difficulty managing oral secretions. A common associated factor in patients with oral cancer is the use of tobacco (both chewing and smoking); therefore, possible underlying lung disease must also be considered. During physical therapy assessment, the patient should be assessed for adventitious breath sounds and effectiveness of airway clearance. Oral secretions should be cleared effectively before assessing breath sounds.
• Proper positioning is important to prevent aspiration and excessive edema that may occur after surgery of the face, neck, and head.
• Patients may also require a tracheostomy, artificial airway, or both to manage the airway and secretions.
• After a surgical procedure, the physician should determine activity and range-of-motion restrictions, especially after skin and muscle flap reconstructions. Physical therapy treatment to restore posture and neck, shoulder, scapulothoracic, and temporomandibular motion is emphasized.
• When treating patients with head, neck, and facial cancers, it is important to consider the potential difficulties with speech, chewing, or swallowing and loss of sensations, including smell, taste, hearing, and sight.
• Because the patient may have difficulty with communicating and swallowing, referring the patient to a speech therapist and registered dietitian may be necessary.

## Neurologic Cancers

Tumors of the nervous system can invade the brain, spinal cord, and peripheral nerves. Brain tumors can occur in astrocytes (astrocytoma), meninges (meningeal sarcoma), and nerve cells (neuroblastoma), or they can be the result of cancer that has metastasized to the brain.[9] Symptoms related to cancers of the nervous system depend on the size of the tumor and the area of the nervous system involved. Neurologic symptoms can persist after tumor excision, owing to destruction of neurologic tissues. Changes in neurologic status due to compression of tissues within the nervous system can indicate further spread of the tumor or may be related to edema of brain tissue. Sequelae include cognitive deficits, skin changes, bowel and bladder control problems, sexual dysfunction, and the need for assistive devices and positioning devices. After resection of a brain tumor, patients may demonstrate many other neurologic sequelae, including hemiplegia and ataxia. Radiation therapy to structures of the nervous system may also cause transient neurologic symptoms.

---

### Clinical Tip

The therapist should assess the patient's need for skin care, splinting, positioning, assistance in activities of daily living, cognitive training, gait training, balance, assistive devices, and special equipment. See Chapter 4 for further treatment considerations.

---

## Skin Cancer

The physical therapist may identify suspicious lesions during examination or treatment, and these should be reported to the medical doctor. Suspicious lesions are characterized by (1) irregular or asymmetric borders, (2) uneven coloring, (3) nodules or ulceration, (4) bleeding or crusting, and (5) change in color, size, or thickness. Cancers of the skin include basal cell cancer, squamous cell cancer, malignant melanoma, and Kaposi's sarcoma.[1]

Basal cell carcinoma is the most common skin cancer.[9] It is usually found in areas exposed to the sun, including the face, ears, neck, scalp, shoulders, and back. Risk factors include chronic exposure to the sun, light eyes, and fair skin. Diagnosis is made with a biopsy or a tissue sample. The following are five warning signs of basal cell carcinoma the physical therapist should look for when working with patients[31]:

- Open sore that bleeds, oozes, or crusts and remains open for 3 or more weeks

- Reddish patch or irritated area, which may crust, itch, or hurt

- Smooth growth with an elevated, rolled border, and an indentation in the center; tiny vessels may develop on the surface

- Shiny bump or nodule that is pearly or translucent and is often pink (can be tan, black, or brown in dark-haired individuals)

- Scar-like area that is white, yellow, or waxy, with poorly defined borders and shiny, taut skin

Squamous cell cancer usually occurs in areas exposed to the sun or ultraviolet radiation. Lesions may be elevated and appear scaly or keratotic (horny growth).[9] Squamous cell lesions can metastasize to the lymph nodes, lungs, bone, and brain.

*Malignant melanoma* is a neoplasm that arises from the melanocytes. Risk factors include previous history or family history of melanoma, immunosuppression, and a history of blistering sunburns before age 20. Malignant melanoma can metastasize to the lymph nodes, lung, brain, liver, bone, and other areas of the skin.[9] Moles or pigmented spots exhibiting the following signs (called the *ABCD rule*) may indicate malignant melanoma[9]:

A = *A*symmetry

B = Irregular *b*order

C = Varied *c*olor

D = *D*iameter of more than 6 mm

---

**Clinical Tip**

- After resection of skin lesions, proper positioning is important to prevent skin breakdown.

- The physical therapist should assess the need for positioning and splinting devices.
- The physical therapist should determine the location of the lesion and the need for range-of-motion exercises to prevent contractures. If the lesion involves an area that will be stressed (e.g., joints), the physical therapist should check the physician's orders for precautions limiting motion.

## General Physical Therapy Guidelines for Patients with Cancer

The following are general goals and guidelines for the physical therapist working with the patient who has cancer. These guidelines should be adapted to a patient's specific needs.

The primary goals of physical therapy in this patient population are similar to those of other patients in the acute care setting; however, because of the systemic nature of cancer, the time frames for achieving goals will most likely be longer. These goals are to (1) optimize functional mobility, (2) maximize activity tolerance and endurance, (3) prevent joint contracture and skin breakdown, (4) prevent or reduce limb edema, and (5) prevent postoperative pulmonary complications.

General guidelines include, but are not limited to, the following:

- Knowing the stage and grade of cancer can help the physical therapist modify a patient's treatment parameters and establish realistic goals and intervention.

- Patients may be placed on bed rest while receiving cancer treatment or postoperatively and will be at risk for developing pulmonary complications, deconditioning, and skin breakdown. Deep-breathing exercises, frequent position changes, and an exercise program that can be performed in bed are beneficial in counteracting these complications.

- Patients who have metastatic processes, especially to bone, are at high risk for pathologic fracture. Pulmonary hygiene is indicated for most patients who undergo surgical procedures. Care should be taken with patients who have metastatic processes during the performance of manual chest physical therapy techniques. Metastatic processes should also be considered when prescribing resistive exercises to patients, as the muscle action on the frail bone may be enough to cause fracture.

• Patient and family education regarding safety management, energy conservation, postural awareness, and body mechanics during activities of daily living should be provided. An assessment of the appropriate assistive devices, prosthetics, and required orthotics should also be performed. Decreased sensation requires special attention when prescribing and fitting adaptive devices.

• If a patient is placed on isolation precautions, exercise equipment, such as stationary bicycles or upper-extremity ergometers (after being thoroughly cleaned with sterile solutions), should be placed in his or her room. Assessment is necessary for the appropriateness of this equipment, along with the safety of independent use.

• When performing mobility or exercise treatments, care should be taken to avoid bruising or bleeding into joint spaces when patients have low platelet counts.

• Emotional support for both the patient and family is at times the most appreciated and effective method in helping to accomplish the physical therapy goals.

• Timely communication with the entire health care team is essential for safe and effective care. Communication should minimally include patient's current functional status, progress toward patient's goals, and any factors that are interfering with the patient's progress.

• Laboratory values, especially hemoglobin/hematocrit, white blood cell count, platelet count, and prothrombin time/international normalized ratio (PT/INR) should be monitored daily.

## References

1. Cotran RS, Kumar V, Robbins S, Schoes FJ (eds). Robbins Pathologic Basis of Disease. Philadelphia: Saunders, 1994.
2. Goodman CC, Boissonnault WG (eds). Pathology: Implications for the Physical Therapist. Philadelphia: Saunders, 1998.

3. Tamparo CD, Lewis MA (eds). Diseases of the Human Body (3rd ed). Philadelphia: FA Davis, 2000.

4. Thomas CL (ed). Taber's Cyclopedic Medical Dictionary (17th ed). Philadelphia: FA Davis, 1993.

5. Baird S (ed). A Cancer Source Book for Nurses (6th ed). Atlanta: American Cancer Society, 1991.

6. American Cancer Society. Cancer Manual (8th ed). Boston: American Cancer Society, 1990;292.

7. Tierney LM, McPhee SJ, Papadakis MA (eds). Current Medical Diagnosis and Treatment. New York: McGraw-Hill, 2000.

8. Moreau D (ed). Nursing '96 Drug Handbook. Springhouse, PA: Springhouse, 1996;657, 944.

9. Wells NJ, Boyle JC, Snelling CF, et al. Lower extremity burns and Unna paste: Can we decrease health care costs without compromising patient care? Can J Surg 1995;38(6):533–536.

10. Poole GH, Mills SM. One hundred consecutive cases of flap lacerations of the leg in ageing patients. N Z Med J 1994;28;107(986 Pt 1):377–378.

11. Budny PG, Lavelle J, Regan PJ, Roberts AH. Pretibial injuries in the elderly: a prospective trial of early mobilisation versus bed rest following surgical treatment. Br J Plast Surg 1993;46(7):594–598.

12. Norris J (ed). Professional Guide to Diseases (5th ed). Springhouse, PA: Springhouse, 1995.

13. Lewis RJ, Caccavale RJ, Bocage JP, Widmann MD. Video-assisted thoracic surgical non-rib spreading simultaneously stapled lobectomy; a more patient-friendly oncologic resection. Chest 1999;116(4):1119–1124.

14. Santambrogio R, Montorsi M, Bianchi P, et al. Intraoperative ultrasound during thoracoscopic procedures for solitary pulmonary nodules. Ann Thorac Surg 1999;68(1):218–222.

15. Matin TA, Goldberg M. Surgical staging of lung cancer. Oncology. 1999;13(5):679–685.

16. Burrell LO (ed). Adult Nursing in Hospital and Community Settings. East Norwalk, CT: Appleton & Lange, 1992;558, 816.

17. Baird S (ed). A Cancer Source Book for Nurses (6th ed). Atlanta: American Cancer Society, 1991.

18. Hicks JE. Exercise for Cancer Patients. In JV Basmajian, SL Wolf (eds), Therapeutic Exercise. Baltimore: Williams & Wilkins, 1990;351.

19. Badger CM, Peacock JL, Mortimer PS. A randomized, controlled, parallel-groups clinical trial comparing multilayer bandaging followed by hosiery versus hosiery alone in the treatment of patients with lymphedema of the limb. Cancer 2000;88(12):2832–2837.

20. Berlin E, Gjores JE, Ivarsson C, et al. Postmastectomy lymphoedema. Treatment and a five-year follow-up study. Int Angiol 1999;18(4):294–298.

21. Johansson K, Albertsson M, Ingvar C, Ekdahl C. Effects of compression bandaging with or without manual lymph drainage treatment in patients with postoperative arm lymphedema. Lymphology 1999;32(3):103–110.

22. Mattiasson A. Discussion: bladder and pelvic floor muscle training for overactive bladder. Urology 2000;55(Suppl 5A):12–16.
23. Lewey J, Lilas L. Electrical stimulation of the overactive bladder. Prof Nurse 1999;15(3):211–214.
24. Cammu H, Van Nylen M, Amy JJ. A 10-year follow-up after Kegel pelvic floor muscle exercises for genuine stress incontinence. BJU Int 2000;85(6):655–658.
25. Gibbons G. Skin care and incontinence. Community Nurse 1996; 2(7):37.
26. Murr MM, Sarr MG, Oishi AJ. Pancreatic cancer. CA Cancer J Clin 1994;44:304–318.
27. Brunner TB, Grabenbauer GG, Baum U, et al. Adjuvant and neoadjuvant radiochemotherapy in ductal pancreatic carcinoma. Strahlenther Onkol 2000 Jun;176(6):265–273.
28. Schwarz A, Beger HG. Biliary and gastric bypass or stenting in nonresectable periampullary cancer: analysis on the basis of controlled trials. Int J Pancreatol 2000;27(1):51–58.
29. Reese JL. Head and Neck Cancers. In R McCorkle, M Grant, M Frank-Stromberg, S Baird (eds), Cancer Nursing: A Comprehensive Textbook (2nd ed). Philadelphia: Saunders, 1996;567.
30. Haskell CM (ed). Cancer Treatment (4th ed). Philadelphia: Saunders, 1995;343, 457.
31. Robins P, Kopf A. Squamous Cell Carcinoma [pamphlet]. New York: Skin Cancer Foundation, 1990;1.

# 6

# Vascular System and Hematology
## *Michele P. West and Jaime C. Paz*

### Introduction

Alterations in the integrity of the vascular and hematologic systems can alter a patient's activity tolerance. The physical therapist must be aware of the potential impact that a change in blood composition or blood flow has on a multitude of body functions, including cardiac output, hemostasis, energy level, and healing. The objectives of this chapter are to provide the following:

1.  A review of the structure and function of blood and blood vessels

2.  A review of vascular and hematologic evaluation, including physical examination and diagnostic and laboratory tests

3.  A description of vascular and hematologic diseases and disorders, including clinical findings, medical and surgical management, and physical therapy intervention

## Structure

The network of arteries, veins, and capillaries comprises the vascular system. Living blood cells and plasma within the blood vessels are the structures that comprise the hematologic system. The lymphatic system assists the vascular system by draining unabsorbed plasma from tissue spaces and returning this fluid (lymph) to the heart via the thoracic duct, which empties into the left jugular vein. The flow of lymph is regulated by intrinsic contractions of the lymph vessels, muscular contractions, respiratory movements, and gravity.[1]

### Vascular System Structure

All blood vessels are composed of three similar layers. Table 6-1 describes the structural characteristics of the three different blood vessel layers. Blood vessel diameter, length, and wall thickness vary according to location and function. Table 6-2 describes the unique characteristics of arteries, veins, and capillaries.

**Table 6-1.** Blood Vessel Layers

| Layer | Description | Function |
|-------|-------------|----------|
| Tunica intima | Innermost layer Endothelial layer over a basement membrane | Provides a smooth surface for laminar blood flow |
| Tunica media | Middle layer Smooth muscle cells and elastic connective tissue with sympathetic innervation | Constricts and dilates for blood pressure regulation |
| Tunica adventitia | Outermost layer Composed of collagen fibers, lymph vessels, and the blood vessels that supply nutrients to the blood vessel | Protects and attaches blood vessels to nearby structures |

Source: Data from The Cardiovascular System: Blood Vessels. In EN Marieb, Human Anatomy and Physiology (3rd ed). Redwood City, CA: Benjamin-Cummings, 1995.

**Table 6-2.** Characteristics of Blood Vessels

| Vessel | Description |
| --- | --- |
| Artery | Small, medium, or large in diameter. Larger arteries are located closer to the heart. Thick tunica media layer allows arteries to readily accommodate to pressure changes from the heart. |
| Vein | Small, medium, or large in diameter. Thin tunica media and thick tunica adventitia. Valves prevent backflow of blood to maintain venous return to the heart. |
| Capillary network | The interface of the arterial and venous systems where blood cells, fluids, and gases are exchanged. Capillary beds can be open or closed, depending on the circulatory requirements of the body. |

Source: Data from The Cardiovascular System: Blood. In EN Marieb, Human Anatomy and Physiology (3rd ed). Redwood City, CA: Benjamin-Cummings, 1995.

## Hematologic System Structure

Blood is composed of living cells in a nonliving plasma solution and accounts for 8% of total body weight, or 4–5 liters in women and 5–6 liters in men. Table 6-3 describes the characteristics of the different blood cells. Plasma is composed almost completely of water and contains more than 100 dissolved substances. The major solutes include albumin, fibrinogen, protein globules, nitrogenous substances, nutrients, electrolytes, and respiratory gases.[2]

## Function

The function of the blood vessels is to carry blood throughout the body to and from the heart. Normal alterations in the vessel diameter will occur depending on circulating blood volume and the metabolic needs of the tissues.

The following are the seven major functions of blood[2]:

1.    The transport of oxygen and nutrients to body cells from the lungs and gastrointestinal organs, respectively

Table 6-3. Blood Cell Types

| Cell | Description |
| --- | --- |
| Erythrocyte (red blood cell) (RBC) | Contains hemoglobin molecules responsible for oxygen transport to tissues. Composed of four protein chains (two alpha and two beta chains) bound to four iron pigment complexes. An oxygen molecule attaches to each iron atom to become oxyhemoglobin. |
| Leukocyte (white blood cell) (WBC) | Five types of WBCs (neutrophils, basophils, eosinophils, lymphocytes, and monocytes) are responsible for launching immune defenses and fighting infection. WBCs leave the circulation to gain access to a site of infection. |
| Thrombocyte (platelet) | Cell fragment responsible for clot formation. |

Source: Data from The Cardiovascular System: Blood. In EN Marieb, Human Anatomy and Physiology (3rd ed). Redwood City, CA: Benjamin-Cummings, 1995.

2.   The transport of carbon dioxide and metabolic waste products to the lungs and kidneys, respectively

3.   The transport of hormones from endocrine glands to target organs

4.   The maintenance of body temperature via conduction and dispersal of heat

5.   The maintenance of pH with buffers freely circulating in the blood

6.   The formation of clots

7.   The prevention of infection with white blood cells (WBCs), antibodies, and complement

The vascular and hematologic systems are intimately linked, and the examination of these systems is often similar. For the purpose of this chapter, however, the evaluation of the vascular and hematologic systems is discussed separately.

## Physical Examination

### *Vascular Evaluation*

#### History

In addition to the general chart review (see Appendix I-A), the following information is important to gather during the examination of the patient with a suspected vascular disorder[3]:

- Relevant medical history that includes diabetes mellitus, hypertension, syncope or vertigo, and nonhealing ulcers.

- Relevant social history that includes exercise and dietary habits, as well as the use of tobacco or alcohol.

- Presence of intermittent claudication (leg pain that occurs with walking). When (onset) and where (location) does it occur, and what makes it better?

- Presence or history of peripheral edema. Is it acute or chronic? If chronic, what is the patient's baseline level of edema?

- Precautions, such as weight bearing or blood pressure parameters after vascular surgery.

---

#### Clinical Tip

Intermittent claudication is often abbreviated in the clinical setting as IC.

---

#### Inspection

Observation of the following features can help delineate the location and severity of vascular disease and help determine whether these manifestations are arterial or venous in origin[1,3]:

- Skin color. (Note the presence of any discoloration of the distal extremities, which is indicative of decreased blood flow—e.g., mottled skin.)

- Hair distribution. (Patchy hair loss on the lower leg may indicate arterial insufficiency.)

- Venous pattern (dilation or varicosities).

- Edema or atrophy. (Peripheral edema from right-sided congestive heart failure occurs bilaterally in dependent areas; edema from trauma, lymphatic obstruction, or chronic venous insufficiency is generally unilateral.) Refer to Table 1-6, Pitting Edema Scale.

- Presence of cellulitis.

- Presence of petechiae (small, purplish, hemorrhagic spots on the skin).

- Skin lesions (ulcers, blisters, or scars).

- Digital clubbing (could be indicative of poor arterial oxygenation or circulation).

- Gait abnormalities.

## Palpation

During the palpation portion of the examination, the physical therapist can assess the presence of pain and tenderness, strength and rate of peripheral pulses, respiratory rate, blood pressure, skin temperature, and limb girth (if edematous). Changes in heart rate, blood pressure, and respiratory rate may correspond to changes in the fluid volume status of the patient. For example, a decrease in fluid volume may result in a decreased blood pressure that results in a compensatory increase in heart and respiratory rates. The decreased fluid volume and resultant increased heart rate in this situation may then result in a decreased strength of the peripheral pulses on palpation. In patients with suspected or diagnosed peripheral vascular disease, monitoring distal pulses is more important than monitoring central pulses in the larger, more proximal vessels.[3]

The following are two systems used to grade peripheral pulses:

1. On the scale of 0–3 as[1]

   0  Absent

   +1  Weak and thready pulse

   +2  Normal

   +3  Full and bounding pulse

2.  On the scale of 0–4 as[4]

   0  Absent

   1  Markedly diminished

   2  Moderately diminished

   3  Slightly diminished

   4  Normal

Peripheral pulses can be assessed in the following arteries (see Figure 1-6):

*   Temporal
*   Carotid
*   Brachial
*   Ulnar
*   Radial
*   Femoral
*   Popliteal
*   Posterior tibial
*   Dorsalis pedis

---

**Clinical Tip**

*   Peripheral pulse grades are generally denoted in the medical record by physicians in the following manner: dorsalis pedis +1.
*   A small percentage of the adult population may normally have absent peripheral pulses—for example, 10–17% lack dorsalis pedis pulses.[1]
*   In patients who have disorders resulting in vascular compromise (e.g., diabetes mellitus, peripheral vascular disease, or hypertension), pulses should be monitored before, during, and after activity not only to determine any rate changes, but, more important, to determine any changes in the strength of the pulse.

- Notation should be made if the strength of pulses is correlated to complaints of pain, numbness, or tingling of the extremity.

---

## Auscultation

Systemic blood pressure and the presence of bruits (whooshing sound indicative of turbulent blood flow from obstructions) are assessed through auscultation.[3] Bruits are typically assessed by physicians and nurses (see Chapter 1 for further details on blood pressure measurement).

## Vascular Tests

Various tests that can be performed clinically to evaluate vascular flow and integrity are described in Table 6-4. These tests can be performed easily at the patient's bedside without the use of diagnostic equipment.

## Diagnostic Studies

### Noninvasive Laboratory Studies

Various noninvasive procedures can examine vascular flow. The phrases lower-extremity noninvasive studies and carotid noninvasive studies are general descriptions that are inclusive of the noninvasive tests described in Table 6-5.

### Invasive Vascular Studies

The most common invasive vascular study is arteriography, typically referred to as contrast angiography. This study provides anatomic and diagnostic information about the arterial system by injecting radiopaque dye into the femoral, lumbar, brachial, or axillary arteries, followed by radiographic viewing. An angiogram is a picture produced by angiography. Angiography is generally performed before or during therapeutic interventions, such as percutaneous angioplasty, thrombolytic therapy, or surgical bypass grafting.

Postangiogram care includes the following[5]:

- Bed rest for 4–8 hours.

- Pressure dressings to the injection site with assessment for hematoma formation.

- Intravenous fluid administration to help with dye excretion. Blood urea nitrogen (BUN) and creatinine are monitored to ensure proper renal function (refer to Chapter 9 for more information on BUN and creatinine).

**Table 6-4.** Vascular Tests

| Test | Indication | Description | Normal Results and Values |
|------|-----------|-------------|---------------------------|
| Capillary refill time | To assess vacular perfusion and indirectly assess cardiac output | Nail beds of fingers or toes are squeezed until blanching (whitening) occurs, and then they are released. | Blanching should resolve (capillary refill) in less than 3 secs. |
| Elevation pallor | To assess arterial perfusion | A limb is elevated 30–40 degrees, and color changes are observed over 60 secs.<br><br>A gray or pale (pallor) discoloration will result from arterial insufficiency or occlusion. | Grading of pallor:<br>0 = no pallor in 60 secs<br>1 = pallor in 60 secs<br>2 = pallor in 30–60 secs<br>3 = pallor in less than 30 secs<br>4 = pallor with limb flat (not elevated or dependent) |
| Trendelenburg's test | To determine if superficial or deep veins are involved in causing varicosities | A tourniquet is applied to the involved lower extremity, which is elevated while the patient is supine. The patient then stands, and the filling of the varicosities is observed. | Greater saphenous veins are involved if the varicosities fill slowly with the tourniquet on and then suddenly dilate when the tourniquet is removed.<br><br>Deep and communicating veins are involved if the varicosities fill immediately with the tourniquet still on. |

Table 6-4. *Continued*

| Test | Indication | Description | Normal Results and Values |
|------|-----------|-------------|---------------------------|
| Allen's test | To assess the patency of the radial and ulnar arteries | The radial and ulnar arteries are compressed at the level of the wrist while the patient clenches his or her fist. The patient then opens his or her hand and either the radial or the ulnar artery is released. The process is repeated for the other artery. | The pale and mottled hand that results from arterial compression and clenching should resolve in the arterial distribution of either the radial or ulnar artery, depending on which was released. |
| Homans' sign* | To detect the presence of deep vein thrombosis | The calf muscle is gently squeezed, or the foot is quickly dorsiflexed. | Pain that is elicited with either squeezing or dorsiflexing may indicate a deep vein thrombosis. |

*A 50% false-positive rate occurs with this test. Vascular laboratory studies are more sensitive.

Sources: Data from JM Black, E Matassarin-Jacobs (eds), Luckmann and Sorensen's Medical-Surgical Nursing: A Psychophysiologic Approach (4th ed). Philadelphia: Saunders, 1993; P Lanzer, J Rosch (eds). Vascular Diagnostics: Noninvasive and Invasive Techniques, Peri-Interventional Evaluations. Berlin: Springer-Verlag, 1994; and JW Hallet, DC Brewster, RC Darling (eds). Handbook of Patient Care in Vascular Surgery (3rd ed). Boston: Little, Brown, 1995.

**Table 6-5.** Noninvasive Vascular Studies

| Test | Description |
| --- | --- |
| Doppler ultrasound | High-frequency and low-intensity (1–10 MHz) sound waves are applied to the skin with a Doppler probe (and acoustic gel) to detect the presence or absence of blood flow, direction of flow, and flow character over arteries and veins with an audible signal. Low-frequency waves generally indicate low-velocity blood flow. |
| Color duplex scanning or imaging | Velocity patterns of blood flow along with visual images of vessel and plaque anatomy can be obtained by combing ultrasound with a pulsed Doppler detector. Distinctive color changes indicate blood flow through a stenotic area. |
| Plethysmography (5 types) Pulse volume recorder (PVR) Ocular pneumoplethysmography (OPG) Impedance plethysmography (IPG) Phleborheography (PRG) Photoplethysmography (PPG) | Plethysmography is the measurement of volume change in an organ or body region (*volume change* in this context refers to blood volume changes that represent blood flow). PVR and OPG are used to evaluate arterial flow, whereas IPG, PRG, and PPG are used to evaluate venous flow. |

**Table 6-5.** *Continued*

| Test | Description |
|------|-------------|
| Ankle-brachial index (ABI) | Systolic blood pressures are taken in both upper extremities at the brachial arteries and both lower extremities above the ankle, followed by Doppler evaluation of dorsalis pedis or posterior tibialis pulses. The higher of the lower-extremity pressures is then divided by the higher of the upper-extremity pressures (e.g., an ankle pressure of 70 mm Hg and a brachial pressure of 140 mm Hg will yield an ABI of 0.5). |
| | Normal ABI for foot arteries is 0.95–1.20, with indexes below 0.95 indicating arterial obstruction. |
| Exercise testing | Exercise testing is performed to assess the nature of claudication by measuring ankle pressures and PVRs after exercise. |
| | A drop in ankle pressures can occur with arterial disease. |
| | This type of testing provides a controlled method to document onset, severity, and location of claudication. |
| | Screening for cardiorespiratory disease can also be performed, as patients with peripheral vascular disease often have concurrent cardiac or pulmonary disorders (see Chapter 1). |
| Computed tomography (CT) | CT is used to provide visualization of the arterial wall and its structures. |
| | Indications for CT include diagnosis of abdominal aortic aneurysms and postoperative complications of graft infections, occlusions, hemorrhage, and abscess. |

| Magnetic resonance imaging (MRI) | MRI has multiple uses in evaluating the vascular system and is now more commonly used to visualize the arterial system than arteriograms. Specific uses for MRI include detection of deep venous thrombosis and evaluation of cerebral edema. Serial MRIs can also be used to help determine the optimal operative time for patients with cerebrovascular accidents by monitoring their progression. |
| Magnetic resonance angiography (MRA) | MRA uses blood as a physiologic contrast medium to examine the structure and location of major blood vessels and the flow of blood through these vessels. The direction and rate of flow can also be quantified. MRA minimizes complications that may be associated with contrast medium injection. |

Sources: Data from JM Black, E Matassarin-Jacobs (eds). Luckmann and Sorensen's Medical-Surgical Nursing: A Psychophysiologic Approach (4th ed). Philadelphia: Saunders, 1993; P Lanzer, J Rosch (eds). Vascular Diagnostics: Noninvasive and Invasive Techniques, Peri-Interventional Evaluations. Berlin: Springer-Verlag, 1994; KL McCance, SE Huether (eds). Pathophysiology: The Biological Basis for Disease in Adults and Children (2nd ed). St. Louis: Mosby, 1994; JL Kee (ed). Laboratory and Diagnostic Tests with Nursing Implications (5th ed). Stamford: Appleton & Lange, 1999, 606; VA Fahey (ed). Vascular Nursing (3rd ed). Philadelphia: Saunders, 1999;76, 86; and LM Malarkey, ME Morrow (eds). Nurses Manual of Laboratory Tests and Diagnostic Procedures (2nd ed). Philadelphia: Saunders, 2000;359.

- Frequent vital sign monitoring with pulse assessments.

- If a patient has been on heparin before angiography, the drug is not resumed for a minimum of 4 hours.[5]

The following are complications associated with angiography[1,5,6]:

- Allergic reactions to contrast dye

- Thrombi formation

- Vessel perforation with or without pseudoaneurysm formation

- Hematoma formation

- Hemorrhage

- Infections at the injection site

- Neurologic deficits from emboli dislodgment

- Contrast-induced renal failure (refer to Chapter 9)

### Hematologic Evaluation

The medical work-up of the patient with a suspected hematologic abnormality emphasizes the patient history and laboratory studies, in addition to the patient's clinical presentation.

### History

In addition to the general chart review (see Appendix I-A), the following questions are especially relevant in the evaluation of the patient with a suspected hematologic disorder[7-9]:

- What are the presenting symptoms?

- Was the onset of symptoms gradual, rapid, or associated with trauma or other disease?

- Is the patient unable to complete daily activities secondary to fatigue?

- Is there a patient or family history of anemia or other blood disorders, cancer, hemorrhage, or systemic infection?

- Is there a history of blood transfusion?

- Is there a history of chemotherapy, radiation therapy, or other drug therapy?

- Has there been an environmental or occupational exposure to toxins?

- Have there been night sweats, chills, or fever?

- Is the patient easily bruised?

- Is wound healing delayed?

- Is there excessive bleeding or menses?

Other relevant data include the patient's diet (for the evaluation of vitamin- or mineral-deficiency anemia), history of weight loss (as a warning sign of cancer or altered metabolism), whether the patient abuses alcohol (a cause of anemia with chronic use), and race (some hematologic conditions have a higher incidence in certain races).

## Inspection
During the hematologic evaluation, the patient is observed for the following[7]:

- General appearance (for lethargy, malaise, or apathy)

- Degree of pallor or flushing of the skin, mucous membranes, nail beds, and palmar creases

- Presence of petechiae (purplish, round, pinpoint, nonraised spots caused by intradermal or subcutaneous hemorrhage)[10] or ecchymosis (bruising)

- Respiratory rate

## Palpation
The examination performed by the physician includes palpation of lymph nodes, liver, and spleen as part of a general physical examination. For specific complaints, the patient may receive more in-depth examination of a body system. Table 6-6 summarizes the abnormal hematologic findings by body system on physical examination. The physical therapist may specifically examine the following:

**Table 6-6.** Signs and Symptoms of Hematologic Disorders by Body System

| Body System | Sign/Symptom | Associated Condition |
|---|---|---|
| Cardiac | Tachycardia | Anemia, hypovolemia |
| | Palpitations | Anemia, hypovolemia |
| | Murmur | Anemia, hypovolemia |
| | Angina | Anemia, hypovolemia |
| Respiratory | Dyspnea | Anemia, hypovolemia |
| | Orthopnea | Anemia, hypovolemia |
| Musculoskeletal | Back pain | Hemolysis |
| | Bone pain | Leukemia |
| | Joint pain | Hemophilia |
| | Sternal tenderness | Leukemia, sickle-cell disease |
| Nervous | Headache | Severe anemia, polycythemia, metastatic tumor |
| | Syncope | Severe anemia, polycythemia |
| | Vertigo, tinnitus | Severe anemia |
| | Paresthesia | Vitamin $B_{12}$ anemia, malignancy |
| | Confusion | Severe anemia, malignancy, infection |
| Visual | Visual disturbances | Anemia, polycythemia |
| | Blindness | Thrombocytopenia, anemia |
| Gastrointestinal, urinary, and reproductive | Dysphagia | Iron-deficiency anemia |
| | Abdominal pain | Lymphoma, hemolysis, sickle-cell disease |
| | Spleno- or hepatomegaly | Hemolytic anemia |
| | Hematemesis, melena | Thrombocytopenia and clotting disorders |
| | Hematuria | Hemolysis and clotting disorders |
| | Menorrhagia | Iron-deficiency anemia |
| Integumentary | Petechiae | Iron-deficiency anemia |
| | Ecchymosis | Hemolytic, pernicious anemia |
| | Flushing | Iron-deficiency anemia |
| | Jaundice | Hemolytic anemia |
| | Pallor | Conditions with low hemoglobin |

Source: Data from JM Black, E Matassarin-Jacobs (eds). Medical-Surgical Nursing Clinical Management for Continuity of Care (5th ed). Philadelphia: Saunders, 1997.

• The presence, location, and severity of bone or joint pain using an appropriate pain scale (See Appendix VI.)

• Joint range of motion and integrity, including the presence of effusion or bony abnormality

• Presence, location, and intensity of parasthesia

• Blood pressure and heart rate for signs of hypovolemia (See Palpation in the Vascular Evaluation section for a description of vital sign changes with hypovolemia.)

### Laboratory Studies

In addition to the history and physical examination, the clinical diagnosis of hematologic disorders is based primarily on laboratory studies.

*Complete Blood Cell Count*

The standard complete blood cell (CBC) count consists of a red blood cell (RBC) count, WBC count, WBC differential, hematocrit (Hct) measurement, hemoglobin (Hgb) measurement, and platelet (Plt) count. Table 6-7 summarizes the CBC. Figure 6-1 illustrates a common method used by physicians to document portions of the CBC in daily progress notes. If a value is abnormal, it is usually circled within this "sawhorse" figure.

---

### Clinical Tip

• Hct is accurate in relation to fluid status; therefore, Hct may be falsely high if the patient is dehydrated and falsely low if the patient is fluid overloaded.
• Hct is approximately three times the Hgb value.
• A low Hct may cause the patient to experience weakness, dyspnea, chills, or decreased activity tolerance, or it may exacerbate angina.
• The term pancytopenia refers to a significant decrease in RBCs, all types of WBCs, and Plts.

---

*Erythrocyte Indices*

RBC, Hct, and Hgb values are used to calculate three erythrocyte indices: (1) mean corpuscular volume (MCV), (2) mean corpuscular Hgb, and (3) mean corpuscular Hgb concentration. At most institu-

Table 6-7. Complete Blood Cell Count: Values and Interpretation*

| Test | Description | Value | Indication/Interpretation |
|---|---|---|---|
| Red blood cell (RBC) count | Number of RBCs per µl of blood | Female: 3.8–5.1 million/µl<br>Male: 4.3–5.7 million/µl | To assess blood loss, anemia, polycythemia. Elevated RBC count may increase risk of venous stasis or thrombi formation.<br>Increased: polycythemia vera, dehydration, severe chronic obstructive pulmonary disease, acute poisoning.<br>Decreased: anemia, leukemia, fluid overload, recent hemorrhage. |
| White blood cell (WBC) count | Number of WBCs per µl of blood | $4.5–11.0 \times 10^3$<br>(4,500–11,000) | To assess the presence of infection, inflammation, allergens, bone marrow integrity.<br>Monitors response to radiation or chemotherapy.<br>Increased: leukemia, infection, tissue necrosis.<br>Decreased: bone marrow suppression. |
| WBC differential | Proportion (%) of the different types of WBCs (out of 100 cells) | Neutrophils 54–62%<br>Lymphocytes 23–33%<br>Monocytes 3–7%<br>Eosinophils 1–3%<br>Basophils 0–0.75% | To determine the presence of infectious states.<br>Detect and classify leukemia. |

| Hematocrit (Hct) | Percentage of RBCs in whole blood | Female: 35–40% Male: 39–49% | To assess blood loss and fluid balance. Increased: Polycythemia, dehydration. Decreased: anemia, acute blood loss, hemodilution. |
|---|---|---|---|
| Hemoglobin (Hgb) | Amount of hemoglobin in 100 ml of blood | Female: 12–16 g/100 ml Male: 13.5–17.5 g/100 ml | To assess anemia, blood loss, bone marrow suppression. Increased: polycythemia, dehydration. Decreased: anemia, recent hemorrhage, fluid overload. |
| Platelets (Plt) | Number of platelets in μl of blood | $150–450 \times 10^3$ 150,000–450,000 μl | To assess thrombocytopenia. Increased: polycythemia vera, splenectomy, malignancy. Decreased: anemia, hemolysis, DIC, ITP, viral infections, AIDS, splenomegaly, with radiation or chemotherapy. |

*Lab values vary among laboratories. RBC, hemoglobin, and platelet values vary with age and gender.
AIDS = acquired immunodeficiency syndrome; DIC = disseminated intravascular coagulopathy; ITP = idiopathic thrombocytopenic purpura.
Sources: Adapted from RJ Elin. Laboratory Reference Intervals and Values. In L Goldman, JC Bennett (eds), Cecil Textbook of Medicine, Vol. 2 (21st ed). Philadelphia: Saunders, 2000;2305; and E Matassarin-Jacobs. Assessment of Clients with Hematologic Disorders. In JM Black, E Matassarin-Jacobs, Medical-Surgical Nursing Clinical Management for Continuity of Care (5th ed). Philadelphia: Saunders, 1997;1465.

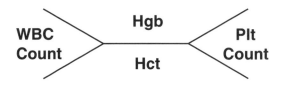

**Figure 6-1.** *Illustration of portions of the complete blood cell count in short-hand format. (Hct = hematocrit; Hgb = hemoglobin; Plt = platelet; WBC = white blood cell.)*

tions, these indices are included in the CBC. Table 6-8 summarizes these indices.

*Erythrocyte Sedimentation Rate*
The erythrocyte sedimentation rate, often referred to as the sed rate, is a measurement of how fast RBCs fall in a sample of anticoagulated blood. Normal values vary widely according to laboratory method. The normal value is 1–20 mm per hour for men and 1–15 mm per hour for women. The sedimentation rate is a nonspecific screening tool used to determine the presence or stage of inflammation, or the need for further medical testing, or it is used in correlation with the clinical course of such diseases as rheumatoid arthritis or temporal arteritis.[11] It may be elevated in systemic infection, collagen vascular disease, and human immunodeficiency virus. Erythrocyte sedimentation rate may be decreased in the presence of sickle-cell disease, polycythemia, or liver disease or carcinoma.

*Peripheral Blood Smear*
A blood sample may be examined microscopically for alterations in size and shape of the RBCs, WBCs, and Plts. RBCs are examined for size, shape, and Hgb distribution. WBCs are examined for proportion and the presence of immature cells. Finally, Plts are examined for number and shape.[11] Peripheral blood smear results are correlated with the other laboratory tests to diagnose hematologic disease.

*Coagulation Profile*
Coagulation tests assess the blood's ability to clot. The tests used to determine clotting are prothrombin time (PT) and partial thromboplastin time (PTT). An adjunct to the measurement of PT is the International Normalized Ratio (INR). The INR was created to ensure reliable and consistent measurement of coagulation levels among all

Table 6-8. Erythrocyte Indices: Values and Interpretation*

| Test | Description | Value | Interpretation |
|------|-------------|-------|----------------|
| Mean corpuscular volume (MCV) (Hct × 10/RBC) | Mean size of a single RBC in a µl of blood | 80–100 µg³ | Increased by macrocytic, folic acid, or vitamin $B_{12}$ deficiency anemias; liver disease; and recent alcohol use. Decreased by microcytic, iron-deficiency, and hypochromic anemias; thalassemia; and lead poisoning. |
| Mean corpuscular hemoglobin (MCH) (Hgb × 10/RBC) | Amount of Hgb in one RBC | 26–34 pg/cell | Increased by macrocytic anemia. Decreased by microcytic anemia. Low mean corpuscular hemoglobin indicates Hgb deficiency. |
| Mean corpuscular hemoglobin concentration (MCHC) (Hgb/Hct × 100) | Proportion of each RBC occupied by Hgb | 31–37 g/dl | Increased by spherocytosis (small round RBC). Decreased by microcytic, hypochromic, and iron-deficiency anemias and thalassemia. |

Hct = hematocrit; Hgb = hemoglobin; RBC = red blood cell.
*Lab values vary among laboratories.
Sources: Adapted from RJ Elin. Laboratory Reference Intervals and Values. In L Goldman, JC Bennett (eds), Cecil Textbook of Medicine, Vol. 2 (21st ed). Philadelphia: Saunders, 2000;2305; and E Matassarin-Jacobs. Assessment of Clients with Hematologic Disorders. In JM Black, E Matassarin-Jacobs (eds), Medical-Surgical Nursing Clinical Management for Continuity of Care (5th ed). Philadelphia: Saunders, 1997;1466.

laboratories. The INR is the ratio of the patient's PT to the standard PT of the laboratory, raised by an exponent (the sensitivity index of the reagent) provided by the manufacturer.[12] Table 6-9 summarizes PT/INR and PTT.

---

**Clinical Tip**

When confirming an order for physical therapy in the physician's orders, the therapist must be sure to differentiate between the order for physical therapy and the blood test (i.e., the abbreviations for both physical therapy and prothrombin time are PT).

---

## Pathophysiology

This section is divided into a discussion of vascular and hematologic disorders.

### Vascular Disorders

Vascular disorders are classified as arterial, venous, or combined arterial and venous disorders. Clinical findings differ between arterial and venous disorders, as described in Table 6-10.

### Arterial Disorders

*Atherosclerosis*
Atherosclerosis is a diffuse and slowly progressive process characterized by areas of hemorrhage and the cellular proliferation of monocytes, smooth muscle, connective tissue, and lipids.* The development of atherosclerosis begins early in life with risk factors that include the following[3,6,13–15]:

---

*Arteriosclerosis* is a general term used to describe any wall thickening or hardening in the arteries. The term *atheroma* is applied to plaque formation with fatty material in the vessel wall.

**Table 6-9.** Coagulation Profile

| Test | Description | Value* (secs) | Indication/Interpretation |
|---|---|---|---|
| Prothrombin time/ international normalized ratio (PT/INR) | Examines the extrinsic and common clotting factors I, II, V, VII, and X | PT 11–15 | Used to assess the adequacy of warfarin (Coumadin) therapy or to screen for bleeding disorders<br>Increased: Coumarin therapy, liver diseases, bile duct obstruction, diarrhea, salicylate intoxication, DIC, hereditary factor deficiency, alcohol use, or drug interaction<br>Decreased: Diet high in fat or leafy vegetables, or drug interaction |
| Partial thromboplastin time (PTT) (activated PTT [APTT] is a rapid version of PTT) | Examines the intrinsic and common clotting factors I, II, V, VIII, IX, X, XI | PTT 60–70<br>APTT 30–40 | Used to assess the adequacy of heparin therapy and to screen for bleeding disorders<br>Increased: Heparin or coumarin therapy, liver disease, vitamin K or congenital clotting factor deficiency, DIC<br>Decreased: Extensive cancer, early DIC |

DIC = disseminated intravascular coagulopathy.

*Values for prothrombin time (PT) and PTT vary between laboratories.

Source: Data from KD Pagana, TJ Pagana. Mosby's Manual of Diagnostic and Laboratory Tests. Blood Studies. St. Louis: Mosby, 1998.

**Table 6-10.** Comparison of Clinical Findings of Arterial and Venous Disorders

| Clinical Finding | Arterial Disorders | Venous Disorders |
|---|---|---|
| Edema | May or may not be present | Present<br>Worse at the end of the day<br>Improve with elevation |
| Muscle mass | Reduced | Unaffected |
| Pain | Intermittent claudication<br>Cramping<br>Worse with elevation | Aching pain<br>Exercise improves pain<br>Better with elevation<br>Cramping at night<br>Paresthesias, pruritus (severe itching)<br>Leg heaviness, especially at end of day<br>Commonly a positive Homans' sign |
| Pulses | Decreased to absent<br>Possible systolic bruit | Usually unaffected but may be difficult to palpate if edema is present |
| Skin | Absence of hair<br>Small, painful ulcers on pressure points, especially lateral malleolus<br>Tight, shiny skin<br>Thickened toenails | Broad, shallow, painless ulcers of the ankle and lower leg<br>Normal toenails |
| Color | Pale<br>Dependent cyanosis | Brown discoloration<br>Dependent cyanosis |
| Temperature | Cool | May be warm in presence of thrombophlebitis |
| Sensation | Decreased light touch<br>Occasional itching, tingling, and numbness | Pruritus |

Source: Data from JM Black, E Matassarin-Jacobs (eds). Luckmann and Sorensen's Medical-Surgical Nursing: A Psychophysiologic Approach (4th ed). Philadelphia: Saunders, 1993;1261.

- Smoking

- Diabetes mellitus

- Hypertension

- Hyperlipidemia (12- to 14-hour fasting blood sample of cholesterol of more than 260 mg/dl or triglyceride of more than 150 mg/dl)

- Low levels of high-density lipoproteins

- High levels of low-density lipoproteins

- Gender (Men are at greater risk than women until women reach menopause; then the risk is equal in both genders.)

- Inactivity

- Family history

In addition to these risk factors, a high level of an inflammatory biomarker, C-reactive protein, has been identified as a good predictive marker for early identification of artherosclerosis.[16]

Clinical manifestations of atherosclerosis result from decreased blood flow through the stenotic areas. Signs and symptoms vary according to the area, size, and location of the lesion, along with the age and physiologic status of the patient. As blood flows through a stenotic area, turbulence will occur beyond the stenosis, resulting in decreased blood perfusion past the area of atherosclerosis. Generally, a 50–60% reduction in blood flow is necessary for patients to present with symptoms (e.g., pain). Turbulence is increased when there is an increase in blood flow to an area of the body, such as the lower extremities during exercise. A patient with no complaint of pain at rest may therefore experience leg pain (intermittent claudication) during walking or exercise as a result of decreased blood flow and the accumulation of metabolic waste (e.g., lactic acid).[3,6,14]

The following are general signs and symptoms of atherosclerosis[17]:

- Peripheral pulses that are slightly reduced to absent

- Presence of bruits on auscultation of major arteries (i.e., carotid, abdominal aorta, iliac, and femoral)

- Coolness and pallor of skin, especially with elevation

- Presence of ulcerations, atrophic nails, and hair loss

• Increased blood pressure

• Subjective reports of continuous burning pain in toes at rest that is aggravated with elevation (ischemic pain) and relieved with walking. Pain at rest is usually indicative of severe, 80–90% arterial occlusion.

• Subjective reports of calf or lower-extremity pain induced by walking (intermittent claudication) and relieved by rest

---

Clinical Tip

Progression of ambulation distance in the patient with intermittent claudication can be optimized if ambulation is performed in short, frequent intervals (i.e., before the onset of claudicating pain).

---

Symptoms similar to intermittent claudication may have a neurologic origin from lumbar canal stenosis or disk disease. These symptoms are referred to as pseudoclaudication or neurologic claudication. Table 6-11 outlines the differences between true claudication and pseudoclaudication.[18] Medications that have been successful in managing intermittent claudication include pentoxifylline and cilostazol.[19]

Treatment of atherosclerotic disease is based on clinical presentation and can range from risk-factor modifications (e.g., low-fat diet, increased exercise, and smoking cessation) to pharmacologic therapy (e.g., anticoagulation and thrombolytics) to surgical resection and grafting. Modification of risk factors has been shown to be the most effective method to lower the risk of morbidity (heart attack or stroke) from artherosclerosis.[15,20]

*Aneurysm*

An aneurysm is a localized dilatation or outpouching of the vessel wall that results from degeneration and weakening of the supportive network of protein fibers with a concomitant loss of medial smooth muscle cells. Aneurysms most commonly occur in the abdominal aorta or iliac arteries, followed by the popliteal, femoral, and carotid vessels.[6,15,21,22] The exact mechanism of aneurysm formation is not fully understood but includes a combination of the following:

Table 6-11. Differentiating True Intermittent Claudication from Pseudoclaudication

| Characteristic of Discomfort | Intermittent Claudication | Pseudoclaudication |
|---|---|---|
| Activity-induced | Yes | Yes or no |
| Location | Unilateral buttock, hip, thigh, calf and foot | Back pain and bilateral leg pain |
| Nature | Cramping Tightness Tiredness | Same as with intermittent claudication or presence of tingling, weakness, and clumsiness |
| Occurs with standing | No | Yes |
| Onset | Occurs at the same distance each time with walking on level surface | Occurs at variable distance each time with walking on level surfaces |
| | Unchanged or decreased distance walking uphill | Increased distance when walking uphill |
| | Unchanged or increased distance walking downhill | Decreased distance walking downhill |
| Relieved by | Stopping activity | Sitting |

Sources: Data from JR Young, RA Graor, JW Olin, JR Bartholomew (eds). Peripheral Vascular Diseases. St. Louis: Mosby, 1991;183; and JM Fritz. Spinal Stenosis. In JD Placzek, DA Boyce (eds). Orthopaedic Physical Therapy Secrets. Philadelphia: Hanley & Belfus, 2001;344.

- Genetic abnormality in collagen (e.g., with Marfan's syndrome)
- Aging and natural degeneration of elastin
- Increased proteolytic enzyme activity
- Atherosclerotic damage to elastin and collagen

A true aneurysm is defined as a 50% increase in the normal diameter of the vessel[22] and involves weakening of all three layers of the arterial wall. True aneurysms are also generally fusiform and circumferential in nature. False and saccular aneurysms are the result of trauma from dissection (weakness or separation of the vascular layers) or clot formation. They primarily affect the adventitial layer.[21] Figure 6-2A and C demonstrate fusiform and saccular aneurysms, and Figure 6-2B illustrates an arterial dissection.

Abdominal aneuryms may present with vague abdominal pain but are relatively asymptomatic until an emboli dislodges from the aneurysm or the aneurysm ruptures.[22] Aneurysms will rupture if the intraluminal pressure exceeds the tensile strength of the arterial wall. The risk of rupture increases with increased aneurysm size.[13]

---

**Clinical Tip**

Abdominal aortic aneurysms are frequently referred to as *AAA* or *Triple A* in the clinical setting.

---

The following are additional clinical manifestations of aneurysms:

- Ischemic manifestations, described earlier, in Atherosclerosis, if the aneurysm impedes blood flow.

- Cerebral aneurysms, commonly found in the circle of Willis, present with increased intracranial pressure and its sequelae (see General Management in Chapter 4 for more information on intracranial pressure).[21]

- Aneurysms that result in subarachnoid hemorrhage are also discussed in Chapter 4.

- Low back pain (aortic aneurysms can refer pain to the low back).

- Dysphagia (difficulty swallowing) and dyspnea (breathlessness) resulting from the enlarged vessel's compressing adjacent organs.

Surgical resection and graft replacement are generally the desired treatments for aneurysms.[23] However, endovascular repair of abdominal aneurysms is demonstrating favorable results. Endovascular repair involves threading an endoprosthesis through the femoral artery to the site of the aneurysm. The endoprosthesis is then attached to the aorta, proximal to the site of the aneurysm, and distal, to the iliac arteries. This effectively excludes the aneurysm from the circulation, which minimizes the risk of rupture.[22] Nonsurgical candidates must have blood pressure and anticoagulation management.[23]

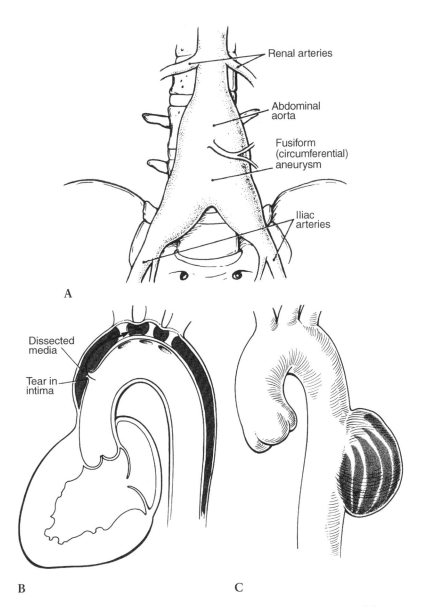

**Figure 6-2.** **A.** *Fusiform aneurysm of the aorta.* **B.** *Consequences of dissection from the ascending aorta across the arch of the aorta.* **C.** *Saccular aneurysm of the descending aorta. (With permission from BL Bullock [ed]. Pathophysiology: Adaptations and Alterations in Function [4th ed]. Philadelphia: Lippincott–Raven, 1996;532.)*

*Arterial Thrombosis*
Arterial thrombosis occurs in areas of low or stagnant blood flow, such as atherosclerotic or aneurysmal areas. The reduced or turbulent blood flow in these areas leads to platelet adhesion and aggregation, which then activates the coagulation cycle to form a mature thrombus (clot). Blood flow may then be impeded, potentially leading to tissue ischemia with subsquent clinical manifestations.[21,23]

*Arterial Emboli*
Arterial emboli arise from areas of stagnant or disturbed blood flow in the heart or aorta. Conditions that predispose a person to emboli formation are (1) atrial fibrillation, (2) myocardial infarction, (3) infective endocarditis, (4) cardiac valve replacement (if not properly anticoagulated), (5) chronic congestive heart failure, and (6) aortic atherosclerosis. Areas in which arterial emboli tend to lodge and interrupt blood flow are arterial bifurcations and areas narrowed by atherosclerosis (especially in the cerebral, mesenteric, renal, and coronary arteries). Signs and symptoms of thrombi, emboli, or both depend on the size of the occlusion, the organ distal to the clot, and the collateral circulation available.[21]

Treatment of thrombi, emboli, or both includes anticoagulation with or without surgical resection of the atherosclerotic area that is predisposing the formation of thrombi, emboli, or both. Medical management of arterial thrombosis can also include antithrombotic drugs (e.g., tissue factor or factor Xa inhibitors) or combined antithrombotic therapy with aspirin, and thienopyridine and warfarin, or both.[24]

*Hypertension*
Hypertension is an elevated arterial blood pressure, both systolic and diastolic, that is abnormally sustained at rest. Table 6-12 outlines normal and hypertensive blood pressures for a given age group. Signs and symptoms that can result from hypertension and its effects on target organs are described in Table 6-13. Two general forms of hypertension exist: essential and secondary.

Essential, or idiopathic, hypertension is an elevation in blood pressure that results without a specific medical cause but is related to the following risk factors[21,25]:

- Genetic predisposition

- Smoking

Table 6-12.  Hypertension as It Relates to Different Age Groups

| Age | Normal Blood Pressure (Systolic/Diastolic) | Hypertensive Blood Pressure (Systolic/Diastolic) |
|---|---|---|
| Infants | 80/40 | 90/60 |
| Children | 100/60 | 120/80 |
| Teenagers (age 12– 17 yrs) | 115/70 | 130/80 |
| Adults | | |
| 20–45 yrs | 120–125/75–80 | 135/90 |
| 45–60 yrs | 135–145/85 | 140–160/90–95 |
| Older than 65 yrs | 150/85 | 160/90 |

Source: Data from B Bullock. Pathophysiology: Adaptations and Alterations in Function (4th ed). Philadelphia: Lippincott–Raven, 1996;517.

• Sedentary lifestyle

• Type A personality

• Obesity

• Diabetes mellitus

• Diet high in fat, cholesterol, and sodium

• Atherosclerosis

• Imbalance of vasomediator production, nitric oxide (vasodilator), and endothelin (potent vasoconstrictor)

Secondary hypertension results from a known medical cause, such as renal disease and others listed in Table 6-14. If the causative factors are treated sufficiently, systolic blood pressure may return to normal limits.[21]

Management of hypertension consists of behavioral (e.g., diet, smoking cessation, activity modification) and pharmacologic intervention to maintain blood pressure within acceptable parameters. The primary medications used are diuretics and angiotensin-converting enzyme inhibitors along with beta blockers, calcium channel blockers, and vasodilators.[21,26–28] A summary of these medications, their actions, and their side effects can be found in Appendix Tables IV-17, IV-2, IV-12, IV-14, and IV-30, respectively.

**Table 6-13.** Hypertensive Effects on Target Organs

| Organ | Hypertensive Effect | Clinical Manifestations |
|---|---|---|
| Brain | Cerebrovascular accident | Area of brain involved dictates presentation. May include severe occipital headache, paralysis, speech and swallowing disturbances, or coma. |
| | Encephalopathy | Rapid development of confusion, agitation, convulsions, and death. |
| Eyes | Blurred or impaired vision | Nicking (compression) of retinal arteries and veins, at the point of their junction. |
| | Encephalopathy | Hemorrhages and exudates on visual examination. |
| | | Papilledema. |
| Heart | Myocardial infarction | Electrocardiographic changes. |
| | | Enzyme elevations. |
| | Congestive heart failure | Decreased cardiac output. |
| | | Auscultation of S3 or gallop. |
| | | Cardiomegaly on radiograph. |
| | Myocardial hypertrophy | Increased angina frequency. |
| | | ST- and T-wave changes on electrocardiogram. |
| | Dysrhythmias | Ventricular or conduction defects. |
| Kidneys | Renal insufficiency | Nocturia. |
| | | Proteinuria. |
| | | Elevated blood urea nitrogen and creatinine levels. |
| | Renal failure | Fluid overload. |
| | | Accumulation of metabolites. |
| | | Metabolic acidosis. |

Source: Data from B Bullock (ed). Pathophysiology: Adaptations and Alterations in Function (4th ed). Philadelphia: Lippincott–Raven, 1996;522.

---

### Clinical Tip

• Knowledge of medication schedule may facilitate activity tolerance by having optimal blood pressures at rest and with activity.

**Table 6-14.** Causes of Secondary Hypertension

| Origin | Description |
|---|---|
| Coarctation of the aorta | Congenital constriction of the aorta at the level of the ductus arteriosus, which results in increased pressure (proximal to the area) of constriction and decreased pressure (distal to the area) of constriction |
| Cushing's disease or syndrome | See Pituitary Gland in Chapter 11 |
| Oral contraceptives | May be related to an increased secretion of glucocorticoids from adrenal or pituitary dysfunction |
| Pheochromocytoma | Tumor of the adrenal medulla causing increased catecholamine secretion |
| Primary aldosteronism | Increased aldosterone secretion primarily as result of an adrenal tumor |
| Renin-secreting tumors | See Adrenal Gland in Chapter 11 |
| Renovascular disease | Parenchymal disease, such as acute and chronic glomerulonephritis |
|  | Narrowing stenosis of renal artery as a result of atherosclerosis or congenital fibroplasia |

Source: Data from B Bullock (ed). Pathophysiology: Adaptations and Alterations in Function (4th ed). Philadelphia: Lippincott–Raven, 1996;517.

- Review and clarify any strict blood pressure parameters that the physician has designated for the patient, as some patients need to have higher or lower systolic pressures than expected normal ranges.

*Systemic Vasculitis*
Systemic vasculitis is a general term referring to the inflammation of arteries and veins that progresses to necrosis, leading to a narrowing of the vessels. The precise etiology is unknown; however, an autoimmune mechanism is suspected and is becoming more delineated. The secondary manifestations of vasculitis are numerous and may include thrombosis, aneurysm formation, hemorrhage, arterial occlusion, weight loss, fatigue, depression, fever, and generalized achiness that is

worse in the morning. The recognized forms of vasculitis are discussed in the following sections.[13,14,29,30]

**Polyarteritis Nodosa** Polyarteritis nodosa (PAN) is a disseminated disease with focal transmural arterial inflammation, resulting in necrosis of medium-sized arteries. Most of the cases present with an unknown etiology; however, the hepatitis B virus has been evolving as one of the more common causative factors.[29] The most frequently involved organs are the kidney, heart, liver, and gastrointestinal tract, with symptoms representative of the dysfunction of the involved organ. Aneurysm formation with destruction of the medial layer of the vessel is the hallmark characteristic of PAN. Pulmonary involvement can occur; however, most cases of vasculitis in the respiratory tract are associated with Wegener's granulomatosis.

Current management of PAN includes corticosteroid therapy with or without concurrent cytoxic therapy with cyclophosphamide (Cytoxan). Antiviral agents may also be used if there is an associated viral infection. Elective surgical correction of PAN is not feasible, given its diffuse nature. Patients diagnosed with PAN have a 5-year survival rate of 12% without medical treatment and 80% with treatment.[13,29]

**Wegener's Granulomatosis** Wegener's granulomatosis is a granulomatous, necrotizing disease that affects small- and medium-sized blood vessels throughout the body, with primary manifestations in the upper respiratory tract, lungs, and kidneys. The etiology is unknown; diagnosis and treatment are still in development. Onset of symptoms generally occurs after 40 years of age and is slightly more common in men. Pulmonary signs and symptoms mimic those of pneumonia (i.e., fever, productive cough at times with negative sputum cultures, and chest pain).[26,29] The 1-year mortality rate is 90% without therapy, 50% with corticosteroid therapy, and 10% with combined corticosteroid and cytotoxic therapy.[29]

Treatment of Wegener's granulomatosis may consist of a combination of immunosuppressive agents and corticosteroids (methotrexate and prednisone, respectively). Anti-infective agents may also be prescribed if there is associated respiratory tract infection.[26,29]

**Thromboangiitis Obliterans** Thromboangiitis obliterans (Buerger's disease) is a clinical syndrome that is found mainly in young men ages 20–45 years and is directly correlated to a heavy smoking history.[3,13,21] The disease is characterized by segmental thrombotic occlusions of the small- and medium-sized arteries in the distal lower and upper extremities. The thrombotic occlusions consist of microabscesses that are inflammatory in nature, suggesting a collagen or autoimmune origin, although the exact etiology is still unknown.[13,21] Rest pain is common, along with intermittent claudication that occurs more in the feet than in the calf region.[3]

Treatment of Buerger's disease can include smoking cessation, corticosteroids, prostaglandin $E_1$ infusion, vasodilators, hemorheologic agents, antiplatelet agents, and anticoagulants.[13,21]

**Giant Cell Arteritis**   Giant cell arteritis (GCA) is another granulomatous inflammatory disorder of an unknown etiology. It predominantly affects the large arteries and is characterized by destruction of the internal elastic lamina. Two clinical presentations of GCA have been recognized: temporal arteritis and Takayasu's arteritis.[21]

Temporal arteritis is a more common and mild presentation of GCA that occurs after 50 years of age. The primary signs and symptoms are persistent headache (temporal and occipital areas), transient visual disturbances (amaurosis fugax and graying or blurring of vision), and jaw and tongue pain. Polymyalgia rheumatica, a clinical syndrome characterized by pain on active motion and acute onset of proximal muscular stiffness, is frequently associated with temporal arteritis. The primary treatment for temporal arteritis is prednisone.[18,29]

Takayasu's arteritis generally affects young Asian women but has been known to occur in both genders of blacks and Hispanics as well. It is a form of generalized GCA that primarily involves the upper extremities and the aorta and its major branches. Lower-extremity involvement is less common. Management of Takayasu's arteritis may consist of prednisone and cyclophosphamide, along with surgical intervention if the disease progresses to aneurysm, gangrene, or both.[18]

*Raynaud's Disease*
Raynaud's disease is a form of intermittent arteriolar vasoconstriction that occurs in patients who have concurrent immunologic disease. The exact etiology is unknown but may be linked to defects in the sympathetic nervous system. Evidence exists for and against the theory of sympathetic overactivity, which is said to lead to Raynaud's disease. Women 16–40 years of age are most commonly affected, especially in cold climates or during the winter season. Other than cold hypersensitivity, emotional factors can also trigger the sudden vasoconstriction. Areas generally affected are the fingertips, toes, and the tip of the nose.[3,18,26]

**Raynaud's Phenomenon** Raynaud's phenomenon may result from Raynaud's disease and is the term used to describe the localized and intermittent episodes of vasoconstriction that cause unilateral color and temperature changes in the fingertips, toes, and tip of nose. The color changes of the affected skin progress from white to blue to red (reflecting the vasoconstriction, cyanosis, and vasodilation process, respectively). Numbness, tingling, and burning pain may also accompany the color changes. However, despite these vasoconstrictive episodes, peripheral pulses remain palpable. Raynaud's phenomenon can also be associated with diseases such as scleroderma, systemic lupus erythematosus, rheumatoid arthritis, and obstructive arterial disease and trauma.[3,18,26]

Management of Raynaud's disease and phenomenon may consist of any of the following: conservative measures to ensure warmth of the body and extremities; regular exercise; diet rich in fish oils and antioxidants (vitamins C and E); pharmacologic intervention, including calcium channel blockers and sympatholytics; conditioning and biofeedback; acupuncture; and sympathectomy.[18,31]

*Reflex Sympathetic Dystrophy*
Reflex sympathetic dystrophy is constant, extreme pain that occurs after the healing phase of minor or major trauma, fractures, surgery, or any combination of these. Injured sensory nerve fibers may transmit constant signals to the spinal cord that result in increased sympathetic activity to the limbs. Affected areas initially present as dry, swollen, and warm but then progress to being cold, swollen, and pale or cyanotic. Raynaud's phenomenon can occur later on.[18] Management of reflex sympathetic dystrophy may consist of any of the following[18,32–35]:

- Physical or occupational therapy, or both

- Pharmacologic sympathetic blocks

- Surgical sympathectomy

- Spinal cord electrical stimulation

- Baclofen drug administration

- Prophylactic vitamin C administration after sustaining fractures

- Biophosphanate administration

## Compartment Syndrome

Compartment syndrome is the swelling in the muscle compartments (myotendon, neural, and vascular structures contained within a fascial compartment of an extremity) that can occur after traumatic injury to the arteries. These injuries include fractures, crush injuries, hematomas, penetrating injuries, circumferential burn injury, electrical injuries, and status post revascularization procedures. External factors, such as casts and circular dressings that are too constrictive, may also lead to compartment syndrome.[6,18,36] Compartment syndrome can also occur as a chronic condition that develops from overuse associated with strenous exercise. Diagnosis of compartment syndrome is established by measuring compartment pressures. Compartment pressures of 25–30 mm Hg can cause compression of capillaries.[36]

A common symptom of compartment syndrome is pain associated with tense, tender muscle groups that worsens with palpation or passive movement of the affected area. Numbness or paralysis may also be accompanied by a gradual diminution of peripheral pulses. Pallor, which indicates tissue ischemia, can progress to tissue necrosis if appropriate management is not performed.[6,18,36]

Management of compartment syndrome consists of preventing prolonged external compression of the involved limb, limb elevation, and, ultimately, fasciotomy (incisional release of the fascia) if compartment pressures exceed 30–45 mm Hg. Mannitol can also be used to help reduce swelling.[6,18,36]

---

### Clinical Tip

• Patient, staff, and family eduction on proper positioning techniques can reduce the risk of swelling and subsequent compartment syndrome.
• The physical therapist should delineate any range-of-motion precautions that may be present after fasciotomies that cross a joint line.

---

### Venous Disorders

#### Varicose Veins

Varicose veins are chronic dilations of the veins that first result from a weakening in the venous walls, which then leads to improper closure of the valve cusps. Incompetence of the valves further exacerbates the venous dilatation. Risk factors for developing varicose veins include increasing age, occupations that require prolonged standing, and obesity (in women).[37] The occurrence of venous thrombosis can also promote varicose vein formation. Patients generally complain of itchy, tired, heavy-feeling legs after prolonged standing.[6,37]

Management of varicose veins may consist of any of the following: behavioral modifications (e.g., avoiding prolonged sitting or standing and constrictive clothing), weight loss (if there is associated obesity), elevating the feet for 10–15 minutes 3 or 4 times a day, gradual exercise, applying well-fitting support stockings in the morning, showering or bathing in the evening, sclerotherapy (to close dilated veins), and surgical ligation and stripping of incompetent veins.[6,37]

*Venous Thrombosis*
Venous thrombosis can occur in the superficial or deep veins (deep venous thrombosis [DVT]) and can result from a combination of venous stasis, injury to the endothelial layer of the vein, and hypercoagulability. The primary complication of venous thrombosis is pulmonary embolism (PE).[6]

The following are risk factors associated with venous thrombosis formation[18,38]:

- Surgery and nonsurgical trauma, such as lower-extremity fracture
- Immobilization
- Limb paresis or paralysis
- Heart failure or myocardial infarction
- Previous DVT
- Increasing age
- Malignancy
- Obesity
- Pregnancy
- Use of oral contraceptives

Signs and symptoms of venous thrombosis can include the following[18,38]:

- Pain and swelling distal to the site of thrombus
- Redness and warmth in the area around the thrombus

- Dilated veins
- Low-grade fever
- A dull ache or tightness in the region of DVT

---

**Clinical Tip**

- Homans' sign (pain in upper calf with forced ankle dorsiflexion) has been used as a screening tool for venous thrombosis, but it is an insensitive and nonspecific test that has a very high false-positive rate.[1,38-40]
- A positive Homans' sign accompanied by swelling, redness, and warmth may be more clinically indicative of a DVT than is a positive Homans' sign alone.
- Ultimately, examination by vascular diagnostic tests, such as venous duplex scanning[38] and laboratory testing of clotting times (PT and PTT), is a better method to evaluate the presence of DVT.
- Physical therapy intervention for patients with suspected DVT should be withheld until cleared by the medical-surgical team.

---

Prevention of venous thrombosis includes avoidance of immobilization; lower-extremity elevation or application of compression stockings (elastic or pneumatic), or both, if bed rest is required; and anticoagulation medications (intravenous heparin or oral warfarin [Coumadin]).

Management of venous thrombosis may also consist of anticoagulation therapy, thrombolytic therapy (streptokinase and urokinase), or both, and surgical thrombectomy (limited uses).[6] Current research has demonstrated that ambulation while wearing compression stockings as early as 24–72 hours after adequate anticoagulation therapy has been attained will prevent extension of the thrombus and formation of PE.[38]

*Pulmonary Embolism*
PE is the primary complication of venous thrombosis, with emboli commonly originating in the lower extremities. Other sources are the upper extremities and pelvic venous plexus. Mechanical blockage of a pulmonary artery or capillary, depending on clot size, results in an acute ventilation-perfusion mismatch that leads to a decrease in partial pressure of oxygen and oxyhemoglobin saturation, which ultimately manifests as tissue hypoxia. Chronic physiologic sequelae

from PE include pulmonary hypertension, chronic hypoxemia, and right congestive heart failure. Refer to Chapter 2 for more details on ventilation-perfusion mismatches, as well as the respiratory sequelae (dyspnea, chest pain, hemoptysis, and tachypnea) from PE.[6,41]

Management of PE consists of prevention of venous thrombosis formation (see Venous Thrombosis), early detection, and thorough anticoagulation therapy with standard or low-molecular-weight heparin. Thrombolytic therapy has also been used in patients with PE. The placement of an inferior vena cava filter is indicated when patients cannot be anticoagulated or where there is recurrence of PE despite anticoagulation.[6,41]

---

### Clinical Tip

Physical therapy intervention should be discontinued immediately if the signs and symptoms of a PE arise during an examination or treatment session.

---

*Chronic Venous Insufficiency and Postphlebitic Syndrome*
Chronic venous insufficiency and postphlebitic syndrome are similar disorders that result from venous outflow obstruction, valvular dysfunction from thrombotic destruction of veins, or both. Valvular dysfunction is generally the most significant cause of either disorder. Within 5 years of sustaining a DVT, approximately 50% of patients develop signs of these disorders. The hallmark characteristics of both are the following[1,6,42]:

- Chronic swollen limbs

- Thickened (induration), coarse, and brownish skin discoloration in the distal lower extremity

- Venous stasis ulceration

Management of these disorders may consist of any of the following: leg elevation above the level of the heart two to four times daily for 10–15 minutes; application of proper elastic supports (knee length preferable); skin hygiene; avoidance of crossing legs, poorly fitting chairs, garters, and sources of pressure above the legs (e.g., tight girdles); elastic compression stockings; pneumatic compression stockings (if the patient needs to remain in bed); exercise to aid muscular pumping of venous blood; surgical ligation of veins; and wound care to venous ulcers. Refer to Chapter 7 for more information on wound care.[1,6,42]

---

### Clinical Tip

Caution should be taken in providing compressive dressings and elevating the lower extremities of patients who have arterial insufficiency, diabetes mellitus, and congestive heart failure.

---

## Combined Arterial and Venous Disorders

*Arteriovenous Malformations*
Arteriovenous malformations (AVMs) involve shunting of blood directly from the artery to the vein, bypassing the capillary bed. The presence of an arteriovenous fistula in the AVM is usually the cause of the shunt. The majority of AVMs occurs in the trunk and extremities, with a certain number of cases also presenting in the cerebrovascular region.[13]

Signs of AVMs may include the following[13]:

- Skin color changes (erythema or cyanosis)

- Venous varices

- Edema

- Limb deformity

- Skin ulceration

- Pulse deficit

- Bleeding

- Ischemic manifestations in involved organ systems

*Congenital Vascular Malformations*
Congenital vascular malformations (CVMs) are rare developmental abnormalities that may involve all components of the peripheral circulation (i.e., arteries, veins, capillaries, and lymphatics). Signs and symptoms of congenital vascular malformations are similar to those of AVMs, with tissue hypoxia being the most significant clinical finding.

Although congenital vascular malformations can be self-limiting or incurable, management of certain cases may consist of arteriogram with embolization, elastic supports, and limb elevation.[13]

## Hematologic Disorders

### Erythrocytic Disorders

Disorders of RBCs are generally categorized as a decrease or an increase in the number of RBCs in the circulating blood.

*Anemia*

Anemia is a decrease in the number of RBCs. Anemia can be described according to etiology as (1) a decrease in RBC production, (2) abnormal RBC maturation, or (3) an increase in RBC destruction.[7] Anemia can also be described according to morphology based on RBC size or color.[43] RBCs that are of normal size are normocytic; RBCs that are smaller than normal are microcytic; and RBCs that are larger than normal are macrocytic. RBCs of normal color are normochromic; RBCs of decreased color are microchromic. Some of the most common anemias are described in this section.

**Posthemorrhagic Anemia** Posthemorrhagic anemia can occur with rapid blood loss from traumatic artery severance, aneurysm rupture, or arterial erosion from malignant or ulcerative lesions, or as a result of surgery. Blood loss results in a normocytic, normochromic anemia. The signs and symptoms of posthemorrhagic anemia depend on the amount of blood loss and may include the following[44]:

- With 20–30% blood volume loss—Dizziness and hypotension when not at rest in a recumbent position, tachycardia with exertion.

- With 30–40% blood volume loss—Thirst, dyspnea, diaphoresis, cold and clammy skin, hypotension and tachycardia, decreased urine output, clouding or loss of consciousness when at rest in a recumbent postion.

- With 40–50% blood volume loss—A severe state of shock with the potential for death ensues.

Management of posthemorrhagic anemia may consist of any of the following: control of bleeding at the source, intravenous and oral fluid administration, blood and blood product transfusion, and supplemental oxygen.[8,43,45]

**Iron-Deficiency Anemia**  Iron-deficiency anemia occurs when decreased iron storage in the bone marrow causes the production of microcytic, microchromic RBCs. Iron deficiency can be caused by chronic blood loss (most commonly from the gastrointestinal tract), pregnancy, excessive menses, frequent blood donation, rapid body development, or the malabsorption of iron. Iron deficiency is diagnosed by clinical presentation and serum ferritin laboratory values. Often, it is asymptomatic if the onset is insidious.[46] Signs and symptoms of iron-deficiency anemia include the following:

- Fatigue, tachycardia, and dyspnea on exertion

- Dizziness

- Headache

- Irritability

- Mouth soreness, difficulty swallowing, and gastritis (severe anemia)

- Softening of nails or pale earlobes, palms, and conjunctivae (severe anemia)

Management of iron-deficiency anemia may consist of a medical work-up to identify a possible blood loss site, iron supplementation, or nutritional counseling.[8,43,45,47]

**Vitamin $B_{12}$ Anemia**  Decreased levels of vitamin $B_{12}$ cause the production of macrocytic, normochromic RBCs. Vitamin $B_{12}$ deficiency is commonly caused by poor absorption of vitamin $B_{12}$ from enteritis or iliac disease. It is less commonly associated with Crohn's disease and pancreatic insufficiency and is rarely caused by dietary insufficiency.[47] Pernicious anemia is a congenital type of vitamin $B_{12}$ anemia caused by the absence of intrinsic factor available to bind to vitamin $B_{12}$. In addition to the general presentation of anemia, the signs and symptoms of vitamin $B_{12}$ deficiency may include the following:

- Anorexia and diarrhea

- Oral ulceration

- Neurologic impairments, such as parasthesia of the extremities, decreased balance, vibratory sense, and proprioception secondary to posterior column degeneration[47]

- Late neurologic manifestations include memory loss, mood changes, and hallucinations[48]

Vitamin $B_{12}$ deficiency is diagnosed by clinical presentation, low serum vitamin $B_{12}$ levels, elevated lactate dehydrogenase and MCV values, and positive urine sampling (Schilling test). Neurologic symptoms are reversible if the onset is less than 6 months.[47] Management of vitamin $B_{12}$ anemia consists of lifelong vitamin $B_{12}$ supplementation and nutritional counseling.[8,43,45]

---

Clinical Tip

Patients who receive monthly vitamin $B_{12}$ injections may have improvements in their alertness and activity tolerance for a few days after the injection. Therefore, physical therapy intervention and goal setting should accommodate these changes.

---

Folic Acid Anemia Decreased folic acid (folate) causes the production of macrocytic, normochromic RBCs. Folic acid deficiency is associated with a diet low in folic acid, impaired intestinal absorption of folic acid, pregnancy, or alcoholism. The presentation of folic acid anemia is similar to vitamin $B_{12}$ deficiency anemia, except there are no neurologic sequelae. Folic acid anemia is diagnosed by clinical presentation, a low serum folate level, and elevated lactate dehydrogenase and MCV values.[49] Management of folic acid anemia consists of folic acid supplementation.[47]

Aplastic Anemia Aplastic anemia is characterized by a decreased RBC production secondary to bone marrow damage. The bone marrow damage either causes irreversible changes to the stem cell population, rendering these cells unable to produce RBCs, or alters the stem cell environment, which inhibits RBC production. The exact mechanism of stem cell damage is unknown; however, present theories include exposure to radiation and chemotherapy or pharmacologic agents, the presence of infection or malignancy, or as an autoimmune response.[50] RBCs are normochromic and normocytic or macrocytic. WBC and Plt counts are also decreased. Definitive diagnosis is by bone marrow biopsy. Signs and symptoms of aplastic anemia may include the following:

- Fatigue and dyspnea

- Fever or infection

- Sore throat

- Petechiae, bleeding gums, hematuria, or fecal blood

Management of aplastic anemia may include any of the following: investigation and removal of causative agent, blood transfusion, bone marrow transplantation, corticosteroids, and antibiotics. Aplastic anemia can be fatal if untreated.[8,43,45,47]

**Hemolytic Anemia**    The two types of hemolytic anemia are extravascular and intravascular hemolytic anemia. Extravascular hemolytic anemia involves the destruction of RBCs outside of the circulation, usually in the spleen. This condition is usually the result of an inherited defect of the RBC membrane or structure, but it can be an autoimmune process in which antibodies in the blood cause RBC destruction through mononuclear phagocytosis.

Intravascular hemolytic anemia is the destruction of RBC membrane within the circulation. It results in the deposition of Hgb in plasma. This may occur because of a genetic enzyme deficit, the attack of oxidants on RBCs, or infection. It may also occur traumatically when RBCs are torn apart at sites of blood flow turbulence, near a tumor, through prosthetic valves, or with aortic stenosis.

Signs and symptoms of hemolytic anemia may include the following:

- Fatigue and weakness

- Nausea and vomiting

- Fever and chills

- Decreased urine output

- Jaundice

- Abdominal or back pain and splenomegaly (intravascular only)

Management of hemolytic anemia may include any of the following: investigation and removal of the causative factor, fluid replacement, blood transfusion, corticosteroids, or splenectomy.[8,43,45]

**Sickle Cell Anemia** Sickle cell anemia is an autosomal homozygous (hemoglobin SS or HgSS) recessive trait characterized by RBCs that become sickle (crescent)-shaped when deoxygenated. Over time, cells become rigid and occlude blood vessels, thus causing tissue ischemia and infarction. The risk of cerebrovascular accident and infarction of other organs or muscles is high. Symptoms and physical findings of sickle cell anemia may include the following:

- Jaundice, nocturia, hematuria, pyelonephritis, renal failure, splenohepatomegaly
- Retinopathy or blindness
- Chronic nonhealing ulcers of the lower extremity
- Systolic murmur and an enlarged heart
- Paresthesias
- Neck, chest, abdominal, bone, and joint pain

A complication of sickle cell anemia that may require hospitalization is pain crisis, the intense pain of any major organ or body area. Pain crisis, lasting from 4 to 6 days to weeks, can be precipitated by infection, dehydration, hypoxia, sleep apnea, exposure to cold, or menstruation, or it may be of unknown etiology.[51] Acute chest syndrome is a situation that requires hospital admission. The patient presents with chest pain, dyspnea, hypoxemia, and infiltrates on chest x-ray, perhaps with pleural effusion.[52] Acute chest syndrome may be caused by intrapulmonary sickling, sickle cell emboli, or bone marrow or fat embolism, or from infection.[52]

Management of sickle cell anemia may include the prevention or supportive treatment of symptoms with rest, hydration, analgesia, supplemental oxygen, and the use of corticosteroids or cytotoxic agents, such as hydroxyurea,[53] partial RBC exchange, and psychosocial support.[8,43,45,50] The average life expectancy of a patient with sickle cell anemia is 40–50 years.[47] Note that sickle cell anemia is differentiated from sickle cell trait. A patient with sickle cell trait has a heterozygous trait of Hgb that is asymptomatic for the signs and symptoms of anemia, although RBCs may sickle under the conditions of high altitude, strenuous exercise, or anesthesia.[50]

Clinical Tip

The use of oximetry can help the physical therapist and patient monitor RBC oxygenation and gauge exercise intensity.

*Polycythemia*
The three types of polycythemia are primary polycythemia (polycythemia vera), secondary polycythemia, and relative polycythemia. They involve the abnormal increase in the number of RBCs and result in increased blood viscosity.

1.    Primary polycythemia, or polycythemia vera, is an increase in the number of RBCs, WBCs, and Plts.[54] The origin of this disease is unknown; however, there is an autonomous overproduction of erythroid stem cells from bone marrow leading to increased blood viscosity and expanded blood volume. Thus, there is a risk for thrombus formation and bleeding.[47] Primary polycythemia may convert to chronic myelogenous leukemia or myelofibrosis.

2.    Secondary polycythemia is the overproduction of RBCs owing to a high level of erythropoietin. The increased erythropoietin level is a result of either altered stem cells (which automatically produce erythropoietin or erythropoietin-secreting tumors, such as hepatoma or cerebellar hemangioblastoma)[46] or chronic low oxygenation of tissues, in which the body attempts to compensate for hypoxia. The latter is common in individuals with chronic obstructive pulmonary disease, cardiopulmonary disease, or exposure to high altitudes.

3.    Relative polycythemia is the temporary increase in RBCs secondary to decreased fluid volume (dehydration), as with excessive vomiting, diarrhea, or excessive diuretic use, or after a burn injury.

Signs and symptoms of polycythemia may include the following:

* Fatigue
* Headache
* Dizziness
* Blurred vision

- Paresthesia in the hands and feet

- Splenomegaly (polycythemia vera only)

Management of polycythemia may include any of the following: myelosuppressive therapy, antiplatelet therapy (this is controversial), radiophosphorus (for primary polycythemia), smoking cessation and phlebotomy (for secondary polycythemia), and fluid resuscitation (for relative polycythemia).

## Thrombocytic Disorders

### Disseminated Intravascular Coagulation

Disseminated intravascular coagulation (DIC) involves the introduction of thromboplastic substances into the circulation that initiate a massive clotting cascade accompanied by fibrin, plasmin, and Plt activation. It is a complex and paradoxic disorder characterized by both hemorrhage and thrombus formation. First, fibrin is deposited in the microcirculation, leading to organ ischemia and the destruction of RBCs as they pass through these deposits. Second, Plts and clotting factors are consumed and hemorrhage occurs. Plasmin is activated to further decrease clotting factor, and fibrin further inhibits Plt function, which further increases bleeding.

DIC, either acute or chronic, is always a secondary process mediated by inflammatory cytokines.[55] The onset of acute DIC usually occurs in the presence of illness within hours or days of the initial injury or event. This condition is associated with infection, trauma, burn injury, shock, tissue acidosis, antigen-antibody complexes, or the entrance of amniotic fluid or placenta into the maternal circulation. It is highly associated with gram-negative sepsis.[46]

Chronic DIC is associated with hemangioma and other cancers (particularly pancreatic or prostate cancer), systemic lupus erythematosus, or missed abortion.

Signs and symptoms of DIC may include the following:

- Abrupt (in acute DIC) or slow (in chronic DIC) blood loss from an injury site, nose, gums, or gastrointestinal or urinary tracts

- Thrombosis (for chronic DIC)

- Tachypnea, tachycardia, hypotension, and dysrhythmia

- Altered consciousness, anxiety, fear, or restlessness

- Ecchymosis, petechiae, and purpura
- Weakness
- Decreased urine output
- Acute renal failure (for acute DIC)

DIC may be mild and self-limiting or severe and is often associated with critical illness.[56] Management of DIC may include any of the following: treatment of the causative condition; blood and blood product transfusion for active bleeding; fluid, hemodynamic, and shock management; heparin therapy (this is controversial); and recombinant protein factor therapy (experimental).[55]

*Hemophilia*
Hemophilia is a disease characterized by excessive spontaneous hemorrhaging at mucous membranes, into joint spaces (hemarthrosis) and muscles, or intracranially. It is the result of a genetic deficiency of a clotting factor. There are four basic types[57]:

1. Hemophilia A is characterized by the lack of factor VIII and is inherited as an X-linked recessive trait.

2. Hemophilia B (Christmas disease) is characterized by the lack of factor IX and is inherited as an X-linked recessive trait.

3. Hemophilia C is characterized by the lack of factor XI and is inherited as an autosomal recessive trait.

4. von Willebrand's disease is characterized by the lack of factor VIII and is inherited as an autosomal dominant trait.

Patients with mild hemophilia experience bleeding only with trauma or after surgical procedures, whereas patients with severe hemophilia may bleed with minor trauma or spontaneously.[47]
Symptoms and physical findings of bleeding episode from hemophilia may include the following:

- Petechiae, purpura, and ecchymosis
- Hematoma
- Disorientation
- Convulsions

- Tachycardia, tachypnea, and hypotension

Management of hemophilia may include any of the following: methods to stop active bleeding (e.g., direct pressure), supportive therapy depending on the location of the bleed (e.g., joint debridement), factor replacement therapy, and pain management.[50]

---

Clinical Tip

Watch for signs of joint effusion (warmth and edema) in patients with hemophilia who are prone to hemarthrosis, especially during weight-bearing activites.

---

*Thalassemia*
Thalassemia is an autosomal-recessive disease characterized by abnormal formation of Hgb chains in RBCs, resulting in RBC membrane damage and abnormal erythropoiesis and hemolysis.

Hgb is composed of two alpha and two beta chains. $\alpha$-Thalassemia is a defect in alpha-chain synthesis in which one (alpha trait), two ($\alpha$-thalassemia minor), or three (Hgb H disease) genes are altered. Each type of $\alpha$-thalassemia varies in presentation from a lack of symptoms (alpha trait and minor) to chronic severe hemolytic anemia (Hgb H) which requires regular blood transfusions.[46] $\beta$-Thalassemia minor is a defect in beta-chain synthesis in one of two beta chains and is usually asymptomatic. $\beta$-Thalassemia major is a severe reduction or absence in beta-chain production that results in severe anemia, growth failure, bony deformities, hepatosplenomegaly, and jaundice with a life expectancy of 20–30 years from complications of heart failure, cirrhosis, and endocrinopathy.[47] Management of the thalassemia may include folate supplementation, blood transfusion, iron-chelating agents, and splenectomy.[47]

*Thrombocytopenia*
Thrombocytopenia is an acute or chronic decrease in the number of Plts (less than 150,000/µl) in the circulation. It can result from decreased Plt production (caused by infection, drug or immune responses, or blood vessel damage), increased Plt destruction (caused by malignancy, antiplatelet antibodies, or the use of myelosuppressive drugs), or altered Plt distribution (caused by cardiac surgery–induced hypothermia, portal hypertension, or splenomegaly).[57]

Signs and symptoms of thrombocytopenia may include the following[58]:

- Bleeding of nose, gums, or puncture sites or blood in emesis, urine, or stool

- Ecchymosis and petechiae

- Tachycardia and tachypnea

- Signs of increased intracranial pressure if a cranial bleed is present

- Renal failure

- Splenomegaly

Management of thrombocytopenia may include any of the following: treatment of the causative factor, immunosuppressive therapy, anticoagulants in plasma transfusion or plasmapheresis, corticosteroids, or splenectomy.[57]

*Heparin-Induced Thrombocytopenia*
Heparin can have a dramatic thrombocytopenic effect, usually 5–10 days after the initiation of heparin therapy. The clinical presentation of heparin-induced thrombocytopenia (HIT) is distinct and may include the following[59]:

- Large, bilateral lower-extremity DVT

- Upper-extremity DVT at a venous catheter site

- Skin lesions at the injection site

- Aortic or ileofemoral thrombus with limb ischemia

- Pulmonary embolism

- An acute systemic reaction to heparin

HIT may be type I (the asymptomatic aggregation of Plts) or type II (an immune response resulting in Plt activation and venous or arterial thrombi).[60] HIT is diagnosed by clinical presentation, a Plt count less than $100 \times 10^9$/L and a positive Plt aggregation test. Management of HIT starts with the immediate discontinuation of heparin and may include plasmapheresis, immunoglobulin therapy, and anticoagulants (experimental), in addition to supportive therapies for alteration in skin integrity and pain.[60]

*Thrombotic Thrombocytopenic Purpura*

Thrombotic thrombocytopenic purpura (TTP) is the rapid accumulation of thrombi in small blood vessels. The etiology of TTP is unknown; however, it is associated with bacterial or viral infections, estrogen use, pregnancy, and autoimmune disorders, such as acquired immunodeficiency syndrome.[47]

Signs and symptoms of TTP may include the following:

• Hemolytic anemia, thrombocytopenia

• Fatigue and weakness

• Fever

• Pallor, rash, petechiae

• Waxing and waning headache, confusion, altered consciousness from lethargy to coma

• Abdominal pain

• Acute renal failure

Management of TTP may include any of the following: emergent plasmaphoresis, plasma exchange, antiplatelet agents, corticosteroids, immunosuppressive agents, or splenectomy if not refractory to initial therapy or if the condition recurs.[47,57]

## Management

The management of vascular disorders includes pharmacologic therapy and vascular surgical procedures. Hematologic disorders may be managed with pharmacologic therapy, as well as with nutritional therapy and blood product transfusion.

### Pharmacologic Therapy

Common drug classifications for the management of vascular and hematologic disorders include (1) anticoagulants (see Appendix Table IV-4), (2) antiplatelet agents (see Appendix Table IV-10), and (3) thrombolytic agents (see Appendix Table IV-29).

## Anticoagulation Therapy

The standard INR goal for anticoagulation therapy with warfarin (Coumadin) is 1.5–2.5 times a control value and is categorized by condition or clinical state according to the following[61]:

INR 2.0–3.0

- DVT

- Pulmonary, systemic, or recurrent systemic embolism

- Valvular heart disease or after tissue heart valve replacement

- Atrial fibrillation

INR 2.5–3.5

- Recurrent systemic emboli while on warfarin.

- Recurrent myocardial infarction.

- Mechanical prosthetic heart valve replacement.

The physical therapist should understand some basic concepts of anticoagulation therapy to intervene safely and estimate length of stay.

- The physician will determine the PT/INR and PTT goal for each patient. This goal is documented in the medical record. The patient remains in a hospital setting until the goal is reached.

- The therapeutic effect of heparin is reached within minutes or hours, whereas the effect of warfarin is reached in 3–5 days; thus, heparin is usually prescribed before warfarin. Both drugs are given simultaneously until the proper PT/INR is achieved, then heparin is discontinued.

- The terms subtherapeutic and supertherapeutic imply a coagulation level below or above the anticoagulation goal, respectively.

- A subtherapeutic PT/INR or PTT indicates a risk for thrombus formation, whereas a supertherapeutic level indicates a risk for hemorrhage.

- Supertherapeutic anticoagulation is rapidly reversed by vitamin K or fresh-frozen plasma.

- Anticoagulant agents are temporarily discontinued before surgery to minimize bleeding intra- or postoperatively.

- The physical therapist should always monitor the patient who is taking anticoagulants for signs and symptoms of bleeding, as bleeding can occur even if the PT/INR is therapeutic.[61]

## Nutritional Therapy

Nutritional therapy is the treatment of choice for anemia caused by vitamin and mineral deficiency. Appendix Table IV-25 describes the indications and general side effects of the agents used to manage iron deficiency, vitamin $B_{12}$, and folic acid anemias.

## Blood Product Transfusion

Blood and blood products are transfused to replete blood volume, maintain oxygen delivery to tissues, or maintain proper coagulation.[62] Table 6-15 lists the most common transfusion products and the rationale for their use. Blood may be autologous (patient donates own blood) or homologous (from a volunteer donor).

Before transfusing blood or blood products, the substance to be given must be typed and crossed. This process ensures that the correct type of blood is given to a patient to avoid adverse reactions. A variety of transfusion reactions can occur during or after the administration of blood products. Transfusion reactions are either immunologic (caused by the stimulation of antibodies in response to antigens on the transfused cells) or nonimmunologic (caused by the physical or chemical properties of the transfused cells).[63] Table 6-16 lists the signs and symptoms of various types of acute adverse transfusion reactions. In addition to these reactions, complications of blood transfusion include air embolism (if the blood is pumped into the patient) or circulatory overload (from a rapid increase in volume). Circulatory overload occurs when the rate of blood (fluid) transfusion occurs faster than the circulation can accommodate. Signs and symptoms include tachycardia, cough, dyspnea, crackles, headache, hypertension, and distended neck veins. To prevent circulatory overload during a transfusion, intravenous fluids may be stopped, or a diuretic (e.g., furosemide [Lasix]) may be given. Delayed adverse transfusion reactions include iron overload, graft-versus-host disease, hepatitis, human immunodeficiency virus-1 infection, or delayed hemolytic reaction (approximately 7–14 days post transfusion).[64]

**Table 6-15.** Common Blood Products and Their Clinical Indications and Outcomes

| Product | Content | Clinical Indications | Outcome |
|---|---|---|---|
| Whole blood | Blood cells and plasma | Acute major blood loss in setting of hypotension, tachycardia, tachypnea, pallor, and decreased Hct and Hgb. To treat oxygen-carrying deficit (RBC) and volume expansion (plasma). Whole blood is rarely used. | Resolution of signs and symptoms of hypovolemic shock or anemia. Hct should increase 3% in a nonbleeding adult (per unit transfused). |
| Red blood cells (RBCs) | RBCs only | Acute or chronic blood loss. To treat oxygen-carrying deficit in setting of tachycardia, tachypnea, pallor, fatigue, and decreased Hct and Hgb. Anemia without need for volume expansion. | Resolution of signs and symptoms of anemia. Hct should increase 3% in a nonbleeding adult (per unit transfused). |
| Platelets (Plts) | Concentrated Plts in plasma | To restore clotting function associated with or after blood loss. To increase Plt count in a bleeding patient with Plt <100,000, in advance of a procedure with Plt <50,000, or prophylactically with Plt <10,000. | Resolution of thrombocytopenia. Prevention or resolution of bleeding. Plt should increase 5,000 in a 70-kg adult (per unit). |

**Table 6-15.** *Continued*

| Product | Content | Clinical Indications | Outcome |
|---------|---------|---------------------|---------|
| Fresh-frozen plasma (FFP) | All plasma components, namely blood factors and protein | To replace or increase coagulation factor levels. Acute disseminated intravascular coagulopathy. Thrombotic thrombocytopenic purpura. Factor XI deficiency. Rapid reversal of warfarin therapy. | Improved or adequate coagulation levels or factor assays. |
| Albumin | Albumin cells with few globulins and other proteins | Volume expansion in situations when crystalloid (saline or Ringers lactate) is inadequate such as shock, major hemorrhage, or plasma exchange. Acute liver failure. Burn injury. See Albumin, above. | Acquire and maintain adequate blood pressure and volume support. |
| Plasma protein fraction (PPF) | Albumin, globulins, and plasma proteins | See Albumin, above. | See Albumin, above. |

| Cryoprecipitate | Factors VIII and XIII, von Willebrand's factor, and fibrinogen in plasma | Replacement of these factor deficiencies. Replacement of fibrinogen when an increase in volume would not be tolerated with FFP. Bleeding associated with uremia. | Correction of these factor or fibrinogen deficiencies. Cessation of bleeding in uremic patients. |

Hct = hematocrit, Hgb = hemoglobin.
Sources: Data from National Blood Resource Education Programs Transfusion Therapy Guidelines for Nurses. US Department of Health and Human Services, National Institutes of Health, September 1990; and adapted from WH Churchill. Transfusion Therapy. New York: Scientific American Medicine, 2001;4.

**Table 6-16.** Acute Adverse Blood Reactions

| Reaction | Cause | Signs and Symptoms |
|---|---|---|
| Febrile reaction | Patient's blood (antileukocyte antibodies) is sensitive to transfused plasma protein, platelets, or white blood cells. | Low-grade fever, headache, chills, flushed skin, muscle pain, anxiety (mild)<br>Hypotension, tachycardia, tachypnea, cough (severe)<br>Onset: during transfusion or up to 24 hrs post transfusion |
| Allergic reaction | Patient's blood (IgE, IgG, or both) is sensitive to transfused plasma protein. | Hives, flushed or itchy skin, and bronchial wheezing (mild)<br>Tachypnea, chest pain, cardiac arrest (severe)<br>Onset: within minutes of transfusion |
| Septic reaction | Transfused blood components are contaminated with bacteria. | Rapid onset of high fever, hypotension, chills, emesis, diarrhea, abdominal cramps, renal failure, shock<br>Onset: within minutes to 30 mins after transfusion |
| Acute hemolytic reaction | Patient's blood and transfused blood are not compatible, resulting in red blood cell destruction. | Tachycardia, hypotension, tachypnea, cyanosis, chest pain, fever, chills, head- or backache, acute renal failure, cardiac arrest<br>Onset: within minutes to hours after transfusion |

| Anaphylactic reaction | Patient is deficient in IgA and develops IgA antibody to transfused components. | Hives (mild) Wheezing or bronchospasm, anxiety, cyanosis, nausea, emesis, bloody diarrhea, abdominal cramps, shock, cardiac arrest (severe) Onset: within a few seconds after exposure |

Ig = immunoglobulin.

Sources: Adapted from B Kozier, G Erb, K Blais, JM Wilkinson (eds). Fundamentals of Nursing: Concepts, Process and Practice (5th ed). Redwood City, CA. Benjamin-Cummings, 1995;110; and data from PJ Larison, LO Cook. Adverse Effects of Blood Transfusion. In DM Harmening (ed), Modern Blood Banking and Transfusion Practices. Philadelphia: FA Davis, 1999; and National Blood Resource Education Programs Transfusion Therapy Guidelines for Nurses. US Department of Health and Human Services, National Institutes of Health. September 1990.

---

Clinical Tip

• If the patient is receiving blood products, the physical therapist should observe the patient for signs or symptoms, or both, of transfusion reaction before initiating physical therapy intervention.
• Depending on the medical status of the patient, the therapist may defer out of bed or vigorous activities until the transfusion is complete. On average, the transfusion of a unit of blood takes 3–4 hours.
• Defer physical therapy intervention during the first 15 minutes of a blood transfusion as most blood transfusion reactions occur within this time frame.
• During a blood transfusion, vital signs are usually taken every 15–30 minutes by the nurse and posted at the bedside.

---

## Vascular Surgical Procedures

Surgical management of coronary vascular disorders, such as angioplasty, arthrectomy, and stent placement, is described in Chapter 1 under Percutaneous Revascularization Procedures. These same techniques are also used in peripheral arteries rather than coronary arteries. This section therefore concentrates on embolization therapy, transcatheter thrombolysis, endarterectomy, bypass grafting, and aneurysm repair and replacement with synthetic grafts. Patients who undergo percutaneous catherization procedures will have similar precautions and considerations, as described earlier in the Invasive Vascular Studies section.

### Embolization Therapy

Embolization* therapy is the process of purposely occluding a vessel with Gelfoam, coils, balloons, polyvinyl alcohol, and various glue-like agents, which are injected as liquids and then solidify in the vessel. Embolization therapy is performed with a specialized intravascular catheter after angiographic evaluation has outlined the area to be treated.

---

*The term *embolization* is general and can refer to a pathologic occlusion of a vessel by fat, air, or a dislodged portion of a thrombus, or to the therapeutic procedure described in this section. The context in which embolization is discussed must be considered to avoid confusion.

Indications for embolization therapy include disorders characterized by inappropriate blood flow, such as AVMs or, less commonly, persistent hemoptysis.

Complications of embolization therapy include tissue necrosis, inadvertent embolization of normal tissues, and passage of embolic materials through arteriovenous communications.[23]

### Transcatheter Thrombolysis

Transcatheter thrombolysis is the process of directly infusing thrombolytic agents (generally, urokinase) into occluded vessels via percutaneous catheter access. Once the catheter is inserted and placed in the area of occlusion, the catheter is left in place for extended periods of time, as long as 3 days, to allow the clot to be properly lysed. This procedure may also include angioplasty, if warranted, to open a stenotic area. By injecting the thrombolytic agent into the area of occlusion, transcatheter thrombolysis has less systemic complications of hemorrhage compared to intravenous infusion of thrombolytic agents.[5]

### Peripheral Vascular Bypass Grafting

To reperfuse an area that has been ischemic from peripheral vascular disease, two general bypass grafting procedures (with many specific variations of each type) can be performed. The area of vascular occlusion can be bypassed with an inverted portion of the saphenous vein or with a synthetic material, such as Gore-Tex, Dacron, or Lycra. (The synthetic graft is referred to as a prosthetic graft.) Vascular surgeons generally describe and illustrate in the medical record what type of procedure was performed on the particular vascular anatomy. The terminology used to describe each bypass graft procedure indicates which vessels were involved. (For example, a fem-pop bypass graft involves bypassing an occlusion of the femoral artery with another conduit to the popliteal artery distal to the area of occlusion.) After a bypass procedure, patients, depending on premorbid physiologic status and extent of surgery, require approximately 24–48 hours to become hemodynamically stable and are usually monitored in an intensive care unit setting. Figures 6-3 and 6-4 illustrate two vascular bypass procedures.

Complications that can occur after bypass grafting include the following[6]:

- Hemorrhage (at graft site or in gastrointestinal tract)
- Thrombosis

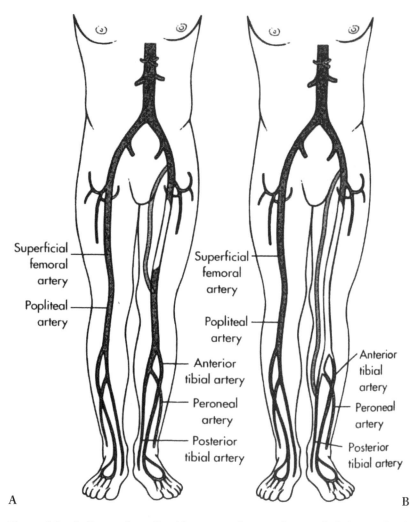

**Figure 6-3.** *A. Femoral-popliteal bypass graft around an occluded superficial femoral artery. B. Femoral-posterior tibial bypass graft around occluded superficial femoral, popliteal, and proximal tibial arteries. (With permission from SM Lewis, MM Heitkemper, SR Dirksen [eds]. Medical-Surgical Nursing, Assessment and Management of Clincal Problems [5th ed]. St. Louis: Mosby, 2000;990.)*

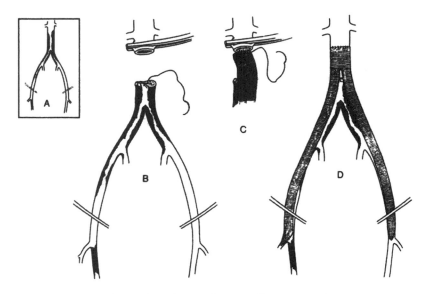

**Figure 6-4.** *Aortofemoral graft. A. Schematic illustration of a preoperative aortogram. B. A segment of diseased aorta is resected, and the distal aortic stump is oversewn. C. End-to-end proximal anastomosis. D. Completed reconstruction. (With permission from RB Rutherford [ed]. Vascular Surgery [5th ed]. Philadelphia: Saunders, 2000;951.)*

- Pseudoaneurysm formation at the anastomosis
- Infection
- Renal failure
- Sexual dysfunction
- Spinal cord ischemia
- Colon ischemia

**Endarterectomy**
Endarterectomy is a process in which the stenotic area of an artery wall is excised and the noninvolved ends of the artery are reanastomosed. It can be used to correct localized occlusive vascular disease, commonly in the carotid arteries, eliminating the need for bypassing the area.[23]

---

**Clinical Tip**

The abbreviation CEA is often used to refer to a carotid endarterectomy procedure.

---

**Aneurysm Repair and Reconstruction**

Aneurysm repair and reconstruction involve isolating the aneurysm by clamping off the vessel proximal and distal to the aneurysm, excising the aneurysm, and replacing the aneurysmal area with a synthetic graft. Performing the procedure before the aneurysm ruptures (elective surgery) is preferable to repairing a ruptured aneurysm (emergency surgery), because a ruptured aneurysm presents an extremely challenging and difficult operative course owing to the hemodynamic instability from hemorrhage. The cross-clamp time of the vessels is also crucial, because organs distal to the site of repair can become ischemic if the clamp time is prolonged. Complications that may occur after aneurysm repair are similar to those discussed in Peripheral Vascular Bypass Grafting.[6] Figure 6-5 illustrates an aneurysm repair and reconstruction.

---

**Clinical Tip**

• Incisions should be inspected before and after physical therapy interventions to assess the patency of the incision, as drainage or weeping may occur during activity. If drainage or weeping occurs, stop the current activity and inspect the amount of drainage. Provide compression, if appropriate, and notify the nurse promptly. Once the drainage is stable or under the management of the nurse, document the incidence of drainage accordingly in the medical record.

• Abdominal incisions or other incisional pain can limit a patient's cough effectiveness and lead to pulmonary infection. Diligent attention to position changes, deep breathing, assisted coughing, and manual techniques (e.g., percussion and vibration techniques as needed) can help prevent pulmonary infections.

• Grafts that cross the hip joint, such as aortobifemoral grafts, require clarification by the surgeon regarding the amount of flexion allowed at the hip.

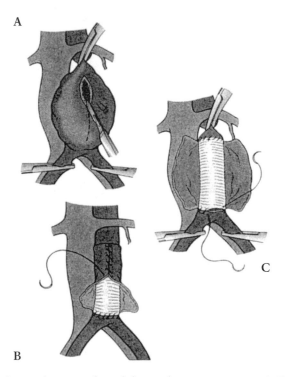

**Figure 6-5.** *Surgical repair of an abdominal aortic aneurysm. A. Incising the aneurysmal sac. B. Insertion of synthetic graft. C. Suturing native aortic wall over synthetic graft. (With permission from SM Lewis, MM Heitkemper, SR Dirksen [eds]. Medical-Surgical Nursing, Assessment and Management of Clinical Problems [5th ed]. St. Louis: Mosby, 2000;981.)*

- After a patient is cleared for out-of-bed activity, specific orders from the physician should be obtained regarding weight bearing on the involved extremities, particularly those with recent bypass grafts.
- Patients may also have systolic blood pressure limitations postoperatively to maintain adequate perfusion of the limb or to ensure the patency of the graft area. Blood pressures that are below the specified limit may decrease perfusion, whereas pressures above the limit may lead to graft damage. Thorough vital sign monitoring before, during, and after activity is essential.[7]

- Patients who are status post bypass grafting procedures should have improved peripheral pulses; therefore, any reduction in the strength of distal peripheral pulses that occurs after surgery should be brought to the attention of the nurse and physician.

### Physical Therapy Interventions for Patients with Vascular and Hematologic Disorders

The primary goal of physical therapy for patients with vascular and hematologic disorders is the optimization of functional mobililty and activity tolerance. In addition to these goals, patients with vascular disorders require patient education to prevent skin breakdown and DVT formation, manage edema, and prevent joint contractures and muscle shortening. Patients with hematologic disorders may require patient education for activity modification, pain management, or fall prevention (especially if the patient is at risk of bleeding or on anticoagulant therapy).

Guidelines for the physical therapist working with the patient who has vascular or hematologic dysfunction include the following:

- Patients with peripheral vascular disease commonly have concurrent coronary artery disease and diabetes mellitus; therefore, being watchful for signs and symptoms of angina in conjunction with monitoring vital signs and blood glucose levels is essential.

- Patients with peripheral vascular disease may also have concurrent chronic obstructive pulmonary disease; therefore, activity tolerance may have pulmonary limitations as well.

- Patients with peripheral vascular disease may have impaired sensation from arterial insufficiency, comorbid diagnosis of diabetes mellitus, or peripheral edema; therefore, sensation testing is an important component of the physical therapy evaluation.

- Peripheral edema can result from a variety of disorders, including venous insufficiency, liver disease, renal insufficiency or renal failure, and heart failure; therefore, the physical therapist should perform a thorough review of the patient's medical history before performing any edema management techniques. For example, limb elevation may be helpful in chronic venous insufficiency but may be detrimental in acute congestive heart failure.

• The physical therapist should monitor a patient's CBC and coagulation profile on a daily basis to determine the potential risk for bruising or bleeding, thrombus formation, and for altered oxygen-carrying capacity with exertion.

• To gain insight into the hemostatic condition of the patient, determine (1) whether the abnormal blood laboratory values are expected or consistent with patients medical-surgical status, (2) the relative severity (mild, moderate, or severe) of the abnormal laboratory values, and (3) whether the patient has a medical history or predisposing condition that could be exacerbated by the abnormal laboratory values.

• The physical therapist must determine the need to modify or defer physical therapy intervention in the setting of abnormal blood laboratory values, most commonly alterations in Hct, Plt, and PT/INR. Often, there is no specific numeric protocol for this purpose; thus, the decision to modify or defer physical therapy must be based on the clinical picture as well as the quantitative data. For example, a patient may have a low Plt count but is hemodynamically stable without signs of active bleeding. The physical therapist may therefore decide to continue to mobilize the patient out of bed. Conversely, if a patient with a low Plt count has new hemoptysis, the physical therapist may then defer manual chest physical therapy techniques, such as percussion.

• Exercise guidelines for patients with thrombocytopenia vary among hospitals. A general rule of thumb regarding exercises that should be performed is the following:  activities of daily living; active range of motion, and ambulation with physician approval for Plt count of less than 20,000 mm$^3$; active range of motion and walking as tolerated for Plt count of 20,000–30,000 mm$^3$; active range of motion, ambulation, or stationary bicycling for Plt count of 30,000–50,000 mm$^3$; and, progressive resistive exercise, ambulation, or stationary bicycling for a Plt count of 50,000–150,000 mm$^3$.[65]

• For an INR greater than 3.5 (the standard highest level for anticoagulation), consult with the nurse or physician before physical therapy intervention and modify treatment accordingly. There is no common protocol for activity guidelines for the patient with an INR greater than 3.5; however, most patients continue out-of-bed activities and activities of daily living with caution or supervision with an INR slightly greater than 3.5. Generally, physical therapy intervention is deferred, and the patient may be on bed rest if the INR is greater than 6.0.

• The monitoring of blood pressure, heart rate, and respiratory rate is recommended at rest and with activity, because the hemodynamic sequelae of alterations in blood volume or viscosity may be subtle or insidious in onset and first noticed in response to exercise by the physical therapist.

• Observe the patient for the signs and symptoms of thrombus formation or bleeding during physical therapy intervention. Immediately report any abnormalities to the nurse.

• Progression of activity tolerance in patients with hematologic disorders does not occur at the same rate as in patients with normal blood composition; therefore, the time frame for goal achievement may need to be lengthened.

## References

1. Black JM, Matassarin-Jacobs E (eds). Luckmann and Sorensen's Medical-Surgical Nursing: A Psychophysiologic Approach (4th ed). Philadelphia: Saunders, 1993;1286.
2. Marieb EN. Blood. In EN Marieb (ed), Human Anatomy and Physiology (3rd ed). Redwood City, CA: Benjamin-Cummings, 1995;584–611.
3. Knight CA. Peripheral Vascular Disease and Wound Care. In SB O'Sullivan, TJ Schmitz (eds), Physical Rehabilitation: Assessment and Treatment (4th ed). Philadelphia: FA Davis, 2001;583–608.
4. Lanzer P, Rosch J (eds). Vascular Diagnostics: Noninvasive and Invasive Techniques, Peri-Interventional Evaluations. Berlin: Springer-Verlag, 1994.
5. Fahey VA (ed). Vascular Nursing (3rd ed). Philadelphia: Saunders, 1999.
6. Hallet JW, Brewster DC, Darling RC (eds). Handbook of Patient Care in Vascular Surgery (3rd ed). Boston: Little, Brown, 1995.
7. Hillman RS, Ault KA (eds). Hematology in Clinical Practice: A Guide to Diagnosis and Management. New York: McGraw-Hill, 1995;17.
8. Goodman CC, Snyder TK. Overview of Hematology: Signs and Symptoms. In CC Goodman, TK Snyder (eds), Differential Diagnosis in Physical Therapy: Musculoskeletal and Systemic Conditions. Philadelphia: Saunders, 1990;114.

9. Matassarin-Jacobs E. Assessment of Clients with Hematologic Disorders. In E Matassarin-Jacobs, JM Black (eds), Medical-Surgical Nursing: Clinical Management for Continuity of Care (5th ed). Philadelphia: Saunders, 1997;1461–1468.

10. Dorland WA. Dorland's Illustrated Medical Dictionary (29th ed). Philadelphia: Saunders, 2000.

11. Perkins SL. Examination of the Blood and Bone Marrow. In GR Lee, J Foerster, J Lukens (eds). Wintrobe's Clinical Hematology, Vol. 1 (10th ed). Baltimore: Williams & Wilkins, 1999;9–35.

12. Zieve PD, Waterbury L. Thromboembolic Disease. In LR Barker, JR Burton, PD Zieve (eds), Principles of Ambulatory Medicine (5th ed). Baltimore: Williams & Wilkins, 1999;642–651.

13. Moore WS (ed). Vascular Surgery: A Comprehensive Review (4th ed). Philadelphia: Saunders, 1993;90.

14. McCance KL, Huether SE (eds). Pathophysiology: The Biologic Basis for Disease in Adults and Children (2nd ed). St. Louis: Mosby, 1994;1001.

15. Weiner SD, Reis ED, Kerstein MD. Peripheral arterial disease: medical management in primary care practice. Geriatrics 2001;56(4):20.

16. Ridker PM, Stampfer MJ, Rifai N. Novel risk factors for systemic atherosclerosis: a comparison of c-reactive protein, fibrinogen, homocysteine, lipoprotein(a), and standard cholesterol screening as predictors of peripheral arterial disease. JAMA 2001;285(19):2481.

17. Thompson JM, McFarland GK, Hirsch JE, et al (eds). Clinical Nursing. St. Louis: Mosby, 1986;85.

18. Young JR, Graor RA, Olin JW, Bartholomew JR (eds). Peripheral Vascular Diseases. St. Louis: Mosby, 1991.

19. Tjon JA, Reimann LE. Treatment of intermittent claudication with pentoxifylline and cilostazol. Am J Health Syst Pharm 2001;58(6):485–493.

20. Tierney S, Fennessy F, Hayes DB. ABC of arterial and vascular disease. Secondary prevention of peripheral vascular disease. BMJ 2000; 320(7244):1262–1265.

21. Bullock BL (ed). Pathophysiology: Adaptations and Alterations in Function (4th ed). Philadelphia: Lippincott–Raven, 1996;524.

22. Thompson MM, Bell PRF. Arterial aneurysms (ABC of arterial and venous disease). BMJ 2000;320(7243):1193.

23. Strandness DE, Breda AV (eds). Vascular Diseases: Surgical and Interventional Therapy, Vols. 1 and 2. New York: Churchill Livingstone, 1994.

24. Rauch U, Osende JI, Fuster V, et al. Thrombus formation on atherosclerotic plaques: pathogenesis and clinical consequences. Ann Intern Med 2001;134(3):224.

25. Brown MJ. Science, medicine, and the future. Hypertension. BMJ 1997;314(7089):1258–1261.

26. Smeltzer SC, Bare BG (eds). Brunner and Suddarth's Textbook of Medical-Surgical Nursing (8th ed). Philadelphia: Lippincott, 1995;722.

27. Mulrow CD, Pignone M. What are the elements of good treatment for hypertension? (Evidence-based management of hypertension.) BMJ 2001;322(7294):1107.

28. Hyman DJ, Pavlik VN. Self-reported hypertension treatment practices among primary care physicians. Arch Intern Med 2000;160(15):2281.

29. Easton DM. Systematic vasculitis: a difficult diagnosis in the elderly. Physician Assistant 2001;25(1):37.
30. Kallenberg CGM, Cohen Tervaert CGM. What is new in systemic vasculitis? Ann Rheum Dis 2000;59(11):924.
31. Mawdsley A. The big freeze. (Treating Raynaud's phenomenon.) Chem Druggist 1998:S4
32. Wittink H. Adjuvant physical therapy versus occupational therapy in patients with reflex sympathetic dystrophy/complex regional pain syndrome type I. Phys Ther 2001;81(1):753.
33. Schwartzman RJ. New treatments for reflex sympathetic dystrophy. N Engl J Med 2000;343(9):654–656.
34. Zollinger PE, Tuinebreijer WE, Kreis RW, Breederveld RS. Effect of vitamin C on frequency of reflex sympathetic dystrophy in wrist fractures: a randomised trial. Lancet 1999;354(9195):2025.
35. Adami S, Fossaluzza V, Gatti D, Fracassi E, Braga V. Bisphosphonate therapy of reflex sympathetic dystrophy syndrome. Ann Rheum Dis 1997:56(3):201–204.
36. Tumbarello C. Acute extremity compartment syndrome. J Trauma Nurs 2000:7(2):30.
37. London NJM, Nash R. ABC of arterial and venous disease. Varicose veins. BMJ 2000;320(7246):1391.
38. Tepper SH, McKeough DM. Deep Venous Thrombosis: Risks, Diagnosis, Treatment Interventions and Prevention. Acute Care Perspectives: American Physical Therapy Association, Vol. 9(1), 2000.
39. Breen P. DVT. What every nurse should know. RN 2000;63(4):58–62.
40. Church, V. Staying on guard for DVT & PE. Nursing 2000;30(2):34–42.
41. Saunders CS. Improving survival in pulmonary embolism. Patient Care 2000;34(16):50.
42. Coats U. Management of venous ulcers. Crit Care Nurse Q 1998;21(2): 14–23.
43. Purtillo DT, Purtillo RP (eds). A Survey of Human Diseases (2nd ed). Boston: Little, Brown, 1989;287.
44. Lee GR. Acute Posthemorrhagic Anemia. In GR Lee, J Foerster, J Lukens, et al. (eds), Wintrobe's Clinical Hematology, Vol. 2 (10th ed). Baltimore: Williams & Wilkins, 1999;1485–1488.
45. Erythrocyte Disease. In AE Belcher (ed), Blood Disorders. St. Louis: Mosby–Year Book, 1993;51.
46. The Hematopoietic and Lymphoid Systems. In Kumar V, Cotran R, Robbins SL (eds), Basic Pathology (6th ed). Philadelphia: Saunders, 1997;340–392.
47. Linker CA. Blood. In LM Tierney, SJ McPhee, MA Papadakis (eds), Current Medical Diagnosis and Treatment 2001. Stamford, CT: Appleton & Lange, 2001;505–558.
48. Lehne RA. Drugs for Deficiency Anemias. In RA Lehne (ed), Pharmacology for Nursing Care (4th ed). Philadelphia: Saunders, 2001;589–602.
49. Roper D, Stein S, Payne M, Coleman M. Anemias Caused by Impaired Production of Erythrocytes. In BF Rodak (ed), Diagnostic Hematology. Philadelphia: Saunders, 1995;181.

50. Sheppard KC. Nursing Management of Adults with Hematologic Disorders. In PG Beare, JL Myers (eds), Adult Health Nursing (3rd ed). St. Louis: Mosby, 1998;670–711.
51. Reid CD, Charach S, Lubin B (eds). Painful Events. In Management and Therapy of Sickle Cell Disease (3rd ed). National Institutes of Health, 1995. Pub. 25-2117;35.
52. Reid CD, Charach S, Lubin B (eds). Acute Chest Syndrome. In Management and Therapy of Sickle Cell Disease (3rd ed). National Institutes of Health, 1995. Pub. 25-2117;47.
53. Day SW, Wynn LW. Sickle Cell Pain and Hydroxyurea. Am J Nurs 2000;100:34–39.
54. Babior BM, Stossel TP. Hematology: A Pathophysiological Approach (3rd ed). New York: Churchill Livingstone, 1994;359.
55. Levi M, De Jonge E. Current Management of Disseminated Intravascular Coagulation. Hosp Pract (Off Ed) 2000;35:59–66.
56. Matassarin-Jacobs E. Nursing Care of Clients with Hematologic Disorders. In E Matassarin-Jacobs, JM Black (eds), Medical-Surgical Nursing: Clinical Management for Continuity of Care (5th ed). Philadelphia: Saunders, 1997;1469–1532.
57. Thrombolytic Disorders. In AE Belcher, Blood Disorders. St. Louis: Mosby, 1993;112.
58. Horrell CJ, Rothman J. Establishing the etiology of thrombocytopenia. Nurse Pract 2000;25:68–77.
59. Warkentin TE. Clinical Picture of Heparin-Induced Thrombocytopenia. In TE Warkentin, A Greinacher (eds), Heparin-Induced Thrombocytopenia. New York: Marcel Dekker, 1999;43–73.
60. Jerdee Al. Heparin-associated thrombocytopenia: nursing implications. Crit Care Nurse 1998;18:38–43.
61. Gibbar-Clements T, Shirrell D, Dooley R, Smiley B. The challenge of warfarin therapy. Am J Nurs 2000;100:38-40.
62. Harkness GA, Dincher JR (eds). Medical-Surgical Nursing: Total Patient Care (9th ed). St. Louis: Mosby, 1996;656.
63. Schroeder ML. Principles and Practice of Transfusion Medicine. In GR Lee, J Foerster, J Lukens, et al. (eds), Wintrobe's Clinical Hematology, Vol. 1 (10th ed). Baltimore: Williams & Wilkins, 1999;817–874.
64. National Blood Resource Education Programs Transfusion Therapy Guidelines for Nurses. US Department of Health and Human Services, National Institutes of Health. September 1990.
65. Goodman CC. The Hematologic System. In: CC Goodman, WG Boissonnault (eds), Pathology: Implications for the Physical Therapist. Philadelphia: Saunders, 1998;381.

# 7

# Burns and Wounds

*Michele P. West, Kimberly Knowlton,
and Marie Jarrell-Gracious*

## Introduction

Treating a patient with a major burn injury or other skin wound is
often a specialized area of physical therapy.* Physical therapists
should, however, have a basic understanding of normal and abnormal
skin integrity, including the etiology of skin breakdown and the factors that influence wound healing. The main objectives of this chapter
are therefore to provide a fundamental review of the following:

> 1.  The structure and function of the skin (integument)
>
> 2.  The evaluation and physiologic sequelae of burn injury,
> including medical-surgical management and physical therapy
> intervention

---

*For the purpose of this chapter, an alteration in skin integrity secondary to a
burn injury is referred to as a *burn*. Alteration in skin integrity from any other
etiology is referred to as a *wound*.

3.   The etiology of different types of wounds and the process of wound healing

4.   The evaluation and management of wounds, including physical therapy intervention

## Structure and Function: Normal Integument

### Structure

The integumentary system consists of the skin and its appendages (hair and hair shafts, nails, and sebaceous and sweat glands), which are located throughout the skin, as pictured in Figure 7-1.

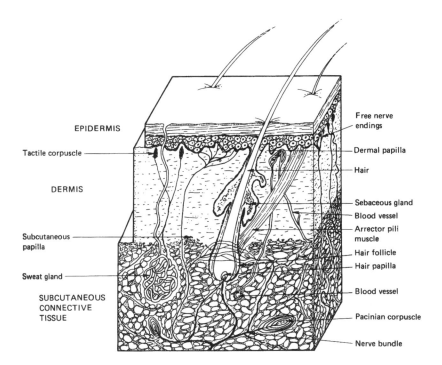

**Figure 7-1.** *Three-dimensional representation of the skin and subcutaneous connective tissue layer showing the arrangement of hair, glands, and blood vessels. (With permission from N Palastanga, D Field, R Soames, et al. Anatomy and Human Movement [2nd ed]. Oxford, UK: Butterworth–Heinemann, 1989;49.)*

Skin is 0.5–4.0 mm thick and is composed of two major layers: the epidermis and the dermis. These layers are supported by subcutaneous tissue and fat that connect the skin to muscle and bone. The thin, avascular epidermis is composed mainly of cells containing keratin. The epidermal cells are in different stages of growth and degeneration. The thick, highly vascularized dermis is composed mainly of connective tissue. Table 7-1 lists the major contents of each skin layer.

The skin has a number of clinically significant variations: (1) Men have thicker skin than women; (2) the young and elderly have thinner skin than adults[1]; and (3) the skin on various parts of the body varies in thickness, number of appendages, and blood flow.[2] These variations affect the severity of a burn injury or skin breakdown, as well as the process of tissue healing.

### Function

The integument has seven major functions[3]:

1.   Temperature regulation. Body temperature is regulated by increasing or decreasing sweat production, superficial blood flow, or both.

2.   Protection. The skin acts as a barrier to protect the body from micro-organism invasion, ultraviolet (UV) radiation, abrasion, chemicals, and dehydration.

3.   Sensation. Multiple sensory cells within the skin detect pain, temperature, and touch.

4.   Excretion. Heat, sweat, and water can be excreted from the skin.

5.   Immunity. Normal periodic loss of epidermal cells removes micro-organisms from the body surface, and immune cells in the skin transport antigens from outside the body to the antibody cells of the immune system.

6.   Blood reservoir. Large volumes of blood can be shunted from the skin to central organs or muscles as needed.

7.   Vitamin D synthesis. Modified cholesterol molecules are converted to vitamin D when exposed to UV radiation.

Table 7-1. Normal Skin Layers: Structure and Function

| Layer | Composition | Function |
|---|---|---|
| **Epidermis** | | |
| Stratum corneum | Dead keratinocytes | Tough outer layer that protects deeper layers of epidermis |
| Pigment layer | Melanocytes | Produces melanin to prevent ultraviolet absorption |
| Stratum granulosum | Mature keratinocytes | Produces keratin to make the skin waterproof |
| | Langerhans' cells | Interacts with immune cells |
| Stratum spinosum | Keratinocytes | Undergoes mitosis to continue skin cell development but to a lesser degree than basal |
| Stratum basale | New keratinocytes | The origin of skin cells, which undergoes mitosis, then moves superficially |
| | Merkel's cells | Detects touch |
| **Dermis** | | |
| Papillary layer | Areolar connective tissue | Binds epidermis and dermis together |
| | Meissner's corpuscles | Detects light touch |
| | Blood and lymph vessels | Provides circulation and drainage |
| | Free nerve endings | Detects heat and pain |
| Reticular layer | Collagen, elastin, and reticular fibers | Provides strength and resilience |
| Hypodermis | Subcutaneous fat | Provides insulation and shock absorption |
| | Pacinian cells | Detects pressure |
| | Free nerve endings | Detects cold |

Source: Data from GA Thibodeau, KT Patton (eds). Structure and Function of the Body (11th ed). St Louis: Mosby, 2000.

## Pathophysiology of Burns

Skin and body tissue destruction occurs from the absorption of heat energy and results in tissue coagulation. This coagulation is depicted in zones (Figure 7-2). The *zone of coagulation*, located in the center of the burn, is the area of greatest damage and contains nonviable tissue referred to as *eschar*. Although eschar covers the surface and may appear to take the place of skin, it does not have any of the characteristics or functions of normal skin. Instead, eschar is constrictive, attracts micro-organisms, and houses burn toxins that may circulate throughout the body.[1] The *zone of stasis*, which surrounds the zone of coagulation, contains marginally viable tissue. The *zone of hyperemia*, the outermost area, is the least damaged and heals rapidly.

### Physiologic Sequelae of Burn Injury

A series of physiologic events occurs after a burn (Figure 7-3). The physical therapist must appreciate the multisystem effects of a burn injury—namely, that the metabolic demands of the body increase dramatically. Tissue damage or organ dysfunction can be immediate or delayed, minor or severe, and local or systemic. A

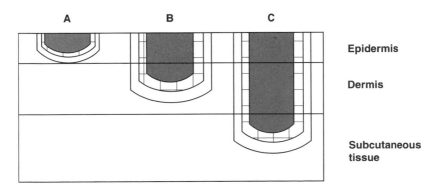

**Figure 7-2.** *The zones of coagulation. Superficial burn (A). Partial-thickness burn (B). Full-thickness burn (C). (Modified from WG Williams, LG Phillips. Pathophysiology of the Burn Wound. In DN Herndon [ed], Total Burn Care. London: Saunders, 1996;65.)*

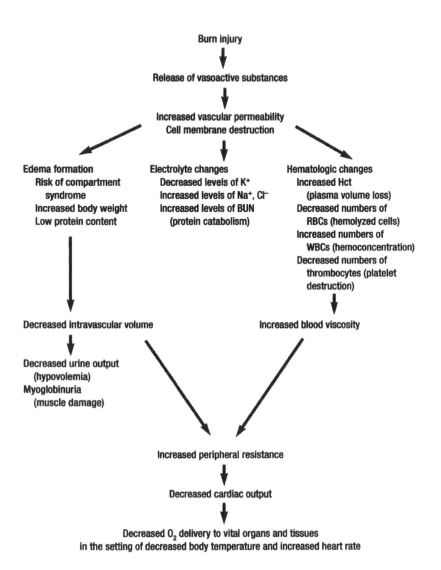

Figure 7-3. *The physiologic sequelae of major burn injury. (BUN = blood urea nitrogen; Cl⁻ = chlorine; Hct = hematocrit; K⁺ = potassium; Na⁺ = sodium; O₂ = oxygen; RBC = red blood cell; WBC = white blood cell.) (Modified from J Marvin. Thermal Injuries. In VD Caradona, PD Hurn, PJ Bastnagel Mason, et al. [eds], Trauma Nursing from Resuscitation through Rehabilitation [2nd ed]. Philadelphia: Saunders, 1994;740; and RH Demling, C LaLonde. Burn Trauma. New York: Thieme, 1989;99.)*

**Table 7-2.** Systemic Complications of Burn Injury

| Body System | Complications |
| --- | --- |
| Respiratory | Inhalation injury, restrictive pulmonary pattern (which may occur with a burn on the trunk), atelectasis, pneumonia, microthrombi, and adult respiratory distress syndrome |
| Cardiovascular | Hypovolemia/hypotension, pulmonary hypertension, subendocardial ischemia, anemia, and disseminated intravascular coagulopathy |
| Gastrointestinal/ genitourinary | Stress ulceration, hemorrhage, ileus, ischemic colitis, cholestasis, liver failure, and urinary tract infection |
| Renal | Edema, hemorrhage, acute tubular necrosis, acute renal failure |

Source: Data from HA Linares. The Burn Problem: A Pathologist's Perspective. In DN Herdon (ed), Total Burn Care. London: Saunders, 1996.

summary of the most common complications of burns is listed in Table 7-2.

### Types of Burns

**Thermal Burns**
Thermal burns can be the result of conduction or convection, as in contact with a hot object, hot liquid, chemicals, flame, or steam. In order of frequency, the most common types of thermal burns are scalds, flame burns, flash burns, and contact burns (Table 7-3).[4] The severity of burn depends on the location of the burn, the temperature of the burn source, and the duration of contact.[5]

**Electrical Burns**
An electrical burn is caused by exposure to a low- or high-voltage current and results in superficial burns, as well as less-visible but massive damage of muscle, nerves, and bone. Tissue necrosis of these deeper structures occurs from the high heat intensity of the current and the electrical disruption of cell membranes.[4] Tissue damage occurs along the path of the current, with smaller distal areas of the body damaged most severely. This pattern of tissue

**Table 7-3.** Thermal Burns: Types and Characteristics

| Burn Type | Description | Characteristics |
|---|---|---|
| Scald burn | Spill of or immersion in a hot liquid, such as boiling water, grease, or tar | Often causes deep partial- or full-thickness burns. Exposure to thicker liquids or immersion causes a deeper burn from increased contact time. Immersion burns commonly cover a larger total body surface area than do spills. |
| Flame burn | Flame exposure from fire or flammable liquids, or ignition of clothing | Often causes superficial and deep partial-thickness burns. Associated with carbon monoxide poisoning. |
| Flash burn | Explosion of flammable liquid, such as gasoline or propane | Often causes partial-thickness burns. Burns may be distributed over all exposed skin. Associated with upper airway thermal damage. Most common in the summer and associated with the consumption of alcohol. |
| Contact burn | Exposure to hot objects, such as glass, plastic, metal, or coal | Often causes deep partial- or full-thickness burns. Associated with crushing injuries, such as motor vehicle accidents. Most common cause of serious burns in the elderly. |

Sources: Data from GD Warden, DM Heimbach. Burns. In SI Schwartz (ed), Principles of Surgery, Vol. 1 (7th ed). New York: McGraw-Hill, 1999; and RF Edlich, JC Moghtader. Thermal Burns. In P Rosen (ed), Emergency Medicine Concepts and Clinical Practice, Vol. 1 (4th ed). St. Louis: Mosby, 1998.

damage accounts for the high incidence of amputation associated with electrical injury.[4,6] The severity of an electrical burn depends primarily on the duration of contact with the source, as well as the voltage of the source, the type and pathway of current, and the amperage and resistance through the body tissues.[6]

Electrical burns are characterized by deep entrance and exit wounds or arc wounds. The *entrance wound* is usually an obvious necrotic and depressed area, whereas the exit wound varies in presentation. The *exit wound* can be a single wound or multiple wounds located where the patient was grounded during injury.[7] An *arc wound* is caused by the passage of current directly between joints in close opposition. For example, if the elbow is fully flexed and an electrical current passes through the arm, burns may be located at the volar aspect of the wrist, antecubital space, and axilla.[4]

Complications specific to electrical injury include the following[4,8]:

- Cardiovascular: Cardiac arrest (ventricular fibrillation for electric current or asystolic for lightning), arrhythmia (usually sinus tachycardia or nonspecific ST changes) secondary to alterations in electrical conductivity of the heart, myocardial contusion or infarction, or heart wall or papillary muscle rupture

- Neurologic: Headache, seizure, brief loss of consciousness or coma, peripheral nerve injury (resulting from ischemia), spinal cord paralysis (from demyelination), herniated nucleus pulposus, or decreased attention and concentration

- Orthopedic: Dislocations or fractures secondary to sustained muscular contraction or from a fall during the burn injury

- Other: Visceral perforation or necrosis, cataracts, tympanic membrane rupture, anxiety, depression, or post-traumatic stress disorder

### Lightning

Lightning, considered a form of very high electrical current, causes injury via four mechanisms[9]:

1. Direct strike, in which the person is the grounding site

2. Flash discharge, in which an object deviates the course of the lightning current before striking the person

3. Ground current, in which lightning strikes the ground and a person within the grounding area creates a pathway for the current

4. Shock wave, in which lightning travels outside the person and static electricity vaporizes moisture in the skin

### Chemical Burns

Chemical burns can be the result of reduction, oxidation, corrosion, or desecration of body tissue with or without an associated thermal injury.[10] The severity of burn depends on the type of chemical and its concentration, duration of contact, and mechanism of action. Unlike thermal burns, chemical burns significantly alter systemic tissue pH and metabolism. These changes can cause serious pulmonary complications (e.g., airway obstruction from bronchospasm, edema, or epithelial sloughing) and metabolic complications (e.g., liver necrosis or renal dysfunction from prolonged chemical exposure).

### Ultraviolet and Ionizing Radiation Burns

A *sunburn* is a superficial partial-thickness burn from the overexposure of the skin to UV radiation. Ionizing radiation burns with or without thermal burn occur when electromagnetic or particulate radiation energy is transferred to body tissues, resulting in the formation of chemical free radicals.[11] Ionizing radiation burns usually occur in laboratory or industrial settings. The severity of the ionizing radiation burn depends on the dose, dose rate, and the tissue sensitivity of exposed cells. Often referred to as *acute radiation syndrome*, complications of ionizing radiation burns include the following[11]:

- Gastrointestinal: Cramps, nausea, vomiting, diarrhea, and bowel ischemia

- Hematologic: Pancytopenia (decreased number of red blood cells, white blood cells, and platelets), granulocytopenia (decreased number of granular leukocytes), thrombocytopenia (decreased number of platelets), and hemorrhage

- Vascular: Endothelium destruction

## Burn Assessment and Acute Care Management of Burn Injury

### Classification of a Burn

The extent and depth of the burn determine its severity and dictate acute care treatment.

### Assessing the Extent of a Burn

The accurate assessment of the extent of a burn is necessary to calculate fluid volume therapy and is a predictor of morbidity.[12] The extent of a burn injury is referred to as *total body surface area* (TBSA) and can be calculated by the rule of nines or the Lund and Browder formula.

### Rule of Nines

The rule of nines divides the body into sections, seven of which are assigned 9% of TBSA. The anterior and posterior trunk are each assigned 18%, and the genitalia is assigned 1% (Figure 7-4). This

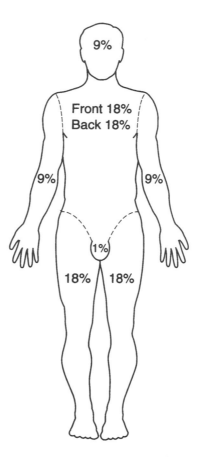

**Figure 7-4.** *The rule of nines method of assessing the extent of a burn injury. (With permission from M Walsh [ed]. Nurse Practitioners: Clinical Skills and Professional Issues. Oxford, UK: Butterworth–Heinemann, 1999;32.)*

formula is quick and easy to use, especially when a rapid initial estimation of TBSA is needed in the field or the emergency room. To use the rule of nines, the area of burn is filled in on the diagram, and the percentages are added for a TBSA. Modifications can be made if an entire body section is not burned. For example, if only the posterior left arm is burned, the TBSA is 4.5%.

*Lund and Browder Formula*

Table 7-4 describes the Lund and Browder formula. The body is divided into 19 sections, and each is assigned a different percentage of TBSA. These percentages vary with age from infant to adult to accommodate for relative changes in TBSA with normal growth. The Lund and Browder formula is a more accurate predictor of TBSA than the rule of nines because of the inclusion of a greater number of body divisions along with the adjustments for age and normal growth.

*Estimating the Extent of Irregularly Shaped Burns*

It is important to note that using the rule of nines or the Lund and Browder formula may not be accurate for irregularly shaped burns. To estimate TBSA with irregularly shaped burns, the patient's palm is used to measure the shape of the burn. The palm represents 1% TBSA.[12]

**Assessing the Depth of a Burn**

The depth of a burn can be described as superficial, moderate partial thickness, deep partial thickness, or full thickness (Figure 7-5). Each type has its own appearance, sensation, healing time, and level of pain, as described in Table 7-5. The assessment of burn depth allows an estimation of the proper type of burn care or surgery and the expected functional outcome and cosmesis.[13] Although clinical observation remains the standard for burn depth estimation, there is often error or underestimation. Experimental technologies for more precise burn depth estimation include cell biopsy, vital dyes, fluorescein fluorometry, laser Doppler flowmetry, thermography, ultrasound, and nuclear magnetic resonance.[4]

A burn wound is considered to be a dynamic wound in that it can normally change in appearance, especially during the first few days. A partial-thickness burn can convert to a full-thickness burn from infection, inadequate fluid resuscitation, or excessive pressure from dressings or splints.[14]

Table 7-4. Lund and Browder Method of Assessing the Extent of Burns*

|  | Birth | 1–4 yrs | 5–9 yrs | 10–14 yrs | 15 yrs | Adult |
|---|---|---|---|---|---|---|
| Head and trunk |  |  |  |  |  |  |
| Head | 19 | 17 | 13 | 11 | 9 | 7 |
| Neck | 2 | 2 | 2 | 2 | 2 | 2 |
| Anterior trunk | 13 | 13 | 13 | 13 | 13 | 13 |
| Posterior trunk | 13 | 13 | 13 | 13 | 13 | 13 |
| Left buttock | 2.5 | 2.5 | 2.5 | 2.5 | 2.5 | 2.5 |
| Right buttock | 2.5 | 2.5 | 2.5 | 2.5 | 2.5 | 2.5 |
| Genitalia | 1 | 1 | 1 | 1 | 1 | 1 |
| Upper extremity |  |  |  |  |  |  |
| Left upper arm | 4 | 4 | 4 | 4 | 4 | 4 |
| Right upper arm | 4 | 4 | 4 | 4 | 4 | 4 |
| Left forearm | 3 | 3 | 3 | 3 | 3 | 3 |
| Right forearm | 3 | 3 | 3 | 3 | 3 | 3 |
| Left hand | 2.5 | 2.5 | 2.5 | 2.5 | 2.5 | 2.5 |
| Right hand | 2.5 | 2.5 | 2.5 | 2.5 | 2.5 | 2.5 |
| Lower extremity |  |  |  |  |  |  |
| Left thigh | 5.5 | 6.5 | 8 | 8.5 | 9 | 9.5 |
| Right thigh | 5.5 | 6.5 | 8 | 8.5 | 9 | 9.5 |
| Left lower leg | 5 | 5 | 5.5 | 6 | 6.5 | 7 |
| Right lower leg | 5 | 5 | 5.5 | 6 | 6.5 | 7 |
| Left foot | 3.5 | 3.5 | 3.5 | 3.5 | 3.5 | 3.5 |
| Right foot | 3.5 | 3.5 | 3.5 | 3.5 | 3.5 | 3.5 |

*Values represent percentage of total body surface area.
Sources: Adapted from WF McManus, BA Pruitt. Thermal Injuries. In DV Feliciano, EE Moore, KL Mattox (eds), Trauma. Stamford, CT: Appleton & Lange, 1996;941; and CC Lund, NC Browder. The estimation of areas of burns. Surg Gynecol Obstet 1944;79:355.

## Acute Care Management of Burn Injury

This section discusses the admission guidelines and resuscitative and reparative phases of burn care.

### Admission Guidelines

In addition to the burn's extent and depth, the presence of associated pulmonary, orthopedic, or visual injuries determines what level of

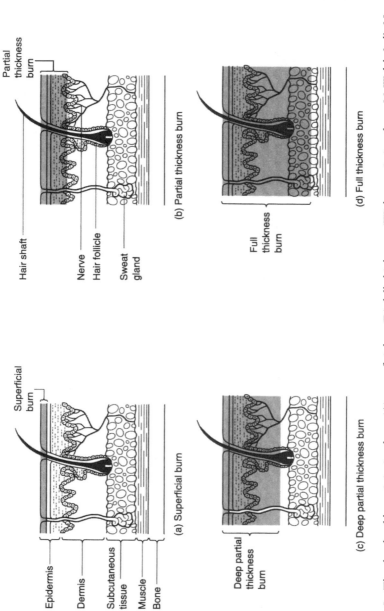

Figure 7-5. *The depth of burn injuries from (A) superficial to (D) full thickness. (With permission from M Walsh [ed]. Nurse Practitioners: Clinical Skills and Professional Issues. Oxford, UK: Butterworth–Heinemann, 1999;28.)*

Table 7-5. Burn Depth Characteristics

| Depth | Appearance | Healing | Pain |
|-------|-----------|---------|------|
| Superficial (first-degree)—epidermis injured | Pink to red<br>With or without edema<br>Dry appearance without blisters<br>Blanches<br>Sensation intact<br>Skin intact when rubbed | 3–5 days by epithelialization<br>Skin appears intact | Tenderness to touch or painful |
| Moderate partial-thickness (second degree)—superficial dermis injured | Pink to mottled red or red with edema<br>Moist appearance with blisters<br>Blanches with slow capillary refill<br>Sensation intact | 5 days to 3 wks by epithelialization<br>Pigmentation changes are likely | Very painful |
| Deep partial-thickness (second degree)—deep dermis injured with hair follicles and sweat glands intact | Pink to pale ivory<br>Dry appearance with blisters<br>May blanch with slow capillary refill<br>Decreased sensation to pinprick<br>Hair readily removed | 3 wks to mos by granulation tissue formation and epithelialization<br>Scar formation likely | Very painful |
| Full-thickness—entire dermis injured (third degree) or fat, muscle, and bone injured (fourth degree) | White, red, brown, or black (charred if fourth degree)<br>Dry appearance without blanching<br>May be blistered<br>Insensate to pinprick<br>Depressed wound | Not able to regenerate | No pain, perhaps an ache |

Source: Data from P Wiebelhaus, SL Hansen. Burns: handle with care. RN 1999;62:52–75.

care is optimal for the patient. The American Burn Association rec-
ommends medical care at a burn center if the patient has any of the
following[15]:

- Second- and third-degree burns that are greater than or equal to
  10% of TBSA in patients younger than 10 years of age or older
  than 50 years of age

- Burns of any type that are greater than 20% of TBSA in patients
  between 10 and 50 years of age

- Full-thickness burns that are greater than or equal to 5% of
  TBSA

- Second- and third-degree burns of the face, hands, feet, genitalia, perineum, or major joints

- High-voltage electrical or lightning injury

- Inhalation injury or other trauma

- A significant chemical burn

- Pre-existing disease in which the burn could increase mortality

**Resuscitative Phase**

The objectives of emergency room management of the patient who has
a major burn injury include simultaneous general systemic stabilization and burn care. The prioritization of care and precautions during
this initial time period have a great impact on survival and illustrate
some key concepts of burn care. General systemic stabilization involves
(1) the assessment of inhalation injury and carbon monoxide (CO)
poisoning and the maintenance of the airway and ventilation with supplemental oxygen (see Appendix III-A) or mechanical ventilation (see
Appendix III-B), (2) fluid resuscitation, (3) the use of analgesia (see
Appendix VI), and (4) the treatment of secondary injuries.[16]

*Inhalation Injury and Carbon Monoxide Poisoning*

The inhalation of smoke, gases, or poisons, which may be related to
burn injuries, can cause asphyxia, direct cellular injury, or both. Inhalation injury significantly increases mortality and varies depending on
the inhalant and exposure time. There is no strict definition of inhalation injury. Inhalation injury is suspected if the patient was exposed to
noxious inhalants, especially in an enclosed space, or if the patient

has one or more of the following: (1) altered mental status; (2) burns on the face, neck, or upper chest; (3) singed eyebrows or nose hairs; (4) laryngeal edema; (5) arterial blood gas levels consistent with hypoxia; (6) abnormal breath sounds; (7) the presence of soot in sputum; or (8) positive blood test results for chemicals.

The oropharynx and tracheobronchial tree are usually damaged by thermal injury, whereas the lung parenchyma is damaged by the chemical effects of the inhalant. Thermal airway injury is characterized by immediate upper-airway mucosal edema, erythema, hemorrhage, and ulceration.[4] Elective endotracheal intubation is indicated with this type of injury, as progressive edema can readily lead to airway obstruction. The patient remains intubated until airway edema is decreased, usually 2–4 days post injury.[17]

The pathophysiology of inhalation injury generally occurs in three stages: (1) inhalation injury (0–36 hours after injury), (2) pulmonary edema (6–72 hours after injury), and (3) bronchopneumonia (3–10 days after injury). Pulmonary edema occurs from increased lung capillary permeability, increased bronchial blood flow, and impaired lymph function.[18] There are de-epithelialization and exudate formation throughout the airways, as well as decreased alveolar surfactant.[4] Decreased lung compliance (functional residual capacity and vital capacity) and hypoxia are the primary effects of inhalation injury, each of which is dependent on the location and severity of the injury. Supplemental oxygen, elective intubation, bronchodilators, and fluid resuscitation are initiated to maximize gas exchange and reverse hypoxia.[19-21]

The inhalation of CO, which is a colorless, odorless, tasteless, combustible, nonirritating gas produced by the incomplete combustion of organic material, results in asphyxia. CO molecules displace oxygen molecules from hemoglobin to form carboxyhemoglobin and shift the oxyhemoglobin curve to the left, thereby decreasing the release of oxygen. Additionally, CO molecules increase pulmonary secretions and decrease the effectiveness of the mucociliary elevator.[22] Elevated carboxyhemoglobin levels cause headache, disorientation, nausea, visual changes, or coma, depending on the percentage. CO poisoning is usually reversible with the use of 100% oxygen if the patient has not lost consciousness.[4]

*Burn Care in the Resuscitative Phase*
During the first 72 hours after a burn injury, medical management consists of continued fluid resuscitation, infection control, body

temperature maintenance, pain and anxiety management, and initial burn care.

## Fluid Resuscitation

After a burn, fluid shifts from vascular to interstitial and intracellular spaces because of increased capillary pressure, increased capillary and venular permeability, decreased interstitial hydrostatic pressure, chemical inflammatory mediators, and increased interstitial protein retention.[23] This is compounded by evaporative water loss from a disruption of the skin.[24] In burns of more than 20% TBSA, this fluid shift becomes massive and requires immediate fluid repletion.[13] This fluid shift, referred to as *burn shock*, is a life-threatening condition because of hypovolemia and the potential for shock induced renal failure (see Figure 7-3). Plasma, sodium-rich solutions, and other fluids are infused over a 48-hour period according to a standard formula derived from individual TBSA and body weight. The formula used varies according to hospital preference.

During and after fluid administration, the patient is monitored closely for adequacy of fluid resuscitation. Heart rate, blood pressure, cardiac output, base deficit, urine output, and bowel sounds provide valuable information about the effectiveness of fluid resuscitation, as do peripheral body temperature, capillary refill, and mental status.[23]

## Infection Control

Prevention of infection at the burn site(s) is crucial in the resuscitative and reparative phases of burn care. The patient with a major burn is considered immunocompromised because of the loss of skin and the inability to keep micro-organisms from entering the body. Infection control is achieved by the following[13]:

- Observation of the patient for signs and symptoms of sepsis (See Sepsis in Chapter 10.)

- Minimization of the presence of micro-organisms in the patient's internal and external environment

- Use of aseptic techniques in all interactions with the patient

- Use of topical antimicrobial agents or antibiotics, as needed

- Tetanus prophylaxis

## Clinical Tip

To minimize the risk of infection, the physical therapist must use sterile techniques according to the burn unit procedures when entering a patient's room or approaching the patient's bedside. The physical therapist should be familiar with the institution's policies regarding the use and disposal of protective barriers, such as gloves, gowns, caps, and masks.

### Body Temperature Maintenance

The patient with a major burn injury is at risk for hypothermia from skin loss and the inability to thermoregulate. Body heat is lost through conduction to the surrounding atmosphere and to the surface of the bed. Initially, dry dressings may be placed on the patient to minimize heat loss. The patient should be placed in a warm atmosphere to maintain body temperature. The patient's room, burn unit, or both may have overhead radiant heat panels and may be humidified in an effort to preserve the patient's body heat.

### Pain Management

A patient with a burn injury can experience pain as a result of any of the following:

- Free nerve ending exposure

- Edema

- Exudate accumulation

- Burn debridement and dressing changes

- Mobility

- Secondary injury, such as fracture

Patients may also experience fear from the injury and burn treatment, which can exacerbate pain. Analgesia, given intravenously, is therefore started as soon as possible (see Appendix VI).

### Initial Burn Care

To neutralize the burn source, the patient's clothing and jewelry are removed, and the burn is rinsed or lavaged (for a chemical burn). Initially, a burn is debrided, cleaned, and dressed with the hospital's or burn unit's antimicrobial agent of choice once the patient is stabilized from a cardiopulmonary perspective. Topical antimicrobial agents attempt to prevent or minimize bacterial growth in a burn and expedite eschar separation. There is a variety of antimicrobial agents, each with its own application, advantages, and disadvantages. Ideally, the antimicrobial agent of choice should penetrate eschar, work against a wide variety of micro-organisms, have minimal systemic absorption, and not impede healing.[25] The physician determines whether to cover the burn or leave it open and estimates the time frame for burn repair, the need for surgical intervention, or both.

### Escharotomy and Fasciotomy

Circumferential burns of the extremities or trunk can create neurovascular complications. Inelastic eschar paired with edema can cause increased tissue swelling in all directions with the result of decreased blood flow, nerve compression, and increased compartment pressures. Tissue ischemia and loss of limb can ensue if these conditions are not treated with escharotomy or fasciotomy. *Escharotomy* is the surgical incision through eschar to decompress tissue below the burn. *Fasciotomy* is the surgical incision through fascia to decompress tissue within a fascial compartment. Both procedures are typically performed at the bedside. Clinical indications for escharotomy or fasciotomy are decreased arterial blood flow, as determined by loss of Doppler flowmetry signal, or increased compartment pressure measurements (greater than or equal to 30 mm Hg).[25]

### Burn Management in the Reparative Phase

Tissue healing at burn sites occurs over weeks to months according to the depth of the burn and is described in Process of Wound Healing. For a discussion of variables that can slow the process of burn healing, see Factors That Can Delay Wound Healing. After the healing process, a scar forms. A burn scar may be *normotrophic,* with a normal appearance from the dermal collagen fibers that are arranged in an organized parallel formation, or *hypertrophic,* with an abnormal appearance as a result of the disorganized formation of dermal collagen fibers.[26]

Burn management can be divided into two major categories: the surgical management of burns, and burn cleansing and debridement. It is beyond the scope of this chapter to discuss in detail the indications, advantages, and disadvantages of specific surgical interventions that facilitate burn closure. Instead, surgical procedures related to burn care are defined below.

*Surgical Procedures*
The cornerstone of present surgical burn management is *early* burn excision and grafting. *Excision* is the surgical removal of eschar and exposure of viable tissue to minimize infection and promote burn closure. *Grafting* is the implantation or transplantation of skin onto a prepared wound bed.[27] Early burn closure minimizes infection, the incidence of multisystem organ failure, and morbidity. Table 7-6 describes the different types of excision and grafting. Table 7-7 describes the different artificial and biological skin substitutes for use when there is a lack of viable autograft sites.

Surgical excision and grafting are completed at any site if patient survival will improve. If morbidity is greater than 50%, the priority is for the excision and grafting of large flat areas to rapidly reduce the burn wound area.[25] Grafting is otherwise performed to maximize functional outcome and cosmesis, with the hands, arms, face, feet, and joint surfaces grafted before other areas of the body.[28] Permanent grafting is ideal; however, grafting may be temporary. Temporary grafting is indicated for small wounds expected to heal secondarily and for large wounds for which an autograft would not last or if permanent coverage is not available.[29]

Grafts, which typically adhere in 2–7 days, may not adhere or "take" in the presence of any of the following[27,28]:

- An incomplete eschar excision
- Movement of the graft on the recipient site
- A septic recipient site
- A hematoma at the graft site
- A recipient site with poor blood supply
- Poor nutritional status

---

**Clinical Tip**

- To promote grafting success, restrictions on weight bearing and movement of a specific joint or entire limb

**Table 7-6.** Types of Excision and Grafting

| Procedure | Description |
|-----------|-------------|
| Tangential excision | Removal of eschar in successive layers down to the dermis |
| Full-thickness excision | Removal of eschar as a single layer down to the subcutaneous tissue |
| Autograft | Surgical harvesting of a patient's own skin from another part of the body (donor site) and placing it permanently on the burn (recipient site) |
| Split-thickness skin graft (STSG) | Autograft consisting of epidermis and a portion of dermis |
| Full-thickness skin graft (FTSG) | Autograft consisting of epidermis and the entire dermis |
| Mesh graft | Autograft placed through a mesher (a machine that expands the size of the graft usually 3–4 times) before being placed on the recipient site |
| Sheet graft | Autograft placed on the recipient site as a single piece without meshing |
| Cultured epidermal autograft (CEA) | Autograft of unburned epidermal cells cultured in the laboratory |
| Composite skin graft | Autograft of unburned epidermal and dermal cells cultured in the laboratory |
| Allogenic graft | Autograft of unburned epidermal cells and cadaver skin cultured in the laboratory |
| Homograft | Temporary graft from cadaver skin |
| Heterograft (xenograft) | Temporary graft from another animal species, typically of porcine skin |
| Amnion graft | Temporary graft from placental membrane |

Source: Data from SF Miller, MJ Staley, RL Richard. Surgical Management of the Burn Patient. In RL Richard, MJ Staley (eds), Burn Care and Rehabilitation: Principles and Practice. Philadelphia: FA Davis, 1994.

**Table 7-7.** Temporary and Permanent Skin Substitutes for the Treatment of Burns

| Product | Description | Use |
|---|---|---|
| Biobrane (Bertex Pharmaceuticals, Morgantown, WV) | Temporary graft option. Two-layered graft composed of nylon mesh impregnated with porcine collagen and silicone; the outer silicone layer is permeable to gases but not to fluid or bacteria. Applied within 24 hours. Spontaneously separates from a healed wound in 10–14 days. | For small to medium superficial-thickness burns or partial-thickness burns Has had limited success on full-thickness burns because of infection May also be used to protect a meshed autograft |
| Dermagraft TC (Advanced Tissue Sciences, La Jolla, CA) | Temporary graft option. Two-layered material composed of biological wound-healing factors (e.g., fibronectin, type I collagen, tenascin) and growth factors (e.g., factor β) on an external synthetic barrier. | For partial-thickness burns |
| TransCyte (Advanced Tissue Sciences, La Jolla, CA) | Temporary graft option. Composed of a polymer membrane and newborn human fibroblast cells cultured on a porcine collagen–coated nylon mesh. The fibroblasts secrete human dermal collagen, matrix proteins, and growth factors. | Used for partial-thickness burns that will require debridement and may heal without surgical intervention, or on excised deep-partial or full-thickness burns prior to autografting |

**Table 7-7.** *Continued*

| Product | Description | Use |
|---|---|---|
| AlloDerm (Life Cell Corp., The Woodlands, TX) | Permanent graft option. Composed of chemically treated cadaver dermis with the epidermal antigenic cellular components removed so that it is immunologically inert. Applied to a debrided burn with an ultrathin split thickness autograft immediately applied over it. | For full-thickness burns Also used in post-burn reconstruction after contracture release |
| Integra (Integra Life Sciences, Plainsboro, NJ) | Permanent graft option. Two-layered material composed of a disposable outer layer of silastic that acts as a barrier to evaporative water loss and bacteria and an inner layer of bovine collagen and chondroitin-6-sulfate that becomes incorporated into the burn to form a *neodermis*. When the neodermis becomes vascularized, the silastic covering can be removed and replaced with thin autografts. | For life-threatening full-thickness burns or deep partial-thickness burns |

Sources: Data from SL Hansen, DW Voigt, P Wiebelhaus, CN Paul. Using skin replacement products to treat burns and wounds. Adv Skin Wound Care 2001;14:37–44; and P Dziewulski, JP Barret. Assessment, Operative Planning, and Surgery for Burn Wound Closure. In SE Wolf, DN Herndon (eds), Burn Care. Austin, TX: Landes Bioscience, 1999.

may be present postoperatively. The therapist should become familiar with the surgeon's procedures and protocols and alter positioning, range of motion (ROM), therapeutic exercise, and functional mobility accordingly.

• The therapist should check with the physician to determine whether the graft crosses a joint and how close the graft borders the joint.

• If possible, observe the graft during dressing changes to get a visual understanding of the exact location of the graft.

• The autograft site or donor site is often more painful than the burn itself.

• Donor sites are oriented longitudinally and are commonly located on the thigh, low back, or outer arm and may be reharvested in approximately 2 weeks.

*Nonsurgical Procedures*

Burn cleansing and debridement may be performed many times a day to minimize infection and promote tissue healing. These procedures, as described in Wound Cleansing and Debridement, may be performed by a physician, nurse, or physical therapist depending on the hospital's or burn unit's protocol. Table 7-8 lists the topical agents used specifically for the treatment of burns.

## Physical Therapy Examination in Burn Care

Physical therapy intervention for the patient with a burn injury is often initiated within 48 hours of hospital admission.

### History

In addition to the general chart review (see Appendix I-A), the following information is especially relevant in the evaluation, treatment planning, and understanding of the physiological status of a patient with a burn.

• How, when, where, and why did the burn occur?

• Did the patient get thrown (as in an explosion) or fall during the burn incident?

**Table 7-8.** Topical Agents Commonly Used for the Treatment of Burns

| Agent | Description | Advantages (A)/Disadvantages (D) |
|---|---|---|
| Silver sulfadiazine (Silvadene) | Antimicrobial cream for use with partial- and full-thickness burns<br>Applied with or without a dressing | A = Painless application, wide spectrum coverage<br>D = Poor eschar penetration, may cause maceration and epithelial retardation, associated with leukopenia, costly |
| Mafenide acetate (Sulfamylon) | Antimicrobial cream for use with partial- and full-thickness burns<br>Applied with a dressing<br>Can be applied directly to burns of the ear | A = Penetrates eschar well, effective against *Pseudomonas*<br>D = Painful, not for use on large areas, can cause acidemia |
| Acticoat (Westaim Biomedical, Exeter, NH) silver dressing | Three-ply gauze dressing consisting of an absorbent rayon/polyester core and upper and lower layers of silver-coated, high-density polyethylene mesh<br>For use with partial- and full-thickness burns and meshed autografts | A = Abrasion resistant, nonadherent, flexible<br>D = Cannot visualize the wound |
| Silver nitrate | Anti-microbial solution or cream applied as a wet dressing<br>Used for partial- and full-thickness burns | A = Wide spectrum coverage, painless<br>D = Poor eschar penetration, frequent reapplication, stains the patient's skin and the environment, can cause electrolyte imbalance |

| | | |
|---|---|---|
| Bacitracin | Ointment effective against gram-positive organisms<br>Used for superficial and partial-thickness burns as well as donor sites | A = Minimal systemic absorption, painless, can be used on the face<br>D = Nephrotoxic in large amounts, no eschar penetration, frequent reapplication |
| Nystatin | Cream or powder mixed to solution and applied with a dressing<br>Used on superficial, partial- or full-thickness burns | A = Effective fungicide against *Candida*, painless<br>D = Frequent reapplication, no eschar penetration |
| Collagenase | Enzyme derived from *Clostridium histolyticum*<br>Digests collagen in necrotic tissue<br>Applied as an ointment with a dressing over it<br>Used on deep partial- and full-thickness burns | A = Penetrates eschar, does not affect healthy tissue<br>D = Painful, no antimicrobial properties |

Sources: Data from ET Kaye, KM Kaye. Topical antibacterial agents. Infect Dis Clin North Am 1995;9:547–559; JO Kucan, EC Smoot. Five percent mafenide acetate solution in the treatment of thermal injuries. J Burn Care Rehabil 1993;14:158–163; RS Ward, JR Saffle. Topical agents in burn and wound care. Phys Ther 1995;75:526–538; and HS Soroff, DH Sasvary. Collagenase ointment and polymyxin B sulfate/bacitracin versus silver sulfadiazine cream in partial thickness burns: a pilot study. J Burn Care Rehabil 1994;15:13–17.

- Is there an inhalation injury or CO poisoning?
- What are the secondary injuries?
- What is the extent, depth, and location of the burn?
- Does the patient have a condition(s) that might impair tissue healing?
- Was the burn self-inflicted? If so, is there a history of self-injury or suicide?
- Were friends or family members also injured?

## Inspection and Palpation

To assist with treatment planning, pertinent data that can be gathered from the direct observation of a patient or palpation include the following:

- Level of consciousness
- Presence of agitation, pain, and stress
- Location of the burn or graft, including the proximity of the burn to a joint
- Presence and location of dressings, splints, or pressure garments
- Presence of lines, tubes, or other equipment
- Presence and location of edema
- Posture
- Position of head, trunk, and extremities
- Heart rate and blood pressure, respiratory rate and pattern, and oxygen saturation

---

### Clinical Tip

- Avoid popping any blisters on the skin during palpation or with manual contacts.
- Do not place a blood pressure cuff over a burn or graft site or area of edema.

---

*Pain Assessment*

Good pain control increases patient participation and activity tolerance; therefore, pain assessment occurs daily. For the conscious patient, the physical therapist should note the presence, quality, and grade of (1) resting pain; (2) pain with passive, active-assisted, or active ROM; (3) pain at the burn site versus the donor site; and (4) pain before, during, and after physical therapy intervention.

### Clinical Tip

• The physical therapist should become familiar with the patient's pain medication schedule and arrange for physical therapy treatment when pain medication is most effective and when the patient is as comfortable as possible.
• Restlessness and vital sign monitoring (i.e., heart rate, blood pressure, and respiratory rate increases) may be the best indicators of pain in sedated or unconscious patients who cannot verbally report pain.

*Range of Motion*

ROM of the involved joints typically requires goniometric measurements. Exact goniometric values can be difficult to measure when the patient has bulky dressings; therefore, some estimation of ROM may be necessary. The uninvolved joints or extremities can be grossly addressed actively or passively, depending on the patient's level of alertness or level of participation.

### Clinical Tip

• The physical therapist should be aware of the presence of tendon damage before ROM assessment. ROM should not be performed on joints with exposed tendons.
• The physical therapist should always have a good view of the extremity during ROM exercise to observe for banding or areas of tissue that appear white when stretched.

- The physical therapist should pay attention to the position of adjacent joints when measuring ROM to account for any length-tension deficits of healing skin or muscle.
- The physical therapist should appreciate the fact that a major burn injury is usually characterized by burns of different depths and types. The physical therapist must be aware of the various qualities of combination burns when performing ROM or functional activities.
- ROM may be decreased by the presence of bulky dressings. Try to evaluate or perform ROM when the dressings are temporarily off or down.

### Strength

Strength on an uninvolved extremity is usually assessed grossly by function. More formal strength testing, such as resisted isometrics or manual muscle testing, is indicated on either the involved or uninvolved side if there is severe edema, electrical injury, or secondary injury.[30]

### Functional Mobility

Functional mobility may be limited depending on state of illness, medication, need for warm or sterile environment, and pain. The physical therapist should evaluate functional mobility, as much as possible, according to medical stability and precautions.

### Clinical Tip

The skin at grafted areas, as well as at donor site areas, is more fragile than normal skin. These areas should be ace wrapped figure-of-eight style to provide support against venous pooling when the patient is being mobilized out of bed. Without this extra support, the skin is more prone to shearing at graft sites and subcutaneous bleeding.

# Physical Therapy Intervention

## Goals

The primary goal of physical therapy intervention for patients with burn injuries is to maximize function with ROM exercise, stretching, positioning, strengthening, and functional activity. General considerations for physical therapy intervention by impairment are listed in Table 7-9.

## Basic Concepts for the Treatment of Patients with Burn Injury

• The patient with a burn can have multisystem organ involvement and a hypermetabolic state; thus, the physical therapist needs to be aware of cardiac, respiratory, and neurologic status, as well as musculoskeletal and integumentary issues.

• Fluid resuscitation and pain medications can affect blood pressure, heart rate, and respiratory pattern and rate, as well as level of alertness. Monitoring these variables will help the therapist gauge pain level and determine how aggressively to intervene during the therapy session.

• The patient with a burn requires more frequent re-evaluations than other patient populations, because the patient's status and therapy intervention can change dramatically as swelling decreases, wound debridement and closure occur, hemodynamic and respiratory stability are achieved, and mental status improves. The goals and plan of care need to be updated throughout the patient's admission, as activity may be temporarily restricted after surgical grafting.

• A portion(s) of the plan of care is often held for 4–7 days after skin grafting to prevent shearing forces on the new graft. Shearing can disrupt the circulation to the graft and cause it to fail. Grafts over joints or areas with bony prominences, as well as grafts on the posterior surfaces of the body, are at greater risk for shear injury.

• Time frames for physical therapy goals vary widely and are based heavily on TBSA, the location of the burn, age, and pre-existing functional status.

**Table 7-9.** Physical Therapy Considerations for Burn Injury

| Variable | Considerations |
| --- | --- |
| Decreased ROM and altered limb position | Most patients have full ROM on admission but may readily begin to exhibit decreased ROM due to edema, pain, and immobilization. |
| | ROM of uninvolved joints may also be decreased secondary to the process of total body edema. |
| | Devices that can help to properly position the patient include splints, abduction pillows, arm boards attached to the bed, pillows, and blanket rolls. |
| | Incorporate the use of a modality (i.e., pulley) into stretching activities. |
| Decreased strength | Active exercise is preferred unless sedation or the patient's level of consciousness prevents it. |
| | Active exercise (i.e., proprioceptive neuromuscular facilitation) provides muscle conditioning, increased blood flow, edema reduction, and contraction prevention and helps reduce hypertrophic scar formation. |
| Decreased endurance and functional mobility | Prolonged bed rest (see Appendix I-B) may be necessary for weeks or months secondary to medical status or to accommodate grafting, especially of the lower extremity. |
| | The use of a tilt table for progressive mobilization from bed rest may be necessary if orthostatic hypotension or decreased lower-extremity ROM exists. |
| | Assistive devices may need adaptations (i.e., platform walker) to accommodate for ROM and strength deficits or weight-bearing restrictions. |
| | Consider the use of active exercise (i.e., restorator) that addresses cardiovascular conditioning while increasing ROM and strength. |
| Risk for scar development | Healing of deeper burns and skin-grafted burns is accompanied by some scarring. |
| | Hypertrophic scarring can be decreased by the use of pressure garments, silicone gel sheets, ROM, and massage. |
| Patient/family knowledge deficit related to burns and physical therapy | Patient/family education emphasizes information about the role of physical therapy, exercise, positioning, pain and edema control, and skin care. |
| | Education before discharge is of the utmost importance to improve compliance, confidence, and independence. |

ROM = range of motion.

- The joints at risk for contracture formation need to be properly positioned (Table 7-10). The positioning needs to be consistently carried out by all caregivers and documented in the patient care plan. Proper positioning will decrease edema and prevent contracture formation to facilitate the best recovery.

- The therapist should be creative in treating the patient with a burn. Traditional exercise works well; however, incorporating recreational activities and other modalities into the plan of care can often increase functional gains and compliance with less pain.

- The plan of care must be comprehensive and address all areas with burns. For example, burns of the face, neck, and trunk require intervention specifically directed to these areas.

- The therapist should attend bedside rounds with the burn team to be involved in multidisciplinary planning and to inform the team of therapy progression.

**Table 7-10.** Preferred Positions for Patients with Burn Injury

| Area of Body | Position |
| --- | --- |
| Neck | Extension, no rotation |
| Shoulder | Abduction (90 degrees) |
| | External rotation |
| | Horizontal flexion (10 degrees) |
| Elbow and forearm | Extension with supination |
| Wrist | Neutral or slight extension |
| Hand | Functional position (dorsal burn) |
| | Finger and thumb extension (palmar burn) |
| Trunk | Straight postural alignment |
| Hip | Neutral extension/flexion |
| | Neutral rotation |
| | Slight abduction |
| Knee | Extension |
| Ankle | Neutral or slight dorsiflexion |
| | No inversion |
| | Neutral toe extension/flexion |

Source: With permission from RS Ward. Splinting, Orthotics, and Prosthetics in the Management of Burns. In MM Lusardi, CC Nielson (eds), Orthotics and Prosthetics in Rehabilitation. Boston: Butterworth–Heinemann, 2000;315.

## Pathophysiology of Wounds

The different types of wounds, their etiologies, and the factors that contribute to or delay wound healing are discussed in the following sections.

### *Types of Wounds*

#### Trauma Wounds

A *trauma wound* is an injury caused by an external force, such as a laceration from broken glass, a cut from a knife, or penetration from a bullet.

#### Surgical Wounds

A surgical wound is the residual skin defect after a surgical incision. For individuals who do not have problems healing, these wounds are sutured or stapled, and they heal without special intervention. As the benefits of moist wound healing become more widely accepted, gels and ointments are now more frequently applied to surgical wounds. When complications, such as infection, arterial insufficiency, diabetes, or venous insufficiency, are present, surgical wound healing can be delayed and require additional care.

#### Arterial Insufficiency Wounds

A wound resulting from arterial insufficiency occurs secondary to ischemia of the tissue, frequently caused by atherosclerosis, which can cause irreversible damage. Arterial insufficiency wounds, described in Table 7-11, occur most commonly in the distal lower leg because of a lack of collateral circulation to this area. Clinically, arterial ulcers frequently occur in the pretibial areas and the dorsum of the toes and feet, but they may be present proximally if the ulcers were initially caused by trauma.[31-33] They show minimal signs of healing and are often gangrenous.

#### Venous Insufficiency Wounds

A wound resulting from venous insufficiency is caused by the improper functioning of the venous system that leads to poor nutrition to the tissues. This lack of nutrition causes tissue damage, and ultimately tissue death, resulting in ulceration. The exact mechanism by which this occurs has not been established, although some theories do exist. One theory is that venous hypertension is transmitted to the

**Table 7-11.** Clinical Indicators of Vascular Insufficiency Wounds
and Diabetic Ulcers

| Wound Etiology | Clinical Indicators |
| --- | --- |
| Arterial insufficiency | Intermittent claudication<br>Extreme pain, decreased with rest and increased with elevation<br>Decreased or absent pedal pulses<br>Decreased temperature of the distal limb<br>Distinct, well-defined wound edges<br>Deep wound bed<br>Cyanosis |
| Venous insufficiency | Localized limb pain, decreased with elevation and increased with standing<br>Pain with deep pressure or palpation<br>Pedal pulses present<br>Increased temperature around the wound<br>Indistinct, irregular edges<br>Edema around the wound<br>Shallow wound bed<br>Substantial drainage |
| Diabetic ulcer | Painless ulcer; however, general lower-limb pain is present<br>Absent pedal pulses<br>Decreased temperature in the distal limb<br>Deep wound bed frequently located at pressure points (e.g., metatarsal heads)<br>Shiny skin on distal limb |

Sources: Data from JM McCulloch. Evaluation of Patients with Open Wounds. In LC Kloth, KH Miller (eds), Wound Healing: Alternatives in Management. Philadelphia: FA Davis, 1995; RG Sibbald. An approach to leg and foot ulcers: a brief overview. Ostomy Wound Manage 1998;44:29; RG Sibbald. Venous leg ulcers. Ostomy Wound Manage 1998;44:53; P Laing. Diabetic foot ulcers. Am J Surg 1994;167(1A):31; and ML Levin, LW O'Neal, JH Bowker (eds). The Diabetic Foot (5th ed). St. Louis: Mosby, 1993.

superficial veins in the subcutaneous tissue and the overlying skin, which causes widening of the capillary pores.[34,35] Clinically, this would result in the first sign of venous disease, which is the presence of a dilated long saphenous vein on the medial aspect of the calf. This dilation allows the escape of large macromolecules, including fibrinogen, into the interstitial space. This results in the development of edema toward the end of the day because of the pooling of fluid in the dermis. In long-standing venous disease, fibrin accumulates in the dermis, creating a fibrin cuff that presents as hard, nonpitting edema, and the surface skin is rigid and fixed. The theory states that this fibrin cuff forms a mechanical barrier to the transfer of oxygen and other nutrients, which progressively leads to cellular dysfunction, cell death and skin ulceration.[34,35]

Another hypothesis is called the *white blood cell–trapping hypothesis.* This theory states that transient elevations in venous pressures decrease capillary blood flow, resulting in trapping of white blood cells at the capillary level, which in turn plugs capillary loops, resulting in areas of localized ischemia.[35] These white blood cells may also become activated at this level, causing the release of various proteolytic enzymes, superoxide free radicals, and chemotactic substances, which can also lead to direct tissue damage, death, and ulceration.[35]

Venous stasis ulcers, described in Table 7-11, are frequently present on the medial malleolus, where the long saphenous vein is most superficial and has its greatest curvature. Venous ulcers may be present on the foot or above the midcalf but are more likely to have another primary etiology, such as trauma or infection. The leakage of red blood cells over time results in the deposit of hemosiderin and stimulated melanin, causing the characteristic hyperpigmentation around the medial ankle. Other characteristics include a thin skin surface with a loss of hair follicles and sweat glands.[34]

### Pressure Wounds

A *pressure ulcer,* sometimes referred to as a *decubitus ulcer,* is caused by ischemia that develops as a result of sustained pressure in excess of capillary pressure on the tissue. The pressure usually originates from prolonged weight bearing on a bony prominence, causing internal ischemia at the point of contact. This initial point of pressure is where tissue death first occurs. The tissue continues to necrotize externally until a wound is created at the skin surface. By this time, there is significant internal tissue damage. Superficial tissue ulceration can be caused by the effect of mechanical forces acting on localized areas of skin and subcutaneous tissue, whether the forces are of low intensity over long periods or are higher forces applied intermittently.[36,37] The relationships between the amount of force applied, the duration of force, and the direction of the force contribute to the occurrence and severity of a pressure ulcer. Not only can direct pressure create tissue ischemia, but friction and shearing forces contribute as well.[36–38,40,41] Refer to Wound Staging and Classification for the pressure ulcer grading system.

All bed- or chair-bound individuals or any individuals who have an impaired ability to reposition themselves or weight shift are at risk of developing pressure ulcers. Common pressure ulcer sites include the back of the head, the scapular spines, spinous processes, elbows, sacrum, and heels when a patient is laying in supine. While side-lying, a patient may experience increased pressure at the ear, acromion process, rib, iliac crest, greater trochanter, medial and lateral condyles, and the malleoli.[38,39] A person's body weight also plays a role in pressure ulcer development. A person who is too thin has more prominent bony prominences, whereas a person who is overweight has increased pressure on weight-bearing surfaces.[39–41]

### Neuropathic or Neurotropic Ulcers

A *neuropathic* or *neurotropic* ulcer (see Table 7-11) is a secondary complication that occurs from a triad of disorders, including peripheral vascular disease, peripheral neuropathy, and infection.[42] Neuropathic ulcers are most commonly associated with diabetes. The development of ulcers and foot injuries are the leading causes of lower-extremity amputation in people with diabetes.[43] Additionally, there is an increased incidence of atherosclerosis, which appears earlier and progresses more rapidly than in patients without diabetes. However, many people with diabetes who develop foot ulcers have palpable pulses and adequate peripheral blood flow.[44]

Individuals with diabetes may also have changes in the mechanical properties of the skin. Insulin is essential for fibroblastic and collagen synthesis. A lack of insulin in type 1 diabetes can lead to diminished collagen synthesis that can cause stiffness and poor tensile strength of tissue, both of which increase the susceptibility of wound development and decrease healing potential.[45]

The peripheral and central nervous systems can be adversely affected in diabetes. Peripheral neuropathy is common, and sensation and strength can be impaired. Diminished light touch, proprioception, and temperature and pain perception decrease the ability of the person with diabetes to identify areas that are being subjected to trauma, shearing forces, excessive pressure, and warm temperatures, all of which can cause ulcers.[44–48]

Structural deformities can occur as the result of the neuropathies that may be present secondary to diabetes. Any structural deformities, such as "hammer toes" or excessive pronation or supination, can create pressure points that lead to ischemia and a subsequent ulcer.[46–48]

Excessive plantar callus formation may form at the sites of increased pressure and in itself can increase the pressure to the affected area.[44] The minor repetitive ischemia that occurs every time the person bears weight on the pressure points in the tissue underlying the callus can eventually cause the tissue to fail, and ulceration occurs.[48]

Peripheral motor neuropathy contributes to the development of an equinus contracture at the ankle as stronger plantarflexors overcome the weaker dorsiflexors. Weakness of the small intrinsic muscles of the foot causes clawing of the toes. These foot deformities lead to increased weight distribution through the forefoot and increased pressure under the metatarsal heads. The abnormal mechanical forces and intermittent forces can stimulate callus formation.[44]

A neuropathy of the autonomic nervous system is present in the majority of individuals with diabetes and neuropathic ulcers. The autonomic nervous system regulates skin perspiration and blood flow to the microvascular system. Lack of sweat production contributes to the development of a callus. Altered cross-linkage between collagen and keratin results in predisposal to hyperkeratosis and callus formation. Beneath the callus, a cavity often forms as a response to the increased pressure and shear forces and fills with serous fluid, causing a seroma. If the deep skin fissure comes in contact with an underlying seroma, it can become colonized with bacteria and result in ulcer formation.[44]

The immune system is also affected by elevated glucose levels and their resultant problems. Edematous tissues and decreased vascularity, which contribute to lack of blood flow, decrease the body's ability to fight infection because of its inability to deliver oxygen, nutrients, and antibiotics to the area.[49–55]

Although neuropathic ulcers are most often associated with diabetes, they may also occur in individuals with spina bifida, neurologic diseases, muscular degenerative disease, alcoholism, and tertiary syphilis because of similar risk factors in these populations.[33]

## Process of Wound Healing

Epidermal wounds heal by re-epithelialization. Within 24–48 hours after an injury, new epithelial cells proliferate and mature. Deeper wounds, which involve the dermal tissues and even muscle, go through a rather complex and lengthy sequence of (1) an inflammatory response, (2) a fibroplastic phase, and (3) a remodeling phase.[37–41]

In the inflammatory phase, platelets aggregate and clots form. Leukocytes, followed by macrophages, migrate to the area, and phagocytosis begins. Macrophages also provide amino acids and sugars that are needed for wound repair. In preparing the wound for healing, they stimulate the fibroplastic phase. During the fibroplastic phase, granulation begins. Granulation is indicative of capillary buds, growing into the wound bed. Concurrently, fibrocytes and other undifferentiated cells multiply and migrate to the area. These cells network to transform into fibroblasts, which begin to secrete strands of collagen, forming immature pink scar tissue. In the remodeling phase, scar tissue matures. New scar tissue is characterized by its pink color, as it is composed of white collagen fibers and a large number of capillaries. The amount of time the entire healing process takes depends on the size and type of wound. It may take from 3 days to several months or more for complete closure to occur.[49–55]

## Factors That Can Delay Wound Healing

In addition to the problems indigenous to the wound, many other factors can delay wound healing. Age, lifestyle, nutrition, cognitive and self-care ability, vascular status, medical complications, and medications all can affect wound healing. These factors may also be risk factors for the development of new wounds. These factors should therefore be included in the physical therapy assessment and considered when determining goals, interventions, and time frames.

### Age

Skin, just like other tissues and organs, changes with age. Decreased cellular activity during the aging process leads to decreased collagen production that results in less collagen organization in older individuals. Reduced collagen organization results in decreased tensile strength of the skin that could result in greater damage after trauma in the older individual. Other examples of skin changes with age include delayed wound contraction, decreased epithelialization, and delayed cellular migration and proliferation.[56] Other comorbidities that delay wound healing, such as diabetes, peripheral neuropathies, and related vascular problems, occur with greater frequency in older individuals.

*Lifestyle*

A patient's lifestyle can have a great impact on the prognosis for healing, decision-making regarding wound management, and preventive care. For example, occupations and hobbies that require prolonged standing may predispose some individuals to varicosities and other venous problems. Individuals exposed to traumatic situations, such as construction workers, are also more likely to reinjure healing wounds. Behaviors such as cigarette smoking can impede wound healing significantly because of the vasoconstriction that nicotine creates.

*Nutrition*

Good nutrition is necessary for the growth and maintenance of all body tissues. Macronutrients, such as carbohydrates, fats, and proteins, and micronutrients, such as vitamins, are necessary for cell metabolism, division, and growth. Therefore, nutrition is closely linked with all phases of healing.[57] Generally, poor nutrition decreases the body's ability to heal. Additionally, patients with burns, wounds, or infection who are adequately nourished at the time of their injury or the development of their wound may also develop protein-calorie malnutrition.

There are major metabolic abnormalities associated with injury that can deplete nutritional stores, including increased output of catabolic hormones, decreased output of anabolic hormones, a marked increase in metabolic rate, a sustained increase in body temperature, marked increase in glucose demands, rapid skeletal muscle breakdown with amino acids used as an energy source, lack of ketosis, and unresponsiveness to catabolism to nutrient intake.[58] Protein-calorie malnutrition can delay wound healing and cause serious health consequences in patients with wounds, especially if infection exists. Poor nutritional status, whether due to decreased intake or the stress response, can set off a series of metabolic events leading to weight loss, deterioration of lean tissues, increased risk of infection, edema, and breathing difficulty.[58]

These events can lead to severe debilitation and even death. Inadequate diet control in patients with diabetes exacerbates all symptoms of diabetes, including impaired circulation, sensation, altered metabolic processes, and delayed healing. A nutritional assessment by a registered dietitian, nutritional supplements, and careful monitoring of the patient's nutritional status and weight are important components of a comprehensive assessment and treatment program for the patient with a wound.

In addition, therapists should work with other health care professionals to curb the systemic stress response. Removing necrotic tissues, treating infections, and ensuring adequate hydration and blood fluid volumes will help to limit physiologic stressors. Premedication before painful procedures and avoiding extreme temperatures help minimize stress. Exercise serves as an anabolic stimulus for muscle, facilitating a reduction of the catabolic state.[58]

### Cognition and Self-Care Ability

There is an increased risk of infection and other wound healing complications if neither the patient nor the caregiver has the cognitive or physical ability, or both, to properly care for a wound, including wound cleansing and dressing removal and application. The patient's or caregiver's abilities, or both, have a great influence in the choice of dressing(s) and on discharge planning. Certain dressings require more skill than others to maintain. Complex wound care can justify a stay at a rehabilitation hospital or skilled nursing facility.

### Vascular Status

Any compromised vascular status may contribute to the development of delayed wound healing owing to a lack of oxygenation and nutrition to the tissues.

### Medical Status

Generally, compromised health causes a decrease in the body's ability to progress through the healing process. Pre-existing infection or a history of cancer, chemotherapy, radiation, acquired immunodeficiency syndrome, or other immunodeficiency disorders can decrease the patient's ability to heal. Congestive heart failure, hypertension, and renal dysfunction can also slow wound healing.

## Medications

Steroids, antihistamines, nonsteroidal anti-inflammatory drugs, and oral contraceptives may delay wound healing, as can chemotherapy and radiation. These medications can decrease the tensile strength of connective tissue, reduce blood supply, inhibit collagen synthesis, and increase the susceptibility to infection.[59] Anticoagulants thin the blood and decrease its ability to clot; therefore, the healthcare provider needs to diligently monitor bleeding during dressing removal and consider debridement methods that will not cause bleeding.

## Chronic Wounds

In healthy individuals without comorbidities, an acute wound should heal within 3 to 6 weeks, with remodeling occurring over the next year. If a wound remains in one of the stages of healing without progression, it becomes a chronic wound.[60] *Chronic wounds* are defined as wounds that have "failed to proceed through an orderly and timely process to produce anatomic and functional integrity, or proceeded through the repair process without establishing a sustained anatomic and functional result."[61] The acute care therapist should be inclined to search for underlying causes of delayed wound healing, especially when treating a wound that has not healed in more than 6 weeks.

# Wound Assessment and Acute Care Management of Wounds

The evaluation of a patient with a skin wound includes a general history (identification of factors that can delay healing), performing a physical examination (sensation, pain, ROM, strength, and functional mobility) and a specific examination of the wound itself.

## History

In addition to the general chart and medical history review (see Appendix I-A), the following information is especially relevant for determining wound etiology and risk factors, an intervention plan, and potential outcomes:

## Wound History

- How and when did the wound occur?

- What interventions have been administered to the wound thus far? What were the results?

- Is there a previous history of wounds? If so, what were the etiology, intervention, and time frame of healing?

## Risk Factors

- How old is the patient?

- Is the patient cognitively intact?

- Where and for how long is the patient weight bearing on areas involving the wound site?

- What is the patient's occupation or hobby? How many hours does the patient spend on his or her feet per day? What positions and postures is the patient in throughout the day?

- Does the patient smoke?

- Is the patient generally well nourished? Is the patient taking any supplements?

- Has the patient experienced any weight loss or gain lately?

- If the patient has diabetes, is it well controlled?

- Does the patient have an immunodeficiency disorder or a medical condition that increases his or her risk of infection?

- Does the patient have a medical condition that causes altered sensation?

- What medications (including anticoagulants) is the patient taking? What are their effects on wound healing?

## Psychosocial Factors

- Does the patient have a good support system, including physical assistance if necessary?

- What are the patient's mobility needs?

A review of vascular tests, radiographic studies, and tissue biopsy results also lends valuable information about the integrity of the vascular and orthopedic systems and the presence of underlying disease.

## Physical Examination

### Sensation
Sensation to light touch, pressure, pinprick, temperature, and kinesthesia or proprioception, or both, should be examined. Impaired or absent sensation should be addressed through instruction in the appropriate prevention techniques, as well as modifications to shoes, weight bearing, and water temperatures in bathing.

### Pain
The evaluation of pain in the patient with a wound is not unlike the evaluation of pain in any other type of patient. The therapist should evaluate the nature of the pain, including the location, onset, severity (using a pain-rating scale), duration, aggravating and alleviating factors, and the impact on activities of daily living. Understanding the nature of the pain will ultimately allow the physical therapist to provide or recommend the appropriate intervention.

The pain experience associated with wounds has been described as having one of three components: a noncyclic acute component, a cyclic acute component, or a chronic wound pain component.

*Noncyclic acute wound pain* is a single episode of acute pain that is likely to occur with treatment (e.g., the pain felt during sharp debridement). *Cyclic acute pain* is wound pain that recurs throughout the day because of repeated treatments. For example, a patient may experience pain after several days of dressing changes, which creates repetitive trauma to the wound. *Chronic wound pain* is persistent wound pain that occurs intrinsically, not as a result of external intervention (e.g., a patient with a neuropathic ulcer who has a constant, dull ache in the foot).[62]

### Range of Motion
Specific measurement of ROM may not be necessary in a patient with a wound. However, specific goniometric measurements are necessary if a wound crosses a joint line, if edema is present at a joint, or if decreased ROM inhibits mobility. Decreased ROM that inhibits mobility or increases weight bearing, pressure, or both may contrib-

ute to wound development. Therefore, passive or active ROM exercise, or both, should be included, as necessary, in the treatment plan.

### Strength
Strength should be evaluated for its impact on the patient's function. The therapist should keep in mind that the patient may have different functional demands secondary to the wound. For example, a patient who needs to be non weight bearing because of a wound on his or her foot requires sufficient upper-extremity strength to use an assistive device to maintain this precaution while ambulating. If the patient does not have adequate upper-extremity strength, then he or she may be nonambulatory until the weight-bearing status is changed.

### Functional Mobility
Functional mobility, including bed mobility, transfers, and ambulation or wheelchair mobility, should be evaluated. The therapist should consider that the patient's function may have changed simply because of the consequences of the presence of the wound. For example, balance may be compromised if the patient requires orthotics or shoe modifications because of a wound. Gait training with an assistive device is often necessary to decrease weight bearing on an affected lower extremity.

### Edema and Circulation
The evaluation of edema is important because it is frequently an indicator of an underlying pathology. Edema is also a critical factor in lowering tissue perfusion of oxygen and increasing susceptibility to infection. In fact, edema is almost equivalent to insufficient blood supply in lowering the oxygen tension in the area of the wound. Ultimately, the presence of edema must be addressed to heal the wound. Refer to Table 1-6 for the scale on how to grade (pitting) edema.

Therapists should also consider that lymphedema and chronic wounds can be closely linked. Lymphedema is commonly associated in individuals who are status post mastectomy; however, it can also occur after other surgeries and traumas. Cellulitis may actually be due to a compromised lymphatic system that creates small, weeping blisters from fluids being literally pushed through the skin. In addition, edema secondary to chronic venous insufficiency frequently also has a lymphatic component.

Circulation can be grossly evaluated and monitored by examining skin temperature, distal limb color, and the presence of pulses. Refer to Vascular Evaluation in Chapter 6 for more information on the evaluation of circulation. The therapist should notify the physician when any significant changes in these indicators occur. The therapist should be aware of any arterial compromise before using compression bandages.

## Wound Inspection and Evaluation

Wound observation and measurements create an objective record of the baseline status of a wound and can help to determine the best intervention to facilitate wound healing.

### Location, Orientation, Size, and Depth

The location of the wound should be documented in relation to anatomic landmarks. The orientation of a wound; its length, width, and depth; or the presence of undermining (*tunneling*); or a combination of these factors, are essential measurements in wound assessment. The orientation of the wound must be determined to ensure consistent length and width measurements, particularly for a wound with an abstract shape or odd location. One method of determining wound orientation is to consider the wound in terms of a clock, with the patient's head being 12 o'clock.

When documenting length, the measurement is the distance of the wound (measured in the direction from the patient's head to toe), and the width is the horizontal measurement. There are a variety of methods for measuring wounds. Tape measurements are one method, but a calibrated grid on an acetate sheet on which the wound can be traced is optimal, especially for irregularly shaped wounds. Polaroid photographs on grid film can also be used.

---

### Clinical Tip

- When taking a photograph of a wound, create or follow a consistent procedure for taking photographs, as changes in the distance of the camera from the wound, as well as the position of the patient, can affect the appearance of the wound.
- Also, to ensure consistency and accuracy in wound assessments, a consistent unit of measure should be used among all individuals measuring the wound. Cen-

timeters, rather than inches, are more universally used in the literature.

• Multiple wounds can be documented relative to each other if the wounds are numbered—for example, "Wound #1: left lower extremity, 3 cm proximal to the medial malleolus. Wound #2: 2 cm proximal to wound #1."

Depth can be measured by placing a sterile cotton-tip applicator perpendicular to the wound bed. The applicator is then grasped or marked at the point of the wound edge and measured. If the wound has varying depths, this measurement is repeated.

*Undermining* or *tunneling* describes a continuation of the wound underneath intact skin and is evaluated by taking a sterile cotton-tip applicator and placing it underneath the skin parallel to the wound bed and grasping or marking the applicator at the point of the wound edge. Assessment of undermining should be done all around the wound. It can be documented using the clock orientation (e.g., "Undermining: 2 cm at 12 o'clock, 5 cm at 4 o'clock").

### Color

The color of the wound should be documented, because it is an indicator of the general condition and vascularity of the wound. Pink indicates recently epithelized tissue. Red indicates healing, possibly granulating tissue. Yellow indicates infection, necrotic material being sloughed off from the wound, or both. Black indicates eschar.

It is important to document the percentage of each color in the wound bed—an increase in the amount of pink and red tissue, a decrease in the amount of yellow and black tissue, or both are indicative of progress. An increase in the amount of black (necrotic) tissue is indicative of regression.

### Drainage

Wound drainage is described by type, amount, and odor. Drainage can be (1) serous (clear, thin; this drainage may be present in a healthy, healing wound), (2) serosanguineous (containing blood; this drainage may also be present in a healthy, healing wound), (3) purulent (thick, white, pus-like; this drainage may be indicative of infection and should be cultured), or (4) green (usually indicative of *Pseudomonas* infection and should also be cultured). The amount of drainage is generally documented as absent, scant, minimal, moderate, large, or copious. (Note: there is no consistent objective measurement that correlates to these descriptions.) A large amount of drainage can indicate infection, whereas a reduction in the amount of drainage can indicate that an infection is resolving. The presence and degree of odor can be documented as absent, mild, or foul. Foul odors can be indicative of an infection.

## Wound Culture

A wound culture is a sampling of micro-organisms from the wound bed that is subsequently grown in a nutrient medium for the purpose of identifying the type and number of organisms present. A wound culture is indicated if there are clinical signs of infection, such as purulent drainage, large amounts of drainage, increased local or systemic temperature, inflammation, abnormal granulation tissue, local erythema, edema, cellulitis, increased pain, foul odor, and delayed healing.[63] Results of aerobic and nonaerobic cultures can determine whether antibiotic therapy is indicated.[64] Methods of culturing include tissue biopsy, needle aspiration, and swab cultures. Physical therapists may administer swab cultures. Otherwise, wound cultures are performed by the nurse or physician, depending on the protocol of the institution.

All wounds are contaminated, which does not necessarily mean they are infected. *Contamination* is the presence of bacteria on the wound surface. *Colonization* is the presence and multiplication of surface microbes without infection. *Infection* is the invasion and multiplication of micro-organisms in body tissues, resulting in local cellular injury.[63,65,66]

---

### Clinical Tip

Unless specifically prescribed otherwise, cultures should be taken after debridement of thick eschar and necrotic material and wound cleansing; otherwise, the culture will reflect the growth of the micro-organisms of the external wound environment rather than the internal environment.

---

### Surrounding Areas

The area surrounding the wound should also be evaluated and compared to noninvolved areas. Skin color, the absence of hair, shiny or flaky skin, the presence of reddened or darkened areas, edema, or changes in the nailbeds should all be examined and documented accordingly.

Clinical Tip

Increased localized temperature can indicate local infection; decreased temperature can indicate decreased blood supply.

### Wound Staging and Classification

*Superficial wounds* involve only the epidermis. *Partial-thickness wounds* further involve the superficial layers of the dermis; *full-thickness wounds* continue through to muscle and potentially to bone. This terminology should be used to describe and classify wounds that are not pressure ulcers. Pressure ulcers have their own classification system because of their unique characteristic of developing from the "inside out." Pressure ulcers are traditionally described by a four-stage system, presented in Table 7-12.

### Wound Cleansing and Debridement

It is beyond the scope of this chapter to discuss in detail the methods of wound cleansing and debridement. Instead, general descriptions and indications of each are provided. Wound cleansing and debridement can be performed by physical therapists, nurses, or physicians,

**Table 7-12.** Four-Stage Pressure Ulcer Classification

| Stage | Description |
| --- | --- |
| I | Reddened area on the skin with an intact epidermis |
| II | Wound similar to a blister or abrasion on which the dermis is exposed |
| III | Wound that exposes subcutaneous tissue down to, but not through, underlying fascia |
| IV | Wound that exposes muscle, bone, or other supporting structures, such as tendon or joint capsule |

Source: Data from The National Pressure Ulcer Advisory Panel's Summary of the AHCPR Clinical Practice Guideline. Pressure Ulcers in Adults: Prediction and Prevention. (AHCPR Publication No. 92-0047). Rockville, MD. May 1992.

depending on the policy of an individual facility. Physical therapists should also verify state practice acts regarding their ability to perform sharp debridement. Specific management considerations for physical therapists who work with patients who have wounds are described at the end of this chapter.

## Wound Cleansing

*Wound cleansing* is not synonymous with *wound debridement* or *wound decontamination*. The purpose of cleansing a wound is to remove loosely attached cellular debris and bacteria from the wound bed. In most cases, the use of sterile saline is effective and safe for cleansing the wound surface.[67,68] Many studies indicate that using unsterile tap water does not increase the rate of infection and is appropriate to use to cleanse wounds.[67] There are many commercial wound cleansers that contain surfactants. Surfactants help to break the bonds between contaminants, debris, and the surface of the wound.[67] The use of antiseptics is appropriate in the early management of acute traumatic wounds but is of little benefit in chronic wounds. They may be cytotoxic to living tissues and can delay healing.[67,69,70]

The most neutral solution that will meet the needs of the patient should be used. Aggressive agents should be used only when indicated. For example, a bleaching agent may help to dry a heavily exudating wound. Cleansing should be discontinued when the majority of a wound bed is granulating or when re-epithelialization is occurring to avoid damaging new tissue.

---

### Clinical Tip

- If the water source is known or suspected to be contaminated, it should not be used for wound cleansing.[67] If the physical therapist is unsure, the water can be cultured in the hospital laboratory.
- Sterile saline expires 24 hours after opening the bottle and must be discarded. A saline solution can be made by adding 2 tablespoons of salt to 1 quart of boiling water.[67,69] This recipe may be an inexpensive alternative to purchasing saline for the patient who will be cleansing wounds at home.
- It is best to use cleansing materials at body temperature. The application of a cold solution will reduce the temperature of the wound and may affect blood flow.[70]

- Whirlpool, although commonly and perhaps habitually used, does not cleanse the wound. The use of whirlpool jets is actually mechanical debridement and therefore should be used only if mechanical debridement is indicated.

## Clean versus Sterile Technique

Although clean versus sterile technique remains somewhat controversial, clean technique is sufficient for local wound care to chronic wounds and is generally accepted in the medical community, because the chronic wound is already contaminated and far from sterile. Sterile technique is typically reserved for surgical and acute traumatic wounds.[71]

Sterile technique, which includes the use of sterile instruments and sterile gloves, should always be used when invading the blood stream, as with sharp debridement. Otherwise, the use of clean gloves is sufficient. Additionally, originally sterile dressings, once opened, can still be used as long as they are kept in a clean, controlled area.[71]

## Wound Debridement

Debridement has three primary purposes. The first is to remove necrotic tissue or foreign matter from the wound bed, optimizing healing potential. The presence of devitalized tissue prevents re-epithelialization and can splint the wound open, preventing contraction and closure. The second purpose is to prevent infection. The necrotic tissue itself can be the source of the pathogenic organisms. The debridement of the slough and eschar also increases the effectiveness of topical agents. The third purpose is to correct abnormal wound repair. Debridement is generally indicated for any necrotic tissue present in a wound, although occasionally it is advantageous to leave eschar in place. For example, eschar on heel ulcers that is firmly adherent to surrounding tissue without inflammation of surrounding tissue and without drainage and tenderness on palpation may not need to be removed.[72]

There are two types of debridement: selective and nonselective. *Selective debridement* removes nonviable tissue only and is indicated for wounds with necrotic tissue adjacent to viable tissue. Methods of selective debridement include sharp, autolytic, and enzymatic debridement. *Nonselective debridement* removes both viable and nonviable tissues. It is indicated in necrotic wounds with minimal to no healthy tissue. Mechanical debridement is a method of nonselective debridement.[72,73]

## Selective Debridement

### Sharp Debridement

*Sharp debridement* involves the use of scalpels, scissors, and forceps to remove necrotic tissue. It is a highly skilled technique best performed by or under the direct supervision of an experienced clinician. (Note: Not all states and facilities allow physical therapists to perform sharp debridement.) Because the true selectivity of sharp debridement depends on the skill of the clinician, sharp debridement can also result in damage to healthy tissues that can cause bleeding and a risk of infection. Sharp debridement is especially expedient in the removal of large amounts of thick, leathery eschar. Removal of eschar is important in the patient who is immunocompromised, because the underside of eschar can provide a medium for bacterial growth. Sharp debridement has been shown to increase the degree of wound healing when combined with the use of a topical growth factor.[74]

Sharp debridement can be painful; it is therefore recommended that pain medications or topical analgesics be administered before treatment. When debriding, the clinician should spare as much tissue as possible and be careful to have the technique remain selective by not removing viable tissue. Because of the potential for excessive bleeding, extra care should be taken with patients who are taking anticoagulants.

### Autolytic Debridement

*Autolytic debridement* is the natural and most selective form of debridement. The body uses its own enzymes to lyse necrotic tissue and this is a normal process that occurs in any wound. It is painless and does not harm healthy tissues. Moist dressings facilitate autolytic debridement, as do films, hydrocolloids, and calcium alginates, which keep the wounds moist with the exudate from the wound.[72,74] When using autolytic debridement, it is important to cleanse the wound to remove partially degraded tissue.[74] Because it takes time for autolytic debridement to occur, sharp debridement of eschar is recommended before autolytic debridement to expedite the removal of the necrotic tissue. Owing to the risk of infection, autolytic debridement is contraindicated as the primary method of debridement in patients who are immunosuppressed or otherwise require quick elimination of necrotic material.

## Nonselective Debridement

### Mechanical Debridement

*Mechanical debridement* removes dead tissue by agitating the necrotic tissue of the wound or adhering it to a dressing and removing it. Dry gauze dressings, scrubbing, whirlpool, and pulsed lavage or irrigation, or both, are all examples of mechanical debridement.

Wet-to-dry dressings mechanically debride the wound by removing the dressing along with the necrotic tissue embedded in it. If mechanical debridement is indicated, and gauze is used, the sponge or gauze with the largest pores is the most effective for debridement.[74] This technique involves applying a saline-moistened gauze dressing to the wound, allowing it to dry, followed by removal of the dressing. The dressing will also adhere to any growing tissue in the wound bed and may inadvertently remove it.[72] Wet-to-dry dressings, therefore, should not be used on clean, granulating wound beds. If saline gauze dressings are used on a clean wound bed, they must continually be kept moist.

Whirlpool may be used to debride loosely adherent tissue and exudate and deodorize the wound. It may also help to prepare a wound for sharp debridement by softening necrotic tissue and separating desiccated tissues from the wound bed. Or it can be used to soak off adhered dressings. If the intention of the therapist is to use a wet-to-dry technique for mechanical debridement, the dressings should not be soaked off, as necrotic tissue will not be removed.[41,73,75]

There are many precautions and contraindications for the therapist to consider before using whirlpool. For example, it may be inappropriate to place the lower extremity of a patient with venous insufficiency in a dependent position with warm water, or perhaps the treatment may need to be modified by decreasing the temperature or length of a treatment. As with wound cleansing, the therapist should carefully weigh the benefits of antibacterial agents that can be added to the whirlpool versus their cytotoxic effects and use a solution that is most neutral and least damaging to viable tissue. Infected wounds that have foul odors, copious amounts of drainage, and a great deal of exudate and necrotic tissue require more aggressive additives.

Whirlpool should be limited to stage III or IV wounds with greater than 50% of necrotic tissue, because, as with gauze debridement, granulating tissue may be damaged. Whirlpool should be discontinued once the objectives of the whirlpool have been achieved.[41,72,75]

Pulsed lavage is now a viable treatment option for wound management, and systems specifically designed for wound care are currently available. Pulsed lavage uses a pressurized, pulsed solution (usually saline) to irrigate and debride wounds of necrotic tissue. Suction may also be used to remove wound debris and the irrigation solution.[76] The pulsatile action is thought to facilitate growth of granulation tissue because of its effective debridement, and the negative pressure created by the suction may also stimulate granulation.[77] Pulsed lavage may be a more appropriate option than whirlpool for patients who are incontinent, have venous insufficiency, should not be in a dependent position, have an intravenous line, or are mechanically ventilated. Pulsed lavage may access narrow wound tunnels that may not be reached with whirlpool.

### Enzymatic Debridement

*Enzymatic debridement* is achieved through the topical application of enzymes that lyse collagen, fibrin, and elastin. The type of enzyme chosen depends on the type of necrotic tissue in the wound. Enzymes are categorized as proteolytics, fibrinolytics, and collagenases.[72] Different enzymatic debriding agents are effective with each of these tissues. Wounds with heavy black eschar are best debrided by proteinases and fibrolytic enzymes. Collagenases are used when necrotic collagen, which generally appears yellowish, is present. Enzymatic debridement agents are available only by prescription. Enzymatic debridement is indicated on stage III and IV wounds with yellow necrotic material but should be discontinued as soon as the wound is clean. Sharp debridement of the wound can be performed before the use of enzymes to facilitate tissue healing.

---

### Clinical Tip

When applying an enzymatic debriding agent to eschar and it cannot be debrided, crosshatch the eschar and pull in the edges to allow the enzymes to penetrate the eschar.

---

### Dressings and Topical Agents

When applying dressings, the therapist should always follow universal precautions and use a clean technique to prevent cross contamination. When choosing a dressing for a wound, four factors related to the wound itself should be considered: (1) the color of the wound, (2) the amount of drainage, (3) the wound depth, and (4) the surrounding skin. Other significant factors include the patient's cognitive and physical ability to apply the dressing and the accessibility of physical therapy or nursing services to the patient. Cost is also a consideration.

A large number of wound care products are available, and it is virtually impossible to be aware of the purpose and application instructions of every available dressing. It is the responsibility of the therapist to read manufacturer's instructions for application, to know the purpose of the dressing, and to make educated decisions when choosing the appropriate dressing for a given wound at each stage of the healing process. Clinicians should not rely on manufacturer's claims of efficacy to justify a dressing's effectiveness. Although it is not possible to identify every dressing, it is possible to catalog *most* dressings into some basic categories: gauze, nonadherent dressings, hydrocolloids, semipermeable films, hydrogels, foams, and calcium alginates. Table 7-13 is a summary of the indications, advantages, and disadvantages of different dressings.[77–80]

### Other Dressings

The V.A.C. (Vacuum Assisted Closure) (Kinetic Concepts, Inc., San Antonio, TX) device assists in wound closure by applying localized negative pressure to a special porous dressing positioned in or over the wound. The porous dressing distributes negative pressure to the wound and helps remove interstitial fluids. The negative pressure applies noncompressive mechanical forces to the wound site and draws the tissue inward, subjecting it to subatmospheric pressure. The distortion causes epithelial cells to multiply rapidly and form granulation tissue. The stretching also increases cell proliferation by activating ion channels within the cells and releasing biochemical mediators from the plasma membrane. It is also thought to stimulate the growth of new blood vessels. This device is worn continuously 24 hours a day. Dressings for noninfected wounds can be changed every 2–3 days or changed daily for infected wounds. Indications for this therapy include diabetic ulcers, pressure ulcers, traumatic wounds, meshed grafts, and flaps. Contraindications include fistulas, necrotic tissue or eschar, untreated osteomyelitis, malignancy in wound, and exposed arteries or veins.[81,82]

   *Cadexomer-iodine* is an iodine-based wound filler (e.g., Iodoflex, iodoform) and is indicated in highly exudating wounds. It is highly absorbent, provides a moist healing environment, and lowers the pH of the wound. The iodine is slowly released, so it is not cytotoxic to good tissue, but the bacteriostatic and bactericidal effects of iodine remain.

### Skin Substitutes and Biologicals

Although these will not be a first line of defense, therapists in the acute care setting should be aware of other agents that may be used to

**Table 7-13.** Indications and Uses of Basic Types of Dressings

| Type of Dressing | Indication | Description | Advantages | Disadvantages |
|---|---|---|---|---|
| Gauze | May be used for any type of wound if properly applied and removed (although other dressings may be more effective) | Highly porous. Applied dry, wet-to-dry (i.e., the dressing is put on wet but will dry before removal), or wet-to-wet (i.e., the dressing is put on wet and removed when wet). | Readily available Inexpensive | May require frequent changes Can cause skin maceration Permeable to bacteria Removal can be painful |
| Nonadherent dressings | Wounds with low-to-moderate drainage, for minor lacerations or abrasions, or as a secondary dressing for deep full-thickness wounds | Nonimpregnated or impregnated (nonadherent substance integrated into dressing) dressings comprised of inert materials that conform to the wound surface. | Generally nonirritating and nontoxic Less likely to adhere to wound, causing less tissue disruption Relatively inexpensive | May still adhere if allowed to get too dry before removing |

| | Indications | Description | Advantages | Disadvantages |
|---|---|---|---|---|
| Hydrocolloids | Partial- or full-thickness wounds with low-to-moderate drainage, including partially necrotic wounds. Provide a moist wound environment and promotes autolysis | Dressings that contain absorptive particles that interact with moisture to form a gelatinous mass. Cause the pH of the wound surface to decrease, thereby inhibiting bacterial growth. | Prevent secondary wound infection. Impermeable to water, oxygen, and bacteria. Available in many forms (pastes, powders, and sheets). Changed infrequently | Not for use with anaerobic wound infections. Removal may cause skin tears on fragile surrounding skin |
| Semipermeable films | Promote a moist wound environment for wounds with minimal drainage | Transparent polyurethane with a water-resistant adhesive on one side. Semipermeable to water and oxygen but impermeable to bacteria. | Conforms well. Allow for visual wound monitoring | Highly adhesive, can be difficult to apply. Can cause skin tears, especially on fragile skin |
| Hydrogels | Partial-thickness wounds with minimal drainage, or as a secondary dressing on a full-thickness wound | Gel composed of 96% water or glycerin. | Highly conformable. Safe for fragile skin. Available in many forms | Do not absorb much |

**Table 7-13.** *Continued*

| Type of Dressing | Indication | Description | Advantages | Disadvantages |
|---|---|---|---|---|
| Foams | Partial- or full-thickness wounds with minimal-to-moderate drainage | Polyurethane foam with two surfaces: a hydrophilic inner surface and a hydrophobic outer surface. | Nonadherent to skin surface<br>Highly absorbable and conformable<br>Permeable to oxygen (reduce risk of anaerobic infection) | Expensive |
| Calcium alginates | Partial- and full-thickness wounds with large amounts of drainage, infected or noninfected wounds<br>Provide a moist wound environment and facilitate autolysis | Fibrous sheets and rope derived from brown seaweed. The main component, alginic acid, is converted to calcium and sodium salts, which in turn convert to a viscous gel after contact with wound exudates. | Highly conformable | Require a secondary dressing to keep from drying out |

Sources: With permission from J Cuzell, D Krasner. Wound Dressings. In PP Gogia (ed). Clinical Wound Management. Thorofare, NJ: Slack, 1995; JS Feedar. Clinical Management of Chronic Wounds. In LC Kloth, KH Miller (eds). Wound Healing: Alternatives in Management. Philadelphia: FA Davis, 1995; ML Levin, LW O'Neal, JH Bower (eds). The Diabetic Foot (4th ed). St. Louis: Mosby, 1993; JC Lawrence. Dressings and wound infection. Am J Surg 1994;167(1A):21; and CT Hess. When to use hydrocolloid dressings. Adv Skin Wound Care 2000;13:63.

treat the chronic, nonhealing ulcer. Frequently a patient may have been receiving treatment for a wound before hospitalization for an acute medical condition and the therapist may be continuing or may need to recommend alternative healing agents. *Platelet-derived growth factor* promotes cellular migration of leukocytes and macrophages and stimulates fibroblasts to produce collagen. An example of platelet-derived growth factor is Regranex gel (becaplermin).[83]

Another possible solution is *skin substitutes* (e.g., Dermagraft), which consist of fibroblasts from a newborn foreskin donor, placed on a polygalactic acid mesh. The fibroblasts multiply, attach to the mesh, and release growth factors.[82] Living skin equivalent (e.g., graftskin [Apligraf]) consists of bovine type I collagen that is acid dissociated and added to a culture system. Human fibroblasts are then added.[84]

These are typically fairly expensive treatments and are reserved for nonhealing foot ulcers that have not responded to other topical agents and treatments.

## Physical Therapy Intervention in Wound Care

The responsibility and autonomy of the physical therapist in the treatment of wounds vary greatly among facilities. The physical therapist can and should play a key role in the patient's clinical course of preventing a wound, initiating wound care, or both. The physical therapist in the acute care setting can also be responsible for making recommendations about wound care on discharge from the hospital. Unless the wound is superficial and caused by trauma, wound closure is not likely to occur during the acute care phase. Therefore, the ultimate long-term goal of complete wound closure, which may occur over many months, occurs at a different level of care, usually outpatient or home care.

The following are the primary goals of physical therapy for wound treatment in the acute care setting:

- To promote wound healing through wound assessment, dressing choice and application, wound cleansing, and debridement

- To educate patients and families about wound care and prevention of further breakdown and future wounds

Table 7-14. Physical Therapy Considerations for Wound Care

| Physical Therapy Intervention | Consideration |
|---|---|
| Pain management | Coordinate physical therapy session with pain premedication to reduce acute cyclic and noncyclic pain. |
| | Consider the use of positioning, relaxation techniques, deep breathing, exercise, or modalities to relieve pain. |
| | Modify wound treatment techniques as able to eliminate the source of pain. |
| Range of motion, strength, and functional mobility | Adequate range of motion is necessary for proper positioning and minimizing the risk of pressure ulcer formation. |
| | Care should be taken with manual contacts with fragile skin, and care should be taken not to disturb dressings during exercise. |
| | Adequate strength is necessary for weight shifting and functional mobility with the maintenance of weight-bearing precautions. |
| Edema management | Depending on the etiology, exercise, compression therapy, lymphatic drainage, limb elevation (used with caution in the patient with cardiac dysfunction), or a combination of these can be used to manage edema. |
| Prevention | Education (e.g., dressing application, infection control, wound inspection, the etiology of wounds) |
| | Positioning (e.g., splints, turning schedule) |
| | Skin care and hygiene (e.g., dressing removal) |
| | Pressure reduction surfaces (e.g., air mattress, wheelchair cushion) |
| | Footwear adaptations (e.g., orthotics, inserts, extra-depth shoes) |

- To maximize patient mobility and function while accommodating needs for wound healing (e.g., maintaining non–weight-bearing status)

- To minimize pain

- To provide recommendations for interdisciplinary acute care

- To provide recommendations and referrals for follow-up care

To fulfill these responsibilities, the therapist must consider all information gathered during the evaluation process and establish appropriate goals and time frames. The etiology of the wound, risk factors, and other data guide the therapist toward the proper intervention. Objective, measurable, and functional goals are as important in wound care as in any other aspect of physical therapy.

Patients with wounds typically have many other medical complications and needs that a physical therapist cannot address alone. To provide optimal care, the physical therapist should function as a part of an interdisciplinary team that may include a physician, nurse, specialized skin and wound care nurse (referred to as an *enterostomal therapist*), dietitian, and others. The physical therapist should be aware of and make proper recommendations to the appropriate personnel for all of the patient's needs for healing.

Specific considerations for physical therapy intervention with a patient who has a wound include pain management, ROM, strengthening, functional mobility, edema management, and wound prevention. Table 7-14 describes these considerations.

## References

1. Williams WG, Phillips LG. Pathophysiology of the Burn Wound. In DN Herndon (ed), Total Burn Care. London: Saunders, 1996;63.
2. Falkel JE. Anatomy and Physiology of the Skin. In RI Richard, MJ Staley (eds), Burn Care Rehabilitation Principles and Practice. Philadelphia: FA Davis, 1994;10.
3. Totora GJ, Grabowski SR (eds). Principles of Anatomy and Physiology (7th ed). New York: Harper-Collins College, 1989;126.
4. Warden GD, Heimback DM. Burns. In SI Schwartz (ed), Principles of Surgery, Vol.1 (7th ed). New York: McGraw-Hill, 1999;223–262.
5. Johnson C. Pathologic Manifestations of Burn Injury. In RI Richard, MJ Staley (eds), Burn Care and Rehabilitation Principles and Practice. Philadelphia: FA Davis, 1994;29.
6. Rai J, Jeschke MG, Barrow RE, Herndon DN. Electrical injuries: a 30-year review. J Trauma 1999;46(5):933–936.
7. High-Tension Electrical Burns. In RH Demling, C LaLonde (eds), Burn Trauma. New York: Thieme, 1989;223.
8. Winfree J, Barillo DJ. Burn management. Nonthermal injuries. Nurs Clin North Am 1997;32(2):275–296.
9. Lightning. In RH Demling, C LaLonde (eds), Burn Trauma. New York: Thieme, 1989;242.
10. Milner SM, Rylah LTA, Nguyen TT, et al. Chemical Injury. In DN Herndon (ed), Total Burn Care. London: Saunders, 1996;424.

11. Milner SM, Nguyen TT, Herndon DN, Rylah LTA. Radiation Injuries and Mass Casualties. In DN Herndon (ed), Total Burn Care. London: Saunders, 1996;425.
12. McManus WF, Pruitt BA. Thermal Injuries. In DV Feliciano, EE Moore, KL Mattox (eds), Trauma. Stamford, CT: Appleton & Lange, 1996;937.
13. Marvin J. Thermal Injuries. In VD Cardona, PD Hurn, PJ Bastnagel Mason, et al. (eds), Trauma Nursing: from Resuscitation through Rehabilitation (2nd ed). Philadelphia: Saunders, 1994;736.
14. Richard R. Assessment and diagnosis of burn wounds. Adv Wound Care 1999;12(9):468–471.
15. American Burn Association. Hospital and prehospital resources for optimal care of patients with burn injury: guidelines for development and operation of burn centers. J Burn Care Rehabil 1990;11(2):98–104.
16. Gordon M, Goodwin CW. Burn management. Initial assessment, management, and stabilization. Nurs Clin North Am 1997;32(2):237–249.
17. Kao CC, Garner WL. Acute burns. Plast Reconstr Surg 2000;101(7): 2482–2493.
18. Schiller WR. Burn Care and Inhalation Injury. In A Grenvik (ed), Textbook of Critical Care (4th ed). Philadelphia: Saunders, 2000;365–377.
19. Desai MH, Herndon DN. Burns. In DD Trunkey, FR Lewis, BC Decker (eds), Current Therapy of Trauma (3rd ed). Philadelphia: Mosby, 1991;315.
20. Abraham E. Toxic Gas and Inhalation Injury. In BE Brenner (ed), Comprehensive Management of Respiratory Emergencies. Rockville, MD: Aspen Publications, 1995;241.
21. Traber DL, Herndon DN. Pathophysiology of Smoke Inhalation. In EF Haponik, AM Munster (eds), Respiratory Injury: Smoke Inhalation and Burns. New York: McGraw-Hill, 1990;61.
22. Crapo RO. Causes of Respiratory Injury. In EF Haponik, AM Munster (eds), Respiratory Injury: Smoke Inhalation and Burns. New York: McGraw-Hill, 1990;47.
23. Ahrns KS, Harkins DR. Initial resuscitation after burn injury: therapies, strategies, and controversies. AACN Clin Issues 1999;10:46–60.
24. Edlich RF, Moghtader JC. Thermal Burns. In P Rosen (ed), Emergency Medicine Concepts and Clinical Practice, Vol. 1 (4th ed). St. Louis: Mosby, 1998;941–953.
25. Jordan BS, Harrington DT. Management of the burn wound. Nurs Clin North Am 1997;32(2):251–271.
26. Linares HA. Pathophysiology of Burn Scar. In DN Herndon (ed), Total Burn Care. London: Saunders, 1996;383.
27. Wild B, Kemp H. Skin cultures in burns care nursing. Nurs Times 1999;95(36):46–49.
28. Miller SF, Staley MJ, Richard RL. Surgical Management of the Burn Patient. In RL Richard, MJ Staley (eds), Burn Care and Rehabilitation Principles and Practice. Philadelphia: FA Davis, 1994;177.
29. Kagan RJ. Skin substitutes: implications for burns and chronic wounds. Adv Wound Care 1999;12(2):94–95.
30. Richard RL, Staley MJ. Burn Patient Evaluation and Treatment Planning. In RL Richard, MJ Staley (eds), Burn Care and Rehabilitation Principles and Practice. Philadelphia: FA Davis, 1994;201.

31. Micheletti G. Ulcers of the Lower Extremity. In PP Gogia. Clinical Wound Management. Thorofare, NJ: Slack, 1995;105–106.
32. McCulloch JM. Evaluation of Patients with Open Wounds In LC Kloth, KH Miller. Wound Healing: Alternatives in Management. Philadelphia: FA Davis, 1995;118.
33. Sibbald RG. An approach to leg and foot ulcers: a brief overview. Ostomy Wound Manage 1998;44(9):28–32, 34–35.
34. Sibbald RG. Venous Leg Ulcers. Ostomy Wound Manage 1998;44(9): 52–64.
35. Donayre CE. Diagnosis and Management of Vascular Ulcers. In C Sussman, B Bates-Jensen. Wound Care: A Collaborative Practice Manual for Physical Therapists and Nurses. Gaithersburg, MD: Aspen Publishers, 1998;310.
36. Kosiak M. Etiology and pathology of ischemic ulcers. Arch Phys Med Rehabil 1959;40:62–69.
37. Feedar JA. Prevention and Management of Pressure Ulcers. In LC Kloth, KH Miller, Wound Healing: Alternatives in Management. Philadelphia: FA Davis, 1995;187–193.
38. Leigh IH. Pressure ulcers: prevalence, etiology, and treatment modalities. A review. Am J Surg 1994;167(1A):25S–30S.
39. Bolander VP (ed). Sorensen and Luckmann's Basic Nursing. Philadelphia: Saunders, 1994;742.
40. Feedar JA. Prevention and Management of Pressure Ulcers. In LC Kloth, KH Miller, Wound Healing: Alternatives in Management. Philadelphia: FA Davis, 1995;193–195.
41. The National Pressure Ulcer Advisory Panel's Summary of the AHCPR Clinical Practice Guideline. Pressure Ulcers in Adults: Prediction and Prevention (AHCPR Publication No. 92-0047). Rockville, MD. May 1992.
42. Brown AC, Sibbald RG. The diabetic neuropathic ulcer: an overview. Ostomy Wound Manage 1999;45(Suppl 1A):6.
43. Levin ME. Preventing amputation in the patient with diabetes. Diabetes Care 1995;18(10);1383–1394.
44. Daniels TR. Diabetic Foot Ulcerations: An Overview. Ostomy Wound Manage 1999;44(9):77.
45. Weiss EL. Connective Tissue in Wound Healing. In LC Kloth, KH Miller, Wound Healing: Alternatives in Management. Philadelphia: FA Davis, 1995;26.
46. Laing P. Diabetic foot ulcers. Am J Surg 1994,167(1A):31.
47. Levin ML, O'Neal LW, Bowker JH. The Diabetic Foot (5th ed). St. Louis: Mosby, 1993.
48. Catanzariti AR, Haverstock BD, Grossman JP, Mendicino RW. Off loading techniques in the treatment of diabetic plantar neuropathic foot ulceration. Adv Wound Care 1999;12(9):452.
49. Kloth LC, McCulloch JM. The Inflammatory Response to Wounding. In LC Kloth, KH Miller (eds), Wound Healing: Alternatives in Management. Philadelphia: FA Davis, 1995;3–15.
50. Weiss EL. Connective Tissue in Wound Healing. In LC Kloth, KH Miller (eds), Wound Healing: Alternatives in Management. Philadelphia: FA Davis, 1995;16–31.

51. Daly TJ. Contraction and Re-Epithelialization. In LC Kloth, KH Miller (eds), Wound Healing: Alternatives in Management. Philadelphia: FA Davis, 1995;32–46.
52. Gogia PP. Physiology of Wound Healing. In PP Gogia (ed), Clinical Wound Management. Thorofare, NJ: Slack, 1995;1–12.
53. Sussman C. Wound Healing Biology and Chronic Wound Healing. In C Sussman, B Bates-Jensen (eds), Wound Care: A Collaborative Practice Manual for Physical Therapists and Nurses. Gaithersburg, MD: Aspen Publishers, 1998;31–47.
54. Keast DH, Orsted H. The basic principles of wound care. Ostomy Wound Manage 1998;44(8):24–31.
55. Kernstein MD. The scientific basis of healing. Adv Wound Care 1997;10(3);30–36.
56. Mulder GD, Brazinsky BA, Seeley JE. Factors Complicating Wound Repair. In LC Kloth, KH Miller (eds), Wound Healing: Alternatives in Management. Philadelphia: FA Davis, 1995;48–49.
57. Bahl SM. Nutritional Considerations in Wound Management. In PP Gogia (ed), Clinical Wound Management. Thorofare, NJ: Slack, 1995;73.
58. DeSanti L. Involuntary Weight Loss and the Nonhealing Wound. Adv Skin Wound Care 2000;13(Suppl 1):11–20.
59. Mulder GD, Brazinsky BA, Seeley JE. Factors Complicating Wound Repair. In LC Kloth, KH Miller (eds), Wound Healing: Alternatives in Management. Philadelphia: FA Davis, 1995;50–51.
60. Keast DH, Orsted H. The Basic Principles of Wound Care. Ostomy Wound Manage 1998;44(8):28.
61. Lazarus G, Cooper DM, Knighton DR, et al. Definitions and guidelines for assessment of wounds and evaluation of healing. Arch Dermatol 1994;130:489–493.
62. Gallagher SM. Ethical dilemmas in pain management. Ostomy Wound Manage 1998;44(9):20.
63. Thomson PD, Smith DJ. What is infection? Am J Surg 1994;167(1A): 7S–11S.
64. Fowler E. Wound infection: a nurse's perspective. Ostomy Wound Manage 1998;44(8):45.
65. Icrow S. Infection Control Perspectives. In D Krasner, D Kan (eds), Chronic Wound Care: A Clinical Source Book for Healthcare Professionals. Wayne, PA: Health Management Publications, 1997;90–96.
66. Thomson PD, Smith DJ. What is infection? Am J Surg 1994; 167(1A):7S–11S.
67. Fowler E. Wound infection: a nurse's perspective. Ostomy Wound Manage 1998;44(8):47.
68. Gilchrist B. Infection and Culturing. In D Krasner, D Kane (eds), Chronic Wound Care: A Clinical Source Book for Healthcare Professionals (2nd ed). Wayne, PA: Health Management Publications, 1997;109–114.
69. Rodheaver GT. Wound Cleansing, Wound Irrigation and Wound Disinfection. In D Krasner, D Kane (eds), Chronic Wound Care: A Clinical

Source Book for Healthcare Professionals (2nd ed). Wayne, PA: Health Management Publications, 1997;97–106.
70. Sussman G. Management of the Wound Environment. In C Sussman, B Bates-Jensen (eds), Wound Care: A Collaborative Practice Manual for Physical Therapists and Nurses. Gaithersburg, MD: Aspen Publishers, 1998;212.
71. Fowler E. Wound infection: a nurse's perspective. Ostomy Wound Manage 1998;44(9):19.
72. Sieggreen MY, Maklebust JM. Debridement: choices and challenges. Adv Wound Care 1997;10(2):32–37.
73. Feedar JS. Clinical Management of Chronic Wounds. In LC Kloth, KH Miller (eds), Wound Healing: Alternatives in Management. Philadelphia, PA: FA Davis, 1995;151–156.
74. Rodeheaver GT. Pressure ulcer debridement and cleansing: a review of current literature. Ostomy Wound Manage 1999;45(1A Suppl):80S–87S.
75. Scott RG, Loehne HB. Five questions—and answers—about pulsed lavage. Adv Skin Wound Care 2000;13(3):133–134.
76. Loehne HB. Pulsatile Lavage with Concurrent Suction. In C Sussman, B Bates-Jensen (eds), Wound Care: A Collaborative Practice Manual for Physical Therapists and Nurses. Gaithersburg, MD: Aspen Publishers, 1998;389–403.
77. Sussman C. Whirlpool. In C Sussman, B Bates-Jensen (eds), Wound Care: A Collaborative Practice Manual for Physical Therapists and Nurses. Gaithersburg, MD: Aspen Publishers, 1998;447–454.
78. Cuzell J, Krasner D. Wound Dressings. In PP Gogia, Clinical Wound Management. Thorofare, NJ: Slack, 1995:131–144.
79. Feedar JS. Clinical Management of Chronic Wounds. In LC Kloth, KH Miller (eds), Wound Healing: Alternatives in Management. Philadelphia: FA Davis, 1995;156–169.
80. Levin ML, O'Neal LW, Bower JH. The Diabetic Foot (4th ed.) St. Louis: Mosby, 1993.
81. Philbeck TE, Whittington KT, Millsap MH, et al. The clinical and cost effectiveness of externally applied negative pressure wound therapy in the treatment of wounds in home healthcare medicare patients. Ostomy Wound Manage 1999;45(11):41–50.
82. Mendez-Eastman S. When wounds won't heal. RN 1998;61:20–23.
83. Sibbald RG. An approach to leg and foot ulcers. Ostomy Wound Manage 1998;44(9):30.
84. Sibbald RG. Venous leg ulcers. Ostomy Wound Manage 1998;44(9):63.

# 8

# Gastrointestinal System
*Jaime C. Paz*

## Introduction

Disorders of the gastrointestinal (GI) system can have numerous effects on the body, such as decreased nutrition, anemia, and fluid imbalances. These consequences may, in turn, affect the activity tolerance of a patient, which will ultimately influence many physical therapy interventions. In addition, physical therapists must be aware of pain referral patterns from the GI system that may mimic musculoskeletal symptoms (Table 8-1). The objectives of this chapter are to provide the following:

    1.    A basic understanding of the structure and function of the GI system

    2.    Information on the clinical evaluation of the GI system, including physical examination and diagnostic studies

    3.    A basic understanding of the various diseases and disorders of the GI system

**Table 8-1.** Gastrointestinal System Pain Referral Patterns

| Structure | Segmental Innervation | Areas of Pain Referral |
|-----------|----------------------|------------------------|
| Esophagus | T4–6 | Substernal region |
| | | Upper abdomen |
| Stomach | T6–10 | Upper abdomen |
| | | Middle and lower thoracic spine |
| Small intestine | T7–10 | Middle thoracic spine |
| Pancreas | T6–10 | Upper abdomen |
| | | Upper and lower thoracic spine |
| Gallbladder | T7–9 | Right upper abdomen |
| | | Right, middle, and lower thoracic spine |
| Liver | T7–9 | Right, middle, and lower thoracic spine |
| | | Right cervical spine |
| Common bile duct | T6–10 | Upper abdomen |
| | | Middle lumbar spine |
| Large intestine | T11–L1 | Lower abdomen |
| | | Middle lumbar spine |
| Sigmoid colon | T11–12 | Upper sacral region |
| | | Suprapubic region |
| | | Left lower quadrant of abdomen |

Source: With permission from WG Boissonault, C Bass. Pathological origins of trunk and neck pain: part I. Pelvic and abdominal visceral disorders. J Orthop Sports Phys Ther 1990;12:194.

4.    Information on the management of GI disorders, including pharmacologic therapy and surgical procedures

5.    Guidelines for physical therapy intervention in patients with GI diseases and disorders

## Structure and Function

The basic structure of the GI system is shown in Figure 8-1, with the primary and accessory organs of digestion and their respective functions described in Tables 8-2 and 8-3.

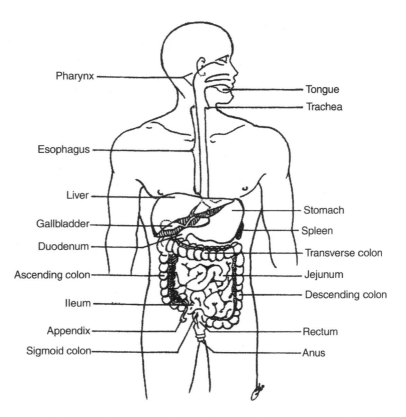

**Figure 8-1.** *Schematic representation of the gastrointestinal system. (Original artwork by Peter Wu.)*

## Clinical Evaluation

Evaluation of the GI system involves combining information gathered through physical examination and diagnostic studies.

### Physical Examination

Physical examination of the abdomen consists of inspection, auscultation, percussion, and palpation. Physicians and nurses usually perform this examination on a daily basis in the acute care setting; however, physical therapists can also perform this examination to help delineate between systemic and musculoskeletal pain.

**Table 8-2.** Structure and Function of the Primary Organs of Digestion

| Structure | Function |
|---|---|
| Oral cavity | Entrance to the gastrointestinal system, mechanical and chemical digestion begins here |
| Pharynx | Involved in swallowing and mechanical movement of food to esophagus |
| Esophagus | Connects mouth to the stomach, transports and disperses food |
| Stomach (cardia, fundus, body, pylorus) | *Mechanical functions*: storage, mixing, and grinding of food and regulation of outflow to small intestine |
| | *Exocrine functions*: secretion of hydrochloric acid, intrinsic factor, pepsinogen, and mucus necessary for digestion |
| | *Endocrine functions*: secretion of hormones that trigger the release of digestive enzymes from the pancreas, liver, and gallbladder into the duodenum |
| Small intestine (duodenum, jejunum, ileum) | *Duodenum*: neutralizes acid in food transported from the stomach and mixes pancreatic and biliary secretions with food |
| | *Jejunum*: absorbs nutrients, water, and electrolytes |
| | *Ileum*: absorbs bile acids and intrinsic factors to be recycled in the body—necessary to prevent vitamin $B_{12}$ deficiency |
| Large intestine (cecum; appendix; ascending, transverse, descending, and sigmoid colon; rectum; anus) | Absorbs water and electrolytes Stores and eliminates indigestible material as feces |

Sources: Data from JC Scanlon, T Sanders (eds). Essentials of Anatomy and Physiology (2nd ed). Philadelphia: FA Davis, 1993;362; and AC Guyton, JE Hall (eds). Textbook of Medical Physiology (9th ed). Philadelphia: Saunders, 1996;803–844.

**Table 8-3.**  Structure and Function of the Accessory Organs of Digestion

| Structure | Function |
|---|---|
| Teeth | Break down food to combine with saliva. |
| Tongue | Provides taste sensations by cranial nerve VII (taste). Keeps the food between the teeth to maintain efficient chewing action for food to mix with saliva. |
| Salivary glands | Produce saliva, which is necessary to dissolve food for tasting and moistens food for swallowing. |
| Liver | Regulates serum levels of fats, proteins, and carbohydrates. Bile is produced in the liver and is necessary for the absorption of lipids and lipid-soluble substances. The liver also assists with drug metabolism and red blood cell and vitamin K production. |
| Gallbladder | Stores and releases bile into the duodenum via the hepatic duct when food enters the stomach. |
| Pancreas | Exocrine portion secretes bicarbonate and digestive enzymes into duodenum. Endocrine portion secretes insulin, glucagons, and numerous other hormones into the bloodstream, all of which are essential in regulating blood glucose levels. |
| Spleen* | Filters out foreign substances and degenerates blood cells from the bloodstream. Also stores lymphocytes. |

*The spleen is not part of the gastrointestinal system but is located near other gastrointestinal components in the abdominal cavity.
Sources: Data from JC Scanlon, T Sanders. Essentials of Anatomy and Physiology (2nd ed). Philadelphia: FA Davis, 1993; and AC Guyton, JE Hall. Textbook of Medical Physiology (9th ed). Philadelphia: Saunders, 1996;803–844.

## History

Before performing the physical examination, the presence or absence of items related to GI pathology is ascertained through patient interview, questionnaire completion, or chart review. For a list of these items, see Table 8-4. Appendix I-A also describes the general medical record review.

## Inspection

Figure 8-2 demonstrates the abdominal regions associated with organ location. During inspection, the physical therapist should note asymmetries in size and shape in each quadrant, umbilicus

Table 8-4. Items Associated with Gastrointestinal Pathology

| Signs and Symptoms | Stool and Urine Characteristics | Associated Disorders |
|---|---|---|
| Nausea and vomiting | Change in stool color | History of hernia |
| Hemoptysis | Change in urine color | History of hepatitis |
| Constipation | Hematochezia (bright | Drug and alcohol |
| Diarrhea | red blood in stool) | abuse |
| Jaundice | Melena (black, tarry | Fatty food intolerance |
| Heartburn | stools) | |
| Abdominal pain | | |

Sources: Data from MB Koopmeiners. Screening for Gastrointestinal System Disease. In WG Boisonnault (ed), Examination in Physical Therapy Practice. New York: Churchill Livingstone, 1991;113; and CC Goodman. The Gastrointestinal System. In CC Goodman, WG Boisonnault (eds), Pathology: Implications for the Physical Therapist. Philadelphia: Saunders, 1998;456–460.

appearance, and presence of abdominal scars indicative of previous abdominal procedures or trauma. The presence of incisions, tubes, and drains should also be noted during inspection, because these may require particular handling or placement during mobility exercises.[1]

| Right upper | Left upper |
|---|---|
| Liver | Stomach |
| Gallbladder | Spleen |
| Colon (hepatic flexure and transverse) | Pancreas |
| Kidney and adrenal gland | Kidney and adrenal gland |
| Duodenum with head of pancreas | Colon (splenic flexure and transverse) |
| Small intestine | Small intestine (jejunum) |

| Right lower | Left lower |
|---|---|
| Colon (ascending) | Colon (descending) |
| Cecum | Sigmoid colon |
| Appendix | |
| Small intestine | Small intestine |

Figure 8-2. The four abdominal quadrants, showing the viscera found in each. (With permission from N Palastanga, D Field, R Soames. Anatomy and Human Movement: Structure and Function [2nd ed]. Oxford, UK: Butterworth–Heinemann, 1989;783.)

## Clinical Tip

Changes in abdominal girth, especially enlargement, should be documented by the physical therapist. In addition, the nurses and physicians should be notified. Abdominal enlargement may hinder the patient's respiratory and mobility status.

### Auscultation

The abdomen is auscultated for the presence or absence of bowel sounds and bruits (murmurs) to help evaluate gastric motility and vascular flow, respectively. Bowel sounds can be altered postoperatively, as well as in cases of diarrhea, intestinal obstruction, paralytic ileus, and peritonitis. The presence of bruits may be indicative of renal artery stenosis.[1]

### Percussion

Mediate percussion is used to evaluate liver and spleen size and borders, as well as to identify ascitic fluid, solid- or fluid-filled masses, and air in the stomach and bowel.[1] The technique for mediate percussion is described in the physical examination section of Chapter 2.

### Palpation

Light palpation and deep palpation are used to identify abdominal tenderness, muscular resistance, and superficial organs and masses. The presence of rebound tenderness (i.e., abdominal pain worsened by a quick release of palpatory pressure) is an indication of peritoneal irritation from possible abdominal hemorrhage and requires immediate medical attention. Muscle guarding during palpation may also indicate a protective mechanism for underlying visceral pathology.[1]

## Diagnostic Studies

Discussion of the diagnostic evaluation for the GI system will be divided into (1) the examination of the GI tract and (2) the examination of the hepatic, biliary, pancreatic, and splenic systems. Examination of the GI tract includes the esophagus, stomach, and the intestines (small and large). Table 8-5 summarizes the laboratory tests

**Table 8-5.** Laboratory Tests for the Gastrointestinal System*

| Test | Description |
|---|---|
| Carcinoembryonic antigen (CEA)<br>Reference value:<br>Adult nonsmoker <2.5 ng/ml<br>Adult smoker: up to 5 ng/ml | Purpose: tumor marker used to monitor recurrence of colorectal cancer.<br>Venous blood is drawn periodically to monitor for increases above the reference range, indicating recurrence of colorectal cancer and presence of metastases. |
| D-Xylose absorption test (xylose tolerance test, xylose absorption test)<br>Reference value:<br>Urine<br>Adult (25-g dose) >4.5 g/5 hrs<br>Whole blood<br>Adult (25-g dose) >25 g/2 hrs | Purpose: investigate the cause of steatorrhea, to diagnose malabsorption syndrome, and to evaluate digestive ability of duodenum and jejunum.<br>A 25-g dose of D-Xylose (carbohydrate) mixed in 250 ml of water is ingested by the patient. Blood samples are drawn periodically in the next 2 hrs. All urine samples for the next 5 hrs are also measured.<br>Decreased levels of D-Xylose recovered in the blood or urine during those time periods could indicate malabsorption. |
| Gastric stimulation test (tube gastric analysis, pentagastrin stimulation test, gastric acid stimulation test)<br>Reference value: gastric pH 1.5–3.5<br>Basal acid output:<br>Male, 0–10.5 mEq/hr; female, 0–5.6 mEq/hr<br>Peak acid output:<br>Male, 12–60 mEq/hr; female, 8–40 mEq/hr | Purpose: to evaluate the ability of the stomach to produce acid secretions in a resting state and after maximal stimulation.<br>Stomach acids are aspirated by a nasogastric tube during resting states (basal output) and after injection of pentagastrin to stimulate gastric acid stimulation (peak output).<br>Increased values can occur with duodenal ulcers and Zollinger-Ellison syndrome.<br>Decreased values can occur with gastric ulcers or cancer. |

Gastrin
Reference value: 25–90 pg/ml

Purpose: used to confirm the diagnosis of Zollinger-Ellison syndrome. Elevated levels of gastrin in venous blood occurs with Zollinger-Ellison syndrome.

*Helicobacter pylori* tests

Purpose: to confirm the diagnosis of *H. pylori* infection, which is the cause of most peptic ulcers and is a proven carcinogen for gastric carcinoma.

Serologic test
Reference value: immunoglobulin G negative

Purpose: identifies the presence of immunoglobulin G antibody to *H. pylori* in the blood.

Urea breath test
Reference value: negative

Purpose: identifies the presence of *H. pylori* in the stomach.

Tissue biopsy
Reference value: negative for *H. pylori*

Purpose: to visualize the *H. pylori* bacteria. A tissue biopsy is obtained during an endoscopy procedure and microscopically examined.

5-Hydroxyindoleacetic acid (5-HIAA)
Reference value: 1–9 mg/24 hrs

Purpose: used to diagnose carcinoid tumor and provide ongoing evaluation of tumor stability. 5-HIAA is a urinary metabolite of serotonin and is produced by most carcinoid tumors.

Lactose tolerance test (oral lactose tolerance test)
Reference value:
Blood glucose >30 mg/dl
Urine lactose 12–40 mg/dl in 24 hrs

Purpose: to identify lactose intolerance–lactase deficiency as a cause of abdominal cramps and diarrhea, as well as to help identify the cause of malabsorption syndrome. An oral dose of lactose is provided to a fasting patient, and serial blood and urine samples are measured. Minimal rise in blood glucose or urine lactose levels indicates lactose intolerance-lactase deficiency.

**Table 8-5.** *Continued*

| Test | Description |
| --- | --- |
| Occult blood (fecal occult blood test, FOBT, FOB)<br>Reference value: negative | Purpose: used as a screening tool for early diagnosis of bowel cancer.<br>Three stool specimens are collected and examined for the presence of occult (nonvisible) blood in the feces, which can be indicative of adenocarcinoma and premalignant polyps in the colon. |
| Serotonin (5-hydroxytryptamine)<br>Reference value: 50–200 ng/ml | Purpose: used to detect carcinoid tumor.<br>Venous blood levels of serotonin are measured, as carcinoid tumors secrete excess amounts of serotonin. |

*Text or abbreviations in parentheses signify synonyms to the test names.
Source: Data from LM Malarkey, ME McMorrow. Nurse's Manual of Laboratory Tests and Diagnostic Procedures. Philadelphia: Saunders, 2000;412–431.

used to measure functional aspects of secretion, digestion, absorption, and elimination within the GI tract.[2] Table 8-6 summarizes diagnostic procedures used to visualize the GI tract.

Examination of the hepatic (liver), biliary (gallbladder and cystic ducts), pancreatic, and splenic systems involves numerous laboratory tests and diagnostic procedures, which are often performed concurrently to fully delineate the etiology of a patient's clinical presentation. Because of the common location of these organs and shared access to the biliary tree, disease or dysfunction in one organ can often extend into the other organs.[3]

---

Clinical Tip

Laboratory tests used to examine the liver are frequently referred to as *liver function tests* or *LFTs*.

---

Hepatocellular injury results in cellular damage in the liver, which causes increased levels of the following enzymes: aspartate aminotransferase (previously called *serum glutamic-oxaloacetic transaminase*), alanine aminotransferase (previously called *serum glutamate pyruvate transaminase*), and lactate dehydrogenase.[4]

Hepatocellular dysfunction can be identified when bilirubin levels are elevated or when clotting times are increased (denoted by an increased prothrombin time). The liver produces clotting factors and, therefore, an increased prothrombin time implicates impaired production of coagulation factors.

*Cholestasis* is the impairment of bile flow from the liver to the duodenum and results in elevations of the following serum enzymes: alkaline phosphatase, aspartate transaminase (previously known as *γ-glutamine-oxaloacetic transaminase* or *γ-glutamyl transpeptidase*), and 5'-nucleotidase.[4]

Table 8-7 summarizes the laboratory tests performed to measure hepatic, biliary, and pancreatic function, whereas Table 8-8 summarizes the diagnostic procedures performed to visualize these organs.

Additional diagnostic procedures used to evaluate the GI system are laparoscopy, magnetic resonance imaging (MRI), and positron emission tomography (PET) scans. These methods are described in the following sections.

**Table 8-6.** Diagnostic Procedures for the Gastrointestinal (GI) System*

| Test | Description |
| --- | --- |
| Barium enema (BE) Reference value: No lesions, deficits, or abnormalities of the colon are noted. | Purpose: To investigate and identify pathologic conditions that change the structure or function of the colon (large bowel). The colon is emptied of feces, and contrast medium (barium) is instilled rectally. Fluoroscopic and x-ray images are then taken to identify the presence of any structural anomalies. |
| Barium swallow (esophagography) Reference value: No structural or functional abnormalities are visualized. | Purpose: To identify pathologic conditions that change the structure or function of the esophagus. The patient takes repeated swallows of barium liquid while x-ray and fluoroscopic images are taken in vertical, semivertical, and horizontal positions to examine the passage of contrast medium during swallowing and peristaltic movement of the esophagus. |
| Colonoscopy (lower panendoscopy) Reference value: No abnormalities of structure or mucosal surface are visualized in the colon or terminal ileum. | Purpose: To perform routine screening of the colon for the presence of polyps or tumors and to investigate the cause of chronic diarrhea or other undiagnosed GI complaints. Patients are sedated, and an endoscope is inserted into the rectum and passed through the various parts of the colon. Tissue biopsy may be performed during this procedure. |
| Computed tomography of the GI tract (CT scan, computerized axial tomography [CAT]) | Purpose: Used to detect intra-abdominal abscesses, tumors, infarctions, perforation, obstruction, inflammation, and diverticulitis. Metastases to the abdominal cavity can also be detected. Intravenous or oral contrast may be used during the procedure. |

Esophageal manometry
Reference value: Lower esophageal sphincter (LES) pressure: 12–25 mm Hg.

Purpose: To evaluate esophageal motor disorders that could be causing dysphagia along with evaluating postoperative outcomes of esophageal surgery. LES pressures are measured with an endoscope that is inserted into the esophagus either nasally or orally.

Esophageal acidity test (Tuttle test)
Reference value: Esophageal pH of 6 or higher.

Purpose: To document gastroesophageal reflux or evaluate the outcomes of medical-surgical antireflux management. The pH of the esophagus is measured with an endoscope.

Acid perfusion test (Bernstein test)
Reference value: Negative.

Purpose: To determine that heartburn is of esophageal rather than cardiac origin. N. hydrochloric acid is instilled into the esophagus through the endoscope. Complaints of heartburn with acid instillation confirm the esophageal origin.

Esophagogastroduodenoscopy (EGD, upper gastrointestinal endoscopy)
Reference value: No abnormal structures or functions are observed in the esophagus, stomach, or duodenum.

Purpose: To identify and biopsy tissue abnormality, to determine the location and cause of upper GI bleeding, to evaluate the healing of gastric ulcers, to evaluate the stomach and duodenum after gastric surgery, and to investigate the cause of dysphagia, dyspepsia, gastric outlet obstruction, or epigastric pain.
An endoscope is passed through the mouth into the esophagus to the stomach, pylorus, and upper duodenum. Tissue biopsy can be performed during the procedure.

Gallium scan (gallium 67 imaging, total body scan)
Reference value: No structural or functional abnormalities are visualized.

Purpose: To locate malignancy, metastases, sites of inflammation, infection, and abscess.
A radionuclide is injected intravenously with images taken in the following time frames:

4–6 hrs later to identify infectious or inflammatory disease
24 hrs later to identify tumors
72 hrs later to identify infectious disease

**Table 8-6.** *Continued*

| Test | Description |
|------|-------------|
| Gastric emptying scan<br>Reference value: No delay in gastric emptying. | Purpose: To investigate the cause of a rapid or slow rate of gastric emptying and to evaluate the effects of treatment for abnormal gastric motility.<br>In a sitting position, the patient ingests a radionuclide mixed with food substances, and images are taken of the stomach and duodenum for the next 3 hrs (15-min intervals). The rate of gastric emptying is then calculated from the images. |
| Gastroesophageal reflux scan (GE reflux scan)<br>Reference value: Reflux is 3% or less. | Purpose: To measure the amount of gastroesophageal reflux.<br>The patient ingests radionuclide-labeled juice in the supine position while wearing an inflatable abdominal binder. Wearing the binder in supine is used to provoke reflux. Amount of reflux is calculated from the images taken during the study. |
| GI bleeding scan (GI scintigraphy)<br>Reference value: No evidence of focal bleeding. | Purpose: To evaluate the presence, source, or both, of GI bleeding.<br>Radionuclide-labeled red blood cells are injected intravenously, followed by intermittent imaging studies of the abdomen and pelvis for up to 24 hrs. |
| GI cytologic studies<br>Reference value: No evidence of abnormal cells or infectious organisms. | Purpose: To identify benign or malignant growth from tissue biopsy of the GI tract.<br>Tissue specimens are obtained during an endoscopic examination. |
| Paracentesis and peritoneal fluid analysis (abdominal paracentesis, abdominal tap)<br>Reference value: Clear, odorless, pale yellow. | Purpose: To help delineate the cause of ascites or suspected bowel perforation along with evaluating the effects of blunt abdominal trauma.<br>The peritoneal cavity is accessed with either a long thin needle or a trocar and stylet with the patient under local anesthesia. Peritoneal fluid is collected and examined.<br>Peritoneal tissue biopsy can also be performed during this procedure for cytologic studies required for the differential diagnosis of tuberculosis, fungal infection, and metastatic carcinoma. |

Roentgenography of the abdomen (abdominal flat plate)
Reference value: No abnormalities visualized.

Sigmoidoscopy and anoscopy
Reference value: No tissue abnormalities are visualized in the sigmoid colon, rectum, or anus.

Upper GI series and small bowel series (small bowel follow-through)
Reference value: No structural or functional abnormalities are found.

Purpose: To provide information about tumors, swelling of the mucosa, abscess formation, fluid in the intestinal lumen, intestinal obstruction, and calcifications in the GI tract. Plain x-ray is taken of the abdomen.

Purpose: Sigmoidoscopy is used as a screening tool for colon cancer and to investigate the cause of rectal bleeding or monitor inflammatory bowel disease. Anoscopy is used to investigate bleeding, pain, discomfort, or prolapse in the anus.

Purpose: Detects disorders of structure or function of the esophagus, stomach and duodenum, and jejunum and ileum (the latter two are for the small bowel series).

Imaging studies of all these areas are performed while the patient drinks a barium solution. Passage of the barium through these structures can range from 30 mins to 6 hrs.

*Text or abbreviations in parentheses signify synonyms to the test names.
Source: Data from LM Malarkey, ME McMorrow (eds). Nurse's Manual of Laboratory Tests and Diagnostic Procedures. Philadelphia: Saunders, 2000;432–468.

**Table 8-7.** Laboratory Tests for the Hepatic, Biliary, and Pancreatic Systems*

| Test | Involved Systems | Purpose |
| --- | --- | --- |
| Alanine aminotransferase (ALT, glutamic-pyruvic transaminase [GPT], SGPT, transaminase)<br>Reference value: 10–35 IU/liter | Hepatic | Used to detect hepatocellular injury.<br>Very specific in detecting acute hepatitis from viral, toxic, or drug-induced causes. |
| Alkaline phosphatase (ALP, total alkaline phosphatase [T-ALP])<br>Reference value: 4.5–13.0 King–Armstrong units/dl | Hepatic, biliary | Nonspecific indicator of liver disease, bone disease, or hyperparathyroidism.<br>Nonspecific tumor marker for liver or bone malignancy. |
| Alkaline phosphatase isoenzymes (I-ALP)<br>Reference value: liver isoenzymes 50–70% | Hepatic, biliary | Used to distinguish between liver and bone pathology when total serum ALP is elevated.<br>There are ALP isoenzymes for both liver and bone. |
| Alpha 1-fetoprotein (AFP1)<br>Reference value: <10 ng/ml | Hepatic, biliary | A tumor marker for hepatocellular carcinoma in nonpregnant adults.<br>AFP normally exists during pregnancy; otherwise, levels are very low. |
| Ammonia (NH$_3$)<br>Reference value: 15–45 µg/dl | Hepatic | To evaluate or monitor liver failure, hepatoencephalopathy, and the effects of impaired portal vein circulation.<br>Ammonia is a by-product of protein metabolism and is converted to urea in the liver. |
| Amylase, serum<br>Reference value: 27–131 U/liter | Pancreatic | Assists in the diagnosis of acute pancreatitis and traumatic injury to the pancreas or as surgical complication of the pancreas. |

| | | |
|---|---|---|
| Amylase, urine<br>Reference values:<br>2–19 U/hr (1-hr test)<br>4–37 U/2 hrs (2-hr test)<br>170–2,000 U/24 hrs (24-hr test) | Pancreatic | Helps to confirm diagnosis of acute pancreatitis when serum amylase levels are normal or borderline elevated. |
| Aspartate aminotransferase (AST, glutamate oxaloacetate transaminase [GOT], SGOT, transaminase)<br>Reference value: 8–20 U/liter | Hepatic | Primarily indicates inflammation, injury, or necrosis of the liver.<br>AST is highly concentrated in the liver, but it is also minimally present in skeletal muscle, kidney, brain, pancreas, spleen, and lungs. |
| Bilirubin<br>Reference values:<br>Total, 0.3–1.2 mg/dl<br>Direct (conjugated), 0–0.2 mg/dl<br>Indirect (unconjugated), <1.1 mg/dl | Hepatic, biliary | Used to evaluate liver function, diagnose jaundice, and monitor progression of jaundice.<br>*Total bilirubin* is the sum of direct and indirect bilirubin.<br>Elevation in direct (conjugated) bilirubin indicates hepatic jaundice, whereas elevation in indirect (unconjugated) bilirubin indicates prehepatic jaundice. |
| Carbohydrate antigen 19-9 (CA 19-9)<br>Reference value: <37 U/ml | Hepatic, pancreatic | A tumor marker used in the preoperative staging of pancreatic cancer.<br>Hepatic cirrhosis can falsely elevate this value in the absence of pancreatic cancer. |

**Table 8-7.** *Continued*

| Test | Involved Systems | Purpose |
|---|---|---|
| Ceruloplasmin<br>Reference value: 18–45 mg/dl | Hepatic | Used to evaluate chronic active hepatitis, cirrhosis, and other liver diseases. |
| Fecal fat (fecal lipids, quantitative fat, 72-hr stool collection, quantitative stool fat)<br>Reference value: <7 g/24 hrs | Hepatic, biliary | The definitive test to identify steatorrhea (high levels of fat in the feces). This can be caused by hepatobiliary, pancreatic, and small intestine disease. |
| Gamma-glutamyltransferase ($\gamma$-glutamyl-transferase [GT], $\gamma$-glutamyl-transpeptidase [GGT, GGTP, GTP])<br>Reference values:<br>Male, 22.1 U/liter<br>Female, 15.4 U/liter | Hepatic, biliary, pancreatic | Used to detect hepatobiliary disease.<br>Levels will rise with posthepatic jaundice and other diseases of the liver and pancreas. |
| Hepatitis virus tests<br>Reference value: negative (no presence of antibodies) | Hepatic | Distinguishes between the six types of viral hepatitis (HAV, HBV, HCV, HDV, HEV, HGV).<br>Presence of distinct antibodies for a specific virus will help confirm the diagnosis and assist with treatment planning. |
| Lactate dehydrogenase (LDH)<br>Reference value: 200–400 U/liter | Hepatic | Can assist in the diagnosis of hepatitis, cirrhosis, congestion of the liver, and hepatic anoxia. However, this is a costly test to perform and not a routine portion of liver function tests. |

| Test | System | Description |
|---|---|---|
| Leucine aminopeptidase (LAP)<br>Reference value: 55.2 U/liter | Hepatic, biliary, pancreatic | Used to detect hepatobiliary disease and biliary obstruction and to assist in differentiating between hepatobiliary and bone diseases. |
| Lipase<br>Reference value: <200 U/liter | Biliary, pancreatic | Used to diagnose pancreatitis and pancreatic disease.<br>Lipase is a digestive enzyme used to digest fatty acids. |
| 5'-Nucleotidase (5'N, 5'-NT)<br>Reference value: 2–17 IU/liter | Hepatic, biliary, pancreatic | Elevated levels help to identify extrahepatic or intrahepatic biliary obstruction and cancer of the liver. |
| Protein electrophoresis<br>Reference value: albumin, 3.5–5.0 g/dl | Hepatic | Separates plasma proteins (albumin and globulins) from the plasma to detect the specific amounts of each protein type.<br>Decreased plasma protein levels are indicative of hepatobiliary disease. |
| Serum proteins (albumin)<br>Reference value: 3.5–5.0 g/dl | Hepatic | Provides general information about the nutritional status, the oncotic pressure of the blood, and the losses of protein associated with liver, renal, skin, or intestinal diseases. |
| Prothrombin time (PT, protime)<br>Reference value: 10–13 secs | Hepatic | Elevated values are indicative of liver disease, as the liver synthesizes clotting factors II, VII, IX and X. |
| Sweat test (sweat chloride, cystic fibrosis sweat test, iontophoresis sweat test)<br>Reference value: 5–40 mEq/liter | Pancreatic | Used to diagnose cystic fibrosis in children, as these children have higher contents of sodium and chloride in their sweat. |

**Table 8-7.** *Continued*

| Test | Involved Systems | Purpose |
|---|---|---|
| Trypsinogen, immunoreactive assay (IRT, immunoreactive trypsin assay)<br>Reference value: <80 µg/liter | Pancreatic | Screening test for cystic fibrosis in newborns of less than 1 mo of age.<br>Elevated levels may indicate presence of disease, but the test has a high false-positive rate; therefore, universal screening with this test is not mandated nationally. |
| Urobilinogen, fecal<br>Reference value: 40–280 mg/day | Hepatic, biliary | Used to confirm the diagnosis of liver disease or biliary tract obstruction as well as identifying disorders of erythrocytes. |
| Urobilinogen, urine<br>Reference value:<br>  Male, 0.3–2.1 mg/2 hrs<br>  Female, 0.1–1.1 mg/2 hrs | Hepatic, biliary | Used to screen for evidence of hemolytic anemia or as an early indicator of liver cell damage. |

*Text or abbreviation in parentheses signifies synonyms to the test names.
Source: Data from LM Malarkey, ME McMorrow (eds). Nurse's Manual of Laboratory Tests and Diagnostic Procedures. Philadelphia: Saunders, 2000;469–524.

**Table 8-8.** Diagnostic Procedure for the Hepatic, Biliary, Pancreatic, and Splenic Systems

| Test | Purpose |
|---|---|
| Cholangiography, percutaneous transhepatic | Visualizes the anatomic structure of intrahepatic and extrahepatic ducts. Evaluates changes in the biliary tree and helps to diagnose causes of obstructive jaundice. Contrast material is injected into the biliary ducts percutaneously. |
| Cholangiography, T-tube, and intravenous | Visualizes the biliary ductal system to help identify stones and other causes of biliary obstruction. Very common after liver transplantation. Contrast material is injected into the biliary ducts intravenously. |
| Cholecystography, oral | Visualizes the gallbladder and biliary ductal system to identify causes of biliary obstruction. Contrast material is ingested, in pill form, by the patient. |
| Computed tomography (CT) of the liver, biliary tract, pancreas, and spleen | Used to identify the presence of tumor, abscess, cyst, sites of bleeding, or hematoma in these organs. Contrast medium may be used with CT scan of the liver and pancreas. |
| Endoscopic retrograde cholangiopancreatography and pancreatic cytology (ECRP)* | Used to investigate the cause of obstructive jaundice, persistent abdominal pain, or both. Generally identifies stones in the common bile duct as well as chronic pancreatitis and cancer. |
| Liver biliary scan | A radionuclide is injected intravenously, and imaging of the hepatobiliary system, gallbladder, and biliary tree is performed to help diagnose acute or chronic biliary tract disorder. |
| Liver biliary biopsy, percutaneous | Used to diagnose pathologic changes in the liver and monitor disease progression. |
| Liver-spleen scan | A radionuclide is injected intravenously, and imaging of the liver and spleen is performed. Used to confirm and evaluate suspected hepatocellular disease and enlargement of the liver or spleen. |

Table 8-8. *Continued*

| Test | Purpose |
| --- | --- |
| Ultrasound of the liver, biliary tract, pancreas and spleen | Primary diagnostic tool for examining the liver, spleen, and pancreas. Cyst, abscess, hematoma, primary neoplasm, and metastatic disease can be detected in the liver. It is the best diagnostic tool to identify gallstones. Pancreatic abscesses and tumors can also be identified. |

*Text or abbreviation in parentheses signifies synonyms to the test names.
Source: Data from LM Malarkey, ME McMorrow (eds). Nurse's Manual of Laboratory Tests and Diagnostic Procedures. Philadelphia: Saunders, 2000;524–549.

### Laparoscopy

*Laparoscopy* is the insertion of a laparoscope (a fiberoptic tube) into the abdominal cavity through a small incision to the left of and above the umbilicus. To perform this procedure, a local anesthetic is given, and gas (i.e., nitric oxide or carbon dioxide) is infused into the abdominal cavity to allow better visualization and manipulation of the scope. Table 8-9 describes the diagnostic and therapeutic interventions that may be performed with a laparoscope.[5,6]

### Magnetic Resonance Imaging

The use of MRI of the GI system is primarily indicated for imaging of the liver for hepatic tumors, iron overload, and hepatic and portal venous occlusion. Otherwise, computed tomography scans are preferred for the visualization of other abdominal organs.[7,8] Good success, however, has been reported recently in using MRI for defining tissue borders for managing and resecting colorectal tumors.[9] MRI has also been successful in helping to delineate the etiology of cirrhosis between alcohol abuse and viral hepatitis.[10]

### Positron Emission Tomography

PET is the use of positively charged ions to create color images of organs and their functions. Clinical uses of PET for the GI system include evaluation of liver disease, pancreatic function, and GI cancer.[7]

**Table 8-9.** Laparoscopic Utilization

---

Diagnostic
  Direct visualization
    Define and examine locations of intra-abdominal hemorrhage after blunt
    trauma
  Tissue biopsy
    Hepatic disease, staging of Hodgkin's disease and non-Hodgkin's lym-
    phoma, metastatic disease, tuberculosis
  Fluid aspiration
    Determination of the etiology of ascites (free fluid in the peritoneal cavity)
    Evaluation of patients with fever of unknown origin
    Evaluation of patients with chronic or intermittent abdominal pain
Therapeutic
  Aspiration of cysts and abscesses
  Lysis of adhesions
  Ligation of fallopian tubes
  Ablation of endometriosis or cancer by laser
  Cholecystectomy (gallbladder removal)
  Appendectomy
  Inguinal herniorrhaphy (hernia repair)
  Gastrectomy
  Colectomy
  Vagotomy

---

Sources: Data from GL Eastwood, C Avunduk (eds). Manual of Gastroenterology (2nd ed). Boston: Little Brown, 1994;27; and LM Malarkey, ME McMorrow (eds). Nurse's Manual of Laboratory Tests and Diagnostic Procedures. Philadelphia: Saunders, 2000;537–540.

## Pathophysiology

GI disorders can be classified regionally by the structure involved and may consist of the following:

- Motility disorders
- Inflammation or hemorrhage
- Enzymatic dysfunction
- Neoplasms

**Table 8-10.** Classification and Common Etiologies of Dysphagia

| Classification | Common Etiologies |
| --- | --- |
| Obstructive | Benign or malignant (squamous cell carcinoma or adenoma) neoplasms, cervical osteophyte or bone spur. Esophageal diverticula, rings, and webs are anatomic abnormalities that disrupt the normal cylindrical shape of the esophagus. Webs and diverticula tend to occur proximally, whereas rings generally occur distally at the gastroesophageal junction. |
| Inflammatory or infectious | Tonsillitis, pharyngitis, epiglottitis, esophagitis, gastroesophageal reflux disease. *Candida* or herpes viruses (herpes simplex, cytomegalovirus) are causative agents in chronically debilitated or immunocompromised patients. |
| Neurologic | Stroke, parkinsonism, amyotrophic lateral sclerosis, multiple sclerosis, myasthenia gravis. |
| Congenital | Tracheoesophageal fistula, esophageal compression by anomalous artery. |

Sources: Data from BJ Bailey. Dysphagia: uncovering the cause when your patient has trouble swallowing. Consultant 1997;37(1):75; TP Gage. Esophageal Rings, Webs, and Diverticula. In MM van Ness, SJ Chobanian (eds), Manual of Clinical Problems in Gastroenterology. Boston: Little, Brown, 1994;32; and SS Shay, MM van Ness. Infectious Esophagitis. In MM van Ness, SJ Chobanian (eds), Manual of Clinical Problems in Gastroenterology. Boston: Little, Brown, 1994;35.

## Esophageal Disorders

### Dysphagia

*Dysphagia*, or difficulty swallowing, can occur from various etiologies and is generally classified by the causative factors (Table 8-10). Dysphagia can also be classified by its location as (1) proximal (cervical) or oropharyngeal dysphagia or (2) distal or esophageal dysphagia.

*Proximal dysphagia* is difficulty swallowing in the upper, or proximal, region of the esophagus and generally results from neurologic or neuromuscular etiologies, such as stroke, myasthenia gravis, or polymyositis.[11–13]

*Distal dysphagia* is difficulty swallowing in the lower, or distal, portion of the esophagus and is usually the result of mechanical obstruction to flow from peptic strictures, mucosal rings, or malignant neoplasms, such as squamous cell carcinoma and adenocarcinoma of the esophagus.[11-13]

Dysphagia can also be characterized by (1) whether it occurs with ingestion of solids, liquids, or both; (2) whether it is accompanied by chest pain or heartburn; (3) whether it is intermittent, constant, or progressive; and (4) whether the patient complains of regurgitation or coughing while eating. The location at which the food becomes stuck should also be noted.[11,12]

### Motility Disorders and Angina-Like Chest Pain

Poor esophageal motility from smooth muscle spasms or abnormal contraction patterns can present as anterior chest pain and mimic anginal symptoms. Systematic cardiac and GI work-up should establish the differential diagnosis. The following are common esophageal motility disorders[14]:

*Achalasia* is a neuromuscular disorder of esophageal motility characterized by esophageal dilation and hypertrophy, along with failure of the lower esophageal sphincter to relax after swallowing. A functional obstruction then results from elevated sphincter pressure. A definitive etiology is currently unknown. Suspected causes include autoimmune dysfunction and genetic predisposition. Clinical manifestations can include episodes of regurgitation, chest pain while eating, and possible aspiration pneumonia.[12,15,16]

*Diffuse esophageal spasm* is characterized by the occurrence of normal peristalsis in the upper one-third of the esophagus and intermittent nonperistaltic, simultaneous contractions of the body of the esophagus. Clinical manifestations include intermittent chest pain with or without eating. Patients will also demonstrate a characteristic "cork-screw" pattern on barium-swallow studies. The etiology is unknown, and management is directed at smooth muscle relaxation with pharmacologic agents.[12,14,15]

### Gastroesophageal Reflux Disease

*Gastroesophageal reflux disease* (GERD) is characterized by gastric acid backflow into the esophagus as a result of improper lower esophageal sphincter relaxation. Clinical manifestations include complaints of heartburn (especially with sour or bitter regurgitation), nausea, gagging, cough, or hoarseness. Although the exact etiology of GERD is unknown, smoking, along with the consumption of fats, alcohol, coffee, or chocolate, has been associated with this inappropriate relaxation. Esophageal and gastric motility disorders may also contribute to GERD. Gastroesophageal reflux is a strong predisposing factor for developing esophageal adenocarcinoma. Depending on the severity of GERD, treatment can range from either dietary modifications (avoid risk factors and eat small, frequent meals in an upright position), antacids, antisecretory agents, or surgery.[12,17,18] However, surgical intervention has not shown positive results in relieving symptoms of GERD.[19]

### Barrett's Esophagus

Barrett's esophagus is a disorder in which columnar epithelium replaces the normal stratified squamous mucosa of the distal esophagus and is generally associated with chronic GERD. The mechanism of cellular metaplasia is thought to occur from chronic inflammatory injury from acid and pepsin that refluxes from the stomach into the distal esophagus.[20] Barrett's esophagus is also a strong predisposing factor for developing esophageal adenocarcinoma, the incidence of which has risen in the 1990s.[19,21]

Associated signs and symptoms include dysphagia, esophagitis, ulceration, perforations, strictures, bleeding, or adenocarcinoma.[22] Treatment for Barrett's esophagus includes controlling symptoms of GERD and promising new therapies that include endoscopic ablation therapy combined with proton pump inhibition (for acid secretion control). Ablation therapy includes such techniques as photodynamic therapy, multipolar polar electrocautery, laser therapy, and, most recently, argon plasma coagulation.[20]

### Esophageal Varices

*Varices* are dilated blood vessels in the esophagus caused by portal hypertension and may result in hemorrhage that necessitates immediate medical and, usually, surgical management. Alcohol abuse is an associated risk factor.[23] Refer to Cirrhosis later in this chapter for more information on portal hypertension and alcoholic cirrhosis.

### Esophageal Cancer

A description of esophageal cancers with respect to evaluation and management can be found in Cancers in the Body Systems in Chapter 5.

---

### Clinical Tip

Physical therapists should be aware of any positioning precautions for patients with esophageal disorders that may exacerbate their dysphagia or GERD.

---

## Stomach Disorders

### Gastrointestinal Hemorrhage

Bleeding in the GI system can occur in either the upper GI system (upper gastrointestinal bleed [UGIB]) or in the lower GI system (lower gastrointestinal bleed [LGIB]). A UGIB can result from one or more of the following: (1) duodenal ulcers, (2) gastric erosion, (3) gastric ulcers, (4) esophageal varices, and (5) use of nonsteroidal anti-inflammatory drug medications (NSAIDs). An LGIB can result from one or more of the following: (1) inflammatory bowel disease, (2) neoplasms, and (3) anal and rectal lesions (e.g., hemorrhoids).[24–26]

GI bleeds can be small and require minimal to no intervention or very severe and constitute medical emergencies because of hemodynamic instability that can lead to shock. *Hematemesis* or dark brown ("coffee-ground") emesis (vomitus), *hematochezia* (passage of blood from the rectum), and *melena* (black, tarry stools) from acid degradation of hemoglobin are the primary clinical manifestations of GI bleeds.

Patients are generally stabilized hemodynamically with intravenous (i.v.) fluids, blood transfusions, or both before the cause of bleeding can be fully delineated. Nasogastric tubes (see Appendix Table III-A.6) are typically used in the stabilization and management of UGIB. Management is targeted at the causative factors that resulted in either UGIB or LGIB. Endoscopy, colonoscopy, or sigmoidoscopy can be performed to help evaluate or treat the source of upper or lower GI hemorrhage.[24,25,27]

### Gastritis

*Gastritis* is the general term used to describe diffuse inflammatory lesions in the mucosal layer of the stomach. Gastritis can be classified as acute, chronic nonerosive, or chronic erosive.

Etiology of *acute gastritis* includes associations with smoking, alcohol abuse, aspirin, NSAIDs, and corticosteroid use, as well as physiologic stress and intense emotional reactions. Clinical manifestations of acute gastritis include nondescript complaints of burning or discomfort in the stomach. Management of acute gastritis involves removing the causative risk factors and relieving the mucosal inflammation.[15,28,29]

The etiology of *chronic nonerosive gastritis* has been definitively linked to *Helicobacter pylori* bacterial infection, which is thought to be transmitted by human-to-human contact.[15,28,30,31] Patients with *H. pylori* gastritis may be asymptomatic until the gastritis leads to gastric ulceration, in which case there will be complaints of dull, gnawing abdominal pain that typically occurs when the stomach is empty.[28] Management of *H. pylori* gastritis includes triple or quadruple antibiotic therapies, in combination with antacid medication, to eradicate the bacterial infection. The primary antibiotics used include metronidazole (Flagyl, Protostat) and clarithromycin (Biaxin) and amoxicillin. Antacid medication can include any one of the following: omeprazole (Prilosec), lansoprazole (Prevacid), and rabeprazole (Aciphex), which is a newer proton pump inhibitor.[28,30,31]

The etiology of chronic erosive gastritis includes NSAIDs and alcohol abuse. Clinical manifestations can range from being asymptomatic to having anorexia nervosa, gastric pain, nausea, and vomiting. Management of chronic erosive gastritis involves removing the causative risk factors and, possibly, antibiotic therapy similar to that used for *H. pylori* gastritis.[28]

### Peptic Ulcer Disease

A peptic ulcer is a loss of the mucosal surface through the muscularis mucosa of the esophagus, stomach, or duodenum that is at least 5 mm in diameter.[32] Peptic ulcers can be classified as acute or chronic. *Acute peptic ulcers* have lesions that involve the full thickness of the mucosa, whereas *chronic peptic ulcers* have lesions of varying depths. Peptic ulcers occur primarily in the stomach or the first part of the duodenum, or both.[15]

#### Gastric Ulcer

Ulceration in the stomach is characterized by a well-defined perforation in the gastric mucosa that extends into the muscularis mucosa.[33] Gastric ulcers are less common than duodenal ulcers; however, patients with gastric ulcers have the highest mortality rate among patients with peptic ulcer disease. Patients with gastric ulcers apparently have normal gastric acid secretion but have lowered defense mechanisms in the mucosal lining to protect against acid secretion. Other highly causative factors for gastric ulcer include *H. pylori* infection and use of NSAIDs.[32] However, high levels of physiologic and emotional stress cannot be ruled out as a contributing factor in the development of gastric ulcer formation.[34]

Symptoms of a gastric ulcer may include abdominal pain during or shortly after a meal, nausea with or without vomiting, or both. Management of gastric ulcers may consist of any or all of the following: modification or elimination of causative agents, antacids, and *H. pylori* therapies (see Gastritis).[32,33]

#### Duodenal Ulcer

*Duodenal ulcers* are more common than gastric ulcers and are defined as a chronic circumscribed break in the mucosa that extends through the muscularis mucosa layer and leaves a residual scar with healing. Duodenal ulcers are linked with gastric acid hypersecretion and genetic predisposition.[35] Other risk factors for developing duodenal ulcers include tobacco use, chronic renal failure, alcoholic cirrhosis, renal transplantation, hyperparathyroidism, and chronic obstructive pulmonary disease.

Clinical manifestations of duodenal ulcer disease may include sharp, burning, or gnawing epigastric pain that may be relieved with food or antacids. Abdominal pain can also occur at night. Management of duodenal ulcers is similar to that of gastric ulcers.[32,33]

### Zollinger-Ellison Syndrome

*Zollinger-Ellison syndrome* is a clinical triad that includes gastric acid hypersecretion, recurrent peptic ulcerations, and a non-beta islet cell tumor (gastrinoma) in the pancreas. Symptoms mimic peptic ulcer disease, but consequences are more severe if left untreated. Patients with Zollinger-Ellison syndrome may also present with diarrhea. Management is primarily directed at surgical resection of the gastrinoma, along with decreasing gastric acid hypersecretion.[32,36,37]

### Gastric Emptying Disorders

Abnormal gastric emptying is described as either decreased or increased emptying. Decreased gastric emptying is also referred to as *gastric retention* and may result from or be associated with (1) pyloric stenosis as a consequence of duodenal ulcers, (2) hyperglycemia, (3) diabetic ketoacidosis, (4) electrolyte imbalance, (5) autonomic neuropathy, (6) postoperative stasis, and (7) pernicious anemia. Pharmacologic intervention to promote gastric motility is indicated for patients with decreased gastric emptying disorders.

Enhanced gastric emptying is associated with an interruption of normal digestive sequencing that results from vagotomy, gastrectomy, or gastric or duodenal ulcers. Gastric peristalsis, mixing, and grinding are disturbed, resulting in rapid emptying of liquids, slow or increased emptying of solids, and prolonged retention of indigestible solids. With enhanced gastric emptying, blood glucose levels are subsequently low and can result in signs and symptoms of anxiety, sweating, intense hunger, dizziness, weakness, and palpitations. Nutritional and pharmacologic management are the usual treatment choices.[38]

### Gastric Cancer

The most common malignant neoplasms found in the stomach are adenocarcinomas, which arise from normal or mucosal cells. Benign tumors are rarely found but include leiomyomas and polyps. For a more detailed discussion of gastric oncology, see Cancers in the Body Systems in Chapter 5.

## Intestinal Disorders

### Appendicitis

Inflammation of the appendix of the large intestine can be classified as simple, gangrenous, or perforated. Simple appendicitis involves an inflamed but intact appendix. Gangrenous appendicitis is the presence of focal or extensive necrosis accompanied by microscopic perforations. Perforated appendicitis is a gross disruption of the appendix wall and can lead to serious complications if it is not managed promptly.[39] The etiology of appendicitis includes a combination of obstruction in the appendix lumen coupled with infection.[15]

Signs and symptoms of appendicitis may include the following[39,40]:

- Right lower quadrant, epigastric, or periumbilical abdominal pain that fluctuates in intensity

- Abdominal tenderness in the right lower quadrant

- Vomiting with presence of anorexia

- Constipation and failure to pass flatus

- Low-grade fever (no greater than 102°F or 39°C)

Management of appendicitis involves timely and accurate diagnosis of acute appendicitis to prevent perforation. Treatment choices include anti-infective agents or surgical appendectomy.[39–41]

### Diverticular Disease

*Diverticulosis* is the presence of *diverticula,* which is an outpocketing, or herniation, of the mucosa of the large colon through the muscle layers of the intestinal wall. *Diverticular disease* occurs when the outpocketing becomes symptomatic. *Diverticulitis* is the result of inflammation and localized peritonitis that occurs after the perforation of a single diverticulum.[15,39,40,42]

Signs and symptoms of diverticular disease include the following:

- Achy, left lower quadrant pain and tenderness (pain intensifies with acute diverticulitis)

- Pain referred to low back region

- Urinary frequency

- Distended and tympanic abdomen
- Fever and elevated white blood cell count (acute diverticulitis)
- Constipation, bloody stools, or both
- Nausea, vomiting, anorexia

Management of diverticular disease includes any of the following[39,40,43,44]:

- Dietary modifications (e.g., increased fiber)
- Insertion of nasogastric tube in cases of severe nausea, vomiting, abdominal distention, or any combination of these
- i.v. fluids
- Pain medications
- Anti-infective agents
- Surgical repair of herniation, resection (colectomy), or both with possible colostomy construction. Video laparoscopic techniques are becoming a more favored surgical approach for these procedures.[42]

## Hernia

### Abdominal Hernia

An abdominal hernia is an abnormal protrusion of bowel that is generally classified by the area where the protrusion occurs. These include the following areas: (1) epigastric, (2) inguinal, (3) femoral, (4) ventral or incisional hernia, and (5) umbilical. Muscle weakening from abdominal distention that occurs in obesity, surgery, or ascites can lead to herniation through the muscle wall. Herniation may also develop congenitally.[39,45]

Signs and symptoms of abdominal herniation include the following[39,45]:

- Abdominal distention, nausea, and vomiting
- Observable bulge with position changes, coughing, or laughing
- Pain of increasing severity with fever, tachycardia, and abdominal rigidity (if the herniated bowel is strangulated)

Management of herniation includes any of the following[39,45]:

- Wearing a binder or corset
- Herniorrhaphy (surgical repair, typically with a laparoscope)
- Hernioplasty (surgical reinforcement of weakened area with mesh, wire, or fascia)
- Temporary colostomy in cases of intestinal obstruction

### Hiatal Hernia

A hiatal hernia is an abnormal protrusion of the stomach upward through the esophageal hiatus of the diaphragm. Causative risk factors for a hiatal hernia are similar to those for abdominal hernia. Clinical manifestations include heartburn-like epigastric pain that usually occurs after eating and with recumbent positioning.

Management of hiatal hernia can include behavior modifications, such as avoiding reclining after meals, eating spicy or acidic foods, drinking alcohol, and smoking tobacco. Eating small, frequent, bland meals containing high fiber content may also be beneficial. Pharmacologic intervention typically includes acid-reducing medications.[45] In certain cases, when these measures have proven ineffective, surgical management of the hiatal hernia can be performed laparoscopically.[46]

---

### Clinical Tip

Positions associated with bronchopulmonary hygiene or functional mobility may exacerbate pain in patients who have a hernia, particularly a hiatal hernia. Therefore, careful modification of these interventions will be necessary for successful completion of these activities.

---

### Intestinal Obstructions

Failure of intestinal contents to propel forward can occur by mechanical or functional obstructions. Blockage of the bowel by adhesion, herniation, volvulus (twisting of bowel on itself), tumor, inflammation, impacted feces, or invagination of an adjacent bowel segment constitutes mechanical obstructions. Loss of the propulsive activity of the intestines leads to functional obstructions (*paralytic ileus*). Obstructions may result from abdominal surgery, intestinal distention, hypokalemia, peritonitis, severe trauma, spinal fractures, ureteral distention, or use of narcotics.[39,40]

Signs and symptoms of intestinal obstructions include the following[39,40]:

- Sudden onset of crampy abdominal pain that may be intermittent in nature as peristalsis occurs

- Abdominal distension

- Vomiting

- Obstipation (inability to pass gas or stool)

- Localized tenderness

- High-pitched or absent bowel sounds (depending on extent of obstruction)

- Tachycardia and hypotension in presence of dehydration or peritonitis

- Bloody stools

Management of intestinal obstructions includes any of the following[39,40]:

- Insertion of a nasogastric tube

- Supportive management of functional etiologies (as able)

- Surgical resection of mechanical obstructions from adhesions, necrosis, tumor, or unresolved inflammatory lesions, particularly if the obstruction is in the large intestine

- Colostomy placement and eventual colostomy closure (Colostomy closure is also referred to as *colostomy takedown*.)

**Intestinal Ischemia**

Ischemia within the intestinal tract, also called *ischemic colitis*, can be acute or chronic and result from many factors, such as thrombosis or emboli to the superior mesenteric artery, intestinal strangulation, chronic vascular insufficiency, hypotension, oral contraceptives, NSAIDs, and vasoconstrictors, such as vasopressin and dihydroergotamine. Methamphetamine and cocaine have vasoconstrictive properties that can also lead to intestinal ischemia. Significant ischemia that is not managed in a timely manner can lead to intestinal necrosis or gangrene and prove to be a life-threatening situation.[39,40,47] Signs and symptoms of intestinal ischemia include the following[39,40]:

- Abdominal pain ranging from colicky pain to a steady severe ache, depending on the severity of ischemia

- Nausea and vomiting

- Diarrhea or rectal bleeding

- Rebound tenderness, abdominal distention, and rigidity (with necrosis)

- Tachycardia, hypotension, and fever (with necrosis)

Management of intestinal ischemia includes any of the following[39,47]:

- Revascularization procedures, including balloon angioplasty, bypass grafting, embolectomy, and endarterectomy

- Resection of necrotic segments with temporary colostomy or ileostomy placement and subsequent reanastomosis of functional segments as indicated

- Anti-infective agents

- Vasodilators or vasopressors (blood perfusion enhancement)

- Anticoagulation therapy

- i.v. fluid replacement

- Insertion of nasogastric tube

- Analgesic agents

**Irritable Bowel Syndrome**
*Irritable bowel syndrome* (IBS), also referred to as *functional bowel disorder* or *spastic colon*, is characterized by inconsistent motility of the large bowel (i.e., constipation or diarrhea). Motility of the large bowel can be affected by emotions; certain foods, such as milk products; neurohumoral agents; GI hormones; toxins; prostaglandins; and colon distention.[39,40] Recent findings now suggest that patients with

IBS may have bacterial overgrowth in their small intestines and are being successfully managed with antibiotic therapy.[48]

Signs and symptoms of IBS include the following[39,40]:

- Diffuse abdominal pain, reports of feeling bloated, or both

- Constipation or diarrhea

- Correlation of GI symptoms with eating, high emotional states, or stress

- No weight loss

- Tender sigmoid colon on palpation

Management of IBS includes any of the following[39,40,49]:

- Laxatives or antidiarrheal (loperamide) agents

- Antispasmodic agents

- Dietary modifications, including a food diary to determine causative risk factors

- Counseling or psychotherapy

- Antibiotic therapy

- Surgery (in rare cases)

## Malabsorption Syndromes

*Malabsorption syndrome* is a general term for disorders that are characterized by the small or large intestine's failure to absorb or digest carbohydrates, proteins, fats, vitamins, and electrolytes. This syndrome is commonly associated with patients who have manifestations of acquired immunodeficiency disease. The nutritional deficits that result from malabsorption can lead to other chronic disorders, such as anemia or osteoporosis. Malabsorption syndromes can result from any of the following[39,50,51]:

- Chronic pancreatitis

- Pancreatic carcinoma

- Crohn's disease (see Crohn's Disease)

- Celiac sprue (small intestine mucosal damage from glutens [wheat, barley, rye, and oats])
- Amyloidosis (disorder of protein metabolism)
- Lactase deficiency
- Zollinger-Ellison syndrome (see Zollinger-Ellison Syndrome)
- Whipple's disease (infection of the small intestine by *Tropheryma whippelii* bacteria)

Signs and symptoms of malabsorption syndromes include the following:

- Diarrhea, steatorrhea (excessive fat excretion), or both
- Anorexia and weight loss
- Abdominal bloating
- Bone pain

Management of malabsorption syndromes includes any of the following[39,51]:

- Antibiotic therapy
- Dietary modifications and nutritional support
- Fluid, electrolyte, vitamin, and mineral support

**Peritonitis**
Peritonitis is general or localized inflammation in the peritoneal cavity as a result of bacterial or chemical contamination. Etiologies can include bacterial infection, ascites, perforation of the GI tract, gangrene of the bowel, trauma, and surgical irritants.[39,40,52]
Signs and symptoms of peritonitis include the following:

- Fever
- Abdominal guarding with diffuse tenderness and rigidity
- Abdominal distention
- Diminished or absent bowel sounds
- Nausea, vomiting, or both

- Pain with deep inspirations (therefore shallow and rapid respirations)

- Tachycardia, hypotension

- Decreased urinary output

Management of peritonitis includes any of the following[39,52,53]:

- Laparoscopic evaluation, with or without subsequent surgical correction of primary etiology

- Antibiotic therapy

- Fluid management with electrolytes and colloids

- Pain management

- Nasogastric suctioning

- Invasive monitoring of central hemodynamic pressures

**Crohn's Disease**
Crohn's disease is a chronic, idiopathic, inflammatory disorder occurring in any part of the GI system. The small intestine, particularly the ileum and the proximal portion of the colon, is most commonly involved, whereas the esophagus and stomach are rarely affected. Suspected causes of Crohn's disease include genetic predetermination, exaggerated immunologic mechanisms, infectious agents, psychological factors, dietary factors, and environmental factors.[39,54,55]

Signs and symptoms of Crohn's disease include the following:

- Constant crampy abdominal pain, often in right lower quadrant, not relieved by bowel movement

- Right lower quadrant abdominal mass

- Diarrhea

- Low-grade fever

- Fistula formation

Management of Crohn's disease includes any of the following[39,54–57]:

- Anti-inflammatory medications (corticosteroids or cytokines)

- Antibiotics

- i.v. fluids and dietary modification and support (possible total parenteral nutrition use)

- Nasogastric suctioning

- Activity limitations (in acute phases)

- Surgical resection, either by open laparotomy or video laparoscopy, of involved area, with or without need for ileostomy

Complications of Crohn's disease can include the following[39,54]:

- Intestinal obstruction, possibly leading to fistula, abscess, or perforations in the intestine

- Inflammation of eyes, skin, and mucous membranes

- Arthritis, ankylosing spondylitis

- Colon cancer

- Gallstones

- Vitamin $B_{12}$ deficiency

- Obstructive hydronephrosis

**Ulcerative Colitis**
Ulcerative colitis is a chronic inflammation of the intestine limited to the mucosal layer of the colon and rectum. The definitive etiology of ulcerative colitis is unknown, but suspected causes are similar to those of Crohn's disease. Inflammation can be mild, moderate, or severe.[39,54,55]

Signs and symptoms of ulcerative colitis include the following[39,54]:

- Crampy lower abdominal pain that is relieved by a bowel movement

- Small, frequent stools to profuse diarrhea (mild to severe)

- Rectal bleeding

- Fever

- Fatigue with anorexia and weight loss

- Dehydration
- Tachycardia

Management of ulcerative colitis includes any of the following[39,54,57]:

- Anti-inflammatory medications, including steroids and mesalamine suppositories
- Surgical resection of involved area with probable ileostomy placement or, more recently, the development of the double-stapled ileal reservoir and ileoanal anastomosis, called the *J pouch*, has been very effective and favored, as this repair keeps the entire anal canal intact and avoids an external bag.
- Dietary modification and support (possible total parenteral nutrition use)
- Activity limitations
- Iron supplements, blood replacement, or both
- Antidiarrheal agents

Related manifestations of ulcerative colitis may include the following[39,54]:

- Arthritis, ankylosing spondylitis
- Inflammation of the eyes, skin, and mucous membranes
- Hepatitis, bile duct carcinoma
- Colon cancer

## Polyps

GI polyps are usually adenomas that arise from the epithelium above the mucosal surface of the colon and rectum. Polyps are generally benign but have the potential to proliferate into carcinoma of the colon.[39,58]

Signs and symptoms of polyps include the following[39,58]:

- Rectal bleeding (occult or overt)
- Constipation or diarrhea

• Lower abdominal crampy pain

Management of polyps includes the following[39,58]:

• Modification of risk factors for colorectal cancer, such as obesity, smoking, and excessive alcohol consumption

• Colonoscopy, proctosigmoidoscopy, endoscopy, or barium enema for detection of the polyp

• Tissue biopsy to determine its malignancy potential

• Polypectomy with electrocautery

• Surgical resection, if indicated, with or without ileostomy

### Intestinal Tumors

Benign or metastatic neoplasms of the intestine include colonic adenomas (polyps), villous or papillary adenomas, lipomas, leiomyomas, and lymphoid hyperplasia. Tumors affect motility and absorption functions in the intestine (see Cancers in the Body Systems in Chapter 5 for further details).

### Anorectal Disorders

Disorders of the anus and rectum generally involve inflammation, obstruction, discontinuity from colon, perforations, or tumors. The most common disorders are (1) hemorrhoids, (2) anorectal fistula, (3) anal fissure, (4) imperforate anus, and (5) rectal prolapse. Signs and symptoms include pain with defecation and bloody stools. Management is supportive according to the disorder, and surgical correction is performed as necessary.

### Liver and Biliary Disorders

### Hepatitis

Hepatic inflammation and hepatic cell necrosis may be acute or chronic and may result from viruses, toxins, alcohol, leukemias, lymphomas, and Wilson's disease (a rare copper metabolism disorder). *Viral hepatitis* is the most common type of hepatitis and can be classified as hepatitis A, B, C, D, E, or G (i.e., HAV, HBV, HCV, HDV, HEV, and HGV, respectively).

Hepatitides A, B, and C are the most common types of viral hepatitis, whereas hepatitis G has recently been discovered. Hepatitis A is transmitted via the fecal-oral route, mostly from contaminated water sources. Hepatitis B is more common than hepatitis C, but both are transmitted through blood and body fluids. Acute viral hepatitis generally resolves with appropriate medical management, but in some cases, hepatitis can become chronic and may ultimately require liver transplantation.[39,59-61]

Signs and symptoms of hepatitis include the following[39,59-61]:

- Abrupt onset of malaise

- Fever

- Anorexia

- Nausea, abdominal discomfort, and pain

- Headache

- Jaundice

- Dark-colored urine

Management of hepatitis includes any of the following[39,59-61]:

- Adequate periods of rest

- Vaccinations (only for HAV, HBV, HDV)

- Fluid and nutritional support

- Removal of precipitating irritants (e.g., alcohol and toxins)

- Anti-inflammatory agents

- Antiviral agents

---

### Clinical Tip

- Health care workers who are exposed to blood and body fluids during patient contact must ensure that they are properly vaccinated against hepatitides B and C. This includes receiving periodic measurements of antibody titers to the viruses and supplementation with booster shots as needed to maintain appropriate immunity against these infections.

• The liver is the only organ in the body with regenerative properties; therefore, patients with acute liver inflammation will heal well if given the proper rest and medical treatment. Physical therapists should aim not to overfatigue these patients with functional activities to help promote proper healing of the liver.

### Cirrhosis

Cirrhosis is a chronic disease state that is characterized by hepatic parenchymal cell destruction and necrosis, and regeneration and scar tissue formation. The scarring and fibrosis that occur in the liver reduce its ability to synthesize plasma proteins (albumin), clotting factors, and bilirubin. The primary complications that can occur from cirrhosis include portal hypertension, ascites, jaundice, and impaired clotting ability.[39,52,61]

Cirrhosis may result from a variety of etiologies, including the following[39,61]:

• Alcohol or drug abuse

• Viral hepatitis B, C, or D

• Hemochromatosis

• Wilson's disease

• Alpha$_1$-antitrypsin deficiency

• Biliary obstruction

• Venous outflow obstruction

• Cardiac failure

• Malnutrition

• Cystic fibrosis

• Congenital syphilis

Signs and symptoms of cirrhosis include the following[39,52,61]:

- Recent weight loss or gain

- Fatigability

- Jaundice

- Lower-extremity edema

- Anorexia, nausea, or vomiting

- Fever

- Decreased urine output (urine dark yellow or amber)

- Associated GI manifestations of esophageal varices, bowel habit changes, and GI bleeding

- Altered mental status

Management of cirrhosis includes the following[39,61]:

- Supportive care, including i.v. fluids, whole blood and blood products, colloid (albumin), vitamin and electrolyte replacement, and dietary and behavioral modifications (eliminate alcohol consumption)

- Medical correction, surgical correction, or both of primary etiology or secondary complications as indicated

- Paracentesis

- Supplemental oxygen

- Liver transplantation (see Chapter 12)

### Hepatic Encephalopathy and Coma

Acute and chronic liver diseases, particularly cirrhosis, may lead to neuropsychiatric manifestations that may progress from hepatic encephalopathy to precoma to coma. The majority of neuropsychiatric manifestations are linked to ammonia intoxication from faulty liver metabolism.[39,52]

Signs and symptoms of hepatic encephalopathy that may progress to coma include the following:

- Altered states of consciousness (e.g., lethargy, stupor, confusion, slowed responses)

- Neuromuscular abnormalities (e.g., tremor, dyscoordination, slurred speech, altered reflexes, ataxia, rigidity, Babinski's sign, and impaired handwriting)

- Altered intellectual function (decreased attention span, amnesia, disorientation)

- Altered personality and behavioral changes (euphoria or depression, irritability, anxiety, paranoia, rage)

Management of hepatic encephalopathy and coma may consist of any of the following[39,52]:

- Administering nonabsorbable disaccharides, such as lactulose, is the mainstay of treatment

- Correction of fluid and electrolyte or acid-base imbalances, or both

- Supplemental oxygen

- Removal of any precipitating substances

- Gastric lavage or enemas

- Ammonia detoxicants

- Anti-infective agents

- Surgical correction of causal or contributing factors (rare)

---

Clinical Tip

Hepatic encephalopathy may also be referred to as *portal systemic encephalopathy* (PSE) because of the association between portal hypertension and cirrhosis in the development of encephalopathy.

---

### Cholecystitis with Cholelithiasis

*Cholecystitis* is acute or chronic inflammation of the gallbladder. It is associated with obstruction by gallstones in 90% of cases. Gallstone formation (cholelithiasis) is associated with three factors: gallbladder hypomobility, supersaturation of bile with cholesterol, and crystal formation from an increased concentration of insoluble bilirubin in the bile. Cholelithiasis can lead to secondary bacterial infection that further exacerbates the cholecystitis.[39,62]

Signs and symptoms of cholecystitis include the following[39,40,62]:

- Severe abdominal pain in right upper quadrant with possible pain referral to interscapular region
- Rebound tenderness and abdominal rigidity
- Jaundice
- Anorexia
- Nausea, vomiting, or both
- Fever

Management of cholecystitis includes any of the following[39,62]:

- Laparoscopic cholecystectomy or cholecystostomy (temporary drain placement in the gallbladder until obstruction is relieved)
- Gallstone dilution therapy with chenodeoxycholic and ursodeoxycholic acid
- Anti-infective agents
- Pain management
- i.v. fluids
- Insertion of nasogastric tube

## Pancreatic Disorders

### Pancreatitis

Inflammation of the pancreas can be acute or chronic. The incidence of acute pancreatitis is rising, and the clinical sequelae are potentially fatal, including adult respiratory distress syndrome (ARDS) and shock. This section therefore focuses on acute pancreatitis. *Acute pancreatitis* can be categorized as necrotizing or interstitial. Pancreatitis involves an exaggerated release and activity of pancreatic enzymes into the peritoneal cavity, along with autodigestion of pancreatic parenchyma. The exact trigger to this process is unknown, but the most common contributing factors are gallstones and alcohol and drug abuse.[39,63] Other contributing factors also include the following[39,63]:

- Trauma
- Endoscopic retrograde cholangiography (see Table 8-8)
- Metabolic disorders
- Vasculitis
- Pancreatic obstruction
- Penetrating peptic ulcer
- Genetic predisposition
- Renal failure
- Hepatitis
- Medications
- Postoperative sequelae from abdominal or cardiothoracic surgery

Signs and symptoms of acute pancreatitis include the following[63-65]:

- Steady, dull abdominal pain in the epigastrium, left upper quadrant or periumbilical area often radiating to back, chest, and lower abdomen. Pain can be exacerbated by food, alcohol, vomiting, and resting in the supine position.
- Nausea, vomiting, and abdominal distention
- Fever, tachycardia, and hypotension (in acute cases)
- Jaundice
- Abdominal tenderness or rigidity
- Diminished or absent bowel sounds
- Associated pulmonary manifestations, such as pleural effusions and pneumonitis
- Decreased urine output
- Weight loss

Management of acute pancreatitis includes any of the following[63–65]:

• Pain management, generally with narcotics, possibly through patient-controlled analgesia (See Appendix VI.)

• i.v. fluid and electrolyte replacement

• Elimination of oral food intake and providing alternative nutritional support, such as total parenteral nutrition

• Surgical correction or resection of obstructions

• Antacids

• Nasogastric suctioning

• Supplemental oxygen and mechanical ventilation (as indicated)

• Invasive monitoring (in more severe cases)

## Management

General management of GI disorders may consist of any of the following: pharmacologic therapy, nutritional support, dietary modifications, and surgical procedures. Nutritional support and dietary modifications are beyond the scope of this book. This section focuses on pharmacologic therapy and surgical procedures. A discussion of physical therapy intervention is also included.

### Pharmacologic Therapy

Medications used to treat GI disorders can be broadly categorized as (1) those that control gastric acid secretion and (2) those that normalize gastric motility. Refer to Appendix IV (Tables IV.19 A-B and IV.20 A-B) for an overview of these medications. Other medications that do not fall into these categories are mentioned in specific sections under Pathophysiology, earlier in the chapter.

### Surgical Procedures

Surgical intervention is indicated in GI disorders when medical intervention is insufficient. The location and extent of incisions depend on the exact procedure. The decision to perform either an open laparotomy or a laparoscopic repair will be dependent on physician preference based on surgical difficulty. However, with the progress of laparoscopic technology, many open laparotomy procedures requiring large abdominal incisions are being replaced with laparoscopic procedures. Laparoscopic procedures have been shown to reduce hospital length of stay, many postoperative complications, or both.[42, 62,66,67] Postoperative complications may include pulmonary infection, wound infection, and bed rest deconditioning. Please refer to Appendix V for further descriptions of the effects of anesthesia.

The following is a description of the more common GI surgical procedures[39,42,62,66–70]:

| | |
|---|---|
| *Appendectomy* | Removal of the appendix. Performed either through open laparotomy or laparoscopically. |
| *Cholecystectomy* | Removal of the gallbladder. Generally performed laparoscopically. |
| *Colectomy* | Resection of a portion of the colon. The name of the surgical procedure generally includes the section removed (e.g., *transverse colectomy* is resection of the transverse colon). A colectomy may also have an associated colostomy or ileostomy. Performed either through open laparotomy or laparoscopically. |
| *Colostomy* | A procedure used to divert stool from a portion of the diseased colon. There are three general types of colostomies: end, double-barrel, and loop colostomy. |
| *End colostomy* | Involves bringing the functioning end of the intestine (the section of bowel that remains connected to the upper GI tract) out onto the surface of the abdomen and forming the stoma by cuffing the intestine back on itself and suturing the end to the skin. |
| *Double-barrel colostomy* | Two separate stomas are formed on the abdominal wall. The proximal stoma is the functional end that is connected to the upper GI tract and will drain stool. The distal stoma, also called a *mucous fistula*, is connected to the rectum to drain small amounts of mucus material. This is most often a temporary colostomy. |

| | |
|---|---|
| *Loop colostomy* | Created by bringing a loop of bowel through an incision in the abdominal wall. An incision is made in the bowel to allow the passage of stool through the loop colostomy. Also used as a temporary colostomy. |
| *Gastrectomy* | Removal of a portion (partial) or all (total) of the stomach. Partial gastrectomy may either be a Billroth I or Billroth II procedure. |
| *Billroth I* | Resection of the pyloric portion of the stomach.[70] |
| *Billroth II* | Resection of the distal portion of the stomach and the duodenum.[70] |
| *Ileostomy* | A procedure similar to a colostomy and is performed in areas of the ileum (distal portion of the small intestine). A *continent ileostomy* is another method of diverting stool that, instead of draining into an external pouch, drains either into more distal and functioning portions of the intestine or into an internal pouch that is surgically created from the small intestines. |
| *Resection and reanastomosis* | The removal (resection) of a nonfunctioning portion of the GI tract and the reconnection (reanastomosis) of proximal and distal GI portions that are functional. The name of the procedure will then include the sections that are resected or reanastomosed—for example, a *pancreaticojejunostomy* is the joining of the pancreatic duct to the jejunum after a dysfunctional portion of the pancreas is resected.[64,65] |
| *Whipple procedure (pancreaticoduo-denectomy)* | Consists of *en bloc* removal of the duodenum, a variable portion of the distal stomach and the jejunum, gallbladder, common bile duct, and regional lymph nodes. This removal is followed by pancreaticojejunostomy and gastrojejunostomy. This procedure is reserved for the patient with severe or unremitting chronic pancreatitis or pancreatic cancer.[64,65,71] |
| *New GI surgical procedures* | Transplantation of various parts of the GI system, including the stomach and intestines, is being investigated as a possible mechanism to alleviate GI dysfunction in various patient populations. |

With all of the above colostomies, an external, plastic pouch is placed over the stoma in which the patient's stool collects. Patients are instructed on proper care and emptying of their colostomy pouch. This procedure can be performed in the ascending, transverse, and sigmoid portions of the colon, with sigmoid colostomies being the most commonly performed.

---

### Clinical Tip

- Before any mobility treatment, the physical therapist should ensure that the colostomy pouch is securely closed and adhered to the patient. When possible, coordinate with the nurse or the patient to empty the colostomy bag before therapy to fully minimize accidental spills.
- Patients who are experiencing abdominal pain from recent surgical incisions may be more comfortable in the side-lying position (if allowed) to help relieve skin tension on the recent incision.
- Instructing the patient to bend his or her knees up while the head of the bed is being lowered may also decrease incisional discomfort.

---

### Physical Therapy Intervention

The following are general goals and guidelines for the physical therapist when working with the patient who has GI dysfunction. These guidelines should be adapted to a patient's specific needs.

### Goals

The primary physical therapy goals for this patient population are similar to those of other patients in the acute care setting: (1) to optimize functional mobility, (2) to maximize activity tolerance and endurance, and (3) to prevent postoperative pulmonary complications.

### Guidelines for Physical Therapy Intervention

General guidelines include, but are not limited to, the following:

1.   Patients with GI dysfunction can have increased fatigue levels as a result of poor nutritional status from malabsorption and

anemia from inflammatory and hemorrhagic conditions of the GI tract. Therefore, consider the patient's fatigue level with treatment planning and setting of goals.

a) Consultation with the nutritionist is helpful in gauging the appropriate activity prescription, which is based on the patient's caloric intake. It is difficult to improve the patient's strength or endurance if his or her caloric intake is insufficient for the energy requirements of exercise.

b) Reviewing the patient's laboratory values to determine hematocrit and hemoglobin levels before treatment may be helpful in planning the patient's activity level for that session. Refer to Hematologic Evaluation in Chapter 6 for more information on hematology

c) Malabsorption syndromes can also lead to altered metabolism of medications and, therefore, the responses to medications will be less predictable and can impact the treatment planning of the therapist.[7]

2. Patients with GI dysfunction may have certain positioning precautions.

a) Dysphagia can be exacerbated in supine positions and may also lead to aspiration pneumonia.[72]

b) Portal hypertension can be exacerbated in the supine position because of gravitational effects on venous flow.

c) If the patient has associated esophageal varices from portal hypertension, then the risk of variceal rupture may be increased in this position as well.

d) Patients with portal hypertension and esophageal varices should also avoid maneuvers that create a Valsalva effect, such as coughing.

e) The increase in intra-abdominal pressure from Valsalva's maneuvers can further exacerbate the esophageal varices. (Huffing, instead of coughing, may be more beneficial in these situations.)

3. Nonpharmacologic pain management techniques from the physical therapist may benefit patients who have concurrent diagnoses of rheumatologic disorders and GI dysfunction.

a) Because NSAIDs are a causative risk factor for many inflammatory and hemorrhagic conditions of the GI system, these medications will typically be withheld from the patient with any exacerbation of these conditions.

b) Therefore, patients who were reliant on NSAIDs for pain management before admission for their rheumatologic conditions may have limitations in functional mobility as a result of altered pain management.

4. Patients with ascites or large abdominal incisions are at risk for pulmonary complications. Ascites and surgical incisions create ventilatory restrictions for the patient.

a) Additionally, these conditions can hinder cough effectiveness and functional mobility, both of which can further contribute to pulmonary infection.

b) Effective pain management before physical therapy intervention, along with diligent position changes, instruction on incisional splinting during deep breathing and coughing, and early mobilization with or without assistive devices, will help prevent the development of pulmonary complications and deconditioning.

## References

1. Koopmeiners MB. Screening for Gastrointestinal System Disease. In WG Boissonnault (ed), Examination in Physical Therapy Practice. New York: Churchill Livingstone, 1991;105.
2. Malarkey LM, McMorrow ME (eds). Nurse's Manual of Laboratory Tests and Diagnostic Procedures. Philadelphia: Saunders, 2000;412–431.
3. Malarkey LM, McMorrow ME (eds). Nurse's Manual of Laboratory Tests and Diagnostic Procedures. Philadelphia: Saunders, 2000;469.
4. Kapelman B. Approach to the Patient with Liver Disease. In DB Sachar, JD Waye, BS Lewis (eds), Pocket Guide to Gastroenterology. Baltimore: Williams & Wilkins, 1991;90.
5. Laparoscopy and Laparoscopic Surgery. In GL Eastwood, C Avunduk (eds), Manual of Gastroenterology (2nd ed). Boston: Little, Brown, 1994;27.
6. Corbett JV. Laboratory Tests and Diagnostic Procedures with Nursing Diagnoses (5th ed). Upper Saddle River, NJ: Prentice Hall Health, 2000;698.

7. Imaging Studies. In GL Eastwood, C Avunduk (eds), Manual of Gastro-enterology (2nd ed). Boston: Little, Brown, 1994;42.
8. MRI and MRC reveals distinct features in rare type of liver cancer. Hepatitis Weekly, April 23, 2001.
9. Beets-Tan RGH, Beets GL, Vliegen RFA, et al. Accuracy of magnetic resonance imaging in prediction of tumour-free resection margin in rectal cancer surgery. Lancet 2001;357(9255):497.
10. Distinctive characteristics on MRI distinguish alcoholic from viral cirrhosis. Hepatitis Weekly, Jan 22, 2001.
11. Chobanian SJ. Dysphagia. In MM van Ness, SJ Chobanian (eds), Manual of Clinical Problems in Gastroenterology. Boston: Little, Brown, 1994;3.
12. Ravich WJ, Hendrix TR. Disorders of Swallowing. In JD Stobo, DB Hellmann, PW Ladenson, et al. (eds), The Principles and Practice of Medicine (23rd ed). Stamford CT: Appleton & Lange, 1996;430–438.
13. Bailey BJ. Dysphagia: uncovering the cause when your patient has trouble swallowing. Consultant 1997;37(1):75.
14. Castell DO. Esophageal Motility Disorders and Angina. In MM van Ness, SJ Chobanian (eds), Manual of Clinical Problems in Gastroenterology. Boston: Little, Brown, 1994;5.
15. Woolf N. Pathology, Basic and Systemic. London: Saunders, 1998;483–562.
16. Wong RKH. Achalasia. In MM van Ness, SJ Chobanian (eds), Manual of Clinical Problems in Gastroenterology. Boston: Little, Brown, 1994;10.
17. Richter JE. Gastroesophageal Reflux. In MM van Ness, SJ Chobanian (eds), Manual of Clinical Problems in Gastroenterology. Boston: Little, Brown, 1994;14.
18. Pace B, Lynm C, Glass RM. Gastroesophageal Reflux Disease. JAMA 2001;285(18):2408.
19. Spechler SJ, Lee E, Ahnen D, et al. Long-term outcome of medical and surgical therapies for gastroesophageal reflux disease: follow-up of a randomized controlled trial. JAMA 2001;285(18):2331.
20. Morales TG, Sampliner RE. Barrett's esophagus. Arch Intern Med 1999;159(13):1411.
21. Jankowski JA, Harrison RF, Perry I, et al. Barrett's metaplasia. Lancet 2000;356(9247):2079.
22. Johnson DA. Barrett's Esophagus. In MM van Ness, SJ Chobanian (eds), Manual of Clinical Problems in Gastroenterology. Boston: Little, Brown, 1994;28.
23. Miller WO, van Ness MM. Esophageal Varices. In MM van Ness, SJ Chobanian (eds), Manual of Clinical Problems in Gastroenterology. Boston: Little, Brown, 1994;195.
24. Jones DM. Upper Gastrointestinal Bleeding. In MM van Ness, SJ Chobanian (eds), Manual of Clinical Problems in Gastroenterology. Boston: Little, Brown, 1994;45.
25. Hendrix TR, Giardiello FM, Herlong HF. Gastrointestinal Bleeding. In JD Stobo, DB Hellmann, PW Ladenson, et al. (eds), The Principles and

Practice of Medicine (23rd ed). Stamford CT: Appleton & Lange, 1996; 458–464.
26. Lucas BD. A practical approach to acute lower GI bleeding. Patient Care 2000;34(4):23.
27. Hines SE. Current management of upper GI tract bleeding. Patient Care 2000;34(2):20.
28. Norris TG. Gastritis. In K Boyden, D Olendorf (eds), Gale Encyclopedia of Medicine. Farmington Hills, MI: Gale Group, 1999;1255.
29. Lawson JM, Johnson DA. Acute and Chronic Gastritis. In MM van Ness, SJ Chobanian (eds), Manual of Clinical Problems in Gastroenterology. Boston: Little, Brown, 1994;48.
30. McManus TJ. *Helicobacter pylori*: an emerging infectious disease. Nurse Pract 2000;25(8):40.
31. de Boer WA, Tytgat GNJ. Treatment of *Helicobacter pylori* infection. BMJ 2000;320(7226):31.
32. Laird TW Jr. Peptic ulcer disease. Physician Assistant 1999;23(12):14.
33. Lawson JM, Johnson DA. Gastric Ulcer. In MM van Ness, SJ Chobanian (eds), Manual of Clinical Problems in Gastroenterology. Boston: Little, Brown, 1994;51.
34. Levenstein S, Ackerman S, Kiecolt-Glaser JK, Dubois A. Stress and peptic ulcer disease. JAMA 1999;281(1):10.
35. Humphries TJ. Duodenal Ulcer. In MM van Ness, SJ Chobanian (eds), Manual of Clinical Problems in Gastroenterology. Boston: Little, Brown, 1994;69.
36. Collen MJ. Zollinger-Ellison Syndrome. In MM van Ness, SJ Chobanian (eds), Manual of Clinical Problems in Gastroenterology. Boston: Little, Brown, 1994;66.
37. Mark DH, Norton JA. Surgery to cure the Zollinger-Ellison syndrome. JAMA 1999;282(14):1316.
38. Dubois A. Disorders of Gastric Emptying. In MM van Ness, SJ Chobanian (eds), Manual of Clinical Problems in Gastroenterology. Boston: Little, Brown, 1994;57.
39. Broadwell DC. Gastrointestinal System. In JM Thompson, JE Hirsch, GK MacFarland, et al. (eds), Clinical Nursing Practice. St. Louis: Mosby, 1986;1105.
40. Hendrix TR, Bulkley GB, Schuster MM. Abdominal Pain. In Stobo JD, Hellmann DB, Ladenson PW, et al. (eds), The Principles and Practice of Medicine (23rd ed). Stamford CT: Appleton & Lange, 1996;442–443.
41. Helwick CA. Appendicitis. In K Boyden, D Olendorf (eds), Gale Encyclopedia of Medicine. Farmington Hills, MI: Gale Group, 1999;315.
42. Cox JA, Rogers MA, Cox SD. Treating benign colon disorders using laparoscopic colectomy. AORN J 2001;73(2):375.
43. Dietary fiber and diverticular disease. Nutr Res Newsletter 1998;17(5): 6(1).
44. Ferzoco LB, Raptopoulous V, Silen W. Acute diverticulitis. N Engl J Med 1998;338(21):1521–1526.
45. Susan Siok JS. Hernia. In K Boyden, D Olendorf (eds), Gale Encyclopedia of Medicine. Farmington Hills, MI: Gale Group, 1999;1442.

46. Gavaghan M. Anatomy and physiology of the esophagus. AORN J 1999;69(2):372(1).
47. Knudsen JF, Friedman B, Chen M, Goldwasser JE. Ischemic colitis and sumatriptan use. Arch Intern Med 1998;158(17):1946–1948.
48. Voelker R. Bacteria and irritable bowel. JAMA 2001;285(4):401.
49. Jailwala J, Imperiale TF, Kroenke K. Pharmacologic treatment of the irritable bowel syndrome: a systematic review of randomized, controlled trials. Ann Intern Med 2000;133(2):136.
50. Bayless TM, Hendrix TR. Malabsorption. In JD Stobo, DB Hellmann, PW Ladenson, et al. (eds), The Principles and Practice of Medicine (23rd ed). Stamford CT: Appleton & Lange, 1996;485–495.
51. Bonci L, Fasano A, Goff JS, et al. Is malabsorption causing your patient's GI symptoms? Patient Care 1998;32(6):93.
52. Krige JEJ, Beckingham IJ. ABC of diseases of liver, pancreas, and biliary system: portal hypertension—2. Ascites, encephalopathy, and other conditions. BMJ 2001;322(7283):416–18.
53. Navez B. Laparoscopic management of acute peritonitis. Br J Surg 1998;85:32–36; Abstract in JAMA 1998;279(12):896U.
54. Bayless TM, Harris ML. Inflammatory Bowel Disease. In JD Stobo, DB Hellmann, PW Ladenson, et al. (eds), The Principles and Practice of Medicine (23rd ed). Stamford CT: Appleton & Lange, 1996;496–503.
55. Blumberg RS, Strober W. Prospects for research in inflammatory bowel disease. JAMA 2001;285(5):643.
56. Schreiber S. Safety and efficacy of recombinant human interleukin 10 in chronic active Crohn's disease. JAMA 2001;285(11):1421.
57. Galper C, Cerda J, Hanauer SB, et al. Inflammatory bowel disease: guidelines for management. Patient Care 1998;32(5):81.
58. Colorectal Polyps: Latest Guidelines for Detection and Follow-up. Consultant 2001;41(3):364.
59. Cramer DA. Hepatitis. In K Boyden, D Olendorf (eds), Gale Encyclopedia of Medicine. Farmington Hills, MI: Gale Group, 1999;1421–1422, 1425–1433.
60. Mitchell MC. Acute Hepatitis. In JD Stobo, DB Hellmann, PW Ladenson, et al. (eds), The Principles and Practice of Medicine (23rd ed). Stamford CT: Appleton & Lange, 1996;516–525.
61. Goodman CC. The Hepatic, Pancreatic, and Biliary Systems. In CC Goodman, WG Boisonnault (eds), Pathology: Implications for the Physical Therapist. Philadelphia: Saunders, 1998;496–531.
62. Beckingham IJ. ABC of diseases of liver, pancreas, and biliary system. Gallstone disease. BMJ 2001;322(7278):91.
63. Aronson BS. Update on acute pancreatitis. Medsurg Nurs 1999;8(1):9–16.
64. Chronic Pancreatitis. In GL Eastwood, C Avunduk (eds), Manual of Gastroenterology (2nd ed). Boston: Little, Brown, 1994;309.
65. Pancreatic Cancer. In GL Eastwood, C Avunduk (eds), Manual of Gastroenterology (2nd ed). Boston: Little, Brown, 1994;313.
66. Pedersen AG. Randomized clinical trial of laparoscopic versus open appendicectomy. JAMA 2001;285(15):1942.

67. McMahon AJ, Fischbacher CM, Frame SH, MacLeod MCM. Impact of laparoscopic cholecystectomy: a population-based study. Lancet 2000; 356(9242):1632.
68. Margolin DA, Beck DE. Surgical therapy for ulcerative colitis. Ostomy Q 1997;34(1):36.
69. Wright KD. Colostomy. In K Boyden, D Olendorf (eds), Gale Encyclopedia of Medicine. Farmington Hills, MI: Gale Group, 1999;760.
70. Madick SS. Stomach tumors and gastric surgery. AORN J 1999;69(4): 824.
71. Mergener K, Baillie J. Chronic pancreatitis. Lancet 1997;350(9088): 1379–1385.
72. Dean E. Oxygen transport deficits in systemic disease and implications for physical therapy. Phys Ther 1997;77(2):187–202.

# 9

# Genitourinary System
*Jaime C. Paz*

## Introduction

The regulation of fluid and electrolyte levels by the genitourinary system is an essential component to cellular and cardiovascular function. Imbalance of fluids, electrolytes, or both can lead to blood pressure changes or impaired metabolism that can ultimately influence the patient's activity tolerance (see Appendix II). Genitourinary structures can also cause pain that is referred to the abdomen and back. To help differentiate neuromuscular and skeletal dysfunction from systemic dysfunction, physical therapists need to be aware of pain referral patterns from these structures (Table 9-1). The objectives for this chapter are to provide the following:

    1.    A basic understanding of the structure and function of the genitourinary system

    2.    Information about the clinical evaluation of the genitourinary system, including physical examination and diagnostic studies

    3.    A basic understanding of the various diseases and disorders of the genitourinary system

**Table 9-1.** Segmental Innervation and Pain Referral Areas of the Urinary System

| Structure | Segmental Innervation | Possible Pain Referral Area |
|---|---|---|
| Kidney | T10–L1 | Lumbar spine (ipsilateral flank) |
| | | Upper abdomen |
| Ureter | T11–L2, S2–S4 | Groin |
| | | Upper and lower abdomen |
| | | Suprapubic region |
| | | Scrotum |
| | | Medial and proximal thigh |
| | | Thoracolumbar region |
| Urinary bladder | T11–L2, S2–S4 | Sacral apex |
| | | Suprapubic region |
| | | Thoracolumbar region |

Source: With permission from WG Boissonault, C Bass. Pathological origins of trunk and neck pain: part 1. Pelvic and abdominal visceral disorders. J Orthop Phys Ther 1990;12:194.

4.   Information about the management of genitourinary disorders, including dialysis therapy and surgical procedures

5.   Guidelines for physical therapy intervention in patients with genitourinary diseases and disorders

## Structure and Function

The genitourinary system consists of two kidneys, two ureters, one urinary bladder, and one urethra. The genitourinary system also includes the reproductive organs: the prostate gland, testicles, and epididymis in men and the uterus, fallopian tubes, ovaries, vagina, external genitalia, and perineum in women. Of these reproductive organs, only the prostate gland is discussed in this chapter.

The anatomy of the genitourinary system is shown in Figure 9-1. An expanded, frontal view of the kidney is shown in Figure 9-2. The structural and functional unit of the kidney is called the *nephron*. The nephron is located in the renal cortex and the medulla and has two parts: a renal corpuscle and a renal tubule. There are approximately 1 million nephrons in each kidney. Urine is formed in the nephron

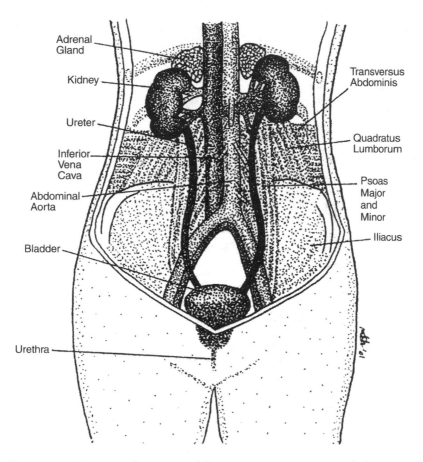

**Figure 9-1.** *Schematic illustration of the genitourinary system, including trunk musculature. (Artwork by Marybeth Cuaycong.)*

through a process consisting of glomerular filtration, tubular reabsorption, and tubular secretion.[1]

The following are the primary functions of the genitourinary system[1,2]:

- Excretion of cellular waste products (e.g., urea, creatinine [Cr], and ammonia) through urine formation and micturition (voiding)
- Regulation of blood volume by conserving or excreting fluids
- Electrolyte regulation by conserving or excreting minerals

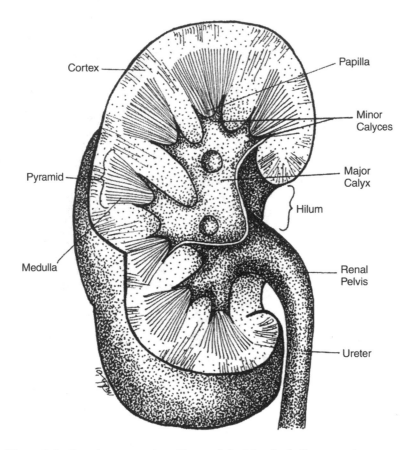

**Figure 9-2.** *Renal cross section. (Artwork by Marybeth Cuaycong.)*

- Acid-base balance regulation ($H^+$ [acid] and $HCO_3$ [base] ions are reabsorbed or excreted to maintain homeostasis.)

- Arterial blood pressure regulation (sodium excretion and renin secretion to maintain homeostasis. Renin is secreted from the kidneys during states of hypotension, which results in formation of angiotensin. Angiotensin causes vasoconstriction to help increase blood pressure.)

- Erythropoietin secretion (necessary for stimulating red blood cell production)

- Gluconeogenesis (formation of glucose)

The brain stem controls micturition through the autonomic nervous system. Parasympathetic fibers stimulate voiding, whereas sympathetic fibers inhibit it. The internal urethral sphincter of the bladder and the external urethral sphincter of the urethra control flow of urine.[2]

## Clinical Evaluation

Evaluation of the genitourinary system involves the integration of physical findings with laboratory data.

### *Physical Examination*

#### History

Patients with suspected genitourinary pathology often present with characteristic complaints or subjective reports. Therefore, a detailed history, thorough patient interview, review of the patient's medical record, or a combination of these provides a good beginning to the diagnostic process for possible genitourinary system pathology. Renal and urinary pains can vary according to their structural origins; however, they are generally described as pain that is colicky, wave-like, or burning, or occurring as dull aches in the abdomen, back, or buttocks.[3]

Changes in voiding habits or a description of micturition patterns are also noted and are listed below[2–4]:

- Decreased force of urinary flow (can indicate obstruction in the urethra or prostate enlargement)

- Increase in urinary frequency (can indicate obstruction from prostate enlargement or an acutely inflamed bladder)

- *Nocturia* (urinary frequency at night, can indicate congestive heart failure or diabetes mellitus)

- *Polyuria* (large volume of urine at one time, can indicate diabetes mellitus, chronic renal failure [CRF], or excessive fluid intake)

- *Oliguria* (usually less than 400 ml of urine in a 24-hour period, can indicate acute renal failure [ARF] or end-stage renal disease [ESRD])

- *Anuria* (less than 100 ml of urine in a 24-hour period, can indicate severe dehydration, shock, transfusion reaction, kidney disease, or ESRD)

• *Dysuria* (pain with voiding, can indicate a wide variety of disorders, including urinary tract infection)

• *Hematuria* (the presence of blood in urine, can indicate serious pathology, e.g., cancer or traumatic Foley catheterization. In either case, the physician should be notified. Refer to Appendix Table III-A.6 for a description of a Foley catheter.)

• Urinary urgency (can indicate bladder, urethral, or prostate infection)

• Incontinence (an inability to control voiding, can indicate sphincter and autonomic dysfunction)

---

### Clinical Tip

• If the patient has a history of urinary incontinence, a condom catheter (for men) or adult diapers (for men and women) can be applied before mobility treatment to aid in completion of the session.
• As a side effect of the medication phenazopyridine (Pyridium), a patient's urine may turn rust-colored and be misinterpreted as hematuria. However, any new onset of possible hematuria should always be alerted to the medical team for proper delineation of the cause.

---

### Observation

The presence of abdominal or pelvic distention, peripheral edema, incisions, scars, tubes, drains, and catheters should be noted when performing patient inspection, because these may reflect current pathology and recent interventions. Patients with genitourinary disorders may also present with skin changes, such as pallor or rough, dry skin.[4] The physical therapist must handle external tubes and drains carefully during positioning or functional mobility treatments.

---

### Clinical Tip

• Securing tubes and drains with a pin or a clamp to a patient's gown during a mobility session can help prevent accidental displacement (see Appendix Table III-A.6).

- Moving tubes and drains out of the way during bed mobility prevents the patient from possibly rolling onto them (see Appendix Table III-A.6).
- Take caution in handling patients with skin changes from dehydration to prevent any skin tears that can lead to infection formation.

## Palpation

The kidneys and a distended bladder are the only palpable structures of the genitourinary system. Distention or inflammation of the kidneys results in sharp or dull pain (depending on severity) with palpation. Kidney enlargement may be indicative of renal carcinoma.[2,4]

## Percussion

Pain and tenderness that are present with fist percussion of the kidneys can be indicative of kidney infection or polycystic kidney disease. Fist percussion is performed by the examiner's striking the fist of one hand against the dorsal surface of the other hand, which is placed along the costovertebral angle of the patient.[4]

## Auscultation

Auscultation is performed to examine the blood flow to the kidneys from the abdominal aorta and the renal arteries. The presence of bruits (*murmurs*) can indicate impaired perfusion to the kidneys, which can lead to renal dysfunction. Placement of the stethoscope is generally in the area of the costovertebral angles and the upper abdominal quadrants. Refer to Figure 8-2 for a diagram of the abdominal quadrants.[4]

## *Diagnostic Tests**

### Urinalysis

Urinalysis is a very common diagnostic tool used not only to examine the genitourinary system, but also to help evaluate for the presence of

---

*The reference range of various laboratory values can vary among different facilities. Be sure to verify the reference values located in the *laboratory test* section of the medical record.

other systemic diseases. Urine specimens can be collected by bladder catheterization or suprapubic aspiration of bladder urine, or by having the patient void into a sterile specimen container. Urinalysis is performed to examine the following[3–5]:

- Urine color, clarity, and odor

- Specific gravity, osmolarity, or both (concentration of urine ranges from 300 [dilute] to 1,300 [concentrated] mOsm/kg)

- pH (4.5–8.0)

- Presence of glucose, ketones, proteins, bilirubin, urobilinogen, occult blood, red blood cells, white blood cells, crystals, casts, bacteria or other microorganisms, enzymes, and electrolytes

Urine abnormalities are summarized in Table 9-2.

---

### Clinical Tip

- If the patient is having his or her urine collected (to measure hormone and metabolite levels), the physical therapist should have the patient use the predesignated receptacle if the patient needs to urinate during a physical therapy session. This will ensure that the collection is not interrupted.
- The predesignated receptacle can be a urinal for men or a collection "hat" placed on the toilet or commode for women.
- Urine may also be collected through the day to measure the patient's urine output relative to the patient's fluid intake (*input*). This provides a general estimate of the patient's renal function. Measurements of the patient's input and output are often abbreviated *I/Os*.

---

### Creatinine Tests

Two measurements of Cr (end product of muscle metabolism) are performed: measurements of plasma Cr and Cr clearance. Plasma Cr is measured by drawing a sample of venous blood. Increased levels are indicative of decreased renal function. The reference range of plasma Cr is 0.5–1.5 mg/dl.

Table 9-2. Urine Abnormalities

| Abnormality | Etiology |
|---|---|
| Glycosuria (presence of glucose) | Hyperglycemia and probable diabetes mellitus. |
| Proteinuria (presence of proteins) | Proteins are usually too large to be filtered; therefore, permeability has abnormally increased. Can occur with acute or chronic renal failure, nephrotic syndrome, high-protein diet, strenuous exercise, dehydration, fever, or emotional stress. |
| Hematuria (presence of blood and red blood cells) | Possible urinary tract bleeding or kidney diseases (calculi, cystitis, neoplasm, glomerulonephritis, or miliary tuberculosis). |
| Bacteriuria (presence of bacteria) | Generally indicates urinary tract infection. Urine is generally cloudy in appearance, with the possible presence of white blood cells. |
| Ketonuria (presence of ketones)* | Can result from diabetes, a high-protein diet, dehydration, vomiting, or severe diarrhea. |
| Bilirubinuria (presence of bilirubin) | Usually an early indicator of liver disease and hepatocellular jaundice. |
| Crystals (end products of food metabolism) | Can occur with urolithiasis, toxic damage to the kidneys, or chronic renal failure. |

*Ketones are formed from protein and fat metabolism, and trace amounts in the urine are normal.
Sources: Data from VC Scanlon, T Sanders (eds). Essentials of Anatomy and Physiology (2nd ed). Philadelphia: FA Davis, 1995;416; P Bates. Nursing Assessment: Urinary System. In SM Lewis, MM Heitkemper, SR Dirksen (eds), Medical-Surgical Nursing: Assessment and Management of Clinical Problems (5th ed). St. Louis: Mosby, 2000;1255; and LM Malarkey, ME McMorrow (eds). Nurse's Manual of Laboratory Tests and Diagnostic Procedures (2nd ed). Philadelphia: Saunders, 2000;38–43.

Cr clearance, also called a *24-hour urine test,* specifically measures glomerular filtration rate. Decreased clearance (indicated by elevated levels) indicates decreased renal function. The normal range of Cr clearance is 75–135 ml per minute.[4–6]

### Blood Urea Nitrogen

As an end product of protein and amino acid metabolism, increased blood urea nitrogen (BUN) levels can be indicative of any of the following: decreased renal function or fluid intake, increased muscle catabolism, increased protein intake, or acute infection. Levels of BUN need to be correlated with plasma Cr levels to implicate renal dysfunction, because BUN level can be affected by decreased fluid intake, increased muscle catabolism, increased protein intake, and acute infection. Alterations in BUN and Cr level can also lead to an alteration in the patient's mental status. Normal BUN levels are 5–30 mg/dl.[4-6]

---

### Clinical Tip

Noting BUN and Cr levels on a daily basis for any changes may help explain changes in the patient's mental status, participation in physical therapy sessions, or both.

---

### Radiographic Examination

*Kidneys, Ureters, and Bladder X-Ray*
An x-ray of the kidneys, ureters, and bladder is generally performed as an initial screening tool for genitourinary disorders. The size, shape, and position of the renal, ureteral, and bladder structures are delineated to help identify renal calculi (*kidney stones*), tumor growth or shrinkage (*chronic pyelonephritis*), and calcifications in the bladder wall. An x-ray of the kidneys, ureters, and bladder can also be performed when internal hemorrhage is suspected after major traumatic incidents. Identification of any of these disorders requires further evaluation.[4,5]

---

### Clinical Tip

This x-ray procedure is often abbreviated KUB.

---

*Pyelography*
Radiopaque dyes are used to radiographically examine the urinary system. Two types of tests are performed: excretory urography (intravenous pyelography) and retrograde urography. Excretory urography is performed more commonly than retrograde urography.

*Excretory urography* consists of (1) taking a baseline radiograph of the genitourinary system, (2) intravenous injection of contrast dye, and (3) sequential radiographs to evaluate the size, shape, and location of urinary tract structures and to evaluate renal excretory function. The location of urinary obstruction or cause of nontraumatic hematuria may be also be identified with this procedure.[4,5]

*Retrograde urography* consists of passing a catheter or cystoscope into the bladder and then proximally into the ureters before injecting the contrast dye. This procedure is usually performed in conjunction with a cystoscopic examination and is indicated when urinary obstruction or trauma to the genitourinary system is suspected. Evaluation of urethral stent or catheter placement can also be performed with this procedure.[3-5]

### Renal Arteriography and Venography

Renal arteriography and venography consist of injecting radiopaque dye into the renal artery (*arteriography*) or vein (*venography*) through a catheter that is inserted into the femoral or brachial artery or femoral vein. Arterial and venous blood supply to and from the kidneys can then be examined radiographically. Indications for arteriography include suspected aneurysm, renovascular hypertension and trauma, palpable renal masses, chronic pyelonephritis, renal abscesses, and determination of the suitability of a (donor) kidney for renal transplantation. Indications for venography include renovascular hypertension, renal vein thrombosis, and renal cell carcinoma.[5,7]

---

### Clinical Tip

Patients who are scheduled for procedures involving contrast dye are generally restricted from eating or drinking 8 hours before the procedure. A patient who is scheduled for an afternoon procedure may therefore be fatigued earlier in the day and may want to defer a scheduled therapy session. Modifying the intended therapy session and respecting the person's wishes at this time are both suitable alternatives.

---

### Bladder Examination: Cystoscopy and Panendoscopy

*Cystoscopy* consists of passing a flexible, fiberoptic scope through the urethra into the bladder to examine the bladder neck, urothelial lining, and ureteral orifices. The patient is generally placed under general or local anesthesia during this procedure. Cystoscopy is performed to examine the causes of hematuria and dysuria, as well as for tumor or polyp removal.[5-7] *Panendoscopy* is a similar procedure to cystoscopy that is used to view the prostatitic urethra (in men), external urinary sphincters, and anterior urethra.[5-7]

---

Clinical Tip

Patients may experience urinary frequency or dysuria after cystoscopic procedures; therefore, the therapist should be prepared for sudden interruptions during a therapy session that is conducted the same day after this diagnostic procedure.

---

## Urodynamic Studies

### Uroflowmetry

In *uroflowmetry*, voiding is analyzed graphically to determine the rate, time, and volume of urinary flow so that ureteral, urethral, and bladder function can be examined and described. Increased flow rates could be indicative of incontinence, whereas decreased flow rates may indicate urethral or bladder neck obstruction.[5,7]

### Cystometrogram

*Cystometrogram* is used to evaluate bladder tone, sensations of filling, and bladder stability. The procedure consists of inserting a catheter into the bladder, followed by saline instillation and pressure measurements of the bladder wall.[4]

## Radioisotope Studies

### Renography

*Renography* consists of injecting a radioisotope intravenously and allowing it to circulate through the urinary system to be excreted in the urine. A renogram (*graphic record*) is taken to assess renal blood flow, glomerular filtration, and tubular secretion.[6]

### Renal Scan

A *renal scan* consists of using an external scanning device, such as a scintillator, to outline the kidneys and ureters after intravenous radioisotope injection. Blood flow, glomerular filtration, tubular function, and excretion can be examined during this procedure. Decreased areas of kidney function, as with abscesses, cysts, or tumors, do not appear on the scan.[4-6]

*Nuclear Cystogram (Radionuclide Cystogram)*
In a *nuclear cystogram*, radioisotope material and normal saline are injected into the bladder through a catheter to assess bladder function. This procedure requires less radiation than does cystography (which requires the use of contrast dye) but does not provide the same anatomic detail.[7] Nuclear cystogram and cystography are indicated for cases in which the structure of the bladder needs to be visualized.

### Ultrasonography Studies
Ultrasound is used to (1) evaluate kidney size, shape, and position; (2) determine the presence of kidney stones, cysts, and prerenal collections of blood, pus, lymph, urine, and solid masses; (3) identify the presence of a dilated collecting system; and (4) help guide needle placement for biopsy or drainage of a renal abscess or for placement of a nephrostomy tube.[5,7]

### Computed Tomography
Indications for computed tomography of the genitourinary system include defining renal parenchyma abnormalities and differentiating solid mass densities as cystic or hemorrhagic. Kidney size and shape, as well as the presence of cysts, abscesses, tumors, calculi, congenital abnormalities, infections, hematomas, and collecting system dilation, can also be assessed with computed tomography.[3,5]

### Magnetic Resonance Imaging
Multiple uses for magnetic resonance imaging include imaging the renal vascular system without the potential adverse effects of contrast dyes, staging of renal cell carcinoma, identifying bladder tumors and their local metastases, and distinguishing between benign and malignant prostate tumors.[5]

### Biopsies

*Renal Biopsy*
A renal biopsy consists of examining a small portion of renal tissue that is obtained percutaneously with a needle to determine the pathologic state and diagnosis of a renal disorder, monitor kidney disease progression, evaluate response to medical treatment, and assess for rejection of a renal transplant. A local anesthetic is provided during the procedure.[4,5]

*Bladder, Prostate, and Urethral Biopsies*

Bladder, prostate, and urethral biopsies involve taking tissue specimens from the bladder, prostate, and urethra with a cystoscope, panendoscope, or needle aspiration via the transrectal or transperineal approach. Biopsy of the prostate can also be performed through an open biopsy procedure, which involves incising the perineal area and removing a wedge of prostate tissue. Examinations of pain, hematuria, and suspected neoplasm are indications for these biopsies.[5,7]

## Pathophysiology

### Renal System Dysfunction

#### Acute Renal Failure

Acute renal failure can result from a variety of causes and is defined as a sudden, rapid deterioration in renal function that results in decreased urine output.[8] There are three types of ARF, which are categorized by their etiology as prerenal, intrarenal, or postrenal.

*Prerenal ARF* is caused by a decrease in renal blood flow from dehydration, hemorrhage, shock, burns, or trauma.

*Intrarenal ARF* involves primary damage to kidneys and is caused by glomerulonephritis, acute pyelonephritis, renal artery or vein occlusion, bilateral renal cortical necrosis, nephrotoxic substances (e.g., aminoglycoside antibiotics or contrast dye), or blood transfusion reactions.

*Postrenal ARF* involves obstruction distal to the kidney and can be caused by urinary tract obstruction by renal stones, obstructive tumors, or benign prostatic hypertrophy.[8-11]

Despite advances in therapies, the mortality rate from ARF is still relatively high, ranging from 40% to 88%.[10,11]

The following are five stages for all three types of ARF[8,9]:

1. *Onset* is the time from the precipitating event to the onset of decreased urine output, or *oliguria.*

2. *Oliguric* or *anuric (no urine) phase* occurs when urine output is less than 400 ml in 24 hours, which can last 8–15 days, with prognosis worsening as the duration increases.

3. *Diuretic phase* is the period from the time urine output is less than 400 ml in 24 hours to the time the BUN level stops rising.

4. The *late* or *recovery period* is the time between falling to stabilizing (i.e., within normal range) BUN levels.

5. The *convalescent phase* occurs when urine output and BUN levels are stable within normal ranges. This phase may last several months and may ultimately progress to CRF.

Clinical manifestations of ARF include the following[8-11]:

- Acid-base imbalance
- Hyperkalemia or hypokalemia
- Infection
- Hyperphosphatemia
- Hemodynamic instability, including hypovolemia and hypertension
- Anemia

Management of ARF includes any of the following[8-11]:

- Treatment of the primary etiology, including anti-infective agents if applicable
- Hydration (intravenous fluids and osmotics [proteins])
- Diuretics
- Peritoneal dialysis, hemodialysis, continuous renal replacement therapy (Refer to Renal Replacement Therapy.)
- Transfusions and blood products
- Nutritional support

### Chronic Renal Failure

CRF is an irreversible reduction in renal function that occurs as a slow, insidious process from the permanent destruction of nephrons. The renal system has considerable functional reserve, and as many as 50% of the nephrons can be destroyed before symptoms occur. Progression of CRF to complete renal failure is termed *end stage renal disease* (ESRD), which requires dialysis for patient survival.[8,9,12]

CRF can result from primary renal disease or other systemic diseases. Primary renal diseases that cause CRF are polycystic kidney disease, chronic glomerulonephritis, chronic pyelonephritis, and chronic urinary obstruction. The two primary systemic diseases that cause CRF are type 2 diabetes and hypertension.[13] Other systemic diseases that can result in CRF include gout, systemic lupus erythematosus, amyloidosis, and nephrocalcinosis. Complications of CRF are similar to those of ARF but can also include decreased bone density as a result of decreased activation of vitamin D, which impairs intestinal absorption of calcium, resulting in low serum calcium levels. Patients with CRF can also experience episodes of ARF in situations when they are noncompliant with their management, when their management proves insufficient, or both.[8,9,12,14,15]

Management of CRF may consist of conservative management or renal replacement therapy.[16]

Conservative management includes the following[8,9,12,16]:

- Nutritional support, dietary modifications

- Antacids, anticonvulsant, antihypertensive, anti-infective, and antiemetic agents for symptomatic management of complications from CRF

Renal replacement therapy consists of the following[8,9,12,16]:

- Peritoneal dialysis or hemodialysis to maintain fluid and electrolyte balance

- Renal transplantation (See Chapter 12.)

### Pyelonephritis

*Pyelonephritis* is an acute or chronic inflammatory response in the kidney, particularly the renal pelvis, from bacterial, fungal, or viral infection. It can be classified as acute or chronic.

#### Acute Pyelonephritis

Acute pyelonephritis is frequently associated with concurrent cystitis (bladder infection). The common causative agents are bacterial, including *Escherichia coli, Proteus, Klebsiella, Enterobacter,* and *Pseudomonas.* Predisposing factors for acute pyelonephritis include urine reflux from the ureter to the kidney (*vesicoureteral reflux*), kidney stones, pregnancy, neurogenic bladder, catheter or endoscope insertion, and female sexual trauma. Women are more prone to acute pyelonephritis than men.[9,16,17] Spontaneous resolution of acute pyelonephritis may occur in some cases without intervention.

Signs and symptoms of acute pyelonephritis may include the following[9,16–18]:

- Sudden onset of fever and chills

- Tenderness with deep palpatory pressure of one or both costovertebral areas

- Flank or groin pain

- Urinary frequency

- Dysuria, hematuria, pyuria (presence of white blood cells [leukocytes])

Management of acute pyelonephritis may consist of any of the following[9,17,18]:

- Antibiotic therapy commonly includes ciprofloxacin (Cipro), ampicillin (Omnipen) or trimethoprim/sulfamethoxazole (Bactrim, Septra). A 7-day course of ciprofloxacin has been shown to be the most effective treatment for women with acute pyelonephritis thus far.[19]

- Ureteral reimplantation for children with chronic vesicoureteral reflux.[20]

*Chronic Pyelonephritis*
Chronic pyelonephritis is recurrent or persistent inflammation and scarring of one or both kidneys as a result of autoimmune infection. Chronic pyelonephritis can also result from kidney stones or acute pyelonephritis and may lead to CRF. Specific etiologies are difficult to diagnose.[9,16–18,21]

Signs and symptoms of chronic pyelonephritis include the following[9,17,18]:

- Hypertension

- Mild and vague dysuria, urinary frequency, and flank pain

- Renal insufficiency (decreased urine output), possibly progressing to failure

- Pyuria (white blood cells in the urine), hematuria (blood in urine)

Management of chronic pyelonephritis includes any of the following[9,17,18,21]:

- Treatment of primary etiology (if diagnosed)

- Anti-infective agents similar to those mentioned with ARF, for a short or prolonged treatment

### Glomerulonephritis

*Glomerulonephritis* is an inflammation of the glomerular portion of the kidney that can result from immunologic abnormalities, drug or toxin effects, vascular disorders, or systemic disorders. Definitive etiology may be difficult to ascertain in some cases. Glomerulonephritis can be classified according to cause, pathologic lesions, disease progression, or clinical presentation. This section discusses the common types of glomerulonephritis.[9]

*Immunoglobulin A Nephropathy (Berger's Disease)*
Immunoglobulin (Ig) A nephropathy is the most common cause of glomerulonephritis, with 25–40% of cases progressing to renal failure within 20 to 25 years of onset.[22,23] IgA nephropathy is an abnormality of immune system regulation that results in deposition of IgA (antibody) complexes within the glomeruli, ultimately resulting in a reduction of glomerular filtration. Hepatic cirrhosis, inflammatory bowel disease, carcinomas, various infections, and rheumatic disorders have been highly associated with the development of IgA nephropathy.[9,18,22,23]

Signs and symptoms of IgA nephropathy include the following[9,18,22,23]:

- Hematuria

- Proteinuria

- Oliguria

Management of IgA nephropathy includes the administration of any of the following[9,18,23]:

- Anti-inflammatory agents, such as oral glucocorticoids (prednisone)

- Angiotensin converting enzyme (ACE) inhibitors

- Cytotoxic agents

- Fish oils (effectiveness is controversial)[23,24]

*Postinfectious Glomerulonephritis*
As the name states, *postinfectious glomerulonephritis* is acute inflammation in the renal system that occurs after infection. Group α- and β-hemolytic streptococci are the common causative pathogens that lead to the damage of surface proteins in the glomeruli.[9,18,22,25] Other organisms that have been associated with this form of acute glomerulonephritis include hepatitis B virus, hepatitis C virus, and human immunodeficiency virus; spirochetes, such as *Treponema pallidum*; protozoa, such as *Plasmodium malariae*; and fungi, such as *Candida albicans*.[22] Prognosis is generally good once the causative agent is identified and appropriate anti-infective and supportive therapies are provided.[22,25]

Signs and symptoms of poststreptococcal glomerulonephritis include the following[9,18,25]:

- Acute onset of fluid retention, hypertension, and peripheral edema

- Oliguria

- Hematuria

- Mild to moderate proteinuria

- Anemia

- Cola-colored urine with red blood cell casts

Management of poststreptococcal glomerulonephritis includes any of the following[9,18,25]:

- Antibiotics

- Antihypertensive agents

- Diuretics

- Fluid and electrolyte support (as needed)

- Hemodialysis (as needed)

### Rapidly Progressive Glomerulonephritis

Rapidly progressive glomerulonephritis (RPGN) is also known as *subacute, crescentic,* or *extracapillary glomerulonephritis.* It involves glomerular inflammation that progresses to renal failure in a few days or weeks.[25] This disease primarily affects adults who are in their fifties and sixties and has a relatively poor prognosis. Early detection is critical to effective therapy and patient survival.[25,26] Causes of RPGN can include acute or subacute infection from β-hemolytic streptococci or from other bacteria, viruses, or parasites. It can also be caused by multisystem or autoimmune disease.[9,18,25]

Signs and symptoms of RPGN include the following[9,18,25]:

- Rapid, progressive reduction in renal function

- Severe oliguria

- Anuria, with irreversible renal failure

Management of RPGN includes any of the following[9,18,26]:

- Anti-inflammatory agents (e.g., prednisone)

- Plasmapheresis

- Anticoagulation treatment

- Hemodialysis

- Renal transplantation

### Chronic Glomerulonephritis

Chronic glomerulonephritis is the culmination of diseases that can affect the glomeruli leading to progressive renal failure in 10–20 years. These diseases include those mentioned in the previous section, along with diabetes, hepatitis, and systemic lupus erythematosus.[27] Chronic glomerulonephritis involves scarring and obliteration of the glomeruli, along with vascular sclerosis of arteries and arterioles.[9,18]

Signs and symptoms of chronic glomerulonephritis include the following[9,18]:

- Uremia
- Proteinuria
- Hypertension
- Azotemia

Management of chronic glomerulonephritis includes any of the following[9,18]:

- Treatment of primary disease or dysfunction
- Administration of steroidal anti-inflammatory agents
- Administration of anti-infective or cytotoxic agents, or both
- Dialysis
- Renal transplantation

Other types of glomerulonephritis are minimal change disease (lipoid nephrosis), focal segmental glomerulonephritis membranous nephropathy, and membranoproliferative glomerulonephritis (slowly progressive glomerulonephritis).[7] These are not discussed in this chapter, because they have similar clinical manifestations as the types of glomerulonephritis discussed previously.

### Nephrotic Syndrome

Nephrotic syndrome is a group of symptoms characterized by an increased permeability of the glomerular basement membrane that results in excessive excretion of protein molecules, which ultimately leads to reduced osmotic pressures that can result in peripheral edema. Many conditions can lead to nephrotic syndrome, including the following[8,9,26]:

- Acute glomerulonephritis (IgA nephropathy)
- Diabetes mellitus
- Amyloidosis
- Infections (human immunodeficiency virus, hepatitides B and C)
- Circulatory diseases

- Allergen or drug reactions (nonsteroidal anti-inflammatory agents, penicillin, captopril, heroin)
- Pregnancy (pre-eclampsia)
- Chronic allograft rejection after renal transplantation

Physical findings of nephrotic syndrome include the following[8,9,26]:

- Hypoalbuminemia
- Generalized edema
- Hyperlipidemia
- Lipiduria (lipid casts or free fat droplets in urine)
- Vitamin D deficiency

Management of nephrotic syndrome includes any of the following[8,9,28,29]:

- Treatment of underlying disease
- Administration of steroidal anti-inflammatory agents
- Albumin replacement
- Diuretics
- Anticoagulation therapy
- Dietary modifications (e.g., normal protein, low fat, salt restrictions)

**Interstitial Nephritis**
Infection, urinary tract obstruction, and reactions to medications, particularly nonsteroidal anti-inflammatory agents, can result in inflammatory, interstitial tissue damage, which is referred to as *interstitial nephritis*.[8,30,31] Scarring from the inflammatory process leads to reduced kidney function that can progress to CRF. Early detection is helpful in treating the inflammatory response.[8]
Physical findings of interstitial nephritis include the following[8]:

- Polyuria
- Nocturia

- Pyuria

- Mild hematuria

- Mild proteinuria

Management of interstitial nephritis includes any of the following[8,32]:

- Fluid and nutritional support

- Anti-infective agents (as indicated)

- Dialysis (as indicated)

- Surgery to relieve obstructions (if present)

- Renal transplantation

### Nephrolithiasis

*Nephrolithiasis* is a condition that occurs more commonly in men and is characterized by renal calculi (*kidney stones*) that form in the renal pelvis. There are three primary types of kidney stones, which are categorized according to the stone-forming substances: calcium oxalate, struvite (composed of magnesium, ammonium, and phosphate), and uric acid. Many factors contribute to stone formation and include the following[8,9,33,34]:

- High urinary concentration of stone-forming substances

- Presence of crystal growth facilitators

- Metabolic abnormalities

- Dietary factors (low fluid and high protein intake)

- Infection may contribute to the formation of kidney stones

- Urinary tract obstruction

- Medications (carbonic anhydrase inhibitors, triamterene, indinavir, and vitamin C)[8,9,33]

Signs and symptoms of kidney stones include the following[8,9]:

- Pain in the flank or groin, depending on the stone location (Pain increases greatly as the stone passes through the ureters.)

- Hematuria

- Fever

- Variable urine pH

- Variable levels of serum calcium, chloride, phosphate, carbon dioxide, uric acid, and Cr

Management of kidney stones includes any of the following[8,9,33–35]:

- Analgesics

- Hydration and diuretics

- Discontinuation of the aforementioned medications

- Anti-infective agents

- Reduction in dietary consumption of predisposing factors, such as salt and protein

- Specific therapies aimed at reducing stone formation, including thiazide diuretics, pyridoxine, magnesium, orthophosphate, and potassium citrate

- Surgery (as a last resort)

**Diabetic Nephropathy**
Approximately 20–30% of people with type 1 or type 2 diabetes will develop diabetic nephropathy,[36] which is characterized by systemic vascular changes in the kidneys that result in scarring (nephrosclerosis) of the glomeruli and, ultimately, in reduced kidney function. Pyelonephritis and necrosis of the renal papillae are also associated with diabetic nephropathy. Patients who demonstrate poor glycemic control with resultant vascular disease and hypertension are more likely to develop diabetic nephropathy. Hypertension can lead to or result from diabetic nephropathy.[8,36,37]

Signs and symptoms of diabetic nephropathy include the following[8,36,37]:

- Microalbuminuria, oliguria, anuria. Microalbuminuria is a critical screening tool for early detection of nephropathy.

- Peripheral edema.

Management of diabetic nephropathy includes any of the following[8,36,37]:

- Strict glycemic control (Refer to Diabetes Mellitus in Chapter 11.)
- Antihypertensive agents (ACE inhibitors, calcium channel blockers)
- Restriction of protein intake
- Hydration
- Diuretics
- Nutritional support
- Dialysis
- Simultaneous pancreas-kidney transplantation (See Chapter 12.)

## *Renal Vascular Abnormalities*

### Renal Artery Stenosis or Occlusion

*Renal artery stenosis* is a narrowing of the renal artery lumen; *renal artery occlusion* is blockage of the renal artery lumen. Renal artery stenosis or occlusion can result from any or all of the following: atherosclerotic disease, diabetes mellitus, subacute bacterial endocarditis, emboli from mitral valve stenosis, and mural thrombi that develop after myocardial infarction. Decreased renal perfusion results in renovascular hypertension as a result of increased renin production.[8,38]

Signs and symptoms of renal artery stenosis or occlusion include the following[8,38]:

- Hypertension
- Microscopic hematuria
- Flank or upper abdominal pain
- Abdominal aortic, renal artery bruits, or both
- Peripheral edema

Management of renal artery stenosis or occlusion includes any of the following[8,38]:

- Antihypertensive agents (ACE inhibitors)

- Anticoagulation agents

- Analgesics

- Dialysis

- Surgery (bypass grafting, angioplasty with possible stent placement, or nephrectomy in unilateral renovascular disease)

### Renal Vein Thrombosis

Renal vein thrombosis is an uncommon disorder, resulting in the accumulation of plaque in the renal vein. Renal vein thrombosis can be caused by dehydration, sepsis, a hypercoagulable state, injury to the abdomen or back, renal tumors extending into the renal vein, and nephrotic syndrome. Sudden occlusion of the renal vein results in renal infarcts.[8,39]

Signs and symptoms of renal vein thrombosis include the following[7,8,39]:

- Flank pain

- Gross hematuria

- Proteinuria

- Oliguria

Renal vein thrombosis can be managed with anticoagulants or thrombolytic agents.[7,8,39]

### Urinary Tract Dysfunction

#### Cystitis

Bacteria, viruses, fungi, chemical agents, radiation exposure, and autoimmune dysfunction are all potential causative factors that can lead to cystitis, which is an inflammation of the bladder wall. *Cystitis* and *urinary tract infections* are not synonymous, as inflammation of the bladder can occur from noninfectious causes. However, cystitis can occur with prostatitis or pyelonephritis.[18] Cystitis that occurs from noninfectious causes is called *interstitial cystitis* and is relatively uncommon.[40,41] People who are sexually active or who have an indwelling catheter, urinary tract obstructions, diabetes mellitus, neurogenic bladder, or poor hygiene are at greater risk of developing cystitis.[18]

Signs and symptoms of cystitis include the following[18,40,41]:

- Urinary frequency and urgency

- Dysuria

- Hematuria (in more serious cases)

- Nocturia

- Suprapubic pain, low back pain, or both

Management of cystitis includes any of the following[18,40,41]:

- Anti-inflammatory agents, tricyclic antidepressants, antihistamines, immunosuppressives, antispasmodics, calcium channel blocking agents, and interstitial cystitis agents.

- Increased fluid intake.

- Therapeutic hydrodistention with or without intravesicular instillation. Therapeutic hydrodistention is performed under general anesthesia, and the bladder is hydrodistended to help identify areas of inflamed epithelium and promote healing of these areas, as well as to help distend the bladder, which may help with pain relief. Intravesicular instillation is commonly performed with therapeutic hydrodistention and involves infusion of agents such as anti-inflammatory analgesic agents into the bladder.

- Surgical management with total or subtotal cystectomy, denervation of the bladder, or procedures that increase bladder capacity (all of these are last-resort measures).

### Urinary Calculi

Urinary calculi are stones (*urolithiasis*) that can form anywhere in the urinary tract outside of the kidneys. Formation of stones, symptoms, and management are similar to that of kidney stones (see Nephrolithiasis for further details on the formation and clinical presentation of kidney stones).[42] Management that may be specific to urinary calculi includes extracorporeal shock wave lithotripsy and ureteroscopy.[43]

### Neurogenic Bladder

A neurogenic bladder is characterized by bladder paralysis that occurs with central nervous system disruption (Parkinson's disease, stroke, brain tumors, multiple sclerosis, or trauma) at the cortical or spinal cord level, resulting in urinary flow disturbances. Lesions above the sacral level of the spinal cord result in loss of voluntary control of voiding; lesions below the sacral level result in the loss of voluntary and involuntary control of voiding. Neurogenic bladders may lead to infection, especially when there is associated bladder distention and urine retention, catheter placement, or stone formation, which can be caused by bone resorption from physical immobility.[9,44]

Symptoms of neurogenic bladders with infection are difficult to assess, because altered sensation from neurologic disturbance often masks pain or other symptoms. However, the patient may report a burning sensation with voiding.[9]

Management consists of addressing the primary neurologic disturbance (as able) and providing anti-infective agents for any associated infection.[9] Anticholinergic agents have also been helpful with this disorder.[44] Table 9-3 provides a summary of the different types of urinary incontinence.

### Prostate Disorders

### Benign Prostatic Hypertrophy

*Benign prostatic hypertrophy* (BPH) is a benign, progressive enlargement of the prostate gland and is the most common benign tumor in men.[45] Almost all men older than age 60 develop BPH, which is associated with the normal aging process. Concern arises when enlargement interferes with normal voiding patterns. Acute urinary retention and urinary tract infection are the primary complications of BPH.[46]

Signs and symptoms of BPH include the following[45,46]:

- Palpable prostate gland lobes with digital rectal examination
- Decreased force of urinary stream
- Straining to void
- Postvoid dribble

**Table 9-3.** Types of Urinary Incontinence

| Type | Description | Common Causes |
|---|---|---|
| Stress | Loss of urine that occurs involuntarily in situations associated with increased intra-abdominal pressure, such as with laughing, coughing, or exercise | Weakness in the bladder outlet region, urethral sphincter, or pelvic floor muscles |
| Urge | Leakage of urine that occurs after a sensation of bladder fullness is perceived | Cystitis, urethritis, tumors, stones, outflow obstructions, stroke, dementia, and parkinsonism |
| Overflow | Leakage of urine from mechanical forces or urinary retention from an overdistended bladder | Obstruction by prostate, stricture or cystocele<br>A noncontractile bladder, as occurs in diabetes mellitus or spinal cord injury<br>A neurogenic bladder, as occurs in multiple sclerosis or other lesions above the sacral portion of the spinal cord |
| Functional | The inability to void because of cognitive or physical impairments, psychological unwillingness, or environmental barriers | Depression, anger, hostility, dementia, and other neurologic disorders |

Source: Adapted from BL Bullock. Disorders of Micturition and Obstruction of the Genitourinary Tract. In BL Bullock (ed), Pathophysiology: Adaptations and Alterations in Function (4th ed). Philadelphia: Lippincott, 1996;648.

- Urinary frequency with incomplete emptying

- Nocturia and dysuria

Management of BPH includes any of the following[45,46]:

- Alpha$_1$-adrenergic blocking agents (doxazosin [Cardura], tamsulosin [Flomax], terazosin [Hytrin]) act to relax the smooth muscle in the prostate and neck of the bladder to facilitate voiding.

- 5α-reductase enzyme inhibitor (finasteride [Proscar]) inhibits male hormones to prostate causing the gland to shrink over time.

- Anti-infective agents (if there is associated infection).

- Intermittent self-catheterization.

- Surgical options include transurethral incision of the prostate, transurethral resection of the prostate (TURP), suprapubic or retropubic prostatectomy (open removal of the prostate), and balloon dilation.

### Prostatitis

Prostatitis is an inflammation of the prostate gland. It can be divided into four categories: (1) acute bacterial, (2) chronic bacterial, (3) nonbacterial, and (4) prostatodynia (presence of prostatitis symptoms without physical findings). Nonbacterial prostatitis and prostatodynia occur more commonly than do acute and chronic bacterial prostatitis. Causative pathogens for acute and chronic bacterial prostatitis can include *E. coli, Pseudomonas aeruginosa, Neisseria gonorrhoeae,* and *Mycobacterium tuberculosis.*[45]

Signs and symptoms of prostatitis include the following[42,45]:

- Fever with rectal, perineal, or low back pain (acute bacterial prostatitis)

- Increased urinary frequency or urgency to void

- Painful urination (dysuria)

- Bladder irritability

- Difficulty initiating a stream

- Nocturia

- Sexual dysfunction

Management of prostatitis includes any of the following[42,45]:

- Dietary modifications (alcohol, chili powder, and other hot spices can aggravate symptoms)

- Anti-infective agents (for bacterial prostatitis)

- Alpha$_1$-adrenergic blocking agents (See Benign Prostatic Hypertrophy.)

- Nonsteroid anti-inflammatory drugs

- Antipyretics

- Surgery (open resection of the prostate or TURP)

## Management

The specific management of various genitourinary disorders is discussed earlier in the respective pathophysiology sections. This section expands on renal replacement therapy and surgical procedures. Guidelines for physical therapy intervention for patients who have genitourinary dysfunction are also discussed.

### Renal Replacement Therapy

The primary method of managing fluid and electrolyte balance in patients with ARF or CRF is peritoneal dialysis or intermittent hemodialysis. Both types of dialysis use the principles of diffusion, osmosis, and ultrafiltration to balance fluid and electrolyte levels. *Diffusion* is the movement of solutes, such as Cr, urea, or electrolytes, from an area of higher concentration to an area of lower concentration. *Osmosis* is the movement of fluid from an area of lesser solute concentration to an area of greater solute concentration. *Ultrafiltration*, the removal of water and fluid, is accomplished by creating pressure gradients between the arterial blood and the dialyzer membrane or compartment.[15]

Another method to manage patients with ARF who are critically ill is continuous renal replacement therapy, either through continuous arteriovenous hemofiltration (CAVH) or continuous venovenous hemofiltration (CVVH).[10,15]

#### Peritoneal Dialysis

*Peritoneal dialysis* (PD) involves using the peritoneal cavity as a semipermeable membrane to exchange soluble substances and water between the dialysate fluid and the blood vessels in the abdominal cavity.[8,10,15]

Dialysate fluid is instilled into the peritoneal cavity through an indwelling catheter that is either placed surgically or nonsurgically. Surgical placement is preferable, as direct visualization during the procedure facilitates better placement. After the dialysate is instilled into the peritoneum, there is an equilibration period when water and solutes pass through the semipermeable membrane. Once equilibration is finished, then the peritoneal cavity is drained of the excess fluid and solutes that the failing kidneys cannot remove. Installation, equilibration, and drainage constitute one *exchange*.[15]

The process of peritoneal dialysis can range from 45 minutes to 9 hours, depending on the method of PD, and patients can have anywhere from four to 24 exchanges per day.[15]

There are two types of PD, automated PD and continuous ambulatory PD. *Automated PD* uses an automatic cycling device to control the installation, equilibration, and drainage phases. *Continuous ambulatory PD* involves manually exchanging dialysate fluids four times a day and is schematically represented in Figure 9-3.[15]

The following are indications for peritoneal dialysis[6,8]:

• Need for less rapid management of fluid and electrolyte imbalances

• Staff and equipment for hemodialysis unavailable

• Inadequate vascular access for hemodialysis

• Shock

• Status post cardiac surgery (e.g., coronary artery bypass grafting)

• Severe cardiovascular disease

• Patient refusal of blood transfusions

The following are contraindications for peritoneal dialysis:

• Peritonitis

• Abdominal adhesions

• Hernias

• Concurrent pulmonary complications, such as atelectasis or pneumonia

• Recent abdominal surgery

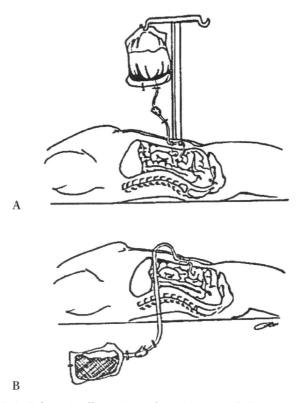

**Figure 9-3.** *Schematic illustration of continuous ambulatory peritoneal dialysis. A. Instillation of dialysate fluid. B. Drainage of excess fluid and solutes. (Artwork by Peter Wu.)*

### Intermittent Hemodialysis

Kidney functions that are controlled by intermittent hemodialysis include (1) fluid volume, (2) electrolyte balance, (3) acid-base balance, and (4) filtration of nitrogenous wastes. The patient's arterial blood is mechanically circulated through semipermeable tubing that is surrounded by a dialysate solution in the dialyzer (artificial kidney). The dialysate fluid contains electrolytes similar to those in normal blood plasma to permit diffusion of electrolytes into or out of the patient's blood.[6,8] As the patient's arterial blood is being filtered through the dialyzer, "clean" blood is returned to the patient's venous circulation. Figure 9-4 illustrates this process.

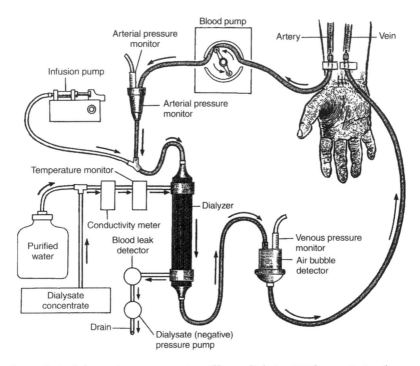

**Figure 9-4.** *Schematic representation of hemodialysis. (With permission from JM Thompson, GK McFarland, JE Hirsch, et al. [eds]. Mosby's Clinical Nursing [3rd ed]. St. Louis: Mosby, 1993;938.)*

Vascular access is attained either through cannula insertion (usually for temporary dialysis) or through an internal arteriovenous fistula (for chronic dialysis use), which is surgically created in the forearm. The arteriovenous fistula is created by performing a side-to-side, side-to-end, or end-to-end anastomosis between the radial or ulnar artery and the cephalic vein. If a native fistula cannot be created, then a synthetic graft is surgically anastomosed between the arterial and venous circulation.[6,8,15] Figure 9-5 illustrates these various types of vascular access.

Patients who require chronic intermittent hemodialysis usually have it administered three to four times per week, with each exchange lasting approximately 3–4 hours. The overall intent of this process is to extract up to 2 days' worth of excess fluid and solutes from the patient's blood.[10]

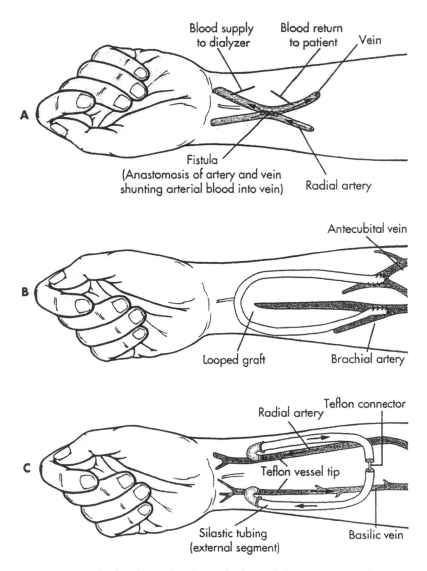

Figure 9-5. *Methods of vascular access for hemodialysis. A. Internal arteriovenous fistula. B. Looped graft in forearm. C. External cannula or shunt. (With permission from SM Lewis, MM Heitkemper, SR Dirsksen [eds]. Medical-Surgical Nursing: Assessment and Management of Clinical Problems [5th ed]. St. Louis: Mosby, 2000;1325.)*

Indications for hemodialysis include the following[6,8]:

• Acute poisoning

• Acute and chronic renal failure

• Severe states of edema

• Hepatic coma

• Metabolic acidosis

• Extensive burns with prerenal azotemia

• Transfusion reactions

• Postpartum renal insufficiency

• Crush syndrome (reduction in circulating plasma volume, hypotension, and hemoconcentration after crush injury)

Contraindications for hemodialysis include the following[8]:

• Associated major chronic illnesses

• No vascular access

• Hemorrhagic diathesis

• Extremes in age

• Poor compliance with treatment regimen

**Continuous Renal Replacement Therapy**
The purpose of *continuous renal replacement therapy* (CRRT) is to provide a slow yet continuous mechanism to remove fluid and electrolytes as well as small and medium solutes from the body in a manner that mimics the natural function of the patient's native kidney. Because of the slow process involved with CRRT, it is frequently used in the critical care setting to stabilize and manage patients without the adverse effects of hypotension that can occur with intermittent hemodialysis. CRRT can be performed for as long as 30 to 40 days, with the hemofilter being changed every 1–2 days. CRRT can also be performed as an adjunct to intermittent hemodialysis. The two main types of CRRT are continuous arteriovenous hemofiltration and continuous venovenous hemofiltration.[10,15]

CAVH uses the femoral artery and vein as common sites for vascular access. Pressure gradients between the arterial and venous system along with oncotic pressures help drive the hemofiltration process, which mimics the urine formation process in the renal glomerulus. Heparin is infused to help prevent clotting in the hemofilter and tubing. Medications and nutrition can also be administered through the circuit.[8,10,15] Figure 9-6 illustrates CAVH.

CVVH is similar to CAVH, except that CVVH only uses the venous system as access sites for blood exchange, and without the arterial system to drive blood flow, CVVH requires a mechanical pump to circulate the blood. CVVH is sometimes preferable to CAVH, as it is difficult to obtain and maintain arterial access for prolonged time periods.[15]

Indications for CRRT include the following:

- Unresponsiveness to diuretic therapy

- Cardiovascular instability

- Parenteral nutrition

- Cerebrovascular or coronary artery disease

- Uncomplicated ARF

- ARF with multiple organ failure

- Inability to tolerate hemodialysis

Contraindications for CRRT include the following:

- Hypercatabolic state

- Hyperkalemia

- Poisoning

- Shock

- Low colloid oncotic pressure

- Congestive heart failure

- Severe arthrosclerosis

- Low blood flow (i.e., mean arterial pressure less than 60 mm Hg)

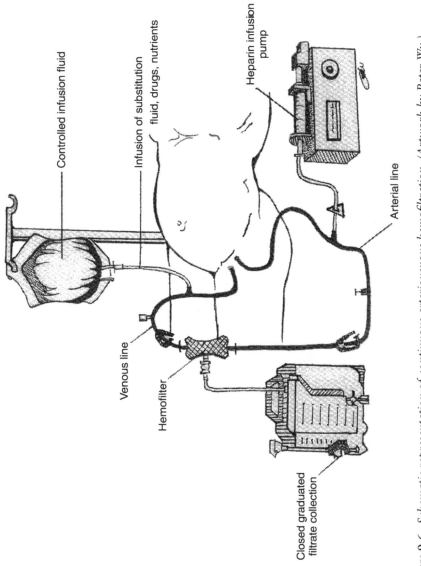

**Figure 9-6.** *Schematic representation of continuous arteriovenous hemofiltration. (Artwork by Peter Wu.)*

---

**Clinical Tip**

- Pulmonary hygiene treatments can be performed during dialysis; however, this depends on the hemodynamic stability of the patient and is at the discretion of the nurse or physician. Extreme caution should be taken with the access site to prevent accidental disruption.
- The dialysis nurse is generally nearby to monitor the procedure and is a valuable source of information regarding the patient's hemodynamic stability.
- Activity tolerance can be altered when fluid and electrolyte levels are unbalanced. Patients will demonstrate variable levels of fatigue; some are more fatigued before a dialysis session, whereas others are more fatigued after a dialysis session.
- Fluid and electrolyte imbalance can also alter the hemodynamic responses to activity; therefore, careful vital sign and symptom monitoring should always be performed.

---

*Surgical Interventions*

Surgical interventions for genitourinary system disorders can be categorized broadly as procedures that remove diseased portions of the genitourinary tract or procedures that restore urinary flow. These interventions are briefly discussed in the following sections. Refer to Appendix V for general postoperative considerations.

**Nephrectomy**
There are three types of nephrectomy. The primary indications for removing a part or all of the kidney include renal tumor, polycystic kidney disease, severe traumatic injury to the kidney, and organ donation, as well as removing a failing transplanted organ.[47,48] Nephrectomy can be performed as an open or laparoscopic procedure. Open nephrectomy is the conventional method that requires an incision of approximately 7 in. Laparoscopic nephrectomy involves five access sites, ranging from less than 0.5 in. to 3 in. Laparoscopic nephrectomy is gaining acceptance as a viable alternative to open nephrectomy, as there have been fewer postoperative complications associated with the procedure.[47-50] The types of nephrectomy and their definitions follow:

*Radical nephrectomy*—removal of the entire kidney, a section of the ureter, the adrenal gland, and the fatty tissue surrounding the kidney.

*Simple nephrectomy*—removal of the entire kidney with a section of the ureter. Generally performed when harvesting donor organs for kidney transplantation.

*Partial nephrectomy*—only the infected or diseased portion of the kidney is removed.

## Open Prostatectomy

*Open prostatectomy* is the surgical removal of a prostate gland with or without its capsule and is primarily indicated for patients with prostate cancer. Five types of surgical approaches can be used: (1) transcoccygeal, (2) perineal, (3) retropubic, (4) transvesical, and (5) suprapubic. This procedure is contraindicated if the prostate is small and fibrous. The suprapubic and retropubic approaches of this procedure are contraindicated in the presence of cancer.[42]

## Transurethral Resection

*Transurethral resection* refers to the surgical approach performed when managing bladder tumors, bladder neck fibrosis, and prostatic hyperplasia. The most common type of transurethral resection is a TURP, which this section focuses on. TURP is indicated for obstructive BPH. Involved tissues are resected with a resectoscope that is inserted through the urethra. Excision and coagulation of tissue are accompanied by continuous irrigation. Contra-indications for TURP include the presence of urinary tract infection and a prostate gland weighing more than 40 g. TURP is also contraindicated with conditions that interfere with operative positioning for the procedure, such as irreversible scrotal hernia or ankylosis of the hip.[42]

## Percutaneous Nephroscopic Stone Removal

Percutaneous nephroscopic stone removal involves the removal of stones formed in the urinary tract with a percutaneous nephrostomy tube that is placed under fluoroscopic monitoring. Depending on the size of the stone, stones may need to be broken up, then removed with a basket. Small fragments can be flushed through the system mechanically or physiologically. Considerations for this procedure include controlling septicemia before removal of the stones.[42]

## Open Urologic Surgery

Open urologic surgery is a large category of surgical procedures that is beyond the scope of this chapter but includes the following[42]:

- *Nephrolithotomy* (renal incisions for kidney stone removal)

- *Pyelolithotomy* (removal of the kidney stone from the pelvis of the kidney)
- *Ureterolithotomy* (removal of a urinary stone from the ureter)
- *Cystectomy* (bladder removal)

### Bladder Neck Suspension

Bladder neck suspension is a procedure used in women to help restore urinary continence by suturing the urethra to the pubic bones, which increases urethral resistance. It is indicated for women with stress incontinence as a result of pelvic relaxation. This procedure may also be called the *Marshall-Marchetti-Krantz procedure* or *retropubic suspension*. Bladder neck suspension is contraindicated in cases of urethral sphincter damage leading to stress incontinence.[42,51,52]

### Urinary Diversion

Obstructed urinary flow can be resolved by diverting urine with any of these four procedures: (1) supravesical diversion, (2) incontinent urinary diversion, (3) continent urinary diversion and, (4) orthotopic bladder substitution.[42,47]

#### Supravesical Diversion

A *supravesical diversion* is one in which the urine is diverted at the level of the kidney by nephrostomy. *Nephrostomy* involves placing a catheter through the renal pelvis and into the renal calyces to temporarily drain urine into an external collection device (Figure 9-7). Complications, such as stone formation, infection, hemorrhage, and hematuria, can be associated with long-term nephrostomy tube placement.[42,47]

#### Incontinent Urinary Diversion

*Incontinent urinary diversion* involves diverting urine flow to the skin through a stoma, which then requires an external appliance to collect urine. Segments of the ileum or colon are generally used as a conduit to bridge the gap from the ureter to the skin when the bladder must be removed or bypassed (see Figure 9-7). Once the diversion is complete, urine drains from the stoma into the collecting device every few seconds. These segments of intestine become totally isolated from the gastrointestinal tract.[3,47] Bladder carcinoma and severe neuropathic bladder dysfunction are common indications for this procedure.

#### Continent Urinary Diversion

*Continent urinary diversions* are internal urine reservoirs that are surgically constructed from segments of the ileum, ileocecal segment, or colon. The internal reservoirs eliminate the need for external appli-

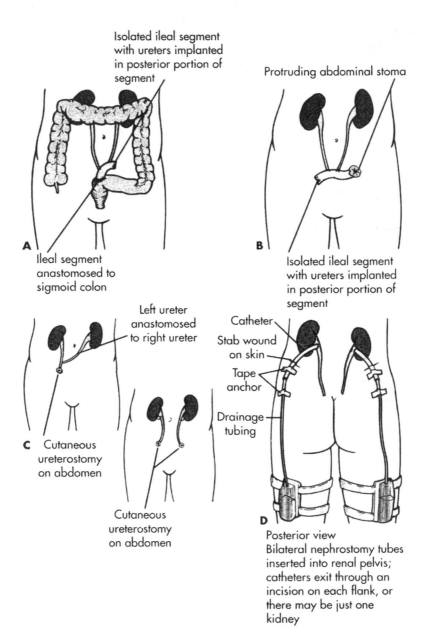

*Figure 9-7. Methods of urinary diversion. A. Ureteroileosigmoidostomy. B. Ileal loop (or ileal conduit). C. Ureterostomy (transcutaneous ureterostomy and bilateral cutaneous ureterostomies). D. Nephrostomy. (With permission from SM Lewis, MM Heitkemper, SR Dirsksen [eds]. Medical-Surgical Nursing: Assessment and Management of Clinical Problems [5th ed]. St. Louis: Mosby, 2000;1292.)*

ances and allow more control for the patient. The internal reservoir is connected to an abdominal stoma, which does not continually drain urine, and patients perform intermittent self-catheterizations through the stoma (see Figure 9-7).[42,47]

*Orthotopic Bladder Substitution*
*Orthotopic bladder substitution* involves reshaping a portion of the distal ileum into a neobladder and connecting the ureters and the urethra to it. Connecting the urethra to the neobladder allows for natural micturition. However, incontinence still may occur occasionally with this procedure, and the patient may also require intermittent catheterization.[47]

*Physical Therapy Intervention*

The following are general goals and guidelines for the physical therapist when working with patients who have genitourinary dysfunction. These guidelines should be adapted to a patient's specific needs.

The primary physical therapy goals in this patient population are similar to those of other patients in the acute care setting. These goals are to (1) optimize safe functional mobility, (2) maximize activity tolerance and endurance, and (3) prevent postoperative pulmonary complications.

General physical therapy management guidelines and considerations revolve around the normal functions of the genitourinary system that are disrupted by the various disorders discussed earlier in this chapter. These include, but are not limited to, the following:

1. Evaluating laboratory values before examination or intervention can help the physical therapist decide which particular signs and symptoms to monitor as well as determine the parameters of the session. Refer to Appendix II for more information on fluid and electrolyte imbalance.

2. The inability to regulate cellular waste products, blood volume, and electrolyte levels can result in:

- Mental status changes from a buildup of ammonia, BUN, Cr, or a combination of these. If this situation occurs, then the therapist may choose to modify or defer physical therapy intervention, particularly educational activities that require concentration.

- Disruption of excitable tissues such as peripheral nerves and skeletal, cardiac, and smooth muscle from altered levels of electrolytes.[53] If this situation occurs, then the therapist may need to reduce exercise intensity during muscle strengthening activities. Additionally, if peripheral neuropathy results in sensory deficits, then the therapist needs to take the appropriate precautions with the use of modalities and educate the patient on protective mechanisms to avoid skin breakdown.

- Peripheral or pulmonary edema from inability to excrete excess body fluids.[53] Pulmonary edema can result in shortness of breath with activities and recumbent positioning. Peripheral edema can result in range-of-motion limitations and skin breakdown. Refer to Table 1-6 for a description of pitting edema, and see Chapter 2 for a description of pulmonary edema.

3.　Blood pressure regulation can be altered by the inability to excrete body fluids and activate the renin-angiotensin system.[53]

4.　Activity tolerance can be reduced by the factors mentioned in this list, as well as anemia that can result from decreased erythropoietin secretion from kidneys, which is necessary for stimulating red blood cell production.[53]

5.　Patients with CRF may present with concurrent clinical manifestations of diabetes mellitus, as diabetes mellitus is a strong contributing factor to this disorder. Refer to Chapter 11 for more information on diabetes mellitus.

6.　As stated in the introduction to this chapter, patients with genitourinary dysfunction may have referred pain (see Table 9-1). Physical therapists can play a role in differentiating the source of a patient's back pain as well as providing symptomatic management of this referred pain.

7.　Patients who are status post surgical procedures with abdominal incisions are less likely to perform deep breathing and coughing because of incisional pain. Diligent position changes, instruction on incisional splinting during deep breathing, and coughing, along with early mobilization, help prevent the development of pulmonary complications.

8.　For patients who are ambulatory and present with urinary urgency, possibly from diuretic therapy, the use of a bedside commode may be a beneficial recommendation to minimize the incidences of incontinence.

9.　Patients who are incontinent may benefit from a home exercise program, referral to a physical therapist who specializes in pelvic floor strengthening, or both on discharge from the hospital.

# References

1. Scanlon VC, Sanders T. Essentials of Anatomy and Physiology (2nd ed). Philadelphia: FA Davis, 1995;416.
2. Bullock BL. Normal Renal and Urinary Excretory Function. In BL Bullock (ed), Pathophysiology: Adaptations and Alterations in Function (4th ed). Philadelphia: Lippincott, 1996;616.
3. McLinn DM, Boissonnault WG. Screening for Male Urogenital System Disease. In WG Boissonnault (ed), Examination in Physical Therapy Practice: Screening for Medical Disease. New York: Churchill Livingstone, 1991;121.
4. Bates P. Nursing Assessment: Urinary System. In SM Lewis, MM Heitkemper, SR Dirksen (eds), Medical-Surgical Nursing: Assessment and Management of Clinical Problems (5th ed). St. Louis: Mosby, 2000; 1241–1255.
5. Malarkey LM, McMorrow ME. Nurse's Manual of Laboratory Tests and Diagnostic Procedures (2nd ed). Philadelphia: Saunders, 2000;38–48, 629–670.
6. Richard CJ. Urinary Function. In GA Harkness, JR Dincher (eds), Medical-Surgical Nursing: Total Patient Care (9th ed). St. Louis: Mosby, 1996;760.
7. Thompson FD, Woodhouse CRJ. Disorders of the Kidney and Urinary Tract. London: Edward Arnold, 1987.
8. Renal System. In JM Thompson, GK McFarland, JE Hirsch, et al. (eds), Mosby's Manual of Clinical Nursing Practice (2nd ed). St. Louis: Mosby, 1989;1021.
9. Huether SE. Alterations of Renal and Urinary Tract Function. In KL McCance, SE Huether (eds), Pathophysiology: The Biologic Basis for Disease in Adults and Children (2nd ed). St. Louis: Mosby, 1994;1212.
10. Dirkes SM. Continuous renal replacement therapy: dialytic therapy for acute renal failure in intensive care. Nephrol Nurs J 2000;27(6):581.
11. Ford-Martin PA. Acute Kidney Failure. In K Boyden, D Olendorf (eds), Gale Encyclopedia of Medicine. Farmington Hills, MI: Gale Group, 1999;33.
12. Ford-Martin PA. Chronic Kidney Failure. In K Boyden, D Olendorf (eds), Gale Encyclopedia of Medicine. Farmington Hills, MI: Gale Group, 1999;716.
13. Boone CA. End-stage renal disease in African-Americans. Nephrol Nurs J 2000;27(6):597.
14. Scott MB. Caring for the orthopaedic patient receiving continuous ambulatory peritoneal dialysis. Orthop Nurs 1999;18(4):59.
15. Brunier B, Bartucci M. Acute and Chronic Renal Failure. In SM Lewis, MM Heitkemper, SR Dirksen (eds), Medical-Surgical Nursing: Assessment and Management of Clinical Problems (5th ed). St. Louis: Mosby, 2000;1310–1330.
16. Boissonault WG. Urinary Tract Disorders. In CC Goodman, WG Boissonnault (eds) Pathology: Implications for the Physical Therapist. Philadelphia: Saunders, 1998;532–546.
17. Wright KD. Pyelonephritis. In K Boyden, D Olendorf (eds), Gale Encyclopedia of Medicine. Farmington Hills, MI: Gale Group, 1999;2422.

18. Bullock BL. Immunologic, Infectious, Toxic and Other Alterations in Function. In BL Bullock (ed), Pathophysiology: Adaptations and Alterations in Function (4th ed). Philadelphia: Lippincott, 1996;633.
19. Talan DA, Stamm WE, Hooton TM, et al. Comparison of ciprofloxacin (7 days) and trimethoprim-sulfamethoxazole (14 days) for acute uncomplicated pyelonephritis in women: a randomized trial. JAMA 2000; 283(12):1583.
20. Ellsworth PI, Cendron M, McCullough MF. Surgical management of vesicoureteral reflux. AORN J 2000;71(3):498.
21. Ershler WB, Konety BR, Wise GJ, D'Epiro P. Underlying disorders and their treatment. Patient Care 1997;31(7):196.
22. Ambrus JL Jr, Sridhar NR. Immunologic aspects of renal disease. JAMA 1997;278(22);1938.
23. Staples BJ. Primary IgA nephropathy: pathophysiology, diagnosis, and clinical management. Nephrol Nurs J 2001;28(2):151.
24. Donadio JV Jr. Use of fish oil to treat patients with immunoglobulin A nephropathy. Am J Clin Nutr 2000;71(1):373S.
25. Couser WG. Glomerulonephritis. Lancet 1999;353(9163):1509.
26. Madaio MP, Harrington JT. The diagnosis of glomerular diseases: acute glomerulonephritis and the nephrotic syndrome. Arch Intern Med 2001;161(1):25.
27. Wright KD. Glomerulonephritis. In K Boyden, D Olendorf (eds), Gale Encyclopedia of Medicine. Farmington Hills, MI: Gale Group, 1999; 1296.
28. Orth SR, Ritz E. The nephrotic syndrome. N Engl J Med 1998;338(17): 1202.
29. Ross JS, Shua-Haim JR. Geriatrics photo quiz. Nephrotic syndrome. Proteinuria characterizes this condition, and treatment targets the underlying pathology. Geriatrics 2000;55(3):80.
30. Schaeffer AJ. What do we know about the urinary tract infection-prone individual? J Infect Dis 2001;183(5):S66.
31. Kumar S, Berl T. NSAID-induced renal toxicity: when to suspect, what to do (nonsteroidal anti-inflammatory drugs). Consultant 1999;39(1): 195(6).
32. Interstitial Nephritis. In WD Glanze, LE Anderson (eds), Mosby's Medical, Nursing, and Allied Health Dictionary (5th ed). St. Louis: Mosby, 1998;48.
33. Pak CYC. Kidney stones. Lancet 1998;351(9118):1797.
34. Bernie JE, Kambo AR, Monga M. Urinary lithiasis: current treatment options. Consultant 2000;40(14):2340.
35. Giannini S, Nobile M, Sartori S, et al. Acute effects of moderate dietary protein restriction in patients with idiopathic hypercalciuria and calcium nephrolithiasis. Am J Clin Nutr 1999;69(2):267.
36. Diabetic nephropathy. Diabetes Care 2001;24(1):S69.
37. Evans TC, Capell P. Diabetic nephropathy. Clin Diabetes 2000;18(1):7.
38. McLaughlin K, Jardine AG, Moss JG. ABC of arterial and venous disease: renal artery stenosis. BMJ 2000;320(7242);1124.
39. Davidson T. Renal Vein Thrombosis. In K Boyden, D Olendorf (eds), Gale Encyclopedia of Medicine. Farmington Hills, MI: Gale Group, 1999;2469.

40. Henderson LJ. Diagnosis, treatment, and lifestyle changes of interstitial cystitis. AORN J 2000;71(3):525.
41. Lamb AR. The ABCs of interstitial cystitis: a primer for midlevel providers. Physician Assistant 2000;24(12):22.
42. Genitourinary System. In JM Thompson, GK Mcfarland, JE Hirsch, et al. (eds), Mosby's Manual of Clinical Nursing Practice (2nd ed). St. Louis: Mosby, 1989;1086.
43. Saunders CS. Urolithiasis: new tools for diagnosis and treatment. Patient Care 1999;33(15):28.
44. Gallo ML, Fallon PJ, Staskin DR. Urinary incontinence: steps to evaluation, diagnosis, and treatment. Nurse Pract 1997;22(2):21.
45. Epperly TD, Moore KE. Health issues in men: part I. common genitourinary disorders. Am Fam Physician 2000;61(12):3657.
46. Bullock BL. Disorders of Micturition and Obstructions of Genitourinary Tract. In BL Bullock (ed), Pathophysiology: Adaptations and Alterations in Function (4th ed). Philadelphia: Lippincott, 1996;646.
47. Bates P. Renal and Urologic Problems. In SM Lewis, MM Heitkemper, SR Dirksen (eds), Medical-Surgical Nursing: Assessment and Management of Clinical Problems (5th ed). St. Louis: Mosby, 2000;1290–1293.
48. Ford-Martin PA. Nephrectomy. In K Boyden, D Olendorf (eds), Gale Encyclopedia of Medicine. Farmington Hills, MI: Gale Group, 1999; 2040.
49. Fornara P, Doehn C, Frese R, Jocham D. Laparoscopic nephrectomy in young-old, old-old, and oldest-old adults. J Gerontol A Biol Sci Soc Sci 2001;56(5):M287.
50. Sasaki TM. Is laparoscopic donor nephrectomy the new criterion standard? JAMA 2000;284(20):2579.
51. Ford-Martin PA. Marshall-Marchetti-Krantz Procedure. In K Boyden, D Olendorf (eds), Gale Encyclopedia of Medicine. Farmington Hills, MI: Gale Group, 1999;1877.
52. McCallig Bates P. Sharing the secret: talking about urinary incontinence. Nurse Pract 2000;25(10):1S8.
53. Dean E. Oxygen transport deficits in systemic disease and implications for physical therapy. Phys Ther 1997;77(2):187.

# 10

# Infectious Diseases
*Jaime C. Paz and V. Nicole Lombard*

## Introduction

A patient may be admitted to the hospital setting with an infectious process acquired in the community or may develop one as a complication from the hospital environment. An infectious disease process generally has a primary site of origin; however, it may result in diffuse systemic effects that may limit the patient's functional mobility and activity tolerance. Therefore, a basic understanding of these infectious disease processes is useful in designing, implementing, and modifying physical therapy treatment programs. The physical therapist may also provide treatment for patients who have disorders resulting from altered immunity. These disorders are mentioned in this chapter because immune system reactions can be similar to those of infectious disease processes (see Appendix 10-A for discussions of three common disorders of altered immunity: systemic lupus erythematosus, sarcoidosis, and amyloidosis). The objectives of this chapter are to provide a basic understanding of the following:

> 1. Clinical evaluation of infectious diseases and altered immune disorders, including physical examination and laboratory studies

2. Various infectious disease processes, including etiology, pathogenesis, clinical presentation, and management

3. Commonly encountered altered immune disorders, including etiology, clinical presentation, and management

4. Precautions and guidelines that a physical therapist should implement when treating a patient with an infectious process or altered immunity

## Definition of Terms

To facilitate the understanding of infectious disease processes, terminology that is commonly used when referring to these processes is presented in Table 10-1.[1–3]

## Overview of the Immune System

A person's immune system is comprised of many complex, yet synergistic, components that defend against pathogens (Table 10-2). Any defect in this system may lead to the development of active infection. Patients in the acute care setting often present with factors that can create some or most of these defects, which can ultimately affect their immune system (Table 10-3).

## Evaluation

When an infectious process is suspected, a thorough patient interview (history) and physical examination are performed to serve as a screening tool for the differential diagnosis and to help determine which laboratory tests are further required to identify a specific pathogen.[4]

### History

Potential contributing factors of the infection are sought out, such as exposure to infectious individuals or recent travel to foreign countries. Also, a qualitative description of the symptomatology is discerned, such as onset or nature of symptoms (e.g., a nonproductive versus productive cough over the past day or weeks).

**Table 10-1.** Terminology Associated with Infectious Disease Processes

| | |
|---|---|
| Antibody | A highly specific protein that is manufactured in response to antigens and defends against subsequent infection |
| Antigen (immunogen) | An agent that is capable of producing antibodies when introduced into the body of a susceptible person |
| Carrier | A person who harbors an infectious agent that can cause a specific disease but who demonstrates no evidence of the disease |
| Colonization | The process of a group of organisms living together; the host can carry the microorganism without being symptomatic |
| Communicable | The ability of an infective organism to be transmitted from person to person, either directly or indirectly |
| Disseminated | Distributed over a considerable area |
| Host | The person whom the infectious agent invades and from whom it gathers its nourishment |
| Immunocompromised | An immune system that is incapable of responding to pathogenic organisms and tissue damage |
| Immunosuppression | The prevention of formation of an immune response |
| Nosocomial infection | Infection that is acquired in the hospital setting |
| Opportunistic | An infectious process that develops in immunosuppressed individuals (Opportunistic infections normally do not develop in individuals with intact immune systems.) |
| Pathogen | An organism capable of producing a disease |
| Subclinical infection | A disease or condition that does not produce clinical symptoms, or the time period before the appearance of disease-specific symptoms |

## *Physical Examination*

### Observation

Clinical presentation of infectious diseases is highly variable according to the specific system that is involved. However, common physical findings that occur with infection include sweating and inflammation, both of which are related to the metabolic response of the body to the antigen. The classic signs of inflammation (redness and edema) in cer-

**Table 10-2.** Components of the Immune System

| Lines of Defense | Components | Description |
|---|---|---|
| First line of defense | Skin, conjunctivae, mucous membranes | Physical barriers to pathogens. |
| Second line of defense | Inflammatory response | If physical barriers are crossed, inflammatory response acts to (1) contain pathogen and (2) bring immune cells to antigen. |
| Third line of defense | Immune response | Specific immune response to pathogens. |
| | Humoral immunity (B cells)* | B cells produce antibodies. |
| | Cellular immunity (T cells)* | T cells: (1) Augment production of antibodies. (2) Directly kill antigens. (3) Turn off immune system. |

*B cells and T cells can also be referred to as *B lymphocytes* or *T lymphocytes*, respectively.
Sources: Data from NS Rote. Immunity. In SE Heuther, KL McCance (eds), Understanding Pathophysiology (2nd ed). St. Louis: Mosby, 2000;125–150; EN Marieb (ed). Human Anatomy and Physiology (2nd ed). Redwood City, CA: Benjamin Cummins, 1992;690–723; and AC Guyton, JE Hall. Textbook of Medical Physiology (9th ed). Philadelphia: Saunders, 1996;445–455.

tain areas of the body can help delineate the source, location(s), or both of infection. Delineating the source of infection is crucial to the diagnostic process.

## Palpation

The presence of warmth and possible pain or tenderness is another typical sign of inflammation that may be consistent with active infection. Lymphoid organs (lymph nodes and spleen) can also be swollen and tender with infection, as lymphocytes (processed in these organs) are multiplying in response to the antigen. Inflammation and tenderness in these or other areas of the body can further help to delineate the infectious process.

**Table 10-3.** Factors Affecting the Immune System

Congenital (rare)
  Disruption in the development of lymphocytes
Acquired
  Pregnancy
  Pre-existing infections
  Malignancies (Hodgkin's disease, acute or chronic leukemia, nonlymphoid
    malignancy or myeloma)
  Stress (emotional or surgical—anesthesia)
  Malnutrition (insufficiency of calories, protein, iron, and zinc)
  Age
  Chronic diseases (diabetes, alcoholic cirrhosis, sickle cell anemia)
  Immunosuppressive treatment (corticosteroids, chemotherapy, or radiation
    therapy)
  Indwelling lines and tubes

Source: Data from NS Rote, SE Heuther, KL McCance. Hypersensitivities, Infection, and Immunodeficiencies. In SE Heuther, KL McCance (eds), Understanding Pathophysiology (2nd ed). St. Louis: Mosby, 2000;204–208.

### Vital Signs

*Heart Rate, Blood Pressure, and Respiratory Rate*
Measurement of heart rate and blood pressure helps in determining whether an infectious process is occurring. (Infections result in an increased metabolic rate, which presents as an increased heart rate and respiratory rate.) Blood pressure may also be elevated when metabolism is increased, or blood pressure can be decreased secondary to vasodilation from inflammatory responses in the body.

*Temperature*
Monitoring the patient's temperature over time (both throughout the day and daily) provides information regarding the progression (a rise in temperature) or a regression (a fall in temperature) of the infectious process. A fall in body temperature from a relatively elevated temperature may also signify a response to a medication.

### Auscultation
Heart and lung sounds are examined to determine whether any infectious processes could be occurring from these areas directly or affecting these areas indirectly.

## Laboratory Studies

Most of the evaluation process for diagnosing an infectious disease is based on laboratory studies. These studies are performed to (1) isolate the microorganisms from various body fluids or sites; (2) directly examine specimens by microscopic, immunologic, or genetic techniques; or (3) assess specific antibody responses to the pathogen.[5] This diagnostic process is essential to prescribing the most specific medical regimen possible for the patient.

### Hematology

During hematologic studies, a sample of blood is taken and analyzed to assist in determining the presence of an infectious process or organism. Hematologic procedures used to diagnose infection include leukocyte count, differential white blood cell (WBC) count, and antibody measurement.[6]

### Leukocyte Count

Leukocyte, or WBC, count is measured to determine whether an infectious process is present and should range between 4,500 and 11,000 cells/μl.[7] An increase in the number of WBCs, termed *leukocytosis*, is required for phagocytosis (cellular destruction of microorganisms) and indicates the presence of an acute infectious process.[7] A decreased WBC count from baseline, termed *leukopenia*, can indicate altered immunity or the presence of an infection that exhausts supplies of certain WBCs.[7] A decreased WBC count relative to a previously high count (i.e., becoming more within normal limits) may indicate the resolution of an infectious process.[7]

### Differential White Blood Cell Count

Five types of WBCs exist: lymphocytes, monocytes, neutrophils, basophils, and eosinophils. Specific types of infectious processes can trigger alterations in the values of one or more of these cells. Detection of these changes can assist in identification of the type of infection present. For example, an infection caused by bacteria can result in a higher percentage of neutrophils, which have a normal range of 2.0–7.5 × 10⁹/liter. In contrast, a parasitic infection will result in increased eosinophils, which have a normal count of 0.0–0.45 × 10⁹/liter.[7]

### Antibody Measurement

Antibodies develop in response to the invasion of antigens from new infectious agents. Identifying the presence and concentration of specific antibodies helps in determining past and present exposure to infectious organisms.[8]

## Microbiology

In microbiology studies, specimens from suspected sources of infection (e.g., sputum, urine, feces, wounds, and cerebrospinal fluid) are collected by sterile technique and analyzed by staining, culture, or sensitivity or resistance testing, or a combination of all of these.

### Staining

Staining allows for morphologic examination of organisms under a microscope. Two types of staining techniques are available: simple staining and the more advanced differential staining. Many types of each technique exist, but the differential Gram's stain is the most common.[8]

Gram's stain is used to differentiate similar organisms by categorizing them as gram-positive or gram-negative. This separation assists in determining subsequent measures to be taken for eventual identification of the organism. A specimen is placed on a microscope slide, and the following six-step process is performed[9]:

1. Crystal violet stain applied to stain all organisms

2. Iodine stain applied to enhance reaction between cell wall and primary stain

3. Ethyl alcohol or acetone applied

4. Safranin O or carbolfuchsin applied to stain gram-negative organisms pink to red

5. Alcohol or acetone applied to decolor gram-negative organisms

6. Safranin reapplied for visualization

A red specimen at completion indicates a gram-negative organism, whereas a violet specimen indicates a gram-positive organism.[9]

### Culture

The purpose of a culture is to identify and produce isolated colonies of organisms found within a collected specimen. Cells of the organism are isolated and mixed with specific mediums that provide the proper nourishment and environment (e.g., pH level, oxygen content) needed for the organism to reproduce into colonies. Once this has taken place, the resultant infectious agent is observed for size, shape, elevation, texture, marginal appearance, and color to assist with identification.[9]

### Sensitivity and Resistance

When an organism has been isolated from a specimen, its sensitivity (susceptibility) to antimicrobial agents or antibiotics is tested. An infectious agent is *sensitive* to an antibiotic when the organism's growth is inhibited under safe dose concentrations. Conversely, an agent is *resistant* to an antibiotic when its growth is not inhibited by safe dose concentrations. Because of a number of factors, such as mutations, an organism's sensitivity, resistance, or both to antibiotics is constantly changing.[10]

## Cytology

*Cytology* is a complex method of studying cellular structures, functions, origins, and formations. Cytology assists in differentiating between an infectious process and a malignancy and in determining the type and severity of a present infectious process by examining cellular characteristics.[8,11] It is beyond the scope of this chapter, however, to describe all of the processes involved in studying cellular structure dysfunction.

## Body Fluid Examination

### Pleural Tap

A *pleural tap*, or *thoracentesis*, is the process by which a needle is inserted through the chest wall into the pleural cavity to collect pleural fluid for examination of possible malignancy, infection, inflammation, or any combination of these. A thoracentesis may also be performed to drain excessive pleural fluid in large pleural effusions.[12]

### Pericardiocentesis

*Pericardiocentesis* is a procedure that involves accessing the pericardial space around the heart with a needle or cannula to aspirate fluid for drainage, analysis, or both. It is primarily used to assist in diagnosing infections, inflammation, and malignancies and to relieve effusions built up by these disorders.[13]

### Synovial Fluid Analysis

*Synovial fluid analysis*, or *arthrocentesis*, involves aspirating synovial fluid from a joint capsule. The fluid is then analyzed and used to assist in diagnosing infections, rheumatic diseases, and osteoarthritis, all of which can produce increased fluid production within the joint.[14]

*Gastric Lavage*
A *gastric lavage* is the suctioning of gastric contents through a nasogastric tube to examine the contents for the presence of sputum in patients suspected of having tuberculosis (TB). The assumption is that patients swallow sputum while they sleep. If sputum is found in the gastric contents, the appropriate sputum analysis should be performed to help confirm the diagnosis of TB.[12,15]

*Peritoneal Fluid Analysis*
*Peritoneal fluid analysis*, or *paracentesis*, is the aspiration of peritoneal fluid with a needle. It is performed to (1) drain excess fluid, or *ascites*, from the peritoneal cavity, which can be caused by infectious diseases, such as TB; (2) assist in the diagnosis of hepatic or systemic malfunctions, diseases, or malignancies; and (3) help detect the presence of abdominal trauma.[12,15]

## Other Studies

Imaging with plain x-rays, computed tomography scans, and magnetic resonance imaging scans can also help identify areas with infectious lesions. In addition, the following diagnostic studies can also be performed to help with the differential diagnosis of the infectious process. For a description of these studies, refer to the sections and chapters indicated below:

- Sputum analysis (see Diagnostic Testing in Chapter 2)

- Cerebrospinal fluid (see Lumbar Puncture in Chapter 4)

- Urinalysis (see Diagnostic Tests in Chapter 9)

- Wound cultures (see Wound Assessment and Acute Care Management of Wounds in Chapter 7)

## Infectious Diseases

Various infectious disease processes, which are commonly encountered in the acute care setting, are described in the following sections. Certain disease processes that are not included in this section are described in other chapters. Please consult the index for assistance.

## Nosocomial Infections

*Nosocomial infection* is a general term that refers to an infection that is acquired in the hospital setting. Many pathogens can cause a nosocomial infection, but the most commonly reported in the past years have been *Escherichia coli, Staphylococcus aureus, Enterococcus faecalis, Pseudomonas aeruginosa*, and coagulase-negative staphylococci.[16] Patients who are at risk for developing nosocomial infections are those who present with the following:

1.   Age; the very young or the very old

2.   Immunodeficiency; chronic diseases (cancer, chronic renal disease, chronic obstructive pulmonary disease, diabetes, or acquired immunodeficiency syndrome [AIDS])

3.   Immunosuppression; chemotherapy, radiation therapy, or corticosteroids

4.   Misuse of antibiotics; overprescription of antibiotics or use of broad-spectrum antibiotics, leading to the elimination of a patient's normal flora, which allows for the colonization of pathogens and development of drug-resistant organisms

5.   Use of invasive diagnostic and therapeutic procedures—indwelling urinary catheters, monitoring devices, intravenous (i.v.) catheters, and mechanical ventilation with intubation

6.   Surgery—incisions provide access to pathogens

7.   Burns—disrupt the first line of defense

8.   Length of hospitalization—increases the exposure to pathogens and medical intervention

The mode of transmission for pathogens that cause nosocomial infections can vary from contact to airborne. Pathogens can also become opportunistic in patients who are immunocompromised or immunosuppressed. Common sites for nosocomial infections are in the urinary tract, surgical wounds, and the lower respiratory tract (e.g., pneumonia). Clinical manifestations and management of nosocomial infections vary according to the type of pathogen and the organ system involved. However, the primary management strategy for nosocomial infections is prevention by following standard and specific precautions outlined in Table 10-4.[5,16,17]

Table 10-4. Summary of Precautions to Prevent Infection

| Precaution | Description |
|---|---|
| Standard | Treat all patient situations as potentially infectious. Wash hands before and after each patient contact. Wear a different set of gloves with each patient. If splashing of body fluids is likely, wear a mask, or face shield, or both, and a gown. |
| Airborne* | A mask is required in situations when contagious pathogens can be transmitted by airborne droplet nuclei, as in the case of measles, varicella (chickenpox), or tuberculosis. |
| Droplet* | A mask or face shield, or both, are necessary when large-particle droplet transmission (usually 3 ft or less) is likely. Droplet transmission involves contact of the conjunctivae or the mucous membranes of the nose or mouth with large-particle droplets (larger than 5 μm in size) generated from coughing, sneezing, talking, and certain procedures, such as suctioning and bronchoscopy. Examples of pathogens requiring droplet precautions are *Haemophilus influenzae*, *Neisseria meningitidis*, mycoplasmal pneumonia, streptococcal pneumonia, mumps, and rubella. |
| Contact* | Gown and gloves are necessary when pathogens are transmitted by direct person-to-person contact or person-to-object contact. Examples of these pathogens include *Clostridium difficile*, *Escherichia coli*, herpes simplex virus, herpes zoster, methicillin-resistant *Staphylococcus aureus*, and vancomycin-resistant *Enterococcus*. |

*These precautions are in addition to practicing standard precautions.
Sources: Data from D Rice, EC Eckstein. Inflammation and Infection. In WJ Phipps, JK Sands, JF Marek (eds), Medical–Surgical Nursing, Concepts and Clinical Practice (6th ed). St. Louis: Mosby, 1999;237–245; and KN Anderson (ed), Mosby's Medical, Nursing, and Allied Health Dictionary (5th ed). St. Louis: Mosby, 1998;2BA5.

## Antibiotic-Resistant Infections

### *Methicillin-Resistant* Staphylococcus aureus *Infection*

Methicillin-resistant *S. aureus* (MRSA) is a strain of *Staphylococcus* that is resistant to methicillin or similar agents, such as oxacillin and nafcillin. *Methicillin* is a synthetic form of penicillin and was developed because *S. aureus* developed resistance to penicillin, which was originally the treatment choice for *S. aureus* infection. However, since the early 1980s, this particular strain of *S. aureus* has become increasingly resistant to methicillin. The contributing factor that is suggested to have a primary role in the increased incidence of this nosocomial infection is the indiscriminate use of antibiotic therapy.[17,18]

Additionally, patients who are at risk for developing MRSA infection in the hospital are patients who[18–20]

- Are debilitated, elderly, or both

- Are hospitalized for prolonged time periods

- Have multiple surgical or invasive procedures, an indwelling cannula, or both

- Are taking multiple antibiotics, antimicrobial treatments, or both

- Are undergoing treatment in critical care units

MRSA is generally transmitted by person-to-person contact or person-to-object-to-person contact. MRSA can survive for prolonged periods of time on inanimate objects, such as telephones, bed rails, and tray tables, unless such objects are properly sanitized. Hospital personnel can be primary carriers of MRSA, as the bacterium can be colonized in healthy adults.

Management of MRSA is difficult and may consist of combining local and systemic antibiotics, increasing antibiotic dosages, and applying whole-body antiseptic solutions. In recent years, vancomycin has become the treatment of choice for MRSA; however, evidence has shown that patients with this strain of *S. aureus* are also developing resistance to vancomycin (vancomycin intermediate *S. aureus*—VISA).[17] Therefore, prevention of MRSA infection is the primary treatment strategy and consists of the following[16,18–20]:

- Placing patients with MRSA infection on isolation or contact precautions

- Strict hand-washing regulations before and after patient care

- Use of gloves, gowns (if soiling is likely), or both

- Disinfection of all contaminated objects

### Vancomycin-Resistant Enterococci Infection

Vancomycin-resistant enterococci (VRE) infection is another nosocomial infection that has become resistant to vancomycin, aminoglycosides, and ampicillin. The infection can develop as endogenous enterococci (normally found in the gastrointestinal or the female reproductive tract) become opportunistic in patient populations similar to those mentioned earlier with MRSA.[16,17,21]

Transmission of the infection can also occur by (1) direct patient-to-patient contact, (2) indirect contact through asymptomatic hospital personnel who can carry the opportunistic strain of the microorganism, or (3) contact with contaminated equipment or environmental surfaces.

Management of VRE infection is difficult, as the enterococcus can withstand harsh environments and survive well on the hands of health care workers and on hospital objects. Treatment options are very limited for patients with VRE, and the best intervention plan is to prevent the spread of the infectious process.[17] Strategies for preventing VRE infection include the following[21]:

• The controlled use of vancomycin

• Timely communication between the microbiology laboratory and appropriate personnel to initiate contact precautions as soon as VRE is detected

• Implementation of screening procedures to detect VRE infection in hospitals where VRE has not yet been detected (i.e., randomly culturing potentially infected items or patients)

• Preventing the transmission of VRE by placing patients in isolation or grouping patients with VRE together, wearing gown and gloves (which need to be removed inside the patient's room), and washing hands immediately after working with an infected patient

• Designating commonly used items, such as stethoscopes and rectal thermometers, to be used only with VRE patients

• Disinfecting any item that has been in contact with VRE patients with the hospital's approved cleaning agent

---

### Clinical Tip

Equipment that is used during physical therapy treatments for patients with MRSA or VRE, such as assistive devices, cuff weights, or goniometers, should be left in the patient's room and not be taken out until the infection is resolved. If there is an equipment shortage, thorough cleaning of the equipment is necessary before using the equipment with other patients.

## Respiratory Tract Infections

Infections of the respiratory tract can be categorized as upper or lower respiratory tract infections. Upper respiratory tract infections that are discussed in this section consist of allergic and viral rhinitis, sinusitis, influenza, and pertussis. Lower respiratory tract infections that are discussed in this section consist of TB, histoplasmosis, and legionellosis. Pneumonia is the most common lower respiratory tract infection and is discussed in Pathophysiology in Chapter 2.

### Upper Respiratory Tract Infections

#### Rhinitis
*Rhinitis* is the inflammation of the nasal mucous membranes and can result from an allergic reaction or viral infection. Allergic rhinitis is commonly a seasonal reaction from allergens, such as pollen, or a perennial reaction from environmental triggers, such as pet dander or smoke. Viral rhinitis, sometimes referred to as the *common cold*, is caused by a wide variety of viruses that can be transmitted by airborne particles or by contact.

Clinical manifestations of allergic and viral rhinitis include nasal congestion, sneezing, watery, itchy eyes and nose, altered sense of smell, and thin, watery nasal discharge. In addition to these, clinical manifestations of viral rhinitis include fever, malaise, headache, and thicker nasal discharge.

Management of allergic rhinitis includes antihistamines, decongestants, and nasal corticosteroid sprays. Management of viral rhinitis includes rest, fluids, antipyretics, and analgesics.[22,23]

#### Sinusitis
*Sinusitis* is the inflammation or hypertrophy of the mucosal lining of any or all of the facial sinuses (frontal, ethmoid, sphenoid, and maxillary). This inflammation can result from bacterial, viral, or fungal infection.

Clinical manifestations of sinusitis include pain over the affected sinus, purulent nasal drainage, nasal obstruction, congestion, fever, and malaise.

Management of sinusitis includes antibiotics (as appropriate), decongestants or expectorants, and nasal corticosteroids.[23]

---

**Clinical Tip**

Despite the benign nature of rhinitis and sinusitis, the manifestations (especially nasal drainage and sinus pain) of these infections can be very disturbing to the patient and therapist during the therapy session and may even lower the tolerance of the patient for a given activity. The therapist should be sympathetic to the patient's symptoms and adjust the activity accordingly.

---

## Influenza

Influenza (the *flu*) is caused by any of the influenza viruses (A, B, or C and their mutagenic strains) that are transmitted by aerosolized mucous droplets. These viruses have the ability to change over time and are the reason why a great number of patients are at risk for developing this infection. Influenza B is the most likely virus to cause an outbreak within a community.

Clinical manifestations of influenza include (1) a severe cough, (2) abrupt onset of fever and chills, (3) headache, (4) backache, (5) myalgia, (6) prostration (exhaustion), (7) coryza (nasal inflammation with profuse discharge), and (8) mild sore throat. Gastrointestinal signs and symptoms of nausea, vomiting, abdominal pain, and diarrhea can also present in certain cases. The disease is usually self-limiting in uncomplicated cases, with symptoms resolving in 7–10 days. A complication of influenza infection is pneumonia, especially in the elderly and chronically diseased individuals.[1,2,12,23]

If management of influenza is necessary, it may consist of the following[1,2,12,23]:

- Anti-infective agents

- Antipyretic agents

- Adrenergic agents

- Antitussive agents

- Active immunization by vaccines

- Supportive care with i.v. fluids and supplemental oxygen, as needed

---

### Clinical Tip

Health care workers should be vaccinated against the influenza virus to decrease the risk of transmission.

---

### Pertussis

*Pertussis*, or *whooping cough*, is an acute bacterial infection of the mucous membranes of the tracheobronchial tree. It occurs most commonly in children younger than 1 year of age and in children and adults of lower socioeconomic populations. The defining characteristics are violent cough spasms that end with an inspiratory "whoop," followed by the expulsion of clear tenacious secretions. Symptoms may last 1–2 months. Pertussis is transmitted through airborne particles.

Management of pertussis may consist of any of the following[12]:

- Anti-infective and anti-inflammatory medications

- Bronchopulmonary hygiene with endotracheal suctioning, as needed

- Supplemental oxygen, assisted ventilation, or both

- Fluid and electrolyte replacement

- Respiratory isolation for 3 weeks after the onset of coughing spasms or 7 days after antimicrobial therapy

### *Lower Respiratory Tract Infections*

### Tuberculosis

*TB* is a chronic pulmonary and extrapulmonary infectious disease caused by the tubercle bacillus. It is transmitted through airborne *Mycobacterium tuberculosis* particles, which are expelled into the air when an individual with pulmonary or laryngeal TB coughs or sneezes.[24] When *M. tuberculosis* reaches the alveolar surface of a new host, it is attacked by macrophages, and one of two outcomes can result: Macrophages kill the particles, terminating the infection, or the particles multiply within the WBCs, eventually causing them to burst. This cycle is then repeated for anywhere between 2 and 12 weeks, after which time the individual is considered to be infected with TB and will test positive on tuberculin skin tests, such as the Mantoux test, which uses tuberculin purified protein derivative,* or the multiple puncture test, which uses tuberculin. At this point, the infection enters a latent period (most common) or develops into active TB.[24,25]

A six-category classification system has been devised by the American Thoracic Society and the Centers for Disease Control and Prevention (CDC) to describe the TB status of an individual[24,26]:

1. No TB exposure, not infected

2. TB exposure, no evidence of infection

3. Latent TB infection, no disease

4. TB, clinically active

5. TB, not clinically active

6. TB suspect (diagnosis pending)

Populations at high risk for acquiring TB include (1) the elderly; (2) Native Americans, Eskimos, and blacks (in particular if they are homeless or economically disadvantaged); (3) incarcerated individuals; (4) immigrants from Southeast Asia, Ethiopia, Mexico, and Latin America; (5) malnourished individuals; (6) infants and children younger than 5 years of age; (7) those with decreased immunity (e.g., from AIDS or leukemia, or after chemotherapy); (8) those with diabetes mellitus, end-stage renal disease, or both; (9) those with silicosis; and (10) those in close contact with individuals with active TB.[3,24]

Persons with normal immune function do not normally develop active TB after acquisition and are, therefore, not considered contagious. Risk factors for the development of active TB after infection include age (children younger than 8 years and adolescents are at greatest risk), low weight, and immunosupression.[27]

---

*A person who has been exposed to the tubercle bacillus will demonstrate a raised and reddened area 2–3 days after being injected with the protein derivative of the bacilli.

When active TB does develop, its associated signs and symptoms include (1) fever, (2) an initial nonproductive cough, (3) mucopurulent secretions that present later, and (4) hemoptysis, dyspnea at rest or with exertion, adventitious breath sounds at lung apices, pleuritic chest pain, hoarseness, and dysphagia, all of which may occur in the later stages. Chest films also show abnormalities, such as atelectasis or cavitation involving the apical and posterior segments of the right upper lobe, the apical-posterior segment of the left upper lobe, or both.[24]

Extrapulmonary TB occurs with less frequency than pulmonary TB but affects up to 70% of human immunodeficiency virus (HIV)–positive individuals diagnosed with TB.[28] Organs affected include the meninges, brain, blood vessels, kidneys, bones, joints, larynx, skin, intestines, lymph nodes, peritoneum, and eyes. When multiple organ systems are affected, the term *disseminated*, or *miliary*, TB is used.[28] Signs and symptoms that manifest are dependent on the particular organ system or systems involved.

Because of the high prevalence of TB in HIV-positive individuals (up to 60% in some states),[28] it should be noted that the areas of involvement and clinical features of the disease in this population differ from those normally seen, particularly in cases of advanced immunosuppression. Brain abscesses, lymph node involvement, lower lung involvement, pericarditis, gastric TB, and scrotal TB are all more common in HIV-positive individuals. HIV also increases the likelihood that TB infection will progress to active TB by impairing the body's ability to suppress new and latent infections.[28]

Management of TB may consist of the following[1,2,12]:

- Anti-infective agents

- Corticosteroids

- Surgical intervention to remove cavitary lesions (rare) and areas of the lung with extensive disease or to correct hemoptysis, spontaneous pneumothorax, abscesses, intestinal obstruction, ureteral stricture, or any combination of these

- Respiratory isolation until antimicrobial therapy is initiated

- Blood and body fluid precautions if extrapulmonary disease is present

- Skin testing (i.e., Mantoux test and multiple puncture test)

- Vaccination for prevention

In recent years, new strains of *M. tuberculosis* that are resistant to antitubercular drugs have emerged. These *multidrug-resistant TB* strains are associated with fatality rates as high as 89% and are common in HIV-infected individuals. Treatment includes the use of direct observational therapy (DOT) and direct observational therapy, short-course (DOTS). These programs designate health care workers to observe individuals to ensure that they take their medications for the entire treatment regimen or for a brief period, respectively, in hopes of minimizing resistance.[28]

---

### Clinical Tip

• Facilities often provide specialized masks to wear around patients on respiratory precautions for TB. The masks are impermeable to the airborne mycobacterium. Always verify with the nursing staff or physician before working with these patients to determine which mask to wear.
• Patients who are suspected of, but not diagnosed with, TB are generally placed on "rule-out TB" protocol, in which case respiratory precautions should be observed.

---

### Histoplasmosis

*Histoplasmosis* is a pulmonary and systemic infection that is caused by infective spores (fungi), most commonly found in the soil of the central and eastern United States. Histoplasmosis is transmitted by inhalation of dust from the soil or bird and bat feces. The spores form lesions within the lung parenchyma that can be spread to other tissues. The incidence of fungal infection is rising, particularly in immunocompromised, immunosuppressed, and chronically debilitated indi-viduals who may also be receiving corticosteroid, antineoplastic, and multiple antibiotic therapy.[29,30]

Different clinical forms of histoplasmosis are (1) acute, benign respiratory disease, which results in flu-like illness and pneumonia; (2) acute disseminated disease, which can result in septic-type fever; (3) chronic disseminated disease, which involves lesions in the bone marrow, spleen, and lungs and can result in immunodeficiency; and (4) chronic pulmonary disease, which manifests as progressive emphysema.

Management of histoplasmosis may consist of the following[12,29,31]:

• Anti-infective agents

• Corticosteroids

• Antihistamines

• Supportive care appropriate for affected areas in the different forms of histoplasmosis

### Legionellosis

*Legionellosis* is commonly referred to as *Legionnaire's disease* and is an acute bacterial infection primarily resulting in patchy pulmonary infiltrate(s) and lung consolidation. However, other organs may also become involved, especially in the immunocompromised patient. Legionellosis is transmitted by inhalation of aerosolized organisms from infected water sources.

Primary clinical manifestations include high fever, malaise, myalgia, headache, and nonproductive cough. Other manifestations can also include diarrhea and other gastrointestinal symptoms. The disease is rapidly progressive during the first 4–6 days of illness, with complications that may include renal failure, bacteremic shock, and respiratory failure.[1,12,32]

Management of legionellosis may consist of the following[1,12,32]:

• Anti-infective agents

• Supplemental oxygen with or without assisted ventilation

• Temporary renal dialysis

• i.v. fluid and electrolyte replacement

## Cardiac Infections

Infections of the cardiac system can involve any layer of the heart (endocardium, myocardium, and pericardium) and generally result in acute or chronic depression of the patient's cardiac output. Those infections that result in chronic cardiomyopathy most likely require cardiac transplantation. Refer to Chapters 1 and 12 for a discussion of cardiomyopathy and cardiac transplantation, respectively. This section focuses on rheumatic fever and resultant rheumatic heart disease.

*Acute rheumatic fever* is a clinical sequela occurring in up to 3% of patients with group A β-streptococcal infection of the upper respiratory tract. It occurs primarily in children who are between the ages of 6 and 15 years. Rheumatic fever is characterized by nonsuppurative inflammatory lesions occurring in any or all of the connective tissues of the heart, joints, subcutaneous tissues, and central nervous system. An altered immune reaction to the infection is suspected as the cause of resultant damage to these areas, but the definitive etiology is unknown. *Rheumatic heart disease* is the term used to describe the resultant damage to the heart from the inflammatory process of rheumatic fever.[12,19,33,34]

Cardiac manifestations can include pericarditis, myocarditis, left-sided endocarditis, and valvular stenosis and insufficiency with resultant organic heart murmurs, as well as congestive heart failure. If not managed properly, all of these conditions can lead to significant morbidity or death.[12,19,33]

Management of rheumatic fever follows the treatment for streptococcal infection. The secondary complications mentioned previously are then managed specifically. The general intervention scheme may include the following[12,19,33]:

- Prevention of streptococcal infection

- Anti-infective agents

- Antipyretic agents

- Corticosteroids

- Bed rest

- i.v. fluids (as needed)

## Neurologic Infections

### Poliomyelitis

*Poliomyelitis* is an acute systemic viral disease that affects the central nervous system. *Polioviruses* are a type of enterovirus that multiply in the oropharynx and intestinal tract. There are three serotypes of poliovirus, types 1, 2, and 3 respectively, with type 1 being the most common cause of polio epidemics in certain areas of the world.[12,35]

Poliomyelitis is usually transmitted directly by the fecal-oral route from person to person but can also be transmitted indirectly by consumption of contaminated water sources.[35]

Clinical presentation can range from subclinical infection, to nonfebrile illness (24–36 hours), to aseptic meningitis, to paralysis (after 4 days), and, possibly, to death. Polio can also be classified as spinal, bulbar, or spinobulbar disease, depending on the areas of the nervous system that are affected. If paralysis does occur, it is generally associated with fever and muscle pain. The paralysis is usually asymmetric and involves muscles of respiration, swallowing, and the lower extremities. Paralysis can resolve completely, have residual deficits, or be fatal.[12,35]

Management of poliomyelitis primarily consists of prevention with inactivated poliovirus vaccine (IPV) given as four doses to children from the ages of 2–6 years of age.[35] If a patient does develop active poliomyelitis, then other management strategies may include the following[12]:

- Analgesics and antipyretics

- Enteric precautions for 7 days after the onset of the disease

- Supplemental oxygen, assisted ventilation, or both

- Bronchopulmonary hygiene

- i.v. fluids and nasogastric feedings

- Bed rest with contracture prevention with positioning and range of motion

### Postpoliomyelitis Syndrome

Postpoliomyelitis syndrome occurs 30–40 years after an episode of childhood paralytic poliomyelitis. It results in muscle fatigue, pain, and decreased endurance. Muscle atrophy and fasciculations may also be present. Patients who are older or critically ill, who have had a previous diagnosis of paralytic poliomyelitis, and who are female are at greater risk for development of this syndrome.[35,36]

### Meningitis

*Meningitis* is an inflammation of the meninges, which cover the brain and spinal cord, that results from acute infection by bacteria, viruses, fungi, or parasitic worms, or by chemical irritation. The route of transmission is primarily inhalation of infected airborne mucous droplets released by infected individuals or through the bloodstream via open wounds or invasive procedures.[37,38]

The more common types of meningitis are (1) meningococcal meningitis, which is bacterial in origin and occurs in epidemic form; (2) *Haemophilus* meningitis, which is the most common form of bacterial meningitis; (3) pneumococcal meningitis, which occurs as an extension of a primary bacterial upper respiratory tract infection; and (4) viral (aseptic or serous) meningitis, which is generally benign and self-limiting.

Bacterial meningitis is more severe than viral meningitis and affects the pia mater, arachnoid and subarachnoid space, ventricular system, and the cerebrospinal fluid. The primary complications of bacterial meningitis include an increase in intracranial pressure, resulting in hydrocephalus. This process frequently results in severe headache and nuchal rigidity (resistance to neck flexion). Other complications of meningitis include arthritis, myocarditis, pericarditis, neuromotor and intellectual deficits, and blindness and deafness from cranial nerve (III, IV, VI, VII, or VIII) dysfunction.[37,38]

Management of any form of meningitis may consist of the following[12,37]:

- Anti-infective agents or immunologic agents [ampicillin, penicillin, cephalosporins (ceftriaxone [Rocephin] or cefotaxime [Claforan])]

- Analgesics

- Mechanical ventilation (as needed)

- Blood pressure maintenance with i.v. fluid and vasopressors (e.g., dopamine)

- Intracranial pressure control

### Encephalitis

*Encephalitis* is an inflammation of the tissues of the brain and spinal cord, commonly resulting from viral or amebic infection. Types of encephalitis include infectious viral encephalitis, mosquito-borne viral encephalitis, and amebic meningoencephalitis.

*Infectious viral encephalitis* is transmitted by direct contact of droplets from respiratory passages or other infected excretions and is most commonly associated with the herpes simplex type 1 virus. Viral encephalitis can also occur as a complication of systemic viral infections, such as poliomyelitis, rabies, mononucleosis, measles, mumps, rubella, and chickenpox. Manifestations of viral encephalitis can be mild to severe, with herpes simplex virus encephalitis having the highest mortality rate among all types of encephalitides.[12,37,38]

*Mosquito-borne viral encephalitis* is transmitted by infectious mosquito bites and cannot be transmitted from person to person. The incidence of this type of encephalitis can be epidemic in nature and typically varies according to geographic regions and seasons.[12,37,38]

*Amebic meningoencephalitis* is transmitted in water and can enter a person's nasal passages while he or she is swimming. Amebic meningoencephalitis cannot be transmitted from person to person.

General clinical presentation of encephalitis may include any of the following[12,37,38]:

- Fever

- Signs of meningeal irritation from increased intracranial pressure (e.g., severe frontal headache, nausea, vomiting, dizziness, nuchal rigidity)

- Altered level of consciousness, irritability, bizarre behaviors (if the temporal lobe is involved)

- Seizures (mostly in infants)

- Aphasia

- Focal neurologic signs

- Weakness

- Altered deep tendon reflexes

- Ataxia, spasticity, tremors, or flaccidity

- Hyperthermia

- Alteration in antidiuretic hormone secretion

Management of encephalitis may consist of the following[12]:

- Anti-infective agents

- Intracranial pressure management

- Mechanical ventilation, with or without tracheostomy (as indicated)

- Sedation

- i.v. fluid and electrolyte replacement
- Nasogastric tube feedings

## Musculoskeletal Infections

*Osteomyelitis* is an acute infection of the bone that can occur from direct or indirect invasion by a pathogen. Direct invasion is also referred to as *exogenous* or *acute contagious osteomyelitis* and can occur any time there is an open wound in the body. Indirect invasion is also referred to as *endogenous* or *acute hematogenous osteomyelitis* and usually occurs from the spread of systemic infection. Both of these types can potentially progress to subacute and chronic osteomyelitis. *Acute osteomyelitis* typically refers to an infection of less than 1 month's duration, whereas *chronic osteomyelitis* refers to infection that lasts longer than 4 weeks' time.[39,40]

*Acute contagious osteomyelitis* is an extension of the concurrent infection in adjacent soft tissues to the bony area. Trauma resulting in compound fractures and tissue infections is a common example. Prolonged orthopedic surgery, wound drainage, and chronic illnesses, such as diabetes or alcoholism, also predispose patients to acute contagious osteomyelitis.[40,41]

*Acute hematogenous osteomyelitis* is a blood-borne infection that generally results from *S. aureus* infection (80%)[1] and occurs mostly in infants, children (in the metaphysis of growing long bones), or patients undergoing long-term i.v. therapy, hyperalimentation, hemodialysis, or corticosteroid or antibiotic therapy. Patients who are malnourished, obese, or diabetic, or who have chronic joint disease, are also susceptible to acute hematogenous osteomyelitis.[39,40]

Clinical presentation of both types of acute osteomyelitis includes (1) delayed onset of pain, (2) tenderness, (3) swelling, and (4) warmth in the affected area. Fever is present with hematogenous osteomyelitis. The general treatment course for acute osteomyelitis is early and aggressive administration of the appropriate antibiotics to prevent or limit bone destruction.[1,31,39,40]

*Chronic osteomyelitis* is an extension of the acute cases discussed above. It results in marked bone destruction, draining sinus tracts, pain, deformity, and the potential of limb loss. Chronic osteomyelitis can also result from infected surgical prostheses or infected fractures. Debridement of dense formations (*sequestra*) may be a necessary adjunct to the antibiotic therapy. If the infection has spread to the surrounding soft tissue and skin regions, then grafting, after debridement, may be necessary. Good results have also been shown with hyperbaric oxygen therapy for chronic osteomyelitis.[39,40]

---

Clinical Tip

Clarify weight-bearing orders with the physician when performing gait training with patients who have any form of osteomyelitis. Both upper and lower extremities can be involved; therefore, choosing the appropriate assistive device is essential to preventing pathologic fracture.

---

## Skin Infections

*Cellulitis*, or *erysipelas*, is an infection of the dermis and the subcutaneous tissue that can remain localized or be disseminated into the bloodstream, resulting in bacteremia (rare). Cellulitis occurs most commonly on the face, neck, and legs.

Groups A and G *Streptococcus* and *S. aureus* are the usual causative agents for cellulitis and generally gain entry into the skin layers when there are open wounds (surgical or ulcers). Patients who are at most risk for developing cellulitis include those who are postsurgical and immunocompromised from chronic diseases or medical treatment.

The primary manifestations of cellulitis are fever with an abrupt onset of hot, stinging, and itchy skin and painful, red, thickened lesions that have firm, raised palpable borders in the affected areas. Identifying the causative agent is often difficult through blood cultures; therefore, localized cultures, if possible in open wounds, may be more sensitive in helping to delineate the appropriate antibiotic treatment.[41–43]

## Gastrointestinal Infections

*Gastroenteritis* is a global term used for the inflammation of the digestive tract that is typically a result of infection. The primary cause of gastroenteritis is viral infection from rotavirus, adenovirus, astrovirus, calicivirus, and small round-structured viruses. Gastroenteritis can also occur from bacterial infection from *E. coli*, *Shigella* (which causes bacterial dysentery), *Clostridium difficile*, and *Salmonella*.

Transmission of these organisms is usually through the ingestion of contaminated food, water, or both or by direct and indirect fecal-oral transmission.

The primary manifestations of any form of gastroenteritis are crampy abdominal pain, nausea, and diarrhea, all of which vary in severity and duration according to the type of infection. Gastroenteritis is generally a self-limiting infection, with resolution occurring in 3–4 days. However, patients in the hospital setting with reduced immunity can have longer periods of recovery, with dehydration being a primary concern.[12,31,44]

Management of acute gastroenteritis may consist of the following[12,31]:

- Anti-infective agents

- i.v. fluid and electrolyte replacement

- Antiemetic agents (if nausea and vomiting occur)

---

### Clinical Tip

Strict contact and enteric precautions should be observed with patients who have a diagnosis of C. *difficile* infection.

---

## Immune System Infections

### Human Immunodeficiency Virus Infection

Two types of HIV exist: HIV-1 and HIV-2, with HIV-1 being the more prevalent and the one discussed here. It is a retrovirus, occurring in pandemic proportions, that primarily affects the function of the immune system. Eventually, however, all systems of the body become affected directly, such as the immune system, or indirectly, as in the cardiac system, or through both methods, as occurs in the nervous system.

The virus is transmitted in blood, semen, vaginal secretions, and breast milk through sexual, perinatal, and blood or blood product contact. Proteins on the surface of the virus attach to CD4+ receptors, found primarily on T4 lymphocytes.[45] Other types of cells found to house the virus include monocytes, macrophages, uterine cervical cells, epithelial cells of the gastrointestinal tract, and microglia cells.[45]

On entering the cell, the viral and cellular DNA combine, making the virus a part of the cell. The exact pathogenesis of cellular destruction caused by HIV is not completely understood, and several methods of destruction may be entailed. It is known that immediately after initial infection, HIV enters a latent period, or asymptomatic stage, in which viral replication is minimal, but CD4+ T cell counts begin to decline.[45] Continued reduction results in decreasing immunity, eventually leading to symptomatic HIV, in which diseases associated with the virus begin to appear.[45] This eventually leads to the onset of AIDS, which the CDC defines as occurring when the CD4+ T-lymphocyte count falls below 200 cells/µl (normal, 650–1,200 cells/µl) or below 14%, when 1 of 26 specific AIDS defining disorders is contracted, or a combination of these factors.[46]

Five laboratory tests are available to detect HIV infection[47,48]:

1. Enzyme-linked immunosorbent assay or enzyme immunoassay test. This procedure tests for the presence of antibodies to HIV proteins in the patient's serum. A sample of the patient's blood is exposed to HIV antigens in the test reagent. If HIV antibodies are identified, it is inferred that the virus is present within the patient.

2. Western blot test. This test detects the presence of antibodies in the blood to two types of HIV viral proteins and is, therefore, a more specific HIV test. It is an expensive test to perform and is used as a confirmatory tool for a positive enzyme-linked immunosorbent assay test.

3. Immunofluorescence assay. In this test, the patient's blood is diluted and placed on a slide containing HIV antigens. The slide is then treated with anti-human globulin mixed with a fluorescent dye that will bind to antigen-antibody complexes. If a fluorescence is seen when the specimen is placed under a microscope, then HIV antibodies are present in the patient's blood.

4. p24 Antigen assay. This test analyzes blood cells for the presence of the p24 antigen located on HIV virions. It can be used to diagnose acute infection, to screen blood for HIV antigens, to determine HIV infection in difficult diagnostic cases, or to evaluate the treatment effects of antiviral agents.

5. Polymerase chain reaction for HIV nucleic acid. This highly specific and extremely sensitive test detects the viral DNA molecule

in lymphocyte nuclei by amplifying the viral DNA. It is used to detect HIV in neonates and when antibody tests are inconclusive.

Once HIV has been detected, it can be classified in a number of ways. The Walter Reed staging system has six categories grouped according to the quantity of helper T cells and characteristic signs, such as the presence of an HIV antigen or antibody.[49] However, a more commonly used classification system was devised by the CDC and was last updated in 1993. In this system, infection is divided into three categories, depending on CD4+ T-lymphocyte counts:

1. Category 1 consists of CD4+ T-lymphocyte counts greater than or equal to 500 cells/μl.

2. Category 2 consists of counts ranging between 200 and 499 cells/μl.

3. Category 3 contains cell counts less than 200 cells/μl.

These groups are then subdivided into A, B, and C, according to the presence of specific diseases.[46]

Advancement in the medical treatment of HIV, in the form of anti-retroviral therapy, has recently been made. This therapy consists of three types of medications[49]:

1. Nucleoside analog reverse transcriptase inhibitors, otherwise known as *nucleoside analogs*. These include zidovudine, didanosine, zalcitabine, stavudine, and lamivudine.

2. Protease inhibitors, including saquinavir, indinavir, ritonavir, and nelfinavir.

3. Non-nucleoside reverse transcriptase inhibitors, including delavirdine and nevirapine.

Each of these therapies assists in limiting HIV progression by helping to prevent viral replication. This prevention is further increased when the drugs are used in combination in a treatment technique termed *highly active antiretroviral therapy* or *HAART*.[49]

As HIV progresses and immunity decreases, the risk for and severity of infections not normally seen in healthy immune systems increase. These opportunistic infections, combined with disorders that result directly from the virus, often result in multiple diagnoses and medically complex patients. These manifestations of HIV can affect every system of the body and present with a wide array of signs and symptoms, many of which are appropriate for physical therapy intervention. Table 10-5 lists common manifestations and complications of HIV and AIDS and the medications generally used in their management.

Disorders affecting the nervous system include HIV-associated dementia complex, progressive multifocal leukoencephalopathy, primary central nervous system lymphoma, toxoplasmosis, and neuropathies. These manifestations may cause paresis, decreased sensation, ataxia, aphagia, spasticity, altered mental status, and visual deficits.[50] In the pulmonary system, TB, cytomegalovirus (CMV), and pneumonia can result in cough, dyspnea, sputum production, and wheezing.[51] In the cardiac system, cardiomyopathy, arrhythmias, and congestive heart failure can cause chest pain, dyspnea, tachycardia, tachypnea, hypotension, fatigue, peripheral edema, syncope, dizziness, and palpitations.[52]

Physical therapy intervention can assist in minimizing the effect of these deficits on functional ability, therefore helping to maximize the independence and quality of life of the individual. However, the course of rehabilitation in HIV-affected individuals can often be difficult owing to coinciding opportunistic infections, an often-rapid downhill disease course, low energy states, and frequent hospitalizations.

## Mononucleosis

Mononucleosis is an acute viral disease that has been primarily linked to the Epstein-Barr virus and less commonly to CMV. Mononucleosis is transmitted generally through saliva from symptomatic or asymptomatic carriers (the Epstein-Barr virus can remain infective for 18 months in the saliva).[12,53]

The disease is characterized by fever, lymphadenopathy (lymph node hyperplasia), and exudative pharyngitis. Splenomegaly, hepatitis, pneumonitis, and central nervous system involvement may occur as rare complications from mononucleosis. The infection is generally self-limiting in healthy individuals, with resolution occurring in approximately 3 weeks without any specific treatment.[12,53]

**Table 10-5.** Common Complications from Human Immunodeficiency Virus (HIV) and Acquired Immunodeficiency Syndrome and Associated Medical Treatment

| Complication | Medication |
| --- | --- |
| Cardiomyopathy | May be reversed with reduction or discontinuation of interleukin-2, adriamycin, $\alpha_2$-interferon, ifosfamide, and foscarnet |
| Cerebral toxoplasmosis | Trimethoprim-sulfamethoxazole |
| Coccidioidomycosis | Amphotericin B, fluconazole, or itraconazole |
| Congestive heart failure | Removal of all nonessential drugs followed by administration of furosemide (Lasix); digoxin; angiotensin-converting enzyme inhibition |
| Cryptococcal meningitis | Amphotericin B or fluconazole |
| Cytomegalovirus | Ganciclovir, foscarnet, cidofovir |
| Distal symmetric polyneuropathy | Pain management using tricyclic antidepressants, gabapentin, and narcotics for severe cases |
| Herpes simplex | Acyclovir, famciclovir, valacyclovir |
| Herpes zoster (shingles) | Acyclovir, valacyclovir, famciclovir, foscarnet |
| HIV-associated dementia complex | Antiretroviral therapy combining at least three drugs, two of which penetrate the blood-brain barrier |
| Histoplasmosis | Amphotericin B or itraconazole |
| Kaposi's sarcoma | Radiotherapy, cryotherapy with liquid nitrogen, daunorubicin hydrochloride, or doxorubicin hydrochloride injections |
| Lymphomas | Chemotherapy: cyclophosphamide, doxorubicin, vincristine, bleomycin, methotrexate, leucovorin |
| *Mycobacterium avium complex* | Clarithromycin, rifabutin, ciprofloxacin, ethambutol |
| Oral hairy leukoplakia | Acyclovir if symptoms present |
| *Pneumocystis carinii pneumonia* | Trimethoprim-sulfamethoxazole, dapsone, clindamycin, pentamidine isethionate |
| Progressive multifocal leukoencephalopathy | Antiretroviral therapy, acyclovir, i.v. cytosine, adenosine-arabinoside, interferon-alphas |
| Pulmonary hypertension | Low-flow $O_2$ if hypoxia present, vasodilators, including nitroglycerin, hydralazine, nifedipine, lisinopril, and prostaglandin E |

Table 10-5.  *Continued*

| Complication | Medication |
|---|---|
| Toxic neuronal neuropathy: neuropathy caused by certain medications | May be reversed with discontinuation or reduction in the following: zalcitabine, didanosine, and stavudine |
| Tuberculosis | Four-drug regimen: isoniazid, rifampin, pyrazinamide, and ethambutol |

Sources: Data from MD Cheitlin. Cardiovascular Complications of HIV Infection. In MA Sande, PA Volberding. The Medical Management of AIDS. Philadelphia: Saunders, 1999;278, 280; CA Kirton. Oncologic Conditions. In CA Kirton, D Talotta, K Zwolski (eds). Handbook of HIV/AIDS Nursing. St. Louis: Mosby, 2001;275, 278–279; RW Price. Management of the Neurologic Complications of HIV-1 Infection and AIDS. In MA Sande, PA Volberding (eds). The Medical Management of AIDS. Philadelphia: Saunders, 1999;227, 229, 231–232; K Zwolski. Fungal Infections. In CA Kirton, D Talotta, K Zwolski (eds). Handbook of HIV/AIDS Nursing. St. Louis: Mosby, 2001;262, 266, 270; K Zwolski. Parasitic Infections. In CA Kirton, D Talotta, K Zwolski (eds). Handbook of HIV/AIDS Nursing. St. Louis: Mosby, 2001;294; K Zwolski, D Talotta. Bacterial Infections. In CA Kirton, D Talotta, K Zwolski (eds). Handbook of HIV/AIDS Nursing. St. Louis: Mosby, 2001:236, 248–49; and K Zwolski. Viral Infections. In CA Kirton, D Talotta, K Zwolski (eds). Handbook of HIV/AIDS Nursing. St. Louis: Mosby, 2001;303, 310–311, 313, 315.

If management of mononucleosis is necessary, it may consist of the following[12,53]:

- Corticosteroids in cases of severe pharyngitis
- Bed rest during the acute stage
- Saline throat gargle
- Aspirin or acetaminophen for sore throat and fever

### Cytomegalovirus Infection

CMV is a member of the herpesvirus group that can be found in all body secretions, including saliva, blood, urine, feces, semen, cervical secretions, and breast milk. CMV infection is a common viral infection that is asymptomatic or symptomatic. CMV infection can remain latent after the initial introduction into the body and can become opportunistic at a later point in time.

If CMV infection is symptomatic, clinical presentation may be a relatively benign mononucleosis in adults, or in patients with HIV infection, manifestations such as pneumonia, hepatitis, encephalitis, esophagitis, colitis, and retinitis can occur.

CMV is usually transmitted by prolonged contact with infected body secretions, as well as congenitally or perinatally.[12,54]

Management of CMV infection may consist of the following[12,54]:

- Antiviral agents

- Corticosteroids

- Immune globulins

- Blood transfusions for anemia or thrombocytopenia

- Antipyretics

### Toxoplasmosis

*Toxoplasmosis* is a systemic protozoan infection caused by the parasite *Toxoplasma gondii,* which is primarily found in cat feces. Transmission can occur from three mechanisms: (1) eating raw or inadequately cooked infected meat or eating uncooked foods that have come in contact with contaminated meat; (2) inadvertently ingesting oocysts that cats have passed in their feces, either in a cat litter box or outdoors in soil (e.g., soil from gardening or unwashed fruits or vegetables); and (3) transmission of the infection from a woman to her unborn fetus. Fetal transmission of *T. gondii* can result in mental retardation, blindness, and epilepsy.[55]

Clinical manifestations can range from subclinical infection to severe generalized infection, particularly in immunocompromised individuals, to death.

The management trend of toxoplasmosis is through prevention by safe eating habits (thoroughly cooking meats, peeling and washing fruits and vegetables) and minimizing the contact with cat feces when pregnant, along with keeping the cat indoors to prevent contamination.[55]

## Sepsis

*Sepsis* is a general term that describes three progressive infectious conditions: bacteremia, septicemia, and shock syndrome (or *septic shock*).[12]

*Bacteremia* is a generally asymptomatic condition that results from bacterial invasion of blood from contaminated needles, catheters, monitoring transducers, or perfusion fluid. Bacteremia can also occur from a pre-existing infection from another body site. Bacteremia can resolve spontaneously or progress to septicemia.

*Septicemia* is a symptomatic extension of bacteremia throughout the body, with clinical presentations that are representative of the infective pathogen and the organ system(s) involved. Sites commonly affected are the brain, endocardium, kidneys, bones, and joints. Renal failure and endocarditis may also occur.

*Shock syndrome* is a critical condition of systemic tissue hypoperfusion that results from microcirculatory failure (i.e., decreased blood pressure or perfusion). Bacterial damage of the peripheral vascular system is the primary cause of the tissue hypoperfusion.

Management of sepsis may consist of any of the following[12]:

- Removal of suspected infective sources (e.g., lines or tubes)

- Anti-infective agents

- Blood pressure maintenance with adrenergic agents and corticosteroids

- i.v. fluids

- Blood transfusions

- Cardiac glycosides

- Supplemental oxygen, mechanical ventilation, or both

- Anticoagulation

## Management

### Medical Intervention

Management of the various infectious diseases discussed in this chapter is described in the specific sections of respective disorders. Appendix IV also lists common anti-infective agents used in treating infectious diseases.

## *Physical Therapy Intervention*

The following are general physical therapy goals and guidelines to be used when working with patients who have infectious disease processes, as well as disorders of altered immunity. These guidelines should be adapted to a patient's specific needs.

### Goals

The primary physical therapy goals in this patient population are similar to those of patient populations in the acute care setting: (1) to optimize the patient's functional mobility, (2) to maximize the patient's activity tolerance and endurance, and (3) to maximize ventilation and gas exchange in the patient who has pulmonary involvement.

### Guidelines for Physical Therapy Intervention

General physical therapy guidelines include, but are not limited to, the following:

1. The best modes of preventing the transmission of infectious diseases are to adhere to the standard precautions established by the CDC and to follow proper hand-washing techniques.

   • Facilities' warning or labeling systems for biohazards and infectious materials may vary slightly.

   • Be sure to check the patient's medical record or signs posted on doors and doorways for indicated precautions.

   • Table 10-4 provides an outline of the types of protective equipment that should be worn with specific precautions.

2. Patients who have infectious processes have an elevated metabolic rate, which will probably manifest as a high resting heart rate. Because of this, the activity intensity level should be modified, or more frequent rest periods should be incorporated during physical therapy treatment to enhance activity tolerance.

   • Patients with infectious processes will also be prone to orthostatic hypotension, hypotension with functional activities, or both as a result of the vasodilation occurring from the inflammation associated with infection.

- Therefore, slow changes in positions, especially from recumbent to upright positions, and frequent blood pressure monitoring are essential to promoting tolerance to functional activities.

3. Monitoring the temperature curve and WBC count of patients with infectious processes helps to determine the appropriateness of physical therapy intervention.

- There will be times when the infectious process worsens, and rest, rather than activity, is indicated. Clarification with the physician or nurse before physical therapy intervention is helpful in making this decision.

## References

1. Smeltzer SC, Bare BG. Brunner and Suddarth's Textbook of Medical-Surgical Nursing (7th ed). Philadelphia: Lippincott, 1992.
2. Thomas CL (ed). Taber's Cyclopedic Medical Dictionary (17th ed). Philadelphia: Davis, 1993.
3. Goodman CC, Snyder TEK. Differential Diagnosis in Physical Therapy: Musculoskeletal and Systemic Conditions. Philadelphia: Saunders, 1995.
4. Kent TH, Hart MN (eds). Introduction to Human Disease (4th ed). Stamford CT: Appleton & Lange, 1998;21–30.
5. Gorbach SL, Bartlett JG, Blacklow NR (eds). Infectious Diseases. Philadelphia: Saunders, 1992.
6. Delost MD. Introduction to Diagnostic Microbiology: A Text and Workbook. St. Louis: Mosby, 1997;1–9.
7. Malarkey LM, McMorrow ME (eds). Nurse's Manual of Laboratory Tests and Diagnostic Procedures (2nd ed). Philadelphia: Saunders, 2000;49–81.
8. Linne JJ, Ringsurd KM (eds). Clinical Laboratory Science: The Basics and Routine Techniques. St. Louis: Mosby, 1999;669–699.
9. Linne JJ, Ringsurd KM (eds). Clinical Laboratory Science: The Basics and Routine Techniques. St. Louis: Mosby, 1999;597–667.
10. Isenburg HD. Clinical Microbiology. In SL Borback, JG Bartlett, NR Blacklow (eds), Infectious Diseases. Philadelphia: Saunders, 1998;123–145.
11. Anderson KN (ed). Mosby's Medical, Nursing, and Allied Health Dictionary (4th ed). St. Louis: Mosby, 1994.
12. Thompson JM, McFarland GK, Hirsch JE, et al (eds). Mosby's Manual of Clinical Nursing (2nd ed). St. Louis: Mosby, 1989.
13. Malarkey LM, McMorrow ME (eds). Nurse's Manual of Laboratory Tests and Diagnostic Procedures (2nd ed). Philadelphia: Saunders, 2000;337–339.

14. Malarkey LM, McMorrow ME (eds). Nurse's Manual of Laboratory Tests and Diagnostic Procedures (2nd ed). Philadelphia: Saunders, 2000;779–782.
15. Malarkey LM, McMorrow ME (eds). Nurse's Manual of Laboratory Tests and Diagnostic Procedures (2nd ed). Philadelphia: Saunders, 2000;457–460.
16. Rice D, Eckstein EC. Inflammation and Infection. In WJ Phipps, JK Sands, JF Marek (eds), Medical-Surgical Nursing, Concepts and Clinical Practice (6th ed). St. Louis: Mosby, 1999;237–245.
17. Donegan NE. Management of Patients with Infectious Diseases. In SC Smeltzer, BG Bare (eds), Brunner and Suddarth's Textbook of Medical-Surgical Nursing (9th ed). Philadelphia: Lippincott, 2000; 1876–1877.
18. Lewis SM. Nursing Management: Inflammation and Infection. In SM Lewis, MM Heitkemper, SR Dirksen (eds), Medical-Surgical Nursing, Assessment and Management of Clinical Problems (5th ed). St. Louis: Mosby, 2000;201–202.
19. Black JM, Matassarin-Jacobs E (eds). Luckmann and Sorenen's Medical-Surgical Nursing: A Psychophysiologic Approach (4th ed). Philadelphia: Saunders, 1993.
20. Shovein J, Young MS. MRSA: Pandora's box for hospitals. Am J Nurs 1992;2:49.
21. The Hospital Infection Control Practices Advisory Committee. Special communication: recommendations for preventing the spread of vancomycin resistance. Am J Infect Control 1995;23:87.
22. Stedman's Medical Dictionary (27th ed). Philadelphia: Lippincott Williams & Wilkins, 1999.
23. Hickey MM, Hoffman LA. Nursing Management, Upper Respiratory Problems. In SM Lewis, MM Heitkemper, SR Dirksen (eds), Medical-Surgical Nursing, Assessment and Management of Clinical Problems (5th ed). St. Louis: Mosby, 2000;582–588.
24. Piessens WF, Nardell EA. Pathogenesis of Tuberculosis. In LB Reichman, ES Hershfield (eds), Tuberculosis: A Comprehensive International Approach (2nd ed). New York: Marcel Dekker, 2000;241–260.
25. Comstock GW. Epidemiology of Tuberculosis. In LB Reichman, ES Hershfield (eds), Tuberculosis A Comprehensive International Approach (2nd ed). New York: Marcel Dekker, 2000;129–56.
26. American Thoracic Society, CDC. Diagnostic standards and classification of tuberculosis in adults and children. Am J Resp Crit Care Med 2000;161:1376–1395.
27. Lobue PA, Perry S, Catanzaro A. Diagnostic of Tuberculosis. In LB Reichman, ES Hershfield (eds), Tuberculosis: A Comprehensive International Approach (2nd ed). New York: Marcel Dekker, 2000;341–376.
28. Hopewell PC, Chaisson RE. Tuberculosis and Human Immunodeficiency Syndrome Virus Infection. In LB Reichman, ES Hershfield (eds), Tuberculosis A Comprehensive International Approach (2nd ed). New York: Marcel Dekker, 2000;525–552.
29. Lewis SM. Nursing Management, Lower Respiratory Problems. In SM Lewis, MM Heitkemper, SR Dirksen (eds), Medical-Surgical Nursing,

Assessment and Management of Clinical Problems (5th ed). St. Louis: Mosby, 2000;629–630.
30. Puhlman M. Infectious Processes. In LC Copstead, JL Banasik (eds), Pathophysiology, Biological and Behavioral Perspectives (2nd ed). Philadelphia: Saunders, 2000;172–173.
31. Rytel MW, Mogabgab WJ (eds). Clinical Manual of Infectious Diseases. Chicago: Year Book, 1984.
32. Smeltzer SC, Bare BG (eds). Brunner and Suddarth's Textbook of Medical-Surgical Nursing (9th ed). Philadelphia: Lippincott, 2000;1884.
33. Kupper NS, Duke ES. Nursing Management, Inflammatory and Valvular Heart Diseases. In SM Lewis, MM Heitkemper, SR Dirksen (eds), Medical-Surgical Nursing, Assessment and Management of Clinical Problems (5th ed). St. Louis: Mosby, 2000;959–964.
34. Banasik JL. Alterations in Cardiac Function. In LC Copstead, JL Banasik (eds), Pathophysiology, Biological and Behavioral Perspectives (2nd ed). Philadelphia: Saunders, 2000;442–443.
35. Poliomyelitis Prevention in the United States: Updated Recommendations of the Advisory Committee on Immunization Practices (ACIP). MMWR Morb Mortal Wkly Rep 2000;49(RR05):1–22.
36. Berkow R, Fletcher AJ (eds). Merck Manual of Diagnosis and Therapy (16th ed). Rahway, NJ: Merck Research Laboratories, 1992.
37. Kerr ME. Nursing Management, Intracranial Problems. In SM Lewis, MM Heitkemper, SR Dirksen (eds), Medical-Surgical Nursing, Assessment and Management of Clinical Problems (5th ed). St. Louis: Mosby, 2000;1638–1643.
38. Boss BJ, Farley JA. Alterations in Neurologic Function. In SE Heuther, KL McCance (eds), Understanding Pathophysiology (2nd ed). St. Louis: Mosby, 2000;403–406.
39. Rhuda SC. Nursing Management, Musculoskeletal Problems. In SM Lewis, MM Heitkemper, SR Dirksen (eds), Medical-Surgical Nursing, Assessment and Management of Clinical Problems (5th ed). St. Louis: Mosby, 2000;1795–1798.
40. McCance KL, Mourad LA. Alterations in Musculoskeletal Function. In SE Heuther, KL McCance (eds). Understanding Pathophysiology (2nd ed). St. Louis: Mosby, 2000;1046–1048.
41. Rowland BM. Cellulitis. In K Boyden, D Olendorf (eds), Gale Encyclopedia of Medicine. Farmington Hills, MI: Gale Group, 1999;616.
42. Cellulitis Fact Sheet. National Institute of Allergy and Infectious Diseases, National Institutes of Health, Bethesda, MD. March 1999.
43. Kirchner JT. Use of blood cultures in patients with cellulitis. Am Fam Physician 2000;61(8):2518.
44. Barret J. Gastroenteritis. In K Boyden, D Olendorf (eds), Gale Encyclopedia of Medicine. Farmington Hills, MI: Gale Group, 1999;1258.
45. Flaskerud JH, Ungvarski PJ. Overview and Update of HIV Disease. In PJ Ungvarski, JH Flaskerud (eds), HIV/AIDS A Guide to Preliminary Care Management. Philadelphia: Saunders, 1999.
46. CDC. 1993 Revised Classification System for HIV Infection and Expanded Surveillance Case Definition for AIDS Among Adolescents and Adults. MMWR Morb Mortal Wkly Rep 1992;41(RR-17):1.

47. Malarkey LM, McMorrow ME (eds). Nurse's Manual of Laboratory Tests and Diagnostic Procedures (2nd ed). Philadelphia: Saunders, 2000.
48. Galantino ML. Clinical Assessment and Treatment of HIV: Rehabilitation of a Chronic Illness. Thorofare, NJ: Slack, 1992.
49. Ungvarski PJ, Angell J, Lancaster DJ, Manlapaz JP. Adolescents and Adults HIV Disease Care Management. In PJ Ungvarski, JH Flaskerud (eds). HIV/AIDS A Guide to Preliminary Care Management. Philadelphia: Saunders, 1999;131–193.
50. Price RW. Neurologic complications of HIV infection. Lancet 1996;348: 445.
51. Rosen MJ. Overview of pulmonary complications. Clin Chest Med 1996;17(4):621.
52. Yunis NA, Stone VE. Cardiac manifestations of HIV/AIDS. J Acquir Immune Defic Syndr Hum Retrovirol 1998;18:145.
53. Auwaerter PG. Infectious mononucleosis in middle age. (Grand Rounds at the Johns Hopkins Hospital). JAMA 1999;281(5):454.
54. Carson-De Witt RS. Cytomegalovirus infection. In K Boyden, D Olendorf (eds), Gale Encyclopedia of Medicine. Farmington Hills, MI: Gale Group, 1999;892.
55. Hughes JM, Colley DG. Preventing congenital toxoplasmosis. MMWR Morb Mortal Wkly Rep 2000;49(RR02):57–75.

# Appendix 10-A:
# Disorders of Altered Immunity

## Systemic Lupus Erythematosus

*Systemic lupus erythematosus* (SLE) is a chronic, multisystem autoimmune disease with strong genetic predisposition. There is also evidence suggesting risk factors that can trigger the onset of this disease, such as physical or emotional stress, pregnancy, sulfa antibiotics, and environmental factors, such as sun exposure. Women who are black, Asian, and Native American, ages 20–40 years, are more susceptible than men in acquiring this disease. SLE is characterized by a systemic, remitting and relapsing clinical presentation.[1-4]

Diagnosis of SLE is confirmed if a patient has four of the following 11 manifestations of SLE: malar rash, discoid rash (individual round lesions), photosensitivity, oral ulcers, arthritis, serositis, renal disorder, neurologic disorder, hematologic disorder, immunologic disorder, and the presence of antinuclear antibodies.[3]

Prognosis for 10-year survival after diagnosis is 90%. The most common cause of death in SLE is renal failure, and the second most common is CNS dysfunction.[1-3]

Clinical presentation of SLE may include the following[1-4]:

- Stiffness and pain in hands, feet, and large joints
- Red, warm, and tender joints

- Butterfly (malar) rash on face

- Fever, fatigue, anorexia, and weight loss

- Raynaud's phenomenon

- Headache, seizures, organic brain syndrome

- Hemolytic anemia, thrombocytopenia, leukopenia

- Renal disease or failure

Management of SLE may consist of nonsteroidal anti-inflammatory drugs, hydroxychloroquine and other antimalarial agents, glucocorticoids, immunosuppressive agents (cyclophosphamide), dialysis, and renal transplantation in severe cases.[1,2,4,5]

## Sarcoidosis

*Sarcoidosis* is a systemic disorder that primarily affects women and nonwhite adults in the third decade of their life. The definitive etiology is unknown, although an autoimmune process that is environmentally triggered is the generally agreed on hypothesis. Sarcoidosis may have periods of progression and remission.[1,5-7]

The lungs are the primary organs affected by sarcoidosis, with dyspnea, dry cough, and chest pain being common symptoms. Pulmonary involvement can be staged according to radiographic evidence[6,7]:

Stage 0—no radiographic abnormalities

Stage I—bilateral hilar lymphadenopathy

Stage II—bilateral hilar adenopathy and parenchymal infiltration

Stage III—parenchymal infiltration without hilar adenopathy

Stage IV—advanced fibrosis with evidence of honey-combing, hilar retraction, bullae, cysts, and emphysema

Other systems of the body can be affected as well, including the following:

- Eye and skin lesions

- Fever, fatigue, and weight loss

- Hepatosplenomegaly

- Hypercalcemia, anemia, and leukopenia

- Arthralgia, arthritis

Management of sarcoidosis usually consists of corticosteroid therapy, ranging from topical to oral administration. Additionally, cytotoxic agents (methotrexate and azathioprine), antimalarial agents (chloroquine and hydroxychloroquine), and nonsteroidal anti-inflammatory drugs may also be used. In severe cases of pulmonary disease, single and double lung transplantation may be performed.[1,5-7]

## Amyloidosis

Amyloidosis is a very rare metabolic disorder characterized by deposition of amyloid (a type of protein) in various tissues and organs. Amyloidosis is classified according to protein type and tissue distribution. The etiology of amyloidosis is not fully understood; however, relation to a disordered reticuloendothelial system and abnormal immunoglobulin synthesis has been shown.

Clinical signs and symptoms are representative of the affected areas. The following areas may be affected:

- Tongue

- Heart

- Gastrointestinal tract

- Liver

- Spleen

- Kidney

- Peripheral nerves

- Pancreas

- Cerebral vessels

- Skin

In general, the deposition of protein in these areas will result in firmer, less distensible tissues that compromise organ function.

Management of amyloidosis consists of controlling any primary disease process that may promote deposition of amyloid into the tissues.[1,8]

# References

1. Bullock BL. Pathophysiology: Adaptations and Alterations in Function (4th ed). Philadelphia: Lippincott, 1996.
2. Kimberly RP. Research advances in systemic lupus erythematosus. JAMA 2001;285(5):650.
3. McConnell EA. About systemic lupus erythematosus. Nursing 1999; 29(9):26.
4. Wallace DJ. Update on managing lupus erythematosus. J Musculoskeletal Med 1999;16(9):531.
5. Chandrasoma P, Taylor CR. Concise Pathology (2nd ed). East Norwalk, CT: Appleton & Lange, 1995.
6. Morey SS. American Thoracic Society issues consensus statement on sarcoidosis. Am Fam Physician 2000;61(2):553.
7. Johns CJ, Michele TM. The clinical management of sarcoidosis a 50-year experience at the Johns Hopkins Hospital. Medicine 1999; 78(2):65.
8. Goodman CC, Snyder TEK. Differential Diagnosis in Physical Therapy: Musculoskeletal and Systemic Conditions. Philadelphia: Saunders, 1995.

# 11

# Endocrine System
*Jaime C. Paz*

## Introduction

The endocrine system consists of endocrine glands, which secrete hormones into the bloodstream, and target cells for those hormones. Target cells are the principal sites of action for the endocrine glands. Figure 11-1 displays the location of the primary endocrine glands.

The endocrine system has direct effects on cellular function and metabolism throughout the entire body, with symptoms of endocrine, metabolic dysfunction, or both often mimicking those of muscle fatigue. Also, the onset of clinical manifestations from endocrine or metabolic dysfunction, or both, can often be insidious and subtle in presentation. Therefore, it is important for the physical therapist to carefully distinguish the source (endocrine versus musculoskeletal) of these symptoms to optimally care for the patient. For example, complaints of weakness and muscle cramps can result from hypothyroidism or inappropriate exercise intensity. If the therapist is aware of the patient's current endocrine system status, then inquiring about a recent medication adjustment may be more appropriate than adjusting the patient's exercise parameters.

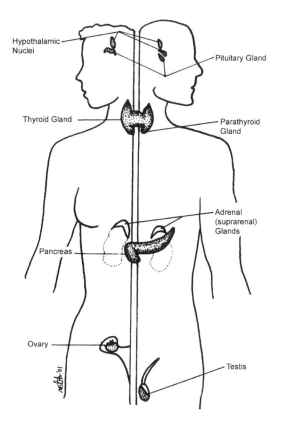

**Figure 11-1.** *Schematic representation of the primary endocrine glands in women and men. (Figure redrawn by Marybeth Cuaycong.)*

The objectives of this chapter are to provide a basic understanding of the following:

1.   Normal functions of the endocrine system, including the thyroid, pituitary, adrenal, and parathyroid glands, as well as the pancreas

2.   Clinical evaluation of these endocrine organs

3.   Endocrine system dysfunction and subsequent medical management

4.   Physical therapy guidelines for working with patients who have endocrine system dysfunction

## Screening for Metabolic and Endocrine Dysfunction

The following questions help to provide a systematic method to differentiate the patient's symptoms and complaints to a specific endocrine gland. Full integration of the patient's signs and symptoms with laboratory data by the physician is, however, necessary to accurately diagnose the disorder. Physical therapists can use these questions to help guide their evaluations and organize inquiries for the medical team regarding treatment parameters. For instance, if the questions lead the therapist to suspect pituitary involvement, seeking clarification from the physician regarding the appropriateness of physical therapy intervention may be necessary.[1]

1. Pituitary

    a. Are menses regular? (If they are irregular, hypopituitarism may be suspected.)

    b. Has there been a change in vision? (Large pituitary tumors can result in vision loss.)

2. Adrenal

    a. Is there skin darkening? (Chronic primary adrenal insufficiency results in hyperpigmentation.)

    b. Is there weight loss, nausea, vomiting, or syncope? (These are suggestive of adrenal insufficiency.)

    c. Have there been episodes of tachycardia, headaches, and sweating? (These are suggestive of pheochromocytoma.)

3. Thyroid

    a. Is there a change in the patient's neck size? (This can indicate the presence of goiter or hyperthyroidism.)

    b. What is the room-temperature preference of the patient? (60°F suggests hyperthyroidism, whereas 80°F suggests hypothyroidism.)

4. Parathyroid

    a. Is there a history of thyroid surgery? (This is the usual cause of hypoparathyroidism.)

    b. Are kidney stones, polyuria, and constipation present? (This could indicate hypercalcemia from hypoparathyroidism.)

5. Pancreas

   a. Is there nocturia or noctidipsia (urination or drinking at night, respectively)? (Both of these can suggest diabetes mellitus.)

   b. Has there been a weight loss or gain and increased appetite? (These also suggest diabetes.)

## General Evaluation of Endocrine Function

Measurement of endocrine function can be performed by examining (1) the endocrine gland itself, using imaging techniques, or (2) levels of hormones or hormone-related substances in the bloodstream or urine. When reviewing the medical record, it is important for the physical therapist to know that high or low levels of endocrine substances can indicate endocrine dysfunction. A common method for assessing levels of hormone is radioimmunoassay (RIA).[2] RIA is an immunologic technique for comparing levels of radiolabeled hormone with unlabeled hormone, which compete for binding sites on a given antibody.

Another method of evaluation, referred to as *provocative testing*, can be classified into suppression or stimulation tests. *Stimulation tests* are used for testing endocrine hypofunction; *suppression tests* are useful in evaluating endocrine hyperfunction.[3] The most commonly used endocrine tests are discussed in this chapter. Clinicians should refer to their particular institution's laboratory values (generally located in the back of the clinical record) for normal ranges of hormone or hormone-related substances referenced in their setting.

---

### Clinical Tip

An imbalance of hormone levels may affect the patient's tolerance to activity. Familiarity with the endocrine tests and values can help the clinician gauge the intended treatment parameters (i.e., type, duration, and intensity) for the next session(s).

---

## Thyroid Gland

### Function

The thyroid gland secretes three hormones: thyroxine (T4), triiodo-thyronine (T3), and calcitionin, with T4 and T3 commonly referred to as the *thyroid hormones*. Thyroxine and triiodothyronine require the presence of adequate amounts of iodine to be properly synthesized. Therefore, dietary deficiencies of iodine can hinder thyroid hormone production. The production and secretion of thyroid hormones are regulated by thyrotropin (also called *thyroid stimulating hormone* [TSH]), which is secreted from the anterior pituitary gland. TSH levels are directly influenced by T4 levels through a negative feedback loop. Thyrotropin is further regulated by thyrotropin releasing hormone, which is secreted from the hypothalamus.[4–6] Table 11-1 summarizes the target sites and actions of the thyroid gland hormones.

### Thyroid Tests

Thyroid hormones T4 and T3 circulate throughout the bloodstream bound to proteins (approximately 99%) or unbound, in which case

**Table 11-1.** Target Sites and Actions of Thyroid Gland Hormones

| Hormone(s) | Target Site(s) | Actions |
| --- | --- | --- |
| Thyroxine (T4) and triiodothy-ronine (T3) | Systemic | Increases metabolic rate, stimulates growth, and development of all cells, particularly of the nervous system, and enhances the effects of catecholamines |
| Thyrocalcitonin | Bone | Inhibits bone resorption Lowers blood levels of calcium |

Sources: Data from BF Fuller. Anatomy and Physiology of the Endocrine System. In CM Hudak, BM Gallo (eds), Critical Care Nursing: A Holistic Approach (6th ed). Philadelphia: Lippincott, 1994;75; M Hartog (ed). Endocrinology. Oxford, UK: Blackwell Scientific, 1987;3; and JV Corbett. Laboratory Tests and Diagnostic Procedures with Nursing Diagnoses (5th ed). Upper Saddle River, NJ: Prentice Hall Health, 2000;409.

**Table 11-2.** Thyroid Hormone Tests

| Hormone | Test Description | Normal Value |
|---|---|---|
| Serum thyroxine | Radioimmunoassay (RIA) measurement. | 4–12 µg/dl |
| Serum triiodo-thyronine | RIA measurement. | 40–204 ng/dl |
| Free thyroxine index | Direct RIA measurement or indirect calculated measurement. | Direct: 0.8–2.7 ng/ml Indirect: 4.6–11.2 ng/ml |
| Thyroid-stimulating hormone (TSH) | Radioisotope and chemical labeling measurement. | 0.4–8.9 µU/ml |
| Thyrotropin-releasing hormone (TRH) TRH augments the function of TSH in patients with hypothyroidism. Only performed in difficult diagnostic cases. | Intravenous administration of TRH to patients. The expected response is a rise in TSH levels. | Normal rise in men and women is 6 µU/ml above baseline TSH levels. Normal rise in men older than 40 years is 2 µU/ml above baseline. Hypothyroidism is indicated by increased response to TRH. Hyperthyroidism is indicated by no response to TRH. |

Sources: Data from WM Burch (ed). Endocrinology for the House Officer (2nd ed). Baltimore: Williams & Wilkins, 1988;1; JV Corbett (ed). Laboratory Tests and Diagnostic Procedures with Nursing Diagnoses (5th ed). Upper Saddle River, NJ: Prentice Hall Health, 2000;409–413; LM Malarkey, ME McMorrow (eds). Nurse's Manual of Laboratory Tests and Diagnostic Procedures. Philadelphia: Saunders, 2000;604–612; and RA Sacher, RA McPherson, JM Campos (eds). Widman's Clinical Interpretation of Laboratory Tests (11th ed). Philadelphia: FA Davis, 2000;786–793.

they are metabolically active by themselves. Thyroxine-binding globulin (TBG) is the major thyroid transport protein. Serum levels of T4 and T3 are usually measured by RIA. Table 11-2 describes the tests used to measure thyroid hormones, and Table 11-3 summarizes other tests used to measure thyroid function.

**Table 11-3.** Thyroid Function Tests

| Test | Description |
|------|-------------|
| Triiodothyronine resin uptake (RT3U) | RT3U indirectly measures the number of unoccupied protein binding sites for serum thyroxine (T4) and serum triiodothyronine (T3) by using radioisotopes. RT3U qualifies levels of bound versus unbound T4 and T3. Thyroid hormone uptake is high with hyperthyroidism and low with hypothyroidism. |
| Thyroidal 24-hr radioactive iodine uptake | Used to determine metabolic activity of the thyroid gland. Radioactive iodine is administered, and the percentage of total administered radioactive iodine taken up by the thyroid in 24 hrs is then calculated. Normal radioactive iodine uptake is 5–30%. Hypothyroidism results in reduced uptake. |
| Thyroid imaging or scan | Intravenous administration of radionuclides allows imaging or scanning of particular areas of the thyroid gland. Increased or decreased uptake of the radionuclide can help diagnose dysfunction. |
| Ultrasound | Nodules of the thyroid gland that are palpable or suspected may be delineated as cystic or solid lesions by ultrasound. |
| Needle biopsy | Fine needle aspiration of thyroid cells may help diagnose a suspected neoplasm. |

Sources: Data from WM Burch (ed). Endocrinology for the House Officer (2nd ed). Baltimore: Williams & Wilkins, 1988;1; M Hartog (ed). Endocrinology. Oxford, UK: Blackwell Scientific, 1987;25; and RA Sacher, RA McPherson, JM Campos (eds). Widman's Clinical Interpretation of Laboratory Tests (11th ed). Philadelphia: FA Davis, 2000;786–793.

---

## Clinical Tip

- Low levels of thyroid hormones T3 or T4 may result in weakness, muscle aching, and stiffness. Based on this information, the physical therapist may decide to alter treatment parameters by decreasing the treatment intensity to optimize activity tolerance, minimize patient discomfort, or both.

- Patients may be on bed rest or precautions after radio-nuclide studies. The physical therapist should refer to the physician's orders after testing to clarify the patient's mobility status.

---

### Thyroid Disorders

Disorders of the thyroid gland result from a variety of causes and can be classified as hyper- or hypothyroidism.

#### Hyperthyroidism

*Hyperthyroidism*, or *thyrotoxicosis*, is characterized by excessive sympathomimetic and catabolic activity resulting from overexposure of tissues to thyroid hormones. The most common causes of hyperthyroidism are outlined in Table 11-4.

General signs and symptoms of hyperthyroidism include the following[1,6]:

- Nervousness, irritation, and emotional lability

- Fatigue, weakness, and weight loss despite normal or increased appetite

- Palpitations, atrial fibrillation (common above the age of 60 years), and tachycardia (heart rate of more than 90 beats per minute at rest)

- Increased perspiration, moist and warm hands, and smooth and velvety skin

- Heat intolerance

- Diarrhea

- Menstrual dysfunction

- Presence of goiter

- Tremor

- Lid lag, retraction, or both

- "Plumber's nails" (onycholysis)

- Thyroid bruit

**Table 11-4.**  Common Causes of Hyperthyroidism

| Cause | Description |
|---|---|
| Graves' disease | A familial, autoimmune disorder responsible for approximately 80–90% of hyperthyroid cases. Occurs more commonly in women than men. Distinguishing features include diffuse thyroid enlargement, ophthalmopathy (double vision and sensitivity to light), exophthalmos (excessive prominence of the eyes), pretibial myxedema (thickening, redness, and puckering of skin in the front of the tibia), atrial fibrillation, fine hand tremors, and weakness of the quadriceps muscle. |
| Thyroiditis | Inflammation of the thyroid gland can result from an acute bacterial infection, a subacute viral infection, or chronic inflammation with unknown etiology. Pain may or may not be present on palpation of the gland. |
| Toxic nodular and multinodular goiter | Areas of the enlarged thyroid gland (goiter) become autonomous and produce excessive amounts of thyroid hormones. |
| Thyroid adenoma | Solitary, benign follicular adenomas that function autonomously result in hyperthyroidism if the adenoma nodule is larger than 4 cm in diameter. May present as a painless lump in the throat. |
| Thyroid carcinoma | Four types of malignancies in the thyroid gland: papillary carcinoma (most common), follicular carcinoma, anaplastic carcinoma, and medullary carcinoma. |
| Exogenous hyperthyroidism | Ingestion of excessive amounts of thyroid hormone or iodine preparation. Can be classified as iatrogenic hyperthyroidism, factitious hyperthyroidism, or iodine-induced hyperthyroidism. |
| Ectopic thyroid hormone production | Thyroid hormone can be produced from the ovaries or from metastatic follicular thyroid carcinoma (rare occurrence). |

Sources: Data from WM Burch (ed). Endocrinology for the House Officer (2nd ed). Baltimore: Williams & Wilkins, 1988;126; and N Woolf (ed). Pathology, Basic and Systemic. London: Saunders, 1998;863–873.

Management of hyperthyroidism may consist of any of the following[7-9]:

- Pharmacologic management with the following:

    Antithyroid medications of the thionamide series (e.g., propylthiouracil, methimazole [Tapazole], carbimazole [used only in Europe and the United Kingdom])

    Beta-adrenergic blockers (e.g., propranolol [Inderal])

    Iodine (e.g., potassium or sodium iodide [strong iodine solution, Lugol's solution])

    Corticosteroids

- Radioiodine-131

- Surgical subtotal-thyroidectomy (indicated for patients who are pregnant, children who have adverse reactions to antithyroid medications, patients with excessively large goiters that are compressive, and patients with thyroid carcinoma)

**Hypothyroidism**
*Hypothyroidism* is the insufficient exposure of peripheral tissues to thyroid hormones. It affects growth and development, as well as many cellular processes. In the majority of cases, hypothyroidism is caused by decreased thyroid hormone production rather than the failure of tissues to respond to thyroid hormones. *Primary hypothyroidism* refers to thyroid gland dysfunction, whereas *secondary hypothyroidism* refers to pituitary disease resulting in reduced TSH levels.

The following are the causes of primary and secondary hypothyroidism[7,10]:

- Maldevelopment, hypoplasia, or aplasia of the thyroid gland

- Inborn deficiencies of biosynthesis or action of thyroid hormone

- Hashimoto's thyroiditis (autoimmune inflammation)

- Lymphatic thyroiditis (autoimmune inflammation that has hyperthyroid symptoms)

- Hypopituitarism or hypothalamic disease

- Severe iodine deficiency

- Thyroid ablation from surgery, radiation of cervical neoplasms, or radioiodine therapy for hyperthyroidism

- Drug toxicity (from amiodarone, antithyroids, or lithium)

General signs and symptoms of hypothyroidism vary according to the degree of thyroid deficiency. Signs and symptoms include the following[1,6]:

- Lethargy, somnolence, and slowness of thought

- Constipation and ileus (decreased motility)

- Rough, scaly, dry, and cool skin and decreased perspiration

- Slow relaxation time of deep tendon reflexes

- Marked cold intolerance

- Weakness, muscle cramps, and aching and stiffness

- Hoarseness and decreased hearing

- Paresthesia

- Pallid and yellow-tinted skin

- Nonpitting edema of eyelids, hands, and feet

- Bradycardia with elevated systolic and diastolic blood pressure

- Cardiac failure

- Pericardial effusion

- Coma and respiratory failure in severe cases

Management of hypothyroidism typically consists of lifelong thyroid hormone replacement. Medications commonly used to treat hypothyroidism are the following[8,9]:

- Synthetic thyroid hormones (e.g., levothyroxine sodium [Cytolen, Levoid, Levothroid, Synthroid], liothyronine [Cytomel, Cytomine], and liotrix [Euthroid, Thyrolar])

- Natural thyroid hormones (e.g., Decloid, Thyrar, Thryrocrine, ThryroTeric, and thyroglobulin [Proloid])

- Adenohypophyseal hormones (e.g., TSH [Thytropar] and thyrotropin-releasing hormone [i.e., protirelin])

---

**Clinical Tip**

Properly managed hyper- or hypothyroidism should not affect physical therapy intervention or activity tolerance. If the signs or symptoms mentioned above are present during physical therapy evaluation, treatment, or both, consultation with the medical team is indicated to help differentiate the etiology of the physical findings. See Screening for Metabolic and Endocrine Dysfunction for more information on screening.

---

## Pituitary Gland

### Function

Hormones secreted by the pituitary gland are responsible for a variety of functions that are summarized in Table 11-5. Secretions of hormones from the pituitary glands are closely regulated by the hypothalamus and by negative feedback from the hormones that are secreted from the pituitary gland.[6]

### Pituitary Tests

Individual pituitary hormone levels can be measured (1) by random blood samples; (2) by blood samples before and after the administration of specific releasing substances, such as serum TSH, during a thyrotropin-releasing hormone test (see Table 11-2); or (3) by blood samples before and after the administration of specific stimuli acting directly on the pituitary or via the hypothalamus, such as serum growth hormone (GH), serum cortisol, and plasma adrenocorticotropic hormone (ACTH).

Table 11-6 describes common tests of pituitary function. Pituitary function can also be evaluated by (1) thyroid function tests, which are an indirect assessment of TSH secretion from the pituitary, and (2) plain x-rays or computed tomography with contrast to highlight a pituitary tumor.[11]

**Table 11-5.** Target Sites and Actions of Pituitary Gland Hormones

| Hormone(s) | Target Site(s) | Action(s) |
|---|---|---|
| **Anterior lobe** | | |
| Growth hormone | Systemic | Growth of bones, muscles, and other organs |
| | Liver | Formation of somatomedin |
| Thyrotropin | Thyroid | Growth and secretion activity of the thyroid gland |
| Adrenocorticotropin | Adrenal cortex | Growth and secretion activity of the adrenal cortex |
| Follicle-stimulating hormone | Ovaries | Development of follicles and secretion of estrogen |
| | Testes | Development of seminiferous tubules and spermatogenesis |
| Luteinizing or interstitial cell stimulating hormone | Ovaries | Ovulation, formation of corpus luteum, and secretion of progesterone |
| | Testes | Secretion of testosterone |
| Prolactin or lactogenic hormone | Mammary glands | Secretion of milk |
| Melanocyte-stimulating hormone | Skin | Pigmentation |
| **Posterior lobe** | | |
| Antidiuretic hormone* (also called *vasopressin*) | Kidney | Reabsorption of water Fluid and electrolyte balance |
| Oxytocin* | Arterioles | Blood pressure regulation |
| | Uterus | Contraction |
| | Breast | Expression of milk |

*Actually produced in the hypothalamus but stored in the pituitary gland.
Sources: Data from BF Fuller. Anatomy and Physiology of the Endocrine System. In CM Hudak, BM Gallo (eds), Critical Care Nursing: A Holistic Approach (6th ed). Philadelphia: Lippincott, 1994;875; and RA Sacher, RA McPherson, JM Campos (eds). Widman's Clinical Interpretation of Laboratory Tests (11th ed). Philadelphia: FA Davis, 2000;744.

Table 11-6. Pituitary Hormone Tests

| Hormone(s) | Test Description |
|---|---|
| Growth hormone (GH) | Serum level measurement by radioimmunoassay (RIA); normal values for men are 0–5 ng/ml; for women, 0–10 ng/ml.<br><br>*Growth hormone stimulation test* (arginine test or insulin tolerance test). Indicated for children with retarded growth and if pituitary tumor is suspected. A baseline level of GH is established, then arginine or insulin is administered to the patient, and serial blood draws are performed to measure GH levels. GH should normally rise. Decreased GH values, despite stimulation, could indicate pituitary dwarfism or tumors.<br><br>*Growth hormone suppression test* (glucose load test). Indicated to confirm diagnoses of gigantism in children and acromegaly in adults. A baseline level of GH is established, followed by patient ingestion of a glucose solution. After 1–2 hrs, levels of GH are remeasured. Normally, glucose inhibits the secretion of GH. If GH levels remain high despite the glucose load, then gigantism or acromegaly can be confirmed. |
| Adrenocorticotropic hormone (ACTH) | Plasma ACTH levels are measured by RIA. Normal values are 25–100 pg/ml in the morning and 0–50 pg/ml in the evening.<br><br>*ACTH stimulation test* (rapid ACTH testing, cosyntropin test, or Cortrosyn stimulating test). Indicated for diagnosing primary and secondary adrenal insufficiency. Cosyntropin (Cortrosyn) (synthetic form of ACTH) is administered to a patient after a baseline level of cortisol is measured. ACTH acts to increase cortisol secretion from the adrenal gland. Normal results show an increased plasma cortisol level to >20 μg/dl after 30–60 mins. |
| Antidiuretic hormone (ADH or vasopressin) | Normal plasma levels of ADH are 2–12 pg/ml if serum osmolality is >290 mOsm/kg and <2 if serum osmolality is <290 mOsm/kg.<br><br>*Water deprivation test* (dehydration test or concentration test). Indicated for diagnosing diabetes insipidus (DI). Normally, if water is withheld, ADH levels rise to help increase water reabsorption in the kidneys. During the test, the patient is deprived of fluids, and serial measurements of urine osmolality are taken. Normally, ADH secretion causes a change in urine osmolality, but |

| Hormone(s) | Test Description |
|---|---|
| | with DI, the osmolality remains unchanged. While the patient is being deprived of water, vasopressin may be administered to help delineate whether the DI is caused by pituitary or renal dysfunction. *Water loading test.* Indicated for diagnosing syndrome of inappropriate antidiuretic hormone (SIADH). During the test, the patient ingests 20–25 ml/kg of fluid, with hourly serum and urine osmolality levels being measured for 4 hrs. Normally, with water ingestion, the plasma and urine osmolality should decrease, and urine output should increase. With SIADH, there is little or no change in these values. |

Source: Data from LM Malarkey, ME McMorrow (eds). Nurse's Manual of Laboratory Tests and Diagnostic Procedures. Philadelphia: Saunders, 2000;580–584, 552–555, 613–614, 616–619.

## Pituitary Disorders

Dysfunction of the pituitary-hypothalamic system generally results from hyper- or hyposecretion of tropic hormones. Hypersecretion of pituitary hormones (*hyperpituitarism*) is most commonly due to benign anterior pituitary tumors. Hyposecretion of pituitary hormones (*pituitary insufficiency*) can result from pituitary disease, diseases affecting the hypothalamus or surrounding structures, or disturbance of blood flow around the hypothalamus and pituitary.[12,13]

### Hyperpituitarism

The overproduction of the pituitary hormones GH, ACTH, and antidiuretic hormone (ADH) is discussed below.

#### Growth Hormone Overproduction

The most common presentation of excessive GH secretion is *acromegaly* in adults or *gigantism* in children. Excessive GH secretion has been linked primarily to anterior pituitary adenomas and not necessarily from excessive hypothalamic stimulation of the pituitary.[13]

Signs and symptoms of acromegaly include the following[1,13]:

- Enlargement of hands and feet, coarse facial features with furrowed brows

- Oligomenorrhea or amenorrhea in women

- Paresthesia of hands, carpal tunnel syndrome

- Sweating

- Headaches

- Impotence in men

- Diabetes mellitus

- Hypertension

- Joint pains, osteoarthritis

Management of acromegaly may consist of the following: transphenoid surgical resection of anterior pituitary adenoma (treatment of choice), GH suppression with somatostatin and its analogs (octreotide), or with dopamine agonists and external irradiation as a last resort.[14]

---

**Clinical Tip**

Given the multisystem effects in patients with acromegaly, activity progression should proceed cautiously, with a focus on energy conservation and joint protection techniques.

---

*Adrenocorticotropic Hormone Overproduction*
An increase in ACTH production by the pituitary gland results in increased levels of serum cortisol, which is a glucocorticoid secreted by the adrenal glands. Glucocorticoids are involved with carbohydrate, protein, and fat metabolism; therefore, excess cortisol levels affect these cellular processes. Any clinical syndrome that results in glucocorticoid excess is called *Cushing's syndrome. Cushing's disease*, however, is specific to pituitary lesions that cause bilateral adrenal hyperplasia and is not discussed in this chapter.[1] Pituitary hypersecretion of ACTH occurs in approximately 70% of the patients with Cushing's syndrome. The hypersecretion of ACTH is mainly from pituitary adenomas or microadenomas.[6]
Signs and symptoms of Cushing's syndrome include the following[6,11,13]:

- Truncal obesity with thin extremities

- Redness and rounding of the face (moon face)

- Easy bruising, thinning of the skin, and presence of striae and darker pigmentation

- Hirsutism, oligomenorrhea, or amenorrhea

- Hypertension

- Osteoporosis (radiographically confirmed)

- Proximal muscle weakness

- Backache

- Glucose intolerance

Management of Cushing's syndrome may consist of any of the following: surgical resection of pituitary lesion, radiation or chemotherapy for the lesion, or medical management with steroidogenic inhibitors (ketoconazole, mitotane, etomidate, metyrapone, and aminoglutethimide) or neuromodulators of ACTH release (valproic acid, bromocriptine, and cyproheptadine). Surgical resection of the adrenal glands is a last-resort measure.[14]

---

**Clinical Tip**

Management of weakness, myopathy, pain, edema, and osteoporosis should be the focus of physical therapy intervention and be complementary to the medical management of the patient. Blood pressure changes during activity should be monitored, given the possibility of hypertension. Caution should also be taken to avoid bruising during mobility. Refer to Diabetes Mellitus for further activity considerations.

---

*Antidiuretic Hormone Overproduction*
The syndrome of inappropriate secretion of ADH (SIADH) is a condition of fluid and electrolyte imbalance resulting in hyponatremia (reduced sodium levels) from excessive water reabsorption. In this condition, ADH is secreted from the posterior pituitary when it should be inhibited.

Numerous etiologies of SIADH exist, with the most frequent cause being small cell or oat cell carcinomas of the lung. Other etiologies include the following[8,15]:

- Bacterial pneumonias, chronic obstructive pulmonary disease, tuberculosis, lung abscesses

- Malignancies of the pancreas, duodenum, colon, lymphoid tissue, and thymus

- Medication side effects from antipsychotics, sedative-hypnotics, diuretics, antihypertensives, analgesics, cardiac drugs, and antibiotics

- Head trauma, central nervous system neoplasms

A mild condition of SIADH is usually asymptomatic. More severe cases, however, can result in fluid and electrolyte imbalances, resulting in interstitial edema from a lack of serum sodium. Many systems will be affected by this edema, with the nervous system being most severely involved. Manifestations can include any of the following: headaches, nausea, confusion, increased blood pressure, peripheral edema, and cerebral edema that leads to seizures and coma (in severe cases).[15]

Management of SIADH may consist of any of the following: treatment of the underlying cause, fluid restriction, intravenous administration of sodium chloride solution, or administration of diuretics (furosemide).[15]

---

Clinical Tip

The physical therapist should be aware of fluid restriction guidelines for patients with SIADH, especially because activity during physical therapy may increase the patient's thirst. These guidelines are often posted at the patient's bedside.

---

Hypopituitarism

There are numerous causes for primary (pituitary directly affected) or secondary (hypothalamus or pituitary stalk affected) hypopituitarism. The most common causes of primary hypopituiatarism are pituitary neoplasms, such as pituitary adenomas and craniopharyngioma, and ischemic necrosis occurring during the late stages of pregnancy (Sheehan's syndrome). Common causes of secondary hypopituitarism include hypothalamic tumors, cranial trauma, sarcoidosis, surgical destruction of the pituitary stalk, or a combination of these.[6,13,16,17]

Symptoms, physical findings, and management depend on the extent of the disorder and the specific hormone and target cells involved. Patients with complete pituitary hormone deficiency (panhypopituitarism) present with the following[11,16]:

- Hypogonadism

- Amenorrhea, regression of secondary sexual characteristics, and infertility

- Dilutional hyponatremia

- Diabetes insipidus (DI)

- Short stature (in children)

- Hypothyroidism

- Glucocorticoid deficiency

Management of panhypopituitarism may consist of any of the following: replacement therapy or pituitary hormones, such as thyroxine, glucocorticoids, and GH for children; desmopressin for DI; androgen therapy for men; or estrogen therapy for women younger than 50 years of age. Management of other clinical sequelae of hypopituitarism will be specific to the involved areas.[11,16]

## Diabetes Insipidus

DI involves the excretion of a large volume (i.e., greater than 30 ml/kg per day) of dilute urine (hypotonic polyuria). DI may result from hypothalamic, pituitary, renal, or psychogenic disorders; however, most incidences of DI are described as idiopathic.[6,18] Pituitary DI involves the failure to synthesize or release vasopressin (ADH). Renal, or nephrogenic, DI is a deficiency of vasopressin receptors in the renal collecting ducts. Psychogenic or dipsogenic DI involves a large intake of fluid that may suppress ADH secretion.[7,8,11,18]

Signs and symptoms of DI may be transient or permanent and include the following[7,8,16,18]:

- Polyuria, nocturia

- Thirst (especially for cold or iced drinks), polydipsia

- Dehydration

- Weight loss

- Dry skin with decreased turgor

- Central nervous system manifestations (e.g., irritability, mental dullness, ataxia, hyperthermia, and coma) if access to water is interrupted

Management of neurogenic (hypothalamic or pituitary dysfunction) DI may consist of pharmacologic treatment, such as the following: aqueous vasopressin or deamino-8-D-arginine vasopressin (Desmopressin), chlorpropamide (Diabinase), and clofibrate (Atromid-S).

Management of nephrogenic (renal) DI may consist of diuretics such as hydrochlorothiazide (HydroDIURIL), in combination with a sodium-restricted diet.[7,8,19]

## Adrenal Gland

### *Function*

The adrenal gland has two distinct areas, the outer cortex and the inner medulla, that differ in their function and embryologic origin.[6] Table 11-7 summarizes the target sites and actions of the adrenal gland.

### *Adrenal and Metabolic Tests*

#### Adrenal Tests

Evaluation of the adrenal cortical (glucocorticoids, androgens, and mineralocorticoids) and medullary (epinephrine and norepinephrine) hormones is described below. Anatomic investigation of the adrenal glands may also be performed to diagnose possible adrenal dysfunction. Common methods to accomplish this are computed tomography scan (to identify adrenal tumors), radioisotope scan using seleno-cholesterol, ultrasound, arteriogram, adrenal venogram (allows measurements of hormone levels), and intravenous pyelogram (see Diagnostic Tests in Chapter 9).[11,20]

**Table 11-7.** Target Sites and Actions of Adrenal Gland Hormones

| Hormone(s) | Target site(s) | Action(s) |
| --- | --- | --- |
| Cortex | | |
| Mineralocorticoids (aldosterone) | Kidney | Reabsorption of sodium and water |
| | | Elimination of potassium |
| Glucocorticoids (cortisol) | Systemic | Metabolism of carbohydrate, protein, and fat |
| | | Response to stress |
| | | Suppresses immune responses |
| | | Anti-inflammation |
| Sex hormones (androgens, progesterone, and estrogen) | Systemic | Preadolescent growth spurt, affects secondary sex characteristics |
| Medulla | | |
| Epinephrine | Cardiac and smooth muscle, glands | Emergency functions |
| | | Stimulates the action of the sympathetic system |
| Norepinephrine | Organs innervated by sympathetic nervous system | Chemical transmitter substance |
| | | Increases peripheral resistance |

Sources: Data from BF Fuller. Anatomy and Physiology of the Endocrine System. In CM Hudak, BM Gallo (eds), Critical Care Nursing: A Holistic Approach (6th ed). Philadelphia: Lippincott, 1994;875; and JV Corbett (ed). Laboratory Tests and Diagnostic Procedures with Nursing Diagnoses (5th ed). Upper Saddle River, NJ: Prentice Hall Health, 2000;391.

*Glucocorticoids*

Glucocorticoids can be evaluated by testing serum and urine cortisol levels, 24-hour urinary corticosteroids, or ACTH. Altered glucocorticoid levels can affect protein and carbohydrate metabolism.

• Serum cortisol levels are measured by RIA, which is indicated for diagnosing Cushing's or Addison's disease. For accuracy, notation should be made as to the time of day the serum was drawn, because levels are highly dependent on the diurnal rhythm of secretion. Normal serum levels are 5–23 µg/dl (8–10 AM) and 3–16 µg/dl (4–6 PM).[21]

• Twenty-four–hour urinary corticosteroids. Analysis of urine over a 24-hour period to determine the urinary levels of corticosteroids will provide a rough outline of cortisol output. Also indicated for diagnosing Cushing's or Addison's disease. Normal urine levels are 20–90 µg/dl for a 24-hour period.[22]

• ACTH levels are usually examined concomitantly with cortisol levels, as ACTH secretion from the pituitary gland is necessary for cortisol secretion from the adrenal glands. Refer to Table 11-6 for details on ACTH measurement.

*Androgens*

Individual androgen levels can be measured by RIA in the serum or by metabolic products (17-ketosteroids) in the urine.[1,6] High concentrations of androgens may result in the following changes in women:

• *Hirsutism,* which is excessive hair growth in skin zones considered male in distribution (i.e., upper lip, side burns, chin, neck, chest, and lower abdomen)

• *Amenorrhea,* which is the absence of menstruation in women older than 16 years of age or the absence of menses for longer than 6 months in women of childbearing age who previously had been menstruating

• Voice change

• Increased muscle mass

*Mineralocorticoids*

Mineralocorticoids can be evaluated by testing serum electrolyte levels or plasma renin activity and aldosterone levels.[11] Abnormalities of serum electrolyte levels, such as an increased potassium level, provide a valuable screening tool for mineralocorticoid secretion disorders. Aldosterone is the primary mineralocorticoid and is controlled by the renin-angiotensin system. A rise in serum potassium and angiotensin II results in aldosterone secretion, which helps to balance fluid and electrolyte levels. Blood samples of aldosterone are usually taken first in the early morning, while the patient is still recumbent, and then again after 4 hours of being awake and active. Normal serum levels of aldosterone range from 2 to 50 ng/dl, depending on whether blood was taken in the supine or upright position.[4,5,11]

*Catecholamines*
Epinephrine and norepinephrine are commonly referred to as *catecholamines*, and their levels are generally measured through 24-hour urine samples. Dopamine, also a catecholamine, is the precursor for epinephrine and norepinephrine and therefore can also be measured to reflect the amount of catecholamines circulating in the body. However, the preferred screening tool is to measure the amount of catecholamine metabolites in the urine. The primary catecholamine metabolite is called *vanillylmandelic acid* (VMA). Normal values for these substances are as follows[4,5]:

Dopamine: 65–100 µg per 24 hours

Epinephrine: 1.7–22.4 µg per 24 hours

Norepinephrine: 12.1–85.5 µg per 24 hours

Vanillylmandelic acid: 1.4–6.5 µg per 24 hours

**Metabolic Tests**

Metabolic tests are described in this section, as glucocorticoids (cortisol) affect carbohydrate, protein, and fat metabolism.

*Glucose Tolerance Test*
A glucose tolerance test was primarily used to diagnose diabetes mellitus; however, because of many confounding variables, it is currently not relied on to establish diabetes mellitus, but rather to help confirm the diagnosis in certain cases. However, the glucose tolerance test is the primary method of establishing the diagnosis of gestational diabetes mellitus.[4,6]

To perform the test, a 75- or 100-g glucose load is given to the subject in the morning after a 10-hour fast. Blood glucose levels are then measured at variable time periods, ranging from every half hour to every hour for the next 2 to 5 hours after the glucose administration. The subject must remain inactive and refrain from smoking throughout the duration of the test. Normally, the blood glucose levels should fall back to baseline values after a 2-hour period. Normal glucose value for a fasting blood sugar (BS) is approximately 70–110 mg/dl.[1,4,6]

## Adrenal Disorders

### Adrenal Insufficiency

Autoimmune dysfunction can lead to destruction of the adrenal cortex (i.e., *primary adrenal insufficiency* or *Addison's disease*). Additionally, ACTH deficiency from the pituitary gland can lead to atrophy of the adrenal cortex (*secondary adrenal insufficiency*). The net result is an impaired adrenal system with decreased levels of glucocorticoids (cortisols), mineralocorticoids (aldosterone), and androgens. Given the systemic functions of these hormones, Addison's disease can have severe consequences if left untreated. Fortunately, the incidence is rare.

Cortisol deficiency results in decreased gluconeogenesis (glucose production), which in turn alters cellular metabolism. Decreased gluconeogenesis also results in hypoglycemia and decreased ability to respond to stress. Aldosterone deficiency causes fluid and electrolyte imbalance, primarily as a result of increased water excretion that leads to dehydration.[23,24]

The following are symptoms and physical findings common to adrenal insufficiency[1,6,25]:

- Weakness, fatigue

- Weight loss, nausea, vomiting, vague abdominal pain

- Muscle and joint pain

- Salt craving in fewer than 20% of patients

- Hyperpigmentation

- Hypotension

Management of adrenal insufficiency typically consists of pharmacologic intervention with any of the following steroids: hydrocortisone (Cortisol, Compound F), hydrocortisone acetate, prednisone (Deltasone), dexamethasone (Decadron, Dexasone), or fludrocortisone (Florinef).[8,18] Caution must be taken, however, with corticosteroid administration, as corticosteroids can suppress the release of endogenous cortisol from the adrenal gland.[26]

### Pheochromocytoma

Pheochromocytoma is a rare adrenomedullary disorder caused by a tumor of the chromaffin cells in the adrenal medulla, which results in excess secretion of the catecholamines, epinephrine, and norepinephrine. The occurrence is equal between men and women during their twenties and thirties. Given the rare occurrence of this tumor, it often goes undiagnosed. However, proper diagnosis is essential, as the sustained release of catecholamines can be life threatening. Early diagnosis generally has favorable results.[6,25,27] Signs and symptoms of pheochromocytoma may include the following[1,23,25,27]:

- Hypertension (sustained or paroxysmal), palpitations, tachycardia, and orthostatic hypotension

- Headache, palpitations, and diaphoresis

- Excessive perspiration

- Nervousness and emotional outbursts or instability

- Elevated blood glucose levels and glucosuria

Management of pheochromocytoma generally consists of surgical excision of the tumor with preoperative pharmacologic management with one of the following medications: alpha-adrenergic blocking agents (e.g., phenoxybenzamine [Dibenzyline], phentolamine [Regitine]), beta-adrenergic blocking agents (e.g., propranolol [Inderal]), or tyrosine inhibitors (alphamethlyparatyrosine).[8,25,28]

### Pancreatic Disorders

### Diabetes Mellitus
Diabetes mellitus is a syndrome with metabolic, vascular, and neural components that originates from glucose intolerance that in turn leads to hyperglycemic states (increased plasma glucose levels). Hyperglycemia can result from insufficient insulin production, ineffective receptive cells for insulin, or both. Insulin promotes storage of glucose as glycogen in muscle tissue and the liver. Deficiency of insulin leads to increased levels of plasma glucose.[1,6,29]

The diagnosis of diabetes is based on the presence of any one of the following three factors[6,30]:

1. Presence of polyuria, polydipsia, weight loss, blurred vision, and random plasma glucose (regardless of last meal) greater than or equal to 200 mg/dl

2.   Fasting plasma glucose greater than or equal to 126 mg/dl (no caloric intake for at least 8 hours)

3.   Two-hour–postload glucose greater than or equal to 200 mg/dl, using a 75-g oral glucose load dissolved in water

The diagnosis is confirmed when one of the above factors is also found on a subsequent day.[6,30]

The two primary types of diabetes mellitus are *type 1* (*insulin-dependent* or *juvenile-onset diabetes*) and *type 2* (*non–insulin-dependent* or *adult-onset diabetes*). After much debate on the classification of diabetes, the current terminology for diabetes uses type 1 and type 2 diabetes to distinguish between the two primary types.[30,31] Other forms of glucose intolerance disorders exist but are not discussed in this text.

### Type 1 Diabetes

*Type 1 diabetes* is an autoimmune disorder with a genetic-environmental etiology that leads to the selective destruction of beta cells in the pancreas. This destruction results in decreased or absent insulin secretion. Type 1 diabetes represents 5–10% of the population with diabetes and generally occurs in individuals under the age of 40 years.[29–33] Other etiologies for type 1 diabetes exist but are not discussed in this text.

Classic signs and symptoms of type 1 diabetes are described in the previous section with the diagnostic criteria for diabetes.[6,29]

Management of type 1 diabetes may consist of any of the following[32–34]:

• Close self- or medical monitoring of blood glucose levels (Table 11-8).

• Insulin administration through oral medications, intramuscular injection, or continuous subcutaneous insulin infusion (CSII) pump. CSII therapy has been shown to be as effective as multiple daily injections of insulin, while also providing the ability to mimic a more natural glycemic response in fasting and postprandial states (Table 11-9).

• Diet modification based on caloric content, proportion of basic nutrients and optimal sources, and distribution of nutrients in daily meals.

• Meal planning.

• Exercise on a regular basis.

**Table 11-8.** Tests to Monitor Control of Diabetes

| Test | Description |
|------|-------------|
| Self-monitoring | |
| Blood glucose finger stick samples | Monitors immediate control of diabetes. Very effective in establishing the correct insulin dosages and preventing complications from diabetes. |
| Reference, 60–110 mg/dl | Capillary blood is obtained by a needle stick of a finger or an earlobe and placed on a reagent strip. The reagent strip is compared to a color chart or placed in a portable electronic meter to read the glucose level. |
| | Patients in the hospital can also have blood drawn from an indwelling arterial line, for ease of use, without compromising accuracy of measurement. |
| Urine testing | A reagent strip is dipped in the patient's urine, and the strip is compared to a color chart to measure glucose levels in the urine. |
| | Provides satisfactory results only for patients who have stable diabetes; otherwise, results can be insensitive for truly delineating hyperglycemia. |
| Medical monitoring | |
| Glycosylated hemoglobin (GHB) | Hyperglycemia results in saturation of hemoglobin molecules during the lifespan of a red blood cell (approximately 120 days). |
| Reference, 7.5–11.4% of total hemoglobin for a patient with controlled diabetes | Measuring the amount of GHB in the blood provides a weighted average of the glucose level over a period of time and is a good indicator of long-term control of diabetes, without confounding factors such as a recent meal or insulin injection. Measurements are performed every 3–6 mos. |
| Fructosamine or glycated protein | Similar to GHB test, hyperglycemia saturates serum proteins, particularly albumin. |
| Reference, 300 mmol/liter = excellent diabetic control | The life span of albumin is approximately 40 days; therefore, this test is performed every 3 wks to monitor short-term control of diabetes. |

Sources: Data from JV Corbett (ed). Laboratory Tests and Diagnostic Procedures with Nursing Diagnoses (5th ed). Upper Saddle River, NJ: Prentice Hall Health, 2000;192–197; LM Malarkey, ME McMorrow (eds). Nurse's Manual of Laboratory Tests and Diagnostic Procedures. Philadelphia: Saunders, 2000;577–580; and RA Sacher, RA McPherson, JM Campos (eds). Widman's Clinical Interpretation of Laboratory Tests (11th ed). Philadelphia: Davis, 2000;817–818.

**Table 11-9.** Summary of Insulin Pump Therapy

| | |
|---|---|
| Patient candidacy | Demonstrated ability to self-monitor glucose and adjust insulin doses based on preprandial blood glucose levels and anticipated future activity level. |
| | Motivated to achieve and maintain improved glycemic control using intensive insulin therapy. |
| | Pregnant patients with type 1 diabetes. |
| | Patients unaware of hypoglycemic episodes with insulin therapy. |
| | Patients who experience wide glycemic variations on a day-to-day basis. |
| | Patients with a significant rise in hyperglycemia in the morning ("dawn phenomenon"). |
| | Patients who need flexibility in their insulin regimen (e.g., erratic work schedules, travel frequently). |
| | Adolescents who experience frequent diabetic ketoacidosis. |
| | Night-time use for children under 10 yrs of age who may not be able to adjust their own insulin requirements. |
| Pump description | Approximately the size of an electronic pager, weighing only 4 oz. |
| | Patients are instructed on how to insert and change (every 2–3 days) infusion catheters into the subcutaneous space of their abdomen. |
| | The catheter can be detached from the insulin pump for bathing or intimate contact. |
| | Two settings: basal rate and bolus doses, both adjustable by the patient depending on needs (e.g., preprandial bolus or decreased basal rate with exercise). |
| | Battery life is approximately 6 wks. |
| Types of insulin | Regular human buffered insulin (short acting). |
| | Insulin analog (rapid acting). |
| Pump complications | Hyperglycemia and diabetic ketoacidosis. |
| | Hypoglycemia and hypoglycemic unawareness. |
| | Skin infections. |
| | Weight gain. |

Sources: Data from J Unger. A primary care approach to continuous subcutaneous insulin infusion. Clin Diabetes 1999;17(3):113; Continuous subcutaneous insulin. Diabetes Care 2001;24(1):S98; and FR Kaufman, M Halvorson, C Kim, P Pitukcheewanont. Use of insulin pump therapy at nighttime only for children 7–10 years of age with type 1 diabetes. Diabetes Care 2000;123(5):579.

Research directed at curing type 1 diabetes is aimed at specifically identifying the causative genes, permanent replacement of lost beta-cell function, which could involve islet cell transplantation, regeneration of beta cells, or development of an immortalized insulin-secreting cell line.[31]

---

### Clinical Tip

• Hypoglycemia may occur during exercise or up to 24 hours after exercise because of an inability to regulate insulin levels. To help prevent this, the patient should consume extra carbohydrates before and during exercise (e.g., 10 g of carbohydrates per 30 minutes of activity), and the nurse or patient may also decrease the dose or rate of insulin infusion, especially with CSII.

• The physical therapist should be aware of the catheter placement on the patient for CSII therapy so the catheter will not be disrupted during intervention.

• Circulation of insulin that is injected into an exercising limb is enhanced as a result of increased blood flow and temperature. The injection into the exercising limb may, therefore, lead to hypoglycemia. Insulin can be injected into the abdomen to help prevent this process.

• Insulin is necessary to modulate lipolysis and hepatic (liver) glucose production during exercise. Performing exercise without adequate insulin can lead to hyperglycemia and ketogenesis.

• The physical therapist should inquire about the patient's blood glucose levels before and after exercise to assist in physical therapy planning.

• Coordinating physical therapy sessions with meals and insulin injections may help optimize exercise tolerance.

• Keeping graham crackers close by when working with diabetic individuals is helpful in case hypoglycemia does occur with activity.

---

### Type 2 Diabetes

Type 2 diabetes is more common in the United States than type 1 diabetes and generally occurs after 40 years of age. Type 2 diabetes is significantly linked to obesity, a sedentary lifestyle, and aging. Genetic predisposition has also been established.[30,31,33]

The mechanism of type 2 diabetes involves increasing cellular resistance to insulin, which results in a compensatory hypersecretion of insulin from the pancreatic beta cells that ultimately leads to a failure in insulin production.[29-33] Other etiologies for type 2 diabetes exist but are not discussed in this text.

Signs and symptoms of type 2 diabetes may be similar to those of type 1 diabetes but can also include the following:

- Recurrent infections and prolonged wound healing

- Genital pruritus

- Visual changes

- Paresthesias

Management of type 2 diabetes is similar to that of type 1 diabetes, with an emphasis on medical nutritional therapy and exercise to control hyperglycemia. Oral hypoglycemic agents and actual insulin administration may also be used.[32,34-36] CSII has been shown to be as effective as multiple dose injections of insulin in patients with type 2 diabetes.[37] Clinical studies are also investigating the use of inhaled insulin for these patients, with preliminary results demonstrating promising results.[38,39]

Listed below are oral hypoglycemic agents that help increase insulin production and belong to the drug class of sulfonylureas[32,33]:

Tolbutamide (Orinase, Oramide)

Tolazamide (Tolinase, Ronase, Tolamide)

Chlorpropamide (Diabinese)

Acetohexamide (Dymelor)

Glyburide (DiaBeta, Micronase)

Glipizide (Glucotrol)

An oral hypoglycemic agent that enhances glucose use in muscle is metformin.[33]

Research direction for type 2 diabetes includes identifying the gene(s) responsible for the predisposition to type 2 diabetes and the mechanisms by which environmental factors trigger this predisposition. Also, identification of the cellular defects responsible for insulin resistance and impaired insulin secretion in type 2 diabetes will, it is hoped, lead to the development of new medications that will be specific and relatively free of unwanted adverse effects.[31]

---

### Clinical Tip

- Glycemic control for patients with type 1 or type 2 diabetes may be altered significantly with the onset of new illnesses, such as systemic infection, because these new processes require added glucose metabolism. It is important for the therapist to carefully monitor the patient's blood glucose levels during therapeutic interventions, because the symptoms of diabetes may be exacerbated in a patient with significant comorbidities.
- Blood glucose levels are denoted in the medical record as *BS levels.*
- Patients with diabetes present with a wide range of their individual "normal" values. Therefore, establishing the tolerable high or low value for each patient during the initial evaluation is very important in determining the parameters for physical therapy intervention.
- Patients with poor glycemic control can have wide fluctuations in the BS levels on a daily basis. Therefore, be sure to always verify their BS level before physical therapy intervention.
- Consult with the nurse or physician regarding whether therapy should be deferred for patients who were recently placed on intravenous insulin to stabilize their glucose levels.
- Patients who were following a regular exercise program for glycemic control before hospital admission will require education about how to modify their exercise parameters during the hospitalization and on discharge. Modification of exercise parameters will be dependent on the nature of concurrent illnesses.

---

### Complications of Diabetes Mellitus

Patients with diabetes mellitus, despite management, can still develop organ and organ system damage linked to lesions of the small and large blood vessels. Complications can manifest 2–15 years after diagnosis. They can be classified as (1) microangiopathy (microvascular disease), which causes retinopathy, nephropathy, and foot ischemia; (2) macroangiopathy (macrovascular disease), which accelerates widespread atherosclerosis; or (3) neuropathy.[32] Another complication from diabetes that is not directly linked to vascular damage is diabetic ketoacidosis (DKA).

### Diabetic Ketoacidosis

The metabolic syndrome of diabetes mellitus gradually progresses from mild to moderate glucose intolerance, to fasting hyperglycemia, to ketosis, and, finally, to ketoacidosis. Most patients do not progress to the ketotic state but have the potential to do so if proper treatment is not administered.[12]

DKA is the end result of ineffective levels of circulating insulin, which lead to elevated levels of ketone bodies in the tissues. This state of an elevated level of ketone bodies is referred to as *ketosis*. Decreased insulin levels lead to uncontrolled lipolysis (fat breakdown), which increases the levels of free fatty acids released from the liver and ultimately leads to an overproduction of ketone bodies. Ketone bodies are acids, and if they are not buffered properly by bases, a state of ketoacidosis occurs. Ketoacidosis almost always results from uncontrolled diabetes mellitus; however, it may also result from alcohol abuse.[6,12,33]

The following are signs and symptoms of DKA[12]:

- Polyuria, polydipsia, dehydration
- Weakness and lethargy
- Myalgia, hypotonia
- Headache
- Anorexia
- Nausea, vomiting, abdominal pain, acute abdomen
- Dyspnea, deep and sighing respirations (Kussmaul's respiration)
- Acetone-smelling ("fruity") breath
- Hypothermia
- Stupor (coma), fixed, dilated pupils
- Uncoordinated movements
- Hyporeflexia

Management of DKA may consist of any of the following: insulin administration, hydration, electrolyte (sodium, potassium, and phosphorus) replacement, supplemental oxygen, and mechanical ventilation.[6,29,33]

### Diabetic Dermopathy

Skin lesions in patients with diabetes, particulary on their feet, are common and multifactorial in nature. Lesions may result from any combination of the following[13,32,40]:

- Loss of sensation from sensory neuropathy

- Skin atrophy from microangiopathy

- Decreased blood flow from macroangiopathy

- Sensory and autonomic neuropathy, resulting in abnormal blood distribution that may cause bone demineralization and Charcot's joint (disruption of the midfoot)[41]

Proper foot care in diabetic individuals helps prevent complications, such as poor wound healing, which can progress to tissue necrosis and ultimately lead to amputation.[40] Table 11-10 describes patient information regarding foot care for patients with diabetes. Refer to Chapter 7 for more details on diabetic ulcers.

### Infection

Individuals with diabetes are at a higher risk for infection because of (1) decreased sensation (vision and touch); (2) poor blood supply, which leads to tissue hypoxia; (3) hyperglycemic states, which promote rapid proliferation of pathogens that enter the body; (4) decreased immune response from reduced circulation, which leaves white blood cells unable to get to the affected area; (5) impaired white blood cell function, which leads to abnormal phagocytosis; and (6) chemotaxis.[29,42]

### Diabetic Neuropathy

The exact link between neural dysfunction and diabetes is unknown; however, the vascular, metabolic, and immunologic changes that occur with diabetes can promote destruction of myelin sheaths and therefore interfere with normal nerve conduction.[43]

Neuropathies can be manifested as (1) focal mononeuropathy and radiculopathy (disorder of single nerve or nerve root); (2) symmetric sensorimotor neuropathy, associated with disabling pain and depression; or (3) autonomic neuropathy.

**Table 11-10.** Foot Care for Patients with Diabetes

| Don't | Do |
|---|---|
| Smoke. | Encourage the patient to have regular |
| Wash feet in cold or hot water. The water temperature should be lukewarm (approximately 85–95°F). | medical or podiatric examinations to determine integrity of his or her feet. |
| Use a heating pad, heating lamp, or hot water bottles to warm the feet. | Inspect feet daily for abrasions, blisters, and cuts. Use a mirror if soles cannot be seen. If vision is poor, another person should check feet. |
| Use razor blades or scissors to cut corns or calluses. Have a podiatrist perform this procedure. | Wash feet daily with lukewarm water and soap. |
| Use over-the-counter medications on corns or calluses. | Dry feet carefully, especially between the toes. |
| Cross legs when sitting. | Apply hand cream or lanolin to feet (dry areas). |
| Wear girdles or garters. | Be careful not to leave cream between |
| Walk barefoot. | the toes. |
| Wear shoes without socks or stockings. | Wear clean socks or stockings daily. |
| Wear sandals with thongs between the toes. | Cut nails straight across and file down edges with an emery board. |
| Wear socks or stocking with raised seams. | Wear comfortable shoes that fit and don't rub. |
| Place hands in shoes for inspection, if sensory neuropathy is present in the hands. Instead shake out the shoes for any objects. | Wear wide toe-box or custom-made shoes if foot deformities exist. |
| | Inspect the inside of shoes for any objects, tacks, or torn linings before putting on the shoes. |

Sources: Data from WM Burch (ed). Endocrinology for the House Officer (2nd ed). Baltimore: Williams & Wilkins, 1988;59; and JA Mayfield, GE Reiber, LJ Sanders. Preventive foot care in people with diabetes. Diabetes Care 2001;24(1):S56.

The most common diabetic neuropathy is peripheral symmetric polyneuropathy. Sensory deficits are greater than motor deficits and occur in a glove-and-stocking pattern, resulting in a loss of pinprick and light-touch sensations in these areas. However, patients will commonly present with a mixture of these three primary types of neuropathies. Foot ulcers and footdrop are common manifestations of diabetic neuropathies.[11,29,32,33,43]

Table 11-11 outlines the signs and symptoms of the different types of diabetic neuropathy.

Management of diabetic neuropathy may include[43]

- Strict glycemic control (primary method)
- Pain relief with:

    Tricyclic antidepressants, such as amitriptyline, nortriptyline, and desipramine

    Anticonvulsants, such as carbamazepine, phenytoin, gabapentin, and clonazepam

    Topical agents, such as capsaicin cream (0.025–0.075%) or lidocaine ointment

    Opioids used as a last resort

    Transcutaneous electrical nerve stimulation

**Table 11-11.** Signs and Symptoms of Diabetic Neuropathy

| Classification of Diabetic Neuropathy | Symptoms | Signs |
|---|---|---|
| Symmetric poly-neuropathies | | |
| Peripheral sensory polyneuropathy | Paresthesias, numbness, coldness, tingling pins and needles (mainly in feet) Pain, often disabling, worse at night | Absent ankle jerk Impairment of vibration sense in feet Foot ulcers (often over metatarsal heads) |
| Peripheral motor neuropathy | Weakness | Bilateral interosseous muscle atrophy, claw or hammer toes, decreased grip strength, decreased manual muscle test grades |
| Autonomic neuropathy | Constipation or diarrhea, nausea or vomiting, tremulousness, impotence, dysphagia | Incontinence, orthostatic hypotension, tachycardia, peripheral edema, gustatory sweating |

Table 11-11. *Continued*

| Classification of Diabetic Neuropathy | Symptoms | Signs |
|---|---|---|
| Focal and multifocal neuropathies | | |
| Cranial neuropathy | Pain behind or above the eye, headaches, facial or forehead pain | Palpebral ptosis Inward deviation of one eye |
| Trunk and limb mononeuropathy | Abrupt onset of cramping or lancinating pain Constricting band-like pain in trunk or abdomen Cutaneous hyperesthesia of the trunk | Peripheral nerve-specific motor loss Abdominal wall weakness |
| Proximal motor neuropathy or diabetic amyotrophy | Pain in lower back, hips, and thighs that is worse at night; loss of appetite, depression | Asymmetric proximal weakness Atrophy in lower limbs Absent or diminished knee jerk |

Sources: Data from JS Boissonault, D Madlon-Kay. Screening for Endocrine System Disease. In WG Boissonault (ed), Examination in Physical Therapy: Screening for Medical Disease. New York: Churchill Livingstone, 1991;159; PA Melvin-Sater. Diabetic neuropathy. Physician Assistant 2000;24(7):63; and CD Saudek. Diabetes Mellitus. In JD Stobo, DB Hellmann, PW Ladenson, et al. (eds), The Principles and Practice of Medicine (23rd ed). Stamford CT: Appleton & Lange, 1996; 330.

- Aldose reductase inhibitors aimed at slowing the progression of nerve damage

- Exogenous nerve growth factors

- Immunotherapy

- Pancreatic transplant

**Coronary Artery Disease**
See Myocardial Ischemia and Infarction in Chapter 1 for a discussion of coronary artery disease.

**Stroke**
See Cerebrovascular Accident in Chapter 4 for a discussion of stroke.

**Peripheral Vascular Disease**
See Atherosclerosis in Chapter 6 for a discussion of peripheral vascular disease.

## Nephropathy

See Chapter 9 for a discussion of nephropathy.

## Hypoglycemia (Hyperinsulinism)

*Hypoglycemia* is a state of decreased BS levels. Excess serum insulin results in decreased BS levels, which leads to symptoms of hypoglycemia. Causes for this imbalance of insulin and sugar levels can be grouped as (1) fasting, (2) postprandial, or (3) induced.

*Fasting hypoglycemia* occurs before eating and can be caused by an insulin-producing islet cell tumor, liver failure, chronic alcohol ingestion, GH deficiency, extrapancreatic neoplasm, or leucine. It can also occur in infants with mothers who have diabetes.

*Postprandial hypoglycemia* occurs after eating and can be caused by reactive hypoglycemia (inappropriate insulin release after a meal), early diabetes mellitus, or rapid gastric emptying.

Hypoglycemia can also be induced by external causes, such as exogenous insulin or oral hypoglycemic overdose.[6,8]

Signs and symptoms of hypoglycemia may include the following:

* Tachycardia and hypertension

* Tremor, irritability, and sweating

* Hunger

* Weight changes

* Headache

* Mental dullness, confusion, and amnesia

* Seizures

* Paralysis and paresthesias

* Dizziness

* Visual disturbance

* Loss of consciousness

Management of hypoglycemia may consist of any of the following: glucose administration (fruit juice or honey); strict monitoring of insulin and oral hypoglycemic administration; dietary modifications; pharmacologic agents, such as glucagon, which is the first agent used in emergency cases of hypoglycemia; diazoxide (Hyperstat) or streptozocin (Zanosar); surgery (e.g., subtotal pancreatectomy, insulinoma resection); or a combination of these.[8,44]

## Parathyroid Gland

### Function

Parathyroid hormone (PTH) is the primary hormone secreted from the parathyroid gland. The target sites are the kidneys, small intestine, and bone. The primary function of PTH is to raise blood calcium levels by mobilizing calcium that is stored in bone, increasing calcium reabsorption from the kidneys, and increasing calcium absorption from the small intestine.[6,45]

### Parathyroid Tests

The primary measurements of parathryoid hormone are summarized in Table 11-12. However, because PTH exerts its effects on the intes-

**Table 11-12.** Primary Tests Used to Evaluate Parathyroid (PTH) Function

| Test | Description |
| --- | --- |
| Serum calcium | Measurement of blood calcium levels indirectly examines parathyroid function. Normally, low calcium levels stimulate parathyroid hormone secretion, whereas high calcium levels could be reflec-tive of high PTH levels. |
| | Reference value for serum calcium is 8.5–11.0 mg/dl in adults. |
| | Calcium levels can also be measured in the urine. Reference value for urinary calcium is 50–300 mg/dl. |
| Parathyroid hormone | Radioimmunoassays and urinalysis are used to measure parathyroid hormone levels. Reference value is 10–60 pg/ml. |

Sources: Data from WM Burch (ed). Endocrinology for the House Officer (2nd ed). Baltimore: Williams & Wilkins, 1988; JV Corbett (ed). Laboratory Tests and Diagnostic Procedures with Nursing Diagnoses (5th ed). Upper Saddle River, NJ: Prentice Hall Health, 2000;167–176; and RA Sacher, RA McPherson, JM Campos (eds). Widman's Clinical Interpretation of Laboratory Tests (11th ed). Philadelphia: FA Davis, 2000;803–804.

tines and kidneys, calcium metabolism can also be evaluated by testing gastrointestinal and renal function. Please refer to Chapters 8 and 9, respectively, for a summary of diagnostic tests for the gastrointestinal and renal systems.

## Parathyroid Disorders

### Hyperparathyroidism

*Hyperparathyroidism* is a disorder caused by overactivity of one or more of the parathyroid glands that leads to increased PTH levels, resulting in increased blood calcium level, decreased bone mineralization, and decreased kidney function. This disorder occurs more frequently in women than in men. Radiation therapy is also a risk factor for developing this disorder.[46]

Hyperparathyroidism can be classified as primary, secondary, or tertiary. Primary hyperparathyroidism represents the most cases and usually results from hyperplasia or an adenoma in the parathyroid gland(s). Secondary hyperparathyroidism results from another organ system disorder, such as renal failure, osteogenesis imperfecta, Paget's disease, multiple myeloma, lymphoma, or bone metastases from primary breast, lung, or kidney tumors. Tertiary hyperparathyroidism occurs when PTH secretion is autonomous despite normal or low serum calcium levels.[6,23,47]

The primary clinical manifestations of hyperparathyroidism are hypercalcemia and hypercalciuria (calcium in urine). Hypercalcemia may then result in the following cascade of signs and symptoms[23,46,47]:

- Bone demineralization and resorption (which causes skeletal changes, such as dorsal kyphosis)
- Backache, joint and bone pain, and pathologic fractures
- Kidney stone formation, abdominal pain, and peptic ulcer disease
- Nausea, thirst, anorexia, and constipation
- Hypertension and dysrhythmias
- Listlessness, depression, and paranoia
- Decreased neuromuscular excitability

Management of hyperparathyroidism may consist of any of the following[8,23,47]:

- Parathyroidectomy (partial or total) is the preferred treatment for patients with moderate to severe hypercalcemia.[46–48] The use of intraoperative, rapid PTH assay has been shown to be effective in fully delineating the areas requiring resection, making for a safer and more specific operative procedure.[48]

- Pharmacologic intervention with the following:

  Parathyroid agents (e.g., calcitonin [Calcimar, Cibacalcin])

  Diuretic agents (e.g., furosemide [Lasix])

  Phosphates

  Bone resorption inhibitors (e.g., mithramycin [Mithracin] and gallium nitrate [Ganite])

- Fluid replacement

- Dietary modification (a diet low in calcium and high in vitamin D)

## Hypoparathyroidism

Hypoparathyroidism is a disorder caused by underactivity of one or more of the parathyroid glands that leads to decreased PTH levels. Decreased levels of PTH occur most commonly as a result of damage to the parathyroid glands during thyroid or parathyroid surgery. Less common causes may include radiation-induced damage, infiltration by metastatic cells, and autoimmune dysfunction.[23,47]

Signs and symptoms of hypoparathyroidism may include the following[23]:

- Hypocalcemia

- Increased neuromuscular irritability (tetany), painful muscle spasms

- Tingling of the fingers

- Laryngospasm

- Dysrhythmias

- Lethargy, personality changes

- Thin, patchy hair; brittle nails; dry, scaly skin

- Convulsions

- Cataracts

Management of hypoparathyroidism may consist of any of the following[8,23,47]:

- Dietary modifications that promote a diet high in calcium and low in phosphate
- Pharmacologic intervention with the following:

  PTH

  Vitamin D supplements: dihydrotachysterol (Hytakerol), dihydroxycholecalciferol, or ergocalciferol (Calciferol) (vitamin $D_2$)

  Nutritional supplements: calcium gluconate, calcium glubionate, calcium lactate, or calcium chloride

### Metabolic Bone Disorders

#### Osteoporosis
*Osteoporosis* is a multifactorial skeletal disorder that leads to decreased bone density and organization, which ultimately reduces bone strength.[49] Bone strength is often measured by bone mineral density studies, which are used in the diagnosis of osteoporosis, as well as monitoring tools for therapeutic improvements. Osteoporosis can be classified as primary or secondary. Primary osteoporosis can occur in both genders at all ages, but often follows menopause in women and occurs later in life in men. Secondary osteoporosis is a result of medications (e.g., glucocorticoids or anticonvulsants), alcoholism, other conditions (e.g., hypogonadism or hypoestrogenism), or diseases (e.g., hyperthyroidism).[49]

There is no clear etiology for osteoporosis. However, many risk factors for women have been elucidated. These risk factors include white or Asian race, petite frame, inadequate dietary intake of calcium, positive family history of osteoporosis, alcohol abuse, cigarette smoking, high caffeine intake, sedentary lifestyle, reduced bone mineral content (most predictive factor), and early menopause or oophorectomy (ovary removal).[1,47,49]

Signs and symptoms of osteoporosis may include the following[1,47]:

- Back pain (aggravated by movement or weight bearing, relieved by rest)
- Vertebral deformity (kyphosis and anterior wedging)

- Presence of vertebral compression fractures, Colles' fracture, hip and pelvic fractures

Management of osteoporosis may consist of any of the following[3,49,50]:

- Daily supplementation with calcium and vitamin D for all women with low bone mineral density

- Hormone replacement therapy with estrogen or estrogen combined with progesterone

- Estrogen receptor modulation therapy with raloxifene hydrochloride

- Bisphosphonate supplementation (inhibits bone resorption) with alendronate sodium or risedronate sodium

- Calcitonin supplementation (increases total body calcium)

- Physical therapy for exercise prescription

- Fracture management (if indicated, refer to Chapter 3)

- Administration of PTH (in research stages)

---

**Clinical Tip**

- Always consult with the physician to determine whether there are any weight-bearing precautions in patients with osteoporosis.
- An abdominal corset can provide additional support for stable vertebral compression fracture(s).
- Also, using a rolling walker that is adjusted higher than normal can promote a more upright posture. Both of these techniques may also help to decrease back pain in patients with osteoporosis.
- Gentle exercises to improve the strength of thoracic extensors can also assist with posture and reduce back pain.
- Caution with resistive exercises and manual contacts should be taken during therapeutic activities to avoid risk of microtrauma or fracture to osteoporotic bones.

---

## Osteomalacia

*Osteomalacia*, or rickets in children, is a disorder characterized by decreased bone mineralization, reduced calcium absorption from the gut, and compensatory hyperparathyroidism. The etiology of osteomalacia stems from any disorder that lowers serum levels of phosphate, calcium, or vitamin D.[11,47]

Signs and symptoms of osteomalacia may include the following[11,47]:

- Bone pain and tenderness

- Softening of cranial vault (in children)

- Swelling of costochondral joints (in children)

- Predisposition to femoral neck fractures (in adults)

- Proximal myopathy

- Waddling gait

Medical management of osteomalacia may consist of treating the underlying or predisposing condition or supplementation with calcium and vitamin D.[11,51]

## Paget's Disease

*Paget's disease* is a bone disease of unknown etiology that usually presents after the age of 55 years. The primary feature is thick, spongy bone that is unorganized and brittle as a result of excessive osteoclastic and subsequent osteoblastic activity. Some evidence points to an inflammatory or viral origin. Fractures and compression of the cranial nerves (especially the eighth nerve) and spinal cord are complications of Paget's disease.[47,52]

Paget's disease is generally asymptomatic; however, the following clinical manifestations may present[47,52]:

- Bone pain that is unrelieved by rest and persists at night

- Bone deformity (e.g., skull enlargement, bowing of leg and thigh)

- Increased warmth of overlying skin of affected areas

- Headaches or hearing loss

Management of Paget's disease consists primarily of bisphosphonate administration (oral etidronate, alendronate, tiludronate, risedronate, or intravenous pamidronate). Other bisphosphonates currently under investigation include zoledronate and ibandronate.[52] Other interventions can include the following[47,52]:

- Administration of calcitonin

- Calcium supplementation (if necessary)

- Promotion of mobility

- Adequate hydration

- Symptomatic relief with nonsteroidal anti-inflammatory agents or acetaminophen

## Management

Clinical management of endocrine dysfunction is discussed earlier in specific endocrine gland and metabolic disorders sections. This section focuses on goals and guidelines for physical therapy intervention. The following are general physical therapy goals and guidelines for working with patients who have endocrine or metabolic dysfunction. These guidelines should be adapted to a patient's specific needs. Clinical tips are provided earlier to address specific situations in which the tips may be most helpful.

### Goals

The primary physical therapy goals in this patient population are the following: (1) to optimize functional mobility, (2) to maximize activity tolerance and endurance, (3) to prevent skin breakdown in the patient with altered sensation (e.g., diabetic neuropathy), (4) to decrease pain (e.g., in patients with osteoporosis or hyperparathyroidism), and (5) to maximize safety for prevention of falls, especially in patients with altered sensation or muscle function.

### Guidelines

Patients with diabetes or osteoporosis represent the primary patient population with which the physical therapist intervenes. Physical therapy considerations for these patients are discussed in the form of clinical tips in earlier sections (Diabetes and Osteoporosis, respectively).

For other patients with endocrine or metabolic dysfunction, the primary physical therapy treatment guidelines are the following:

1.    To improve activity tolerance, it may be necessary to decrease exercise intensity when the patient's medication regimen is being adjusted. For example, a patient with insufficient thyroid hormone replacement will fatigue more quickly than will a patient with adequate thyroid hormone replacement. In this example, knowing the normal values of thyroid hormone and reviewing the laboratory tests helps the therapist gauge the appropriate treatment intensity.

2.    Consult with the clinical nutritionist to help determine the appropriate activity level based on the patient's caloric intake, because caloric intake and metabolic processes are affected by endocrine and metabolic disorders.

## References

1. Burch WM (ed). Endocrinology for the House Officer (2nd ed). Baltimore: Williams & Wilkins, 1988.
2. Bullock BL (ed). Pathophysiology: Adaptations and Alterations in Function (4th ed). Philadelphia: Lippincott, 1996.
3. Diagnostic Procedures. In JM Thompson, GK McFarland, JE Hirsch, et al. (eds), Mosby's Manual of Clinical Nursing Practice (2nd ed). St. Louis: Mosby, 1989;1594.
4. Corbett JV. Laboratory Tests and Diagnostic Procedures with Nursing Diagnoses (5th ed). Upper Saddle River, NJ: Prentice Hall Health, 2000.
5. Malarkey LM, McMorrow ME (eds). Nurse's Manual of Laboratory Tests and Diagnostic Procedures. Philadelphia: Saunders, 2000;604–612.
6. Sacher RA, McPherson RA, Campos JM (eds). Widman's Clinical Interpretation of Laboratory Tests (11th ed). Philadelphia: FA Davis, 2000; 741–823.
7. Lavin N (ed). Manual of Endocrinology and Metabolism (2nd ed). Boston: Little, Brown, 1994.
8. Allen MA, Boykin PC, Drass JA, et al. Endocrine and Metabolic Systems. In JM Thompson, GK McFarland, JE Hirsch, et al. (eds), Mosby's Manual of Clinical Nursing Practice (2nd ed). St. Louis: Mosby, 1989; 876.
9. Woeber KA. Update on the management of hyperthyroidism and hypothyroidism. Arch Intern Med 2000;160(8):1067.

10. Elliot B. Diagnosing and Treating Hypothyroidism. Nurse Pract 2000;25(3):92.
11. Hartog M (ed). Endocrinology. Oxford, UK: Blackwell Scientific, 1987.
12. Hershman JM (ed). Endocrine Pathophysiology: A Patient-Oriented Approach (3rd ed). Philadelphia: Lea & Febiger, 1988;225.
13. Woolf N. Pathology, Basic and Systemic. London: Saunders, 1998;820–873.
14. Drug therapy usually secondary to surgery in the treatment of pituitary adenomas. Drug Ther Perspect 2001;17(3):5–10.
15. Terpstra TL, Terpstra TL. Syndrome of inappropriate antidiuretic hormone secretion: recognition and management. Medsurg Nurs 2000; 9(2):61.
16. Beers MH, Berkow R (eds). Merck Manual of Diagnosis and Therapy (17th ed). Whitehouse Station, NJ: Merck, 1999.
17. Burch WM (ed). Endocrinology for the House Officer (3rd ed). Baltimore: Williams & Wilkins, 1994;97.
18. Wand GS. Pituitary Disorders. In JD Stobo, DB Hellmann, PW Ladenson, et al. (eds), The Principles and Practice of Medicine (23rd ed). Stamford CT: Appleton & Lange, 1996;274–281.
19. Heater DW. Diabetes insipidus. RN 1999;62(7):44.
20. Malarkey LM, McMorrow ME (eds). Nurse's Manual of Laboratory Tests and Diagnostic Procedures. Philadelphia: Saunders, 2000;619–620.
21. Malarkey LM, McMorrow ME (eds). Nurse's Manual of Laboratory Tests and Diagnostic Procedures. Philadelphia: Saunders, 2000;564–566, 570–571.
22. Malarkey LM, McMorrow ME (eds). Nurse's Manual of Laboratory Tests and Diagnostic Procedures. Philadelphia: Saunders, 2000;555–556.
23. Black JM, Matassarin-Jacobs E (eds). Luckmann and Sorensen's Medical Surgical Nursing: A Psychophysiologic Approach (4th ed). Philadelphia: Saunders, 1993.
24. Baker JR Jr. Autoimmune endocrine disease. JAMA 1997;278(22): 1931–1937.
25. Wand GS, Cooper DS. Adrenal Disorders. In JD Stobo, DB Hellmann, PW Ladenson, et al. (eds), The Principles and Practice of Medicine (23rd ed). Stamford, CT: Appleton & Lange, 1996;282–292.
26. Krasner AS. Glucocorticoid-induced adrenal insufficiency. JAMA 1999; 282(7):671.
27. Kizer JR, Koniaris JS, Edelman JD, et al. Pheochromocytoma crisis, cardiomyopathy, and hemodynamic collapse. Chest 2000;118(4):1221.
28. O' Connell CB. A young woman with palpitations and diaphoresis. Physician Assistant 1999;23(4):94.
29. McCance KL, Huether SE (eds). Pathophysiology: The Biologic Basis for Disease in Adults and Children (2nd ed). St. Louis: Mosby, 1994;674.
30. Report of the Expert Committee on the Diagnosis and Classification of Diabetes Mellitus. Diabetes Care 2001;24(1):S5.
31. Olefsky JM. Prospects for research in diabetes mellitus. JAMA 2001; 285(5):628.

32. Lorenzi, M. Diabetes Mellitus. In PA Fitzgerald (ed), Handbook of Clinical Endocrinology (2nd ed). East Norwalk, CT: Appleton & Lange, 1992;463.
33. Saudek CD. Diabetes Mellitus. In JD Stobo, DB Hellmann, PW Ladenson, et al. (eds), The Principles and Practice of Medicine (23rd ed). Stamford, CT: Appleton & Lange, 1996;321–331.
34. Standards of medical care for patients with diabetes mellitus. Diabetes Care 2001;24(1):S33.
35. Nutrition recommendations and principles for people with diabetes mellitus. Diabetes Care 2001;24(1):S44.
36 Zinran B, Ruderman N, Phil O, et al. Diabetes mellitus and exercise. Diabetes Care 2001;24(1):S51
37. Saudek CD, Duckworth WC, Giobbie-Hurder A, et al. Implantable insulin pump vs multiple-dose insulin for non-insulin dependent diabetes mellitus: a randomized clinical trial. Department of Veterans Affairs Implantable Insulin Pump Study Group. JAMA 1997;276(16): 1322–1327.
38. Cefalu WT. Inhaled human insulin treatment in patients with type 2 diabetes mellitus (Abstract). JAMA 2001;285(12):1559.
39. Skyler JS, Cefalu WT, Kourides IA, et al. Efficacy of inhaled human insulin in type 1 diabetes mellitus: a randomised proof-of-concept study. Lancet 2001;357(9253):331.
40. Mayfield JA, Reiber GE, Saunders LJ, et al. Preventive foot care in people with diabetes. Diabetes Care 2001;24(1):S56.
41. Houston DS, Curran J. Charcot foot. Orthop Nurs 2001;20(1):11.
42. Frykberg RG. Diabetic foot infections: evaluation and management. Advances in wound care. J Prev Healing 1998;11(7):329.
43. Melvin-Sater PA. Diabetic neuropathy. Physician Assistant 2000;24(7): 63.
44. Cooper PG. Insulin-reaction hypoglycemia. Clin Reference Syst Ann 2000:919.
45. Hudak CM, Gallo BM (eds). Critical Care Nursing: A Holistic Approach (6th ed). Philadelphia: Lippincott, 1994;874.
46. Trotto NE, Cobin RH, Wiesen M. Hypothyroidism, hyperthyroidism, hyperparathyroidism. Patient Care 1999;33(14):186.
47. Levine MA. Disorders of Mineral and Bone Metabolism. In JD Stobo, DB Hellmann, PW Ladenson, et al. (eds), The Principles and Practice of Medicine (23rd ed). Stamford, CT: Appleton & Lange, 1996;312–320.
48. Irvin GL III, Carneiro DM. Management changes in primary hyperparathyroidism. JAMA 2000;284(8):934.
49. NIH Consensus Development Panel. Osteoporosis prevention, diagnosis, and therapy. JAMA 2001;285(6):785.
50. Altkorn D, Voke T. Treatment of postmenopausal osteoporosis. JAMA 2001;285(11):1415.
51. Vieth R. Vitamin D supplementation, 25-hydroxyvitamin D concentrations, and safety. Am J Clin Nutr 1999;69(5):842.
52. Hines SE. Paget's disease of bone: a new philosophy of treatment. Patient Care 1999;33(20):40.

# 12

# Organ Transplantation
*Jennifer Lee Hunt*

## Introduction

With advances in technology and immunology, organ and tissue transplantation is becoming more common. Approximately 35,000 organ transplants are performed in the world annually, and as increasing numbers of hospitals perform transplantations, physical therapists are involved more frequently in the rehabilitation process for pre- and post-transplant recipients.[1] Owing to limited organ donor availability, physical therapists often treat more potential recipients than post-transplant recipients. Patients awaiting transplants often require admission to an acute care hospital as a result of their end-stage organ disease. They may be very deconditioned and may benefit from physical therapy during their stay. The goal of physical therapy for transplant candidates is reconditioning in preparation for the transplant procedure and postoperative course and increasing functional mobility and endurance in an attempt to return patients to a safe functional level at home. Other transplant candidates may be too acutely sick and may no longer qualify for transplantation during that particular hospital admission. These patients are generally unable to work and may need assistance at home from family members or even require transfer to a rehabilitation facility.

Whether the patient is pre- or post-transplantation, physical therapists focus on reconditioning patients to their maximum functional level and should have a basic knowledge of the patient's end-stage organ disease. The objectives for this chapter are to provide information on the following:

1. The transplantation process, including criteria for transplantation, organ donation, and postoperative care

2. Complications after organ transplantation, including rejection and infection

3. The various types of organ transplantation procedures

4. Guidelines for physical therapy intervention with the transplant recipient

## Types of Organ Transplants

The kidney, liver, pancreas, heart, and lung are organs that are procured for transplantation. The most frequent of those are the kidney, liver, and heart.[2] Double transplants, such as liver-kidney, kidney-pancreas, and heart-lung, are performed if the patient has multiorgan failure. Although bone marrow is not an organ, bone marrow transplantation (BMT) is a common type of tissue transplant that will be discussed.

## Criteria for Transplantation

Transplantation is offered to patients who have end-stage organ disease for which alternative medical or surgical management has failed. The patient typically has a life expectancy of less than 1–3 years.[3–5] Criteria for organ recipients vary, depending on the type of organ transplant needed and the transplant facility.

The basic criteria for transplantation include the following[6]:

• The presence of end-stage disease in a transplantable organ

• The failure of conventional therapy to treat the condition successfully

- The absence of untreatable malignancy or irreversible infection

- The absence of disease that would attack the transplanted organ or tissue

In addition to these criteria, transplant candidates must demonstrate emotional and psychological stability, have an adequate support system, and be willing to comply with lifelong immunosuppressive drug therapy. Other criteria, such as age limits and absence of drug or alcohol abuse, are specific to the transplant facility. To determine whether transplantation is the best treatment option for the individual, all transplant candidates are evaluated by a team of health care professionals consisting of a transplant surgeon, transplant nurse coordinator, infectious disease physician, psychiatrist, social worker, and nutritionist. The patient undergoes many laboratory and diagnostic studies during the evaluation process. Acceptable candidates for organ transplantation are placed on a waiting list. Waiting times for an organ may range between 1 and 4 years.[3,7] Many patients die waiting for a suitable organ to become available.

## Transplant Donation

### Cadaveric Donors

Cadaveric donors are brain-dead individuals who have had severe neurologic trauma, such as from head or spinal cord injury, cerebral hemorrhage, or anoxia.[8] Death must occur at a location where cardiopulmonary support is immediately available to maintain the potential organ donor on mechanical ventilation, cardiopulmonary bypass, or both; preserve organ viability; and prevent ischemic damage to vital organs.[8] The cadaveric donor must have no evidence of malignancy, sepsis, or communicable diseases, such as hepatitis B or human immunodeficiency virus.[6,9,10]

### Living Donors

Because there are not enough cadaveric organs donated to meet the needs of all potential recipients, living donor transplantation offers an alternative means of organ donation. Living donors are always used for bone marrow transplants, often used for kidney transplants, and sometimes used for liver, lung, and pancreas transplantation. They may be genetically or emotionally related to the recipient—that is, they are a blood relative (e.g., sister) or non–genetically related individual (e.g., spouse or close friend). Living donors also are evaluated by the transplant team to determine medical suitability.

The age of a potential donor can range from a term newborn to 65 years, depending on the organ considered for donation and the recipient. Donors do not have a history of drug or alcohol abuse, chronic disease, malignancy, syphilis, tuberculosis, hepatitis B, or human immunodeficiency virus infection. Ideally, the donor's height and weight approximate those of the recipient for the best "fit."

### Donor Matching

The matching of a cadaveric or living donor with a recipient depends on the following factors:

- ABO blood typing
- Histocompatibility typing
- Size

The donor and recipient must be ABO blood type identical or compatible.[11] The process of finding compatible donors and recipients is called *tissue typing* or *histocompatibility typing*. Histocompatibility typing attempts to match the human leukocyte antigens (HLAs), which are the antigens that cause graft rejection. It is performed serologically by adding a standard panel of typing antisera, complement, and tryphan blue stain to purified lymphocytes and then observing the lymphocytotoxicity.[12] The better the histocompatibility match and degree of genetic similarity between the donor and the recipient, the less severe is the rejection response. In living related donors, an identical match is ideal; however, a half match is acceptable.[9] Also, a white cell crossmatch is performed in which the lymphocytes from the donor are mixed with the serum from the recipient and then observed for immune responses. A negative crossmatch indicates no antibody reaction and that the recipient's antibodies are compatible with the donor. A negative crossmatch is required for successful kidney and kidney-pancreas transplants.[7]

Although pretransplant tissue typing is ideal, it is not always performed. Sometimes, there is insufficient time to perform HLA typing between donor and recipient because of the short cold ischemic times for different organs.[12] Owing to the short ischemic time of less than 6 hours for orthotopic cardiac transplants, ABO blood type compatibility, body weight, and accrued waiting time are used for allocation of the donor heart.[8,10] A lung transplant recipient is matched on the basis of ABO blood type and size, because the ischemic time is less than 4 hours.[8] A size match is based on the donor's height, weight, and thoracic dimensions as determined by chest radiograph.[13]

In the United States, organ procurement and distribution for transplantation are administered by the United Network for Organ Sharing (UNOS). UNOS sets the standards for transplant centers, transplant physicians, tissue typing laboratories, and organ procurement organizations. UNOS distributes organs based on the severity of the recipient's illness, blood type, donor-recipient weight match, and length of recipient waiting time.[14]

## General Post-Transplantation Care and Complications

### Postoperative Care for Living Donors

Postoperative care for living donors is similar to that of any patient who has undergone major abdominal or cardiothoracic surgery. These patients are taken off mechanical ventilation in the recovery room and transferred to the general surgery or transplant ward. Vital signs and blood counts are monitored closely for possible postoperative bleeding. Patients are usually out of bed and ambulating on postoperative day 1. On average, the duration of donor hospitalization may range from 3 days for a kidney donor to 8 days for a simultaneous pancreas-kidney (SPK) donor.[7,15]

### Postoperative Care for Transplant Recipients

Once an organ is transplanted, the postoperative care focuses on the monitoring and treatment of the following[14]:

- Allograft function
- Rejection

- Infection

- Adverse effects of immunosuppressive drugs

General postoperative care for transplant recipients is also similar to the care patients receive after major abdominal or cardiothoracic surgery. Except for kidney transplant recipients, who are normally extubated before leaving the operating room, most patients are transferred from the operating room to the surgical intensive care unit, where they are weaned from mechanical ventilation within 24 to 48 hours.[11,16,17] Once extubated and hemodynamically stable, recipients are transferred to specialized transplant floors. Nursing staff monitors the recipient closely for signs and symptoms of infection and rejection, which are the leading causes of morbidity and mortality in the first year after transplantation.

Complications from postoperative transplantation may contribute to an increased length of hospital stay or hospital readmissions. They can be grouped to include the following types:

- Surgical

- Medical

- Rejection

- Infection

Surgical complications include vascular problems, such as thrombosis, stenosis, leakage at anastomotic sites, and postoperative bleeding. Medical complications may include fluid overload or dehydration, electrolyte imbalance, or hypertension.

*Rejection*

The major problem in organ transplantation is not the technical difficulties of surgery, but rather *organ rejection*, or the tendency of the recipient's body to immediately reject anything that is "nonself." Graft rejection is actually a normal immune response to invasion of foreign matter, the transplanted organ or tissue. Some degree of rejection is normal; however, if the patient is not treated with immunosuppressive drugs, the donor organ would be completely rejected and cease to be viable in 10 days.[18] Transplant recipients must receive immunosuppressive drugs for the rest of their lives to suppress or minimize rejection of their transplanted organs. The pharmacologic agents most often used to prevent organ rejection include a double or triple drug therapy, consisting of a combination of tacrolimus or cyclosporine with methylprednisolone, and azathioprine or mycophenolate mofetil.[19] See Table 12-1 for common immunosuppressive medications used in organ transplantation.

These immunosuppressive drugs decrease the body's ability to fight infection. A delicate balance must be reached between suppressing rejection and avoiding infection. Insufficient immunosuppression may result in rejection that threatens the allograft and patient survival, whereas excessive immunosuppression increases the risk of infection and malignancy.[14] If detected early, rejection can be minimized or reversed with an increase in daily doses of immunosuppressive drugs.

When treating postoperative transplant recipients, it is important to monitor for adverse side effects of the immunosuppressive drugs. Immunosuppression protocols now promote the rapid tapering of steroids post transplantation, which diminishes the harsh side effects of the drug.[20]

*Types of Graft Rejection*

There are three types of graft rejection: hyperacute, acute, and chronic.

1. *Hyperacute rejection* is characterized by ischemia and necrosis of the graft that occurs from the time of transplant to 48 hours after transplant.[6] It is believed to be caused by ABO incompatibility and by cytotoxic antibodies present in the recipient that respond to tissue antigens on the donor organ. The manifestations of hyperacute rejection include general malaise and high fever. Rejection occurs before vascularization of the graft takes place. Hyperacute rejection is unresponsive to treatment and removal of the rejected organ is the only way to stop the reaction. Therefore, the recipient will need immediate retransplantation to survive.[6,12,21]

2. *Acute rejection* is a treatable and reversible form of rejection that occurs within the first year after transplantation. Almost every patient has some degree of acute rejection after transplantation. T lymphocytes detect foreign antigens from the graft, become

Table 12-1. Immunosuppressive Drugs Used in Organ Transplantation

| Immunosuppressive Drug | Action | Possible Adverse Effects |
| --- | --- | --- |
| Corticosteroids (methyl-prednisolone [Solu-Medrol], prednisone) | Inhibit gene transcription for cytokines, which affect all immune responses<br>Inhibit T-cell activation<br>Used to reverse early rejection | Muscle loss and weakness, hypertension, hyperglycemia, delayed wound healing, osteoporosis, weight gain, peptic ulcers, cataracts, hypokalemia, mood swings, congestive heart failure |
| Cyclosporine (Neoral, Sandimmune) | Inhibits immune responses by inhibiting T-cell lymphokine production and cell-mediated immunity by blocking transcription of early activation genes<br>Used to prevent, rather than reverse, acute rejection | Hypertension, elevated cholesterol, renal dysfunction, tremor, sodium retention, hyperkalemia, hyperglycemia, pares-thesias, hepatic dysfunction, seizures, hirsutism, gum hyperplasia, malignancy; long-term side effects: diabetic neurotoxicity, decreased bone density |
| Tacrolimus (FK506, Prograf) | Inhibits T-lymphocyte activation<br>Used to prevent acute rejection | Tremors, headache, hepatotoxicity, hypertension, hyperglycemia, hyperkalemia, constipation, diarrhea, nausea, vomiting, renal dysfunction, mental status changes |
| Azathioprine (Imuran) | Inhibits lymphocyte proliferation<br>Inhibits DNA and RNA synthesis<br>Blocks antibody production<br>Suppresses entire immune system | Bone marrow suppression, hepatotoxicity, leukopenia, pancreatitis, cholestasis |

| Mycophenolate mofetil (CellCept) | Inhibits T- and B-lymphocyte proliferation<br>Suppresses antibody formation<br>Inhibits de novo pathway for purine synthesis | Nausea, vomiting, diarrhea, leukopenia, neutropenia, sepsis, abdominal pain |
| --- | --- | --- |
| Muromonab-CD3 (Orthoclone OKT3) | Inhibits T-cell function and proliferation<br>Used only for acute rejection that is refractory to other agents | Chest pain, fever, nausea, vomiting, diarrhea, pulmonary edema, dyspnea, malignant lymphoma, rigors, malaise, meningitis |

Sources: Adapted from JM Black, E Matassarin-Jacobs (eds). Medical-Surgical Nursing: Clinical Management for Continuity of Care (5th ed). Philadelphia: Saunders, 1997;644–645; L Bucher, S Melander. Critical Care Nursing. Philadelphia: Saunders, 1999;343; and data from E Winkel, VJ DiSesa, MR Costanzo. Advances in heart transplantation. Dis Mon 1999;45(3):77–79.

sensitized, and set the immune response into action. Phagocytes, which are attracted to the graft site by the T lymphocytes, damage the inner lining of small blood vessels in the organ. This causes thrombosis of the vessels, resulting in tissue ischemia and eventual death of the graft if left untreated.[9]

The first signs of acute rejection may be detected within 4 to 10 days postoperatively.[6,7,9] The actual manifestations of rejection vary with the affected organ. General signs and symptoms of acute rejection include the following[9]:

- Sudden weight gain (6 lb in less than 3 days)

- Peripheral edema

- Fever, chills, sweating, malaise

- Dyspnea

- Decreased urine output, increased blood urea nitrogen (BUN) and serum creatinine levels

- Electrolyte imbalances

- Increased blood pressure

- Swelling and tenderness at the graft site

Early intervention is the key to reversal of acute rejection. Depending on the severity of rejection, treatment varies from a new dose of intravenous steroids, to a change in current immunosuppressive therapy, to a 10-day course of the murine monoclonal antibody muromonab-CD 3 (Orthoclone OKT3).[19] Some immunosuppressant medications used to treat acute rejection include corticosteroids (prednisone), cyclosporine (Neoral), tacrolimus (Prograf), azathioprine (Imuran), muromonab-CD 3 (Orthoclone OKT3), cyclophosphamide, antithymocyte globulin, and antilymphocyte globulin.[4]

3.   *Chronic rejection* of the graft occurs after the first year of transplantation. It is believed to result from immune complexes of immunoglobulin M and complement that form in the blood vessels of the organ. Deterioration of the graft is gradual and progressive. Immunosuppressive drugs do not stop this type of rejection. The more frequent and severe the rejection episode, the poorer the prognosis. Increasing immunosuppressive medications may slow the pro-

cess, and it may take years before the organ fails, but eventually retransplantation is required.

Chronic rejection in patients with renal transplants presents as a gradual increase in serum creatinine and BUN, electrolyte imbalance, weight gain, new-onset hypertension, decrease in urine output, and peripheral edema.[6,9]

In patients with liver transplants, chronic rejection is seen as a gradual rise in serum bilirubin and elevation of serum glutamic-oxaloacetic transaminase.[19] Progressive thickening of the hepatic arteries and narrowing of the bile ducts occur and eventually lead to progressive liver failure.

In patients with cardiac transplants, chronic rejection manifests in the form of coronary allograft vasculopathy, in which there is accelerated graft atherosclerosis or myocardial fibrosis and increasing blockage of the coronary arteries, which leads to myocardial ischemia and infarction.[6]

Chronic rejection in patients with lung transplants is manifested as bronchiolitis obliterans with symptoms of progressive dyspnea secondary to increasing airflow obstruction and a progressive decline in the forced expiratory volume in one second ($FEV_1$).[3,4]

In patients with pancreas transplants, the pancreatic vessels thicken, leading to fibrosis, and there is a decrease in insulin secretion with resultant hyperglycemia.[6]

## Infection

Suppression of the immune response prevents rejection of the transplanted organ; however, the recipient is more susceptible to infection. Infection may occur in the lungs, liver, colon, and oral mucous membrane. In addition to a surgical wound infection, the recipient is at risk for bacterial, fungal, and viral infections. Bacterial infections may occur in the urinary tract, respiratory tree, and indwelling devices, such as a central venous catheter.[17] The highest risk for infection is during the first 3 months after transplantation.[22] If infection is noted, fewer immunosuppressive drugs are given, and antibiotic treatment is initiated. Antibacterial, antiviral, and antifungal medications are often given prophylactically. Bacterial infections are treated using antibiotics. The use of trimethoprim/sulfamethoxazole (Bactrim) in prophylactic doses has been effective in preventing *Pneumocystis car-*

*inii* pneumonia in cardiac transplant recipients. Fungal infection is caused by yeast and can be treated with amphotericin. Nystatin, an oral antifungal mouthwash, is used for prevention of mucosal candidiasis that often occurs due to immunosuppression. Viral infection, such as cytomegalovirus, is very problematic. Cytomegalovirus causes different clinical syndromes, including pneumonitis, hepatitis, nephritis, and gastrointestinal ulceration.[17] If not detected and treated early with ganciclovir, it can result in the loss of the graft. While in the hospital, proper hand washing, before and after direct contact with transplant recipients, is the most important and effective way to prevent infection.

General signs and symptoms of infection include the following[7]:

• Temperature greater than 38°C (100.5°F)

• Fatigue

• Shaking chills

• Sweating

• Diarrhea lasting longer than 2 days

• Dyspnea

• Cough or sore throat

## Renal Transplantation

Renal or kidney transplants are the most common organ transplant procedure.[6] Renal transplantation is a means of restoring normal renal function to patients with irreversible end-stage renal failure.

The most frequent causes of end-stage renal disease requiring transplantation include the following[8,12]:

• Primary uncontrolled hypertension

• Glomerulonephritis

• Chronic pyelonephritis

• Diabetic nephropathy

• Polycystic kidney disease

Contraindications to renal transplantation include the following[12]:

- Advanced cardiopulmonary disease
- Active vasculitis
- Morbid obesity

### Cadaveric versus Living Donor Renal Transplantation

Kidney transplants may be cadaveric or living donor. Cadaveric kidneys may be maintained for as long as 72 hours before transplantation and, as a result, are the last organs to be harvested. Although less commonly performed, living donor kidney transplants are preferred to cadaveric transplantation. Because the body can function well with one kidney, the kidney donor can lead a normal, active life after recovering from the surgery. There is no increased risk of kidney disease, hypertension, or diabetes, and life expectancy does not change for the donor.[7]

The benefits for the recipient include a longer allograft and patient survival from a living donor kidney transplant. The recipients of living donor kidney transplants have higher survival rates (11–15 years) than the cadaveric transplant (7–8 years).[7] The higher success rate of the recipients of living donor transplants can be attributed to the following[7,23]:

- The renal allograft from a living donor can be more thoroughly evaluated before transplantation than the cadaveric allograft. This results in closer genetic matches between the donor and recipient.

- There is a lower chance of damage to the donor organ during preservation and transport.

- The incidence of acute tubular necrosis (ATN) in the postoperative period is 30–40% when a cadaveric donor is used but is infrequent with a living donor.

- Recipients of living donor transplants require less immunosuppressive medications and may have less risk of subsequent infection or malignancy.

- Living donor transplant recipients undergo transplantation as an elective procedure and may be healthier when they receive their transplant.

## Renal Transplant Procedure

The renal allograft is not placed in the same location as the native kidney. It is placed extraperitoneally in the iliac fossa through an oblique lower abdominal incision.[24,25] The renal artery and vein of the donated kidney are attached to the iliac artery and vein of the recipient. The ureter of the donated kidney is sutured to the bladder. The recipient's native kidney is not removed unless it is a source of infection or uncontrolled hypertension. The residual function may be helpful if the transplant fails and the recipient requires hemodialysis.[25,26]

The advantages of renal allograft placement in the iliac fossa versus placement in the correct anatomic position include the following[27]:

- A decrease in the postoperative pain, because the peritoneal cavity is not entered

- Easier access to the graft postoperatively for biopsy or any reoperative procedure

- Ease of palpation and auscultation of the superficial kidney to help diagnose postoperative complications

- The facilitation of vascular and ureteral anastomoses, because it is close to blood vessels and the bladder

## Indication of Renal Function Post Transplant

Restoration of renal function is characterized by immediate production of urine, massive diuresis, and declining levels of BUN and serum creatinine. Excellent renal function is characterized by a urine output of 800–1,000 ml per hour.[17] However, there is a 20–30% chance that the kidney will not function immediately, and dialysis will be required for the first few weeks.[25] Dialysis is discontinued once urine output increases and serum creatinine and BUN begin to normalize. With time, normal kidney function is restored, and the dependence on dialysis and the dietary restrictions associated with diabetes are eliminated.[25]

## Postoperative Care and Complications

Volume status is strictly assessed. Intake and output records are precisely recorded. Daily weights should be measured at the same time using the same scale. When urine volumes are extremely high, intravenous fluids may be titrated. Other volume assessment parameters include inspection of neck veins for distention, skin turgor and mucous membranes for dehydration, and extremities for edema. Auscultation of the chest is performed to determine the presence of adventitious breath sounds, such as crackles, which indicate the presence of excess volume.[12]

The most common signs of rejection specific to the kidney are an increase in BUN and serum creatinine, decrease in urine output, increase in blood pressure, weight gain greater than 1 kg in a 24-hour period, and ankle edema.[7,12,25] A percutaneous renal biopsy under ultrasound guidance is the most definitive test for acute rejection.[25] Sometimes, ATN occurs post transplantation. Twenty percent to 30% of patients receiving cadaveric kidneys preserved for longer than 24 hours experience delayed graft function.[25] This ischemic damage from prolonged preservation results in ATN. The delayed kidney function may last from a few days to 3 weeks. Therefore, dialysis is required until the kidney starts to function.[7]

Ureteral obstruction may occur owing to compression of the ureter by a fluid collection or by blockage from a blood clot in the ureter. The obstruction can cause hydronephrosis (dilation of the renal pelvis and calyces with urine), which can be seen by ultrasound.[25] The placement of a nephrostomy tube or surgery may be required to repair the obstruction and prevent irreversible damage to the allograft.[25]

Urine leaks may occur at the level of the bladder, ureter, or renal calyx. They usually occur within the first few days of transplantation.[25] Renal ultrasounds are performed to assess for fluid collections, and radionucleotide scans view the perfusion of the kidney. Other potential complications include post-transplant diabetes, renal artery thrombosis or leakage at the anastomosis, hypertension, hyperkalemia, renal abscess or decreased renal function, and pulmonary edema.[6,13,25] Thrombosis most often occurs within the first 2 to 3 days after transplantation.[25] The most common cause of decreased urine output in the immediate postoperative period is occlusion of the urinary catheter due to clot retention, in which case aseptic irrigation is required.[12]

---

### Clinical Tip

Physical therapists should closely monitor blood pressure with exercise. To ensure adequate perfusion of the newly grafted kidney, the systolic blood pressure is maintained at greater than 110 mm Hg. Kidney transplant recipients may be normotensive at rest; however, they respond to exercise with a higher-than-normal blood pressure.[1]

## Liver Transplantation

Indications for liver or hepatic transplantation include the following[6,28]:

- End-stage hepatic disease

- Primary biliary cirrhosis

- Chronic hepatitis B or C

- Fulminant hepatic failure (FHF) resulting from an acute viral, toxic, anesthetic-induced, or medication-induced liver injury

- Congenital biliary abnormalities

- Sclerosing cholangitis

- Wilson's disease

- Budd-Chiari syndrome

- Biliary atresia

- Confined hepatic malignancy (hepatocellular carcinoma)

If the cause of liver failure is alcoholic cirrhosis, the patient must be free from alcohol use for a period determined by the transplant center, which is typically 6 months or more.

Contraindications to hepatic transplantation include the following[19,28]:

- Uncontrolled extrahepatic bacterial or fungal infections

- Extrahepatic malignancy

- Advanced cardiac disease

- Myocardial infarction within the previous 6 months

- Severe chronic obstructive pulmonary disease

- Active alcohol use or other substance abuse

## Pretransplantation Care

Many transplant candidates are debilitated and malnourished secondary to many years of chronic liver failure. Table 12-2 provides some characteristics of liver failure, their clinical effects, and their implications to physical therapy.

## Types of Liver Transplants

1.  *Orthotopic cadaveric liver transplantation.* Orthotopic liver transplantation involves removal of the diseased liver and insertion of a cadaveric liver into the normal anatomic position via a midline sternotomy and continuous laparotomy.

2.  *Living adult donor liver transplant.* A single lobe of the liver from a living adult is transplanted into the recipient. The removal of the lobe does not cause any decrease in liver function to the living donor.[7] Because of the unique ability of the liver to regenerate, the donor's and recipient's livers will grow back to normal size within several months.[7]

3.  *Split liver transplant.* Split liver transplants are sometimes used to expand the donor pool. Surgeons divide an adult cadaveric liver *in situ* into two functioning allografts.[29] Usually, the smaller left lobe is donated to a child, and the larger right lobe is given to an adult.[30]

4.  *Domino liver transplant.* Domino liver transplants are currently rare and are still experimental transplantations. They involve patients with familial amyloidotic polyneuropathy (FAP). Patients with FAP have a metabolic defect within the liver. The liver is structurally and functionally normal, but it synthesizes an abnormal protein, transthyretin, that forms amyloid fibrils and deposits them in the peripheral and autonomic nerves, heart, kidney, and intestine. The domino liver transplant involves three people: the donor, the patient with FAP, and a patient listed on the liver transplant waiting list. The patient with FAP receives the donated liver. The removed liver (from the patient with FAP) is then transplanted into the other transplant recipient, hence the term *domino transplant*. Liver transplantation for patients with FAP leads to normal transthyretin protein production. The recipient who received the FAP liver will likely never experience any of the symptoms associated with FAP, because they take 40–60 years to manifest.[7]

**Table 12-2.** Medical Characteristics of Liver Failure, Their Related Clinical Effects, and Physical Therapy Implications

| Medical Characteristics of Liver Failure | Clinical Effects | Physical Therapy Implications |
| --- | --- | --- |
| ↑ Bilirubin level | Jaundice. Dark, tea-colored urine. May induce nausea and anorexia. | None. |
| ↓ Albumin synthesis | Accumulation of ascites fluid in the peritoneal cavity causes abdominal swelling and increased abdominal girth. May promote protein loss and a negative nitrogen balance. May lead to anasarca (total body edema). | May cause pressure on the diaphragm, leading to respiratory and nutritional difficulties. Monitor for dyspnea with activity. Patient may have an altered center of gravity and decreased balance. |
| Altered clotting ability | Increased prothrombin time and partial thromboplastin time. | Prolonged bleeding time. Patient bruises easily. Monitor patient safety and prevention of falls. |
| Impaired glucose production | Low blood sugar. | Patient may have decreased energy. |
| Portal hypertension | Presence of esophageal varices. May lead to hepatic encephalopathy. | Bleeding may occur spontaneously. Patient may have altered mental status and decreased safety awareness. |
| Diminished phagocytic activity | Spontaneous bacterial peritonitis or cholangitis. | None. |
| Failure to absorb vitamin D | Osteoporosis may result. | May develop compression or pathologic fractures. |

↑ = elevated; ↓ = decreased.
Sources: Data from KM Sigardson-Poor, LM Haggerty. Nursing Care of the Transplant Recipient. Philadelphia: Saunders, 1990;149–151; and RL Braddom (ed). Physical Medicine and Rehabilitation (2nd ed). Philadelphia: Saunders, 2000;1397.

## Indication of Liver Function Post Transplant

1. Once the graft is vascularized in the operating room, the functioning liver starts to produce bile.[12] Thus, prompt outflow of bile through the biliary T tube, which is inserted at the time of surgery, is an early indicator of proper function of the transplanted liver.[9] Thick, dark-green bile drainage indicates good liver function. A sudden drop in amount of bile or change to a light yellow color indicates an alteration in liver function.[9]

2. The most sensitive laboratory indices of liver function are the coagulation factors, prothrombin time (PT) and partial thromboplastin time (PTT). Alteration in liver function is reflected very early by prolonged coagulation times. A steady downward trend to normalization of the PT and PTT should occur postoperatively.[12]

3. The liver function tests (LFTs) should reveal a progressive decline after transplantation. The exact values can vary from patient to patient. For example, if the recipient required large amounts of blood transfusion, the initial LFT levels may be low secondary to hemodilution. More accurate levels are determined 6–12 hours after surgery.[12]

4. In the immediate postoperative period, hypokalemia is another sign that the liver is functional. Once the graft is vascularized, hepatocytes extract potassium from the blood. On the other hand, hyperkalemia often signifies cell death and that the hepatocytes are nonfunctional.[12]

5. Hyperglycemia also indicates that the liver is able to store glycogen and convert it to glucose.

### Postoperative Care and Complications

Postoperatively, liver transplant recipients may emerge with three Jackson-Pratt (JP) suction drains and a biliary T tube. The JP drains lie over the superior surface of the liver and drain blood-tinged fluid. Two of the JP drains are removed within the first 48 hours of surgery. The last JP drain is removed approximately 7 days after surgery, in the absence of a biliary leak.[7,19] The T tube, which is placed in the bile duct, remains in place for up to 12 weeks postoperatively. The amount, color, and consistency of the bile are monitored. The T tube is clamped once the bilirubin level falls below 2.5 mg/dl.[7,19] (The reference range of total bilirubin is 0.1–1.0 mg/dl.)

Primary graft failure is a sign of acute hepatic failure that may be seen immediately postoperatively. It is characterized by a markedly abnormal liver function; prolonged PT, PTT, or both; oliguria; metabolic acidosis; hyperkalemia; hypoglycemia; and coma. In the event of primary graft failure, retransplantation is immediately required.

Potential medical complications include post-transplant diabetes, abscess, atelectasis, and pneumonia secondary to ascites or peritonitis.[6] Acute rejection specific to a transplanted liver includes elevated LFTs (especially an increase in bilirubin and prolonged PT, PTT, or both); jaundice; right upper quadrant pain; clay-colored stools; tea-colored urine; decreased quantity of bile; thin, watery, light-colored bile through the T tube; and increased ascitic drainage. If rejection is identified, immunosuppressive drug doses are increased.

A liver biopsy is the definitive diagnostic test for rejection and is performed at bedside. It can distinguish between early rejection and ischemic injury. Mild rejection will result in elevated serum transaminase or alkaline phosphatase, whereas an elevated serum glutamicoxaloacetic transaminase and serum glutamate-pyruvate transaminase may indicate hepatocellular damage associated with rejection.[19]

Surgical complications include hepatic artery thrombosis, biliary leak, or stricture. These complications present with a rising bilirubin level and are identical in appearance to an acute rejection episode.[19] Consequently, recipients undergo routine Doppler ultrasound of the abdomen to check for fluid collections and patency of the hepatic artery and portal vein.[19] A cholangiogram, which examines the patency of the biliary tree drainage system, may be performed to rule out bile duct obstruction. Surgical intervention is indicated if the biliary obstruction cannot be corrected by a percutaneous transhepatic cholangiogram. Portal vein thrombosis is evident if ascites persists or variceal hemorrhage develops.[13]

---

### Clinical Tip

- Postoperatively, many recipients still have ascites from weeping of sodium- and albumin-rich fluid from the liver's surface.[9] Along with ascites and postsurgical fluid retention, liver transplant recipients have an increased abdominal girth and lower-extremity edema that lead to a shift in the patient's center of gravity and impaired balance. Often, patients have an increase in lumbar lordosis and complain of low back pain.

- Deep breathing and physical activity are beneficial during the early postoperative course. Liver transplant recipients are susceptible to atelectasis and pneumonia because of the long operative procedure and large incision that hinders full chest expansion and cough effectiveness.

## Pancreas Transplantation

### Indication for Pancreas Transplant

Pancreas transplant candidates have insulin-dependent, type 1 diabetes mellitus and are preuremic (without urea in the blood). These patients have severe brittle diabetes and metabolic imbalances, such as hypoglycemic unawareness and subcutaneous insulin resistance.[31,32] Pancreas transplantation attempts to stabilize or prevent the devastating target organ complications of type 1 diabetes by returning the patient to normoglycemia and improving the patient's quality of life.[33] Ideally, pancreas transplantation should be performed before secondary complications of diabetes, such as retinopathy, peripheral neuropathy, vasculopathy, and end-stage renal disease, develop. Pancreas transplantation has been demonstrated to inhibit the progression of neuropathy and reverse diabetic nephropathic lesions in native kidneys after 5–10 years, but it has not been shown to stop severe retinopathy or vascular disease.[32] Because pancreas transplantation is not a life-saving procedure, the patient's condition is evaluated carefully to determine whether the benefits outweigh the risks of transplantation.

Contraindications to pancreas transplantation include the following[32]:

- Severe cardiovascular disease

- Major amputation

- Complete blindness

- Morbid obesity

- Active smoking

Living donor pancreas transplantation, in which the segment of the body and tail of the pancreas are used from a living donor, may be performed; however, whole-organ cadaveric pancreas transplantation is preferred. The donor pancreas is placed intraperitoneally through an oblique lower abdominal incision.[13]

### Enteric Drainage versus Bladder Drainage

The pancreas can be transplanted with a segment of the duodenum to facilitate drainage of pancreatic exocrine secretions.[32] *Enteric drainage* involves anastomosis of the donor duodenum to a loop of the recipient's small bowel.[34] *Bladder drainage* is obtained by anastomosing the donor duodenum with the recipient's urinary bladder.[32] This permits exocrine secretions to be expelled with the urine and allows monitoring of urine amylase as a marker for rejection.[32,34] The disadvantage of bladder drainage is that urologic and metabolic complications are common. Large quantities of sodium bicarbonate that are produced by the pancreas and duodenum are lost, which can result in metabolic acidosis.[35] The pancreas also secretes 1 to 2 liters of fluid each day; thus, if the patient is not adequately hydrated, the loss of this additional fluid results in volume depletion or dehydration. Reflux of the urine into the transplanted organ may cause pancreatitis, and irritation of the bladder mucosa from the digestive enzymes of the pancreas often results in urinary tract infections and urethral stricture formation.[35] Enteric conversion after transplantation may be required if there are persistent poor bladder function and recurrent urinary infections.[32,34] Despite its disadvantages, the bladder drainage technique is more common than the enteric drainage technique, because it allows monitoring of urine amylase for detection of rejection.[31] Enteric drainage is more difficult to monitor for acute rejection and has more episodes of infection post procedure. Ultimately, bladder, rather than enteric, drainage is the choice of the transplant surgeon.[32]

### Indication of Pancreatic Function Post Transplant

Within 24 hours, the transplanted pancreas should be producing insulin. Analysis of blood glucose response and C-peptide levels is used to determine a successful pancreatic transplant. Immediately after transplantation, blood sugar levels are monitored every hour, because glucose levels typically drop 50 mg/dl each hour, and dextrose infusion may be necessary.[34] The blood glucose level should range between 80 and 150 mg/dl within a few hours after the transplantation.[13] C-peptide levels are elevated, and blood sugar level returns to normal within 2 to 3 days postoperatively.[6] After a diet is started, serum glucose is monitored four times a day. Recipients should return to normal or near-normal fasting plasma glucose levels, glycosylated hemoglobin levels (which represent the average blood glucose level over the previous several weeks), and glucose tolerance tests.[31,36] The recipient weans from insulin and becomes insulin independent with normal carbohydrate metabolism for an indefinite period.[13,36] The need for strict adherence to a diet and constant blood sugar monitoring should diminish.[6] Long-term follow-up studies indicate the insulin independence can be sustained for at least 5 years.[36]

## Postoperative Care and Complications

The recipient is often placed on strict bed rest for a few days postoperatively to prevent kinking of the vascular allografts that may result from a position shift of the pancreas.[13] A Foley catheter is left in place for at least the first week to prevent distention of the bladder and leakage from the bladder anastomosis.[13] During the first postoperative day, a baseline radionuclide blood flow study of the pancreas and a Doppler ultrasonography of the allograft vasculature are performed. Repetition of these studies and operative intervention are performed urgently with any sign of pancreatic dysfunction.[13]

Acute rejection after pancreas transplantation is difficult to diagnose. Nonspecific clinical criteria, such as fever, allograft tenderness, ileus, abdominal pain, hematuria, leukocytosis, and hyperglycemia, can be used in combination to detect acute pancreas rejection.[32,35] Hyperglycemia does not occur until 80–90% of the graft has been destroyed.[17] A decrease in bicarbonate, urine pH, or urine amylase levels of more than 25% from baseline, an elevation of serum amylase, or a combination of these factors also indicates acute pancreas rejection in a bladder-drained pancreas transplant recipient.[12,13,15,35] Percutaneous ultrasound-guided or cystoscopic biopsy of the transplanted pancreas is used as a sensitive histologic method to confirm acute graft rejection.[15,32]

Complications related to the bladder drainage procedure in pancreas transplantation include urinary tract infections, dysuria, urethritis, duodenocystostomy fistulas, duodenal-bladder anastomotic leak, duodenal stump leak, chronic hematuria, allograft pancreatitis, metabolic acidosis, dehydration, and hyperkalemia.[23,31] Severe dehydration and acidosis can occur secondary to large losses of bicarbonate in the urine.[13] Other potential complications include graft thrombosis, decreased pancreatic function, peritonitis, pancreatic abscess, intra-abdominal bleeding, and infections.[6,32]

---

Clinical Tip

Remind pancreas transplant recipients to drink enough flu-ids to rehydrate themselves during and after exercise. Hydration is critical in patients with a bladder-drained pan-creas. Recipients must take in 3–4 liters of fluid per day.[34]

---

## Pancreas-Kidney Transplantation

### Types of Pancreas-Kidney Transplants

1. *Simultaneous Pancreas-Kidney (SPK) transplants.* Typically, SPK transplants are offered to patients who have type 1 diabetes mellitus with diabetic nephropathy and renal insufficiency. SPK transplants are more common than a non–life saving pancreas transplantation alone, as physicians are reluctant to use potent immunosuppressive drugs in patients with diabetes before they need a concomitant renal transplant.[36] The benefits of a successful SPK transplant include normoglycemia, elim-ination of dialysis, and prevention of reoccurring diabetic nephropathy in the kidney graft.[31,36]

SPK transplants may be cadaveric or from living donors, in which case a segmental pancreas transplant is performed. Using an abdomi-nal midline incision, the pancreatic graft is implanted first on the right side, and then the kidney graft is implanted on the left side.[15]

2. *Pancreas after kidney (PAK) transplants.* A pancreas trans-plant is performed on a patient who has already received a cadaveric or a living donor kidney transplant.

### Postoperative Care and Complications

In SPK transplants, pancreas rejection episodes frequently occur con-currently with renal allograft rejection. Rejection of the donor pan-creas is more difficult to diagnose; therefore, acute rejection of both allografts is recognized by a deterioration in kidney function (i.e., an increase in serum creatinine).[34,36] When rejection is clinically sus-pected, kidney biopsy specimens are obtained.

The SPK transplant involves a more complex surgical procedure, with more complications and rehospitalizations and a higher incidence of rejection and immunosuppression required than renal transplant alone.[34] The advantage of near-perfect glucose metabolism and the prevention of further secondary diabetic complications help to justify the increased risk.[34] However, graft survival after SKP transplant is higher than graft survival after solitary pancreas transplantation, because renal allograft rejection is easier to detect.

## Cardiac Transplantation

Candidates for heart transplantation have irreversible end-stage cardiac disease, no other surgical or medical options, and a poor prognosis for survival longer than 6 months.[9] Patients typically present with low exercise tolerance, cachexia, generalized weakness, decreased muscle mass, marginal blood pressure, dyspnea, and poor peripheral perfusion.[37]

Common indications for heart transplants include the following[5,9,21]:

- Cardiomyopathy

- Severe left ventricular disease (ejection fraction less than 20%)

- Ischemic heart disease

- Congenital heart disease

- Valvular disease

- Inoperable coronary artery disease, with angina refractory to medical management

- Malignant ventricular dysrhythmias unresponsive to medical or surgical therapy, or both

- Primary cardiac tumors with no evidence of spread to other systems

Contraindications to cardiac transplantation include the following[5,12,21,22]:

- Fixed pulmonary hypertension

- Unresolved pulmonary infarction

- Active peptic ulcer disease

- Type 1 diabetes mellitus with secondary complications

- Chronic obstructive pulmonary disease (COPD) with an $FEV_1$ of less than 50%

### Orthotopic and Heterotopic Heart Transplantation

Orthotopic and heterotopic transplantation are the two types of heart transplant procedures. The more common orthotopic procedure involves a median sternotomy with removal of the recipient's heart (with the exception of the posterior right atrium with sinoatrial node, left atrium, aorta, and pulmonary artery) and the insertion of the donor heart in the normal anatomic position.[5,10,38,39]

In a *heterotopic* or "piggy-back" transplantation, the diseased heart is left intact, and the donor heart is placed in the right side of the thorax adjacent to the native heart with anastomosis between the two hearts. The purpose of the heterotopic transplant is for the donor heart to assist the failing heart. The donor left ventricle supports most of the systemic circulation, and the native right ventricle supports the pulmonary circulation.[13] The heterotopic transplant recipient has two distinct electrocardiograms with different heart rates.[13] Heterotopic transplantation is rare, but it may be used in cases in which there is a size mismatch between the donor and recipient hearts or the recipient has moderate to severe pulmonary hypertension.[5,11,39]

Whether orthotopic or heterotopic heart transplantation is performed, epicardial pacing wires and mediastinal and pleural chest tubes are inserted before closure of the chest wall (see Appendix III-A).

### Indication of Cardiac Function Post Transplant

Postoperatively, patients have a pulmonary artery catheter (that indirectly assesses left ventricular function and cardiac output) and an arterial line (that monitors peripheral arterial pressure) for hemodynamic monitoring. Immediately after surgery, the patient's complete blood count, arterial blood gas, serum electrolyte, metabolic functions, and cyclosporine levels are monitored closely.[5] In addition, an echocardiogram is performed immediately postoperatively to evaluate heart function and left ventricular ejection fraction. Pulmonary artery pressures and fluid balance are monitored closely.[5] Depending on the hemodynamic values, lab values, and ejection fraction, pharmacologic agents and mechanical support are initiated or weaned. Heart rate and rhythm disturbances are treated pharmacologically or by use of epicardial pacing wires.

The new heart takes a few days to achieve a stable intrinsic rhythm.[22] Isoproterenol hydrochloride is typically used for its inotropic and chronotropic effects. The inotropic effect of the drug decreases the peripheral vascular resistance (PVR) and systemic vascular resistance, thus assisting the recovery of the donor heart.[22] The chronotropic effect increases the heart rate and is typically required for the first 3 postoperative days to increase preload and cardiac output and maintain a heart rate of approximately 110 beats per minute.[11,22] Systolic blood pressure should be maintained at 90–110 mm Hg, with afterload reduction agents, such as nitroglycerin, to help reduce the PVR.[5] Sometimes an intra-aortic balloon pump (IABP) must be used to decrease afterload.[5]

Sinus node dysfunction, resulting from donor heart ischemia, atrial stretch, or intraoperative trauma, may cause a slow junctional rhythm. It is treated with bipolar atrial pacing or with a chronotropic drug, such as dobutamine.[5] Ideally, the heart rate should be maintained at 90 to 110 beats per minute to optimize cardiac output.[5] Cardiac function usually returns to normal within 3 to 4 days, at which time intravenous medications, mechanical support, and pacing mechanisms are weaned.[5]

## Postoperative Care and Complications

Immediate postoperative care for cardiac transplant recipients is similar to that of patients who have undergone cardiothoracic surgery. Chest tubes are typically removed 2 days postoperatively once chest drainage is less than 25 ml per hour, and pacing wires are removed 7 days after transplantation if there were no events of bradycardia.[5]

During the early hours after the transplant, the patient may manifest a variable global myocardial depression.[5] This may result from prolonged administration of high levels of vasopressors, an elevated PVR in the recipient, or a prolonged ischemic time.[5] Ischemic time is the time from the cross-clamp of the donor organ to the removal of the recipient's new heart from cardiopulmonary bypass.[22] Ideally, the ischemic time for a heart transplant should be less than 6 hours.[8]

With myocardial depression, the transplanted heart may be affected temporarily by bradycardia, decreased diastolic compliance, diminished systolic function, and impaired contractility.[5,13]

Other potential complications after heart transplant include mediastinal bleeding, cyclosporine-induced hypertension, post-transplant diabetes, thrombosis or leakage of anastomosis, right heart failure, biventricular heart failure, pulmonary hypertension, pericardial effusion, and renal dysfunction.[5,10,14,22] Biventricular failure is a potential complication that is seen in the first 24–48 hours after transplantation. Most patients have some degree of pulmonary hypertension because of native left ventricular failure. Right heart failure is the most common cause of cardiac dysfunction postoperatively.[22] It may be caused by a pre-existing elevated PVR, donor size mismatch in which the donor heart is too small for the recipient, long ischemic time of more than 4 hours, and acute rejection.[22] Clinical evidence of right ventricular heart failure includes hypotension, low cardiac output, an elevated central venous pressure, and low urinary output.[13] Right atrial pressures, pulmonary artery pressure, PVR, cardiac output, and signs of right-sided heart failure are monitored closely.[5] Medications, such as isoproterenol hydrochloride or milrinone, are used to reduce pulmonary pressures and make it easier for the right heart to pump.[22]

Many cardiac transplant recipients have pre-existing renal insufficiency due to their low cardiac output, congestive heart failure, and long-term diuretic use.[5,22] After transplantation, cardiopulmonary bypass and the use of cyclosporine, which is a nephrotoxic agent, can cause renal failure in the transplant recipient.[5] Dopamine is administered to improve renal blood flow, and diuretics are used to maintain adequate urine output.[5] In addition, intravenous cyclosporine may be held postoperatively, and, instead, less-nephrotoxic agents may be administered.[22]

Heart transplant recipients have an increased risk of excessive postoperative bleeding and cardiac tamponade.[13] Owing to chronic congestive heart failure, patients usually have passive liver congestion, which increases the risk of bleeding.[22] Many patients also receive anticoagulation therapy preoperatively to prevent thrombus formation. However, inadequate heparin reversal may occur and, depending on the severity of anticoagulation, treatment includes transfusion of platelets or fresh-frozen plasma.[22]

Objective characteristics of acute rejection specific to cardiac transplant recipients include new cardiac arrhythmias, hypotension, pericardial friction rub, ventricular $S_3$ gallop, decreased cardiac output, peripheral edema, pulmonary crackles, and jugular vein distention.[10-12] Subjectively, recipients may report vague symptoms of decreased exercise tolerance, fatigue, lethargy, or dyspnea. However, the most reliable technique to diagnose rejection is by performing periodic endomyocardial biopsy. The initial biopsy is performed 5–10 days after transplantation. Under local anesthesia, a bioptome catheter is advanced through the right internal jugular vein into the right ventricle under fluoroscopy. Because rejection usually occurs in small areas throughout the heart, three to five tissue specimens are obtained from different sites for histologic and immunologic studies.[11,22] The presence of lymphocytic infiltration, polymorphonuclear leukocytes, interstitial hemorrhage, and myocytic necrosis is an indicator of cardiac rejection, the latter being the most severe.[12] The frequency of surveillance endomyocardial biopsies varies between transplant institutions. They are usually performed weekly for the first month, biweekly for the second and third months, monthly for the next 6 months, every 3 months up to the first 2 years, and then annually.[11,13] If rejection is identified, immunosuppressive agents are intensified by administration of high-dose oral or intravenous corticosteroids, antilymphocyte antibodies, or both.[14] If the cardiac transplant recipient has frequent arrhythmias (which often indicate ischemia), periodic coronary angiography is performed to detect allograft coronary disease.[10,12]

---

### Clinical Tip

• The patient is placed in a protective isolation room. Positive-pressure flow rooms are recommended to limit the transfer of airborne pathogens. The use of a face mask and strict hand washing are required.[39]

• In the initial postoperative period, mediastinal drainage is promoted by elevating the head of the bed to a 30-degree angle and turning the patient every 1–2 hours.[5]

• Phase I cardiac rehabilitation usually begins 2–3 days postoperatively, once the patient is hemodynamically stable. Exercise is progressive and based on the patient's activity tolerance. Exercise is progressed from active supine exercises without resistance to ambulation and stationary biking. Vital signs are monitored before, during, and immediately after exercise.

- The cardiac transplant recipient has a resting heart rate that is higher than normal, owing to the absence of parasympathetic nervous system or vagal tone that would normally slow the heart rate.[5] The rate is usually between 90 and 110 beats per minute, and it does not vary with the recipient's respirations. The transplanted heart is denervated because the extrinsic nervous supply to the donor heart was severed during the procurement surgery.[11] Therefore, it no longer has autonomic nervous system connection to the recipient's body. Consequently, it is unaffected by the recipient's sympathetic and parasympathetic nervous system, which normally controls the rate and contractility.[5,9]
- Patients should gradually increase and decrease demands on the transplanted heart by extending their warm-up and cool-down periods to 5–10 minutes.[9,11,39] In the absence of neural regulation, heart rate increases during exercise, but the increase at the onset of exercise is delayed by 3–5 minutes.[1,40] The denervated heart depends on circulating catecholamines to increase the rate and force of contractions.[5] With exercise, heart rate and cardiac output increase gradually over 3–5 minutes and remain elevated for a longer period of time at the completion of activity.[1] As well, after cessation of exercise, there is a slower-than-normal return to pre-exercise heart rate level.[1,9–11]
- The peak heart rate achieved during maximal exercise is significantly lower in cardiac transplant recipients than in age-matched patients. As a result, exercise prescriptions that are based on target heart rate are not recommended.[11] Instead, the Borg scale, which uses the rate of perceived exertion (RPE), is frequently used during exercise for self-monitoring. The recipients exercise at an RPE between 11 and 13.[11]
- Physical therapists should monitor blood pressure before, during, and after activity. At rest, systolic and diastolic blood pressures of heart transplant recipients are higher than normal.[11,40] The systolic blood pressure should be between 80 and 150 mm Hg, and the diastolic blood pressure should be less than 90 mm Hg.[39]
- Orthostatic hypotension is common in the early postoperative phase, owing to the absence of compensatory reflex tachycardia.[5] Allow the patient time to change position slowly and adapt to the new position.[41]

- Because the transplanted heart is denervated, the recipient does not experience anginal chest pain or pressure. Myocardial ischemia is silent but can manifest as atrial or ventricular arrhythmias and with symptoms of dyspnea, lightheadedness, or an increased RPE.[42] While the patient exercises, a cardiac nurse should closely monitor the telemetry for arrhythmias.[10,12] Complaints of chest pain from the recipient may be due to the sternal incision and musculoskeletal manipulation during surgery.[42]
- The electrocardiogram of a heart transplant recipient has two P waves, as both donor and recipient sinoatrial nodes remain functional. The retained atria of the recipient generates a P wave; however, it does not cross the surgical suture line and therefore does not produce a ventricular contraction. Only the donor P wave can conduct an electrical response leading to a contraction of the heart (i.e., the donor P wave is followed by a QRS complex from the donor heart).[22,24]
- Because fatigue is a sign of rejection or ischemia, it is important to monitor day-to-day changes in a patient's exercise tolerance and keep the patient's nurse or physician notified of any significant changes.[39]
- Patients should follow sternotomy precautions; they are not allowed to push, pull, or lift anything heavier than 10 lb for 2 months after their surgery.

## Lung Transplantation

Major indications for lung transplantations include the following[3,4,16]:

- COPD (with $FEV_1$ of less than 20% of predicted value)
- Cystic fibrosis (with $FEV_1$ of less than 30% of predicted value)
- Emphysema
- Bronchiectasis
- Primary pulmonary hypertension
- Pulmonary fibrosis

- Eisenmenger's syndrome (a congenital heart disease in which there is a defect of the ventricular septum, a malpositioned aortic root that over-rides the interventricular septum, and a dilated pulmonary artery)

- Alpha$_1$-antitrypsin deficiency

Less-frequent indications include the following[4]:

- Sarcoidosis (see Appendix 10-A)

- Eosinophilic granuloma (growth in the bone or lung characterized by eosinophils and histocytes)

- Scleroderma

Contraindications to lung transplantation include the following[16]:

- Poor left ventricular cardiac function

- Significant coronary artery disease

- Significant dysfunction of other vital organs (e.g. liver, kidney, central nervous system)

- Active cigarette smoking

There are three types of surgical procedures for lung transplantation:

1.  *Single-lung transplantation.* This is the most common surgical technique and is indicated for all types of end-stage lung disease, except cystic fibrosis and bronchiectasis.[3] It involves a single anterolateral or posterolateral thoracotomy in which the right or left cadaveric lung is transplanted into the recipient.[16]

2.  *Double-lung* or *bilateral lung transplantation.* With double-lung transplantation, the left and right lungs are transplanted sequentially into one recipient, with the least functional lung resected and replaced first.[16] The incision used is a bilateral anterior thoracotomy in the fourth or fifth intercostal space. Some surgeons also may perform a transverse sternotomy to create a "clamshell" incision.[16] Patients with cystic fibrosis and bronchiectasis require double-lung transplantation to remove both infected lungs. It is also the preferred procedure for patients with pulmonary hypertension.[3,17]

3.  *Living donor lobar transplantation.* Transplantation of lobes involves bilateral implantation of lower lobes from two blood-group-compatible, living donors.[3] The donor's lungs are larger than the recipients for the donor lobes to fill each hemithorax.[3] This procedure is performed primarily for patients with cystic fibrosis. In addition, patients with bronchopulmonary dysplasia, primary pulmonary hypertension, pulmonary fibrosis, and obliterative bronchiolitis may benefit from a lobar transplantation.[8,13]

### Indication of Lung Function Post Transplant

For patients with pulmonary vascular disease, single- and double-lung transplantation results in an immediate and sustained normalization of pulmonary vascular resistance and pulmonary arterial pressures.[3] This is accompanied by an immediate increase in cardiac output. Arterial oxygenation generally returns to normal, and supplemental oxygen is no longer required, usually by the time of hospital discharge.[3]

The maximum improvement in lung function and exercise capacity is achieved within 3 to 6 months after transplantation, once the limiting effects of postoperative pain, altered chest wall mechanics, respiratory muscle dysfunction, and acute lung injury have subsided.[3,4] After double-lung transplantation, normal pulmonary function is usually achieved. However, in single-lung transplantation, lung function improves but does not normalize fully, owing to the disease and residual impairment of the remaining nontransplanted lung. Lung volumes and flow rates improve to two-thirds of normal in single-lung transplantation.[4] Most lung transplant recipients are therefore able to resume an active lifestyle, free of supplemental oxygen, with less dyspnea and improved exercise tolerance.

### Postoperative Care and Complications

Ineffective postoperative airway clearance occurs after lung transplantation. Recipients present with an impaired cough reflex, incisional pain, altered chest wall musculoskeletal function, and diminished mucociliary clearance. Coughing and deep breathing must be relearned, because the lung is denervated.[42] After extubation, aggressive bronchopulmonary hygiene is performed every 2–4 hours, while the patient is awake.[12] Physical therapists, respiratory therapists, and nursing staff provide this intensive pulmonary care. This includes postural drainage, airway suctioning, vibration, gentle percussion, diaphragmatic breathing, coughing exercises, and use of an incentive spirometer and flutter valve device to maximize lung expansion and prevent atelectasis and pneumonia. The large quantity of secretions (20–60 ml per day) is generally thick and blood tinged, and can lead to volume loss and consolidation in the transplanted lung if not suctioned or expectorated.[12] Bronchopulmonary hygiene is a crucial part of the postoperative care, as it helps mobilize secretions and prevent atelectasis and mucous plugging.

Postoperative complications that may develop in the denervated transplanted lung include pulmonary edema or effusion, acute respiratory distress syndrome, dehiscence of the bronchial anastomosis, and anastomotic stenosis.[3] Single-lung transplant recipients may experience complications of ventilation-perfusion mismatch and hyperinflation owing to the markedly different respiratory mechanics in each hemithorax.[13] The rate of infection in lung transplant recipients is higher than that of other organ transplant recipients, because the graft is exposed to the external environment through the recipient's native airway. The patient's white blood cell (WBC) and absolute neutrophil count are monitored closely.[6] Bacterial pneumonia and bronchial infections are very common complications that usually occur in the first 30 days.[3,13] Bronchoalveolar lavage is used to diagnose opportunistic infections.[17]

Clinical manifestations of acute pulmonary rejection in lung transplant recipients include dyspnea, nonproductive cough, leukocytosis, hypoxemia, pulmonary infiltrates as seen on chest x-ray, sudden deterioration of pulmonary function tests (PFTs), elevated WBC count, need for ventilatory support, fever, and fatigue.[6,12,16] The rejection typically presents with a sudden deterioration of clinical status over 6–12 hours.[17] Daily documentation of the oxygen saturation and the $FEV_1$ is used to monitor and detect early rejection, especially in bilateral lung transplant recipients, because a decline in oxygen saturation or spirometry values in excess of 10% commonly accompany episodes of rejection or infection.[3,4,43]

Bronchoscopic lung biopsy and bronchiolar lavages are used to diagnose acute rejection. The presence of perivascular lymphocytic infiltrates is the histologic hallmark of acute rejection.[3,17] Transbronchial biopsies often do not supply enough pulmonary parenchyma for histologic testing.[43] Instead, cytoimmunologic monitoring of the peripheral blood may be used as a specific diagnostic test for acute pulmonary rejection. Bronchoscopy is performed routinely and whenever rejection is suspected to assess airway secretions, healing of the anastomosis, and the condition of the bronchial mucous membrane.[12] The first bronchoscopy is performed in the operating room to inspect the bronchial anastomosis.[17] To prevent infection and atelectasis, routine fiberoptic bronchoscopy with saline lavage and suctioning are used to reduce accumulation of secretions that the recipient is unable to clear.[13]

---

### Clinical Tip

- If the recipient is intubated, suctioning may be performed with a premeasured catheter to prevent damage to the anastomosis. Suctioning removes secretions and helps maintain adequate oxygenation.
- After lung transplantation, recipients should sleep in reverse Trendelenburg position to aid in postural drainage, as long as they are hemodynamically stable.
- In the intensive care unit, during the first 24 hours after surgery, patients with double-lung transplants should be turned side to side. Turning is initiated gradually, beginning with 20- to 30-degree turns and assessing vital signs, and then increasing gradually to 90 degrees each way, every 1–2 hours. Prolonged periods in supine position are avoided to minimize secretion retention.[12]
- Patients with single-lung transplants should lie on their nonoperative side to reduce postsurgical edema, assist with gravitational drainage of the airway, and promote optimal inflation of the new lung.[12]
- Bronchopulmonary hygiene before exercise may enhance the recipient's activity tolerance.
- Schedule physical therapy visits after the patient receives his or her nebulizer treatment and after the patient is premedicated for pain control. Incisional pain can limit activity progression, deep breathing exercises, and coughing. Also, splinting the incision with the use of a pillow can help reduce incisional pain while coughing.
- Lung transplant recipients follow strict thoracotomy precautions. They are not allowed to lift anything heavier than 10 lb. They are restricted to partial weight bearing of their upper extremities, which may limit the use of an assistive device.

- Patients are on respiratory isolation precautions; exercise is performed in the recipient's room. All staff must mask, gown, and glove on entering the patient's room for approximately 1 week. However, the recipient may ambulate in the hallway, if a protective mask is worn.
- Always monitor the recipient's oxygen saturation before, during, and after exercise. If the patient is on room air at rest, supplemental oxygen may be beneficial during exercise to reduce dyspnea and improve activity tolerance. The lung transplant recipient should maintain an arterial oxyhemoglobin saturation greater than 90% with activity.[41]
- Multiple rest periods may be required during activity at the beginning of the postoperative period to limit the amount of dyspnea and muscle fatigue. Rest periods can be gradually decreased so that the patient advances toward periods of continuous exercise as endurance improves.

## Heart-Lung Transplantation

Heart-lung transplantation is performed on patients who have a coexistence of end-stage pulmonary disease and advanced cardiac disease that produces right-sided heart failure.[12]

Indications for HLT include the following[3,8,24]:

- Primary pulmonary hypertension

- COPD

- Cystic fibrosis

- Pulmonary fibrosis

- Eisenmenger's syndrome

- Irreparable cardiac defects or congenital heart disease

- Advanced lung disease and coexisting left ventricular dysfunction or extensive coronary artery disease

The heart and lung of the donor are removed en bloc and placed in the recipient's chest. The anastomosis to join the donor organs is at the trachea, right atrium, and aorta.[8,13] Postoperative HLT care is similar to the heart and lung post-transplant care previously discussed. Rejection of the heart and lung allografts occurs independent of each other.[24] Bacterial pneumonia from contamination in the donor tracheobronchial tree is the most common cause of morbidity and mortality after HLT.[8]

## Bone Marrow Transplantation

BMTs are performed only after conventional methods of treatment fail to replace defective bone marrow. BMT recipients receive healthy marrow from a living donor in an attempt to restore hematologic and immunologic functions. The three types of BMTs are allogeneic, syngeneic, and autologous transplants.

1.    An *allogeneic transplant* is one in which bone marrow is harvested from an HLA-matched donor and immediately infused into the recipient after cytoreduction therapy. The donor may be related or unrelated.

2.    A *syngeneic transplant* is one in which bone marrow is harvested from an identical twin.

3.    An *autologous transplant* is one in which the donor and recipient are the same. Bone marrow is harvested from the patient when he or she is healthy or in complete remission. The marrow is then frozen and stored for future reinfusion.

One type of autologous BMT is the peripheral blood stem cell (PBSC) transplant. Stem cells are primitive cells found in bone marrow or circulating blood that evolve into mature blood cells (white cells, red cells, and platelets). The patient's PBSCs are harvested by leukapheresis. During leukapheresis, the patient's blood is circulated through a high-speed cell separator in which the peripheral stem cells are frozen and stored, and the plasma cells and erythrocytes are reinfused into the patient. The patient may require three to seven harvests to achieve an adequate number of stem cells.[6] The PBSCs are reinfused after the patient receives lethal doses of chemotherapy, radiation, or both. Allogenic PBSC transplant may be performed from a donor or by using umbilical cord blood from a newborn.[6] The hematologic recovery after PBSC transplant is 10–12 days, which is approximately a week earlier than in BMTs.[42] This is because the stem cells procured from the peripheral blood are more mature than in the bone marrow.

Indications for BMT include the following[9,42,44,45]:

- Severe aplastic anemia
- Acute lymphocytic or myelogenous leukemia
- Chronic myelogenous leukemia
- Non-Hodgkin's lymphoma
- Relapsed Hodgkin's disease
- Multiple myeloma
- Neuroblastoma
- Testicular cancer
- Small cell lung cancer
- Breast cancer

Contraindications to BMT include the following[45]:

- Inadequate cardiac function (left ventricular ejection fraction less than 45%)
- Inadequate pulmonary function (forced expiratory capacity and forced vital capacity less than 50%)
- Inadequate renal function (creatinine greater than 2 mg/dl)
- Inadequate hepatic function (bilirubin greater than 2 mg/dl)

*Patient Preparation*

Before the BMT, the recipient's body is deliberately immunosuppressed to gain the greatest acceptance of the graft. The recipient undergoes a 2- to 4-day cytoreduction protocol, consisting of ablative chemotherapy, radiation, or both, designed to destroy malignant cells and create space in the bone marrow for the engraftment of new marrow.[6,9,44]

*Harvesting Procedure and Indication of Post-Procedure Function*

Bone marrow is harvested by multiple aspirations, most commonly from the posterior and anterior iliac crests of the donor or, less commonly, from the sternum. Five hundred to 2,500 ml of aspirated marrow is filtered, heparinized, mixed with peripheral blood, frozen, and stored.[9] One to three days after the last dose of chemotherapy or radiation, the marrow is then infused into the patient, much like a blood transfusion, through a central venous access device or Hickman right atrial catheter.[6,46] The most common side effects of reinfusion are fever, chills, nausea, headache, and flushing. The stem cells from the marrow that were infused migrate to the recipient's marrow cavities, mature, and begin to function 10–28 days post BMT.[44,46] A successful engraftment, which is indicated by an increase in the platelet and WBC count, is decided 10–20 days after BMT.[8,24,46]

*Post-Procedure Care and Complications*

All recipients undergoing BMT experience a period of bone marrow failure, which generally begins within 10 days after the start of chemotherapy or radiation and can last up to 3 weeks after BMT.[44] During this time, recipients may receive daily transfusions of platelets, lymphocytes, and granulocytes (preferably from the donor), and antimicrobial therapy to counteract the side effects of hemorrhage and infection.[8,44] Daily bone marrow aspirations and complete blood counts are performed to monitor the progress of the grafts and to check for recurrence of malignancy.

---

Clinical Tip

- BMT recipients are very susceptible to infection. When the patient's neutrophil count is less than 1,000/mm$^3$, the patient is placed on *reverse protective isolation* or *neutropenic precautions*. Patients are placed in reverse isolation in a private, sterile, laminar airflow room. In the laminar airflow rooms, an air filtration system preserves a sterile environment, and all items entering the room must be sterile. Before entering the patient's room, physical therapists and other hospital staff must thoroughly wash their hands, gown, and mask to maintain precautions. Live plants and floral arrangements are not permitted in the patient's room, because they may harbor bacteria and molds that may be harmful to the patient during neutropenic episodes. Any exercise equipment brought into the patient's room must be cleaned before entering the room.

- When the patient's platelet count is 50,000/mm$^3$ or less, the patient is placed on *thrombocytopenic precautions*. Thrombocytopenic precautions are observed (sometimes for months) until the platelet count returns to normal. The physical therapist should be aware of the recipient's platelet count before any treatment is initiated. Thrombocytopenia, which occurs from chemotherapy, radiation, and the underlying disease process, can cause spontaneous bleeding. The most common bleeding sites include the oral and nasal mucosa, the optic sclera, and the epidermis (petechiae).[44] Generally, patients with platelet counts of 30,000/mm$^3$ or greater are able to tolerate moderate exercise if they are asymptomatic and have no spontaneous hemorrhage.[42] A patient with platelet counts between 20,000/mm$^3$ and 30,000/mm$^3$ should only perform light exercise consisting of active range of motion exercises and ambulation as tolerated. Heavy resistance work is contraindicated.[42]

---

BMT recipients are at risk for fatal infection. Patients' blood counts drop secondary to the cytoreduction therapy. *Pancytopenia*, which is a marked reduction in red blood cells, WBCs, and platelets, persists for at least 3–4 weeks after BMT. Normal immune function may not be regained for 12–18 months, as it can take that long for the transplanted immune system to mature and develop normal function.[9,46]

Some major complications of BMT include infection, pneumonia, hemorrhage, marrow failure, veno-occlusive disease of the liver, interstitial pneumonitis, and graft-versus-host disease (GVHD).[6,9,17,38]

*Veno-occlusive disease* is characterized by obstruction of the hepatic venules by deposits of collagen and fibrin. Clinical manifestations of veno-occlusive disease include sudden weight gain, increased LFTs, hepatomegaly, right upper quadrant pain, ascites, and jaundice.[44] Veno-occlusive disease is related to the amount of chemotherapy and radiation the patient received before transplantation. Veno-occlusive disease may occur 1–3 weeks after BMT and spontaneously resolves within 2–3 weeks in approximately half of those affected.[9]

GVHD is a complication that occurs in approximately 20–50% of allogeneic transplant recipients.[17] It does not occur in patients with autologous BMT or PBSC transplants.[42] It is caused by the donor marrow's production of T lymphocytes that react immunologically to the host recipient. The peak onset is at 30–50 days after BMT. The major organs affected by GVHD are the skin, liver, gastrointestinal tract, and lymphoid system.[6,44] Skin involvement manifests as an erythematous rash that can progress to blistering and desquamation. Liver manifestations include increased liver enzymes and bilirubin, right upper quadrant pain, hepatomegaly, and jaundice. Gastrointestinal tract manifestations include nausea, vomiting, diarrhea, malabsorption, ileus, sloughing of intestinal mucosa, abdominal pain, cramping, and bloody stools.[6,44] GVHD is treated with immunosuppressive medications, such as intravenous methylprednisolone and oral prednisone.[46]

### Physical Therapy for Bone Marrow Transplantation Recipients

Physical therapy is beneficial to BMT recipients during their long hospital stay. Discharge from the hospital typically occurs 2–4 weeks post transplantation. Prolonged bouts of malaise, fever, diarrhea, nausea, and pain from inflammation of mucous membranes of the mouth and digestive tract that usually accompany BMT can be debilitating to patients. Initially, physical therapists provide a gentle exercise program to prevent deconditioning and muscle atrophy from disuse and improve functional mobility as patients slowly regain their strength. When patients are confined to their rooms because of protective isolation, they often use a stationary bicycle or restorator (a portable device that a patient can pedal seated at the bedside or in a chair) as part of their exercise prescription. BMT recipients typically require 6 months to a year before they recover full strength and return to a normal lifestyle.[46]

## General Physical Therapy Guidelines for Transplant Recipients

Physical therapists play an integral role in the rehabilitation of transplant recipients. With the exception of BMT recipients, the length of stay in an acute care hospital, depending on the type of organ transplantation and barring any complications, ranges from 3 to 16 days:

kidney, 3–7 days; liver, heart, and lung, 10–14 days; pancreas, 5–12 days; kidney-pancreas, 10–16 days.[7,13,15,39] Given the short length of stay for transplant recipients, physical therapists are consulted in the early postoperative period to provide treatment and assist the transplant team with a safe discharge plan. If patients are medically stable but need assistance for activities of daily living and ambulation, they will require transfer to a rehabilitation facility for further physical and occupational therapy before discharge home.

## Goals

In the acute care setting, the primary physical therapy goals are similar to those of postoperative abdominal or cardiothoracic surgical patients. They include maximizing functional mobility and endurance; improving range of motion, strength, balance, and coordination; and progressing the recipient to his or her maximum independent functional level safely.

Many transplant recipients have experienced end-stage organ disease for multiple years before receiving their transplant and may present with other medical comorbidities. As a result, they are usually physically deconditioned and present with a marked reduction in exercise capacity and skeletal muscle strength owing to long-standing pretransplant physical inactivity. For example, extreme fatigue and weakness are exhibited in patients with chronic liver disease, reduced muscle endurance is seen in patients with chronic heart failure, and decreased oxygen uptake capacity is exhibited in heart and lung disease.[1] Generalized weakness results from the disease process, fluid and electrolyte imbalance, and poor nutrition. After their transplant, recipients generally require a longer time frame to regain their strength and endurance and to achieve their goals.

## Basic Concepts for the Treatment of Transplant Recipients

- Coordinate the best time for physical therapy with the patient's nurse each day. The patient may be fatigued after nursing intervention or medically inappropriate for exercise owing to a decline in medical status, especially in the intensive care unit or early in the postoperative course.

• Analyze laboratory values daily, as they may change dramatically from day to day. Many recipients have very low platelet counts immediately post transplantation. Patients with low platelet counts or increased PT, PTT, or both are at risk for bleeding. It is usually contraindicated to perform percussion on patients with a platelet count less than 50,000/mm³. Therefore, in this situation, bronchopulmonary hygiene consists of coughing and performing deep-breathing exercises, using the incentive spirometer, and encouraging the patient to splint their incision to cough and mobilize to prevent pneumonia.

• Supine therapeutic exercise in the acute care setting is implemented only if necessitated by the recipient's condition, such as high fever, chills, bed rest restriction secondary to ventilator use, or low platelet count. (A high temperature will result in elevated respiratory and heart rates; therefore, it is important to avoid strenuous cardiovascular and resisted exercise during this time.)

• Generally, patients with an uncomplicated postoperative course should be out of bed to chair and ambulating in their rooms with assistance 24–48 hours after surgery, with close monitoring of vital signs. Early ambulation helps to decrease the risk of cardiovascular and pulmonary infection, increase blood circulation, stimulate gastrointestinal function, relieve gas pains, and maintain muscle tone.[7,18] Many post-transplant patients retain fluid, especially in the lower extremities. Weight bearing may be painful; however, ambulation for short periods of time should still be encouraged. The recipient's balance may be altered secondary to increased fluid retention, and he or she may require the use of an assistive device. The physical therapist will be required to provide assistance or appropriate guarding to maintain maximum safety.

• Always monitor and document vital signs, oxygen saturation, and RPE (for cardiac transplant recipients) before, during, and after physical therapy intervention. Report any abnormal change in the patient's response to activity to the patient's nurse. An activity log or flow sheet may be used to document daily progress or decline and vital sign responses.

• Many patients experience some form of organ rejection. If approved by the transplant team, exercise generally continues if their rejection episode is mild to moderate.[11,41]

- The adverse effects of corticosteroids produce delayed wound healing and can contribute to osteoporosis. Upper-extremity resistive training (for cardiac and lung transplant recipients) should be delayed until 6 weeks post transplant, when wound and tissue healing is complete.[41] Patients should be instructed in postural awareness, alignment, exercise, and optimal body mechanics to combat the effects of osteoporosis.[37]

- In addition to the recipient's current medical status, other pre-existing impairments or medical conditions, such as low back pain, peripheral neuropathy, or arthritis, may affect the recipient's activity tolerance. Thus, exercise should be modified according to the patient's ability.

### Activity Progression

- Activity is increased gradually, and treatment continues until the patient is ambulating independently with sufficient endurance to function safely at home. At first, recipients will fatigue easily and require frequent rest periods. Thus, shorter and more frequent treatment sessions are beneficial to patients.

- Ambulation is progressed in terms of frequency, pace, and duration. Stair climbing is progressed with the goal of achieving one to two flights of reciprocal stair climbing.

### Patient Education

- Physical therapists assist in the education of transplant recipients. Recipients must assume an active role in their health care post transplantation. Patients are educated about what to expect after transplantation. Initially, the recipient is very weak and may have difficulty learning during the early post-transplant rehabilitation phase. The physical therapist reinforces the activity protocol with the patient. The transplant team usually provides the recipient with a comprehensive guide that includes information on medications, proper diet, exercise, and psychosocial changes. The patient must adhere to the medication protocol post transplant and be able to monitor for signs and symptoms of infection, rejection, and toxicity to the medications. Patients are instructed to monitor daily their temperature and weight, inspect mouth and gums, maintain proper oral hygiene, and report fever or infectious symptoms.

• On discharge to home, transplant recipients should participate in a daily home exercise routine. The physical therapy department or the organ transplant team may have preprinted exercise protocols. Otherwise, the physical therapist should customize an individual exercise program that consists of stretching and strengthening exercises and a walking or aerobic program that includes a warm-up and cool-down period. A gradual increase in ambulation to at least 30 minutes a day is recommended. An activity log may be used to document the patient's progress.

• Strenuous exercise and activities that stretch or put pressure on the incision should be avoided until approximately 2 months after discharge from the hospital. In addition, transplant recipients should avoid pushing, pulling, and lifting more than 10 lb until then. Contact sports should be avoided for life after transplantation to prevent trauma to the transplanted organ.[7]

Organ transplantation provides a patient with end-stage organ disease an opportunity to improve his or her quality of life by receiving a donated organ, "the gift of life." With ongoing commitment and hard work, transplant recipients can regain an independent, healthy, and active lifestyle. The number and success rate of organ transplantations will continue to grow with continued advances in organ preservation, surgical techniques, tissue matching, immunosuppression protocols, management and monitoring of rejection, and antibiotic protocols.

# References

1. Kjaer M, Beyer N, Secher NH. Exercise and organ transplantation. Scand J Med Sci Sports 1999;9:1–14.
2. Doenges ME, Moorhouse MF, Geissler AC (eds). Nursing Care Plans: Guidelines for Individualizing Patient Care (4th ed). Philadelphia: FA Davis, 1997;774.
3. Arcasoy SE, Kotloff RM. Lung transplantation. N Engl J Med 1999;340(14):1081–1091.
4. Kesten S. Advances in lung transplantation. Dis Mon 1999;45(3):101–114.
5. Becker C, Petlin A. Heart transplantation: minimizing mortality with proper management. Am J Nurs 1999;(Suppl 5):8–14.

6. Black JM, Matassarin-Jacobs E (eds). Medical-Surgical Nursing: Clinical Management for Continuity of Care (5th ed). Philadelphia: Saunders, 1997;584–585, 641–651, 1148, 1352–1353, 1898–1901, 1931.
7. Jenkins RL (ed). A Guide for Transplant Recipients. Burlington, MA: Lahey Clinic, 2000.
8. Atkinson LJ, Howard Fortunato N (eds). Operating Room Technique (8th ed). Boston: Mosby, 1996;897–912.
9. Monahan FD, Neighbors M. Medical-Surgical Nursing (2nd ed). Philadelphia: Saunders, 1998;227–229, 480–483, 1196–1198, 1408–1411, 1448–1455, 1488–1491.
10. Winkel E, DiSesa VJ, Costanzo MR. Advances in heart transplantation. Dis Mon 1999;45(3):62–87.
11. Sadowsky HS. Cardiac transplantation: a review. Phys Ther 1996;76(5): 498–515.
12. Smith SL. Tissue and Organ Transplantation. St. Louis: Mosby, 1990, 27–28, 179, 183, 202–203, 218, 220, 245, 257, 267, 287, 309.
13. Grenvik A, Ayres SM et al. (eds). Textbook of Critical Care (4th ed). Philadelphia: Saunders, 2000;1938–1985.
14. O'Connell JB, Bourge RC, Costanzo-Nordin MR, et al. Cardiac transplantation: recipient selection, donor procurement, and medical follow-up. Circulation 1992;86(3):1061–1075.
15. Gruessner RWG, Kendall DM, Drangstveit MB, et al. Simultaneous pancreas-kidney transplantation from live donors. Ann Surg 1997; 226(4):471–482.
16. Meyers BF, Patterson GA. Lung transplantation: current status and future prospects. World J Surg 1999;23:1156–1162.
17. Hall JB, Schmidt GA, Wood LDH (eds). Principles of Critical Care (2nd ed). New York: McGraw-Hill, 1998;1093–1094, 1325–1339.
18. Luckmann J (ed). Medical-Surgical Nursing. Philadelphia: Saunders, 1980;167, 1011.
19. Jenkins RL (ed). Liver Transplantation Protocol Manual. Burlington, MA: Lahey Clinic, 1999;7, 8, 33, 37–41.
20. Sheiner PA, Magliocca JF, Bodian CA, et al. Long-term medical complications in patients surviving ≥ 5 years after liver transplant. Transplantation 2000;69(5):781–789.
21. Zavotsky KE, Sapienza J, Wood D. Nursing implications for ED care of patients who have received heart transplants. J Emerg Nurs 2001:33–39.
22. Lynn-McHale D, Dorozinsky C. Cardiac Surgery and Heart Transplantation. In Bucher L, Melander S (eds), Critical Care Nursing. Philadelphia: Saunders, 1999;330–348.
23. Manske CL. Risks and benefits of kidney and pancreas transplantation for diabetic patients. Diabetes Care 1999;22(Suppl 2):B114–B119.
24. Sigardson-Poor KM, Haggerty LM (eds). Nursing Care of the Transplant Recipient. Philadelphia: Saunders, 1990;124, 149–151, 187, 208, 210–211, 287.
25. Bartucci MR. Kidney transplantation: state of the art. AACN Clin Issues 1999;10(2):153–163.
26. Pizer HF (ed). Organ Transplants: A Patient's Guide. Cambridge, MA: Harvard University Press, 1991;155.

27. Nolan MT, Augustine SM (ed). Transplantation Nursing: Acute and Long-Term Management. Stamford, CT: Appleton & Lange, 1995;201, 213–226.

28. Schluger LK, Klion FM. The indications for and timing of liver transplantation. J Intensive Care Med 1999;14(3):109–116.

29. Busuttil RW, Goss JA. Split liver transplantation. Ann Surg 1999; 229(3):313–321.

30. Neuberger J. Liver transplantation. QJM 1999;92:547–550.

31. Shapira Z, Yussim A, Mor E. Pancreas transplantation. J Pediatr Endocrinol Metab 1999;12(1):3–15.

32. Cicalese L, Giacomoni A, Rastellini C, Benedetti E. Pancreatic transplantation: a review. Int Surg 1999;84:305–312.

33. Berkow R, Fletcher AJ. (eds). The Merck Manual (16th ed). Rathway, NJ: Merck & Co, 1992;360–361.

34. Freise CE, Narumi S, Stock PG, Melzer JS. Simultaneous pancreas-kidney transplantation: an overview of indications, complications, and outcomes. West J Med 1999;170(1):11–18.

35. McChesney LP. Advances in pancreas transplantation for the treatment of diabetes. Dis Mon 1999;45(3):88–100.

36. Hricik DE. Combined kidney-pancreas transplantation. Kidney Int 1998;53:1091–1097.

37. Arthur EK. Rehabilitation of potential and cardiac transplant recipients. Cardiopulmonary Rec APTA Section 1986;1:11–13.

38. Hillegass EA, Sadowsky HS (eds). Essentials of Cardiopulmonary Physical Therapy. Philadelphia: Saunders, 1994;165–166, 314–315.

39. Edinger KE, McKeen S, Bemis-Dougherty A, et al. Physical therapy following heart transplant. Phys Ther Pract 1992;1(4):25–33.

40. Young MA, Stiens SA. Rehabilitation Aspects of Organ Transplantation. In Braddom RL (ed), Physical Medicine and Rehabilitation (2nd ed). Philadelphia: Saunders, 2000;1385–1400.

41. Frownfelter D, Dean E (eds). Principles and Practice of Cardiopulmonary Physical Therapy (3rd ed). St. Louis: Mosby, 1996;703–719.

42. Goodman CC, Boissonnault WG (eds). Pathology: Implications for the Physical Therapist. Philadelphia: Saunders, 1998;120, 340–344, 363–366, 381, 437–438.

43. Reichenspurner H, Dienemann H, Rihl M, et al. Pulmonary rejection diagnosis after lung and heart-lung transplantation. Transplant Proc 1993;25(6):3299–3300.

44. James MC. Physical therapy for patients after bone marrow transplantation. Phys Ther 1987;67(6):946–952.

45. Nettina SM (ed). The Lippincott Manual of Nursing Practice (6th ed). Philadelphia: Lippincott–Raven, 1996;791–797.

46. McGlave P. Hematopoietic stem-cell transplantation from an unrelated donor. Hosp Pract (Off Ed) 2000;35(8):46, 49, 50.

# I-A

# Medical Record Review
*Michele P. West*

The medical record, whether paper or electronic, is a legal document that chronicles a patient's clinical course during hospitalization and is the primary means of communication between the various clinicians caring for a single patient. More specifically, the medical record contains information about past or present symptoms and disease(s), test and examination results, interventions, and medical-surgical outcome.[1] The medical record should be kept confidential, and all health care providers should safeguard the availability and integrity of health care information in oral, written, or electronic forms.[2] Specific topics, such as human immunodeficiency virus status, substance abuse, domestic abuse, or psychiatric history, are privileged information and discussion of them is subject to ethical and regulatory guidelines.[3] The physical therapist should comply with the American Physical Therapy Association's *Guide for Professional Conduct*[4] and any policies and procedures of the facility or state in regard to sharing medical record information with the patient, family, visitors, or third parties.

The organization of the medical record can vary from institution to institution; however, the medical record is typically composed of the following basic sections:

## Orders

The order section is a log of all instructions of the plan of care for the patient, including medications, diagnostic or therapeutic tests and procedures, vital sign parameters, activity level, diet, the need for consultation services, and resuscitation status. Orders may be written by a physician, physician assistant, or nurse practitioner. A verbal or telephone order may be taken by a nurse or other health care provider, including a physical therapist, according to departmental, facility, and state policies. All orders should be dated, timed, and signed or cosigned by the appropriate personnel.

## History

The history portion of the record includes an admission note and progress notes (a shortened version of the initial note, with emphasis on the physical findings, assessment, and plan), a nursing admission assessment and problem list, consult service notes from physicians and allied health professionals, and operative and procedural notes. Medication sheets, flow sheets, and clinical pathways are also included in this section.

## Reports

A variety of reports are filed chronologically in individual sections in the medical record (e.g., radiologic or laboratory reports). Each report includes an interpretation or normal reference ranges, or both, for various diagnostic or laboratory test results.

### Admission Note Format

The following outline summarizes the basic format of the admission (initial) note written by a physician, physician assistant, or nurse practitioner in the medical record.[5,6] The italicized items indicate the standard information the physical therapist should review before beginning an intervention.

I.   History (subjective information)

    A.   Data that identify the patient, including the source and degree of reliability of the information.

    B.   *History of present illness* (HPI), including the chief complaint and a chronologic list of the problems associated with the chief complaint.

    C.   *Medical or surgical history, risk factors* for disease, and *allergies.*

    D.   Family health history, including age and health or age and cause of death for immediate family members as well as a relevant familial medical history.

    E.   Personal and social history, including *occupation, lifestyle, functional mobility status, the need for home or outpatient services,* and *architectural barriers at home.*

    F.   *Current medications,* including level of *compliance.*

II.   The physical examination (objective information). Negative (normal) or positive (abnormal) findings are described in detail according to the following outline:

    A.   General information, including *vital signs, laboratory findings, mental status,* and *appearance.*

    B.   Head, *e*yes, *e*ars, *n*ose, *t*hroat, (HEENT) and neck

    C.   Chest

    D.   Heart (Cor)

    E.   Abdomen

    F.   Extremities

    G.   Neurologic system

III.   Assessment. The assessment is a statement of the condition and prognosis of the patient in regard to the chief complaint and medical-surgical status. If the etiology of the problem(s) is unclear, then differential diagnoses are listed.

IV.   Plan.   The plan of care includes further observation, tests, laboratory analysis, consultation with additional specialty services or providers, pharmacologic therapies, other interventions, and discharge planning.

# References

1. Wood DL. Documentation guidelines: evolution, future direction, and compliance. Am J Med 2000;110:332–334.
2. Ziel SE. Federal regulations governing health information security published. AORN J 1998;68:866–867.
3. Rutberg MP. Medical records confidentiality. In MI Weintraub (ed). Neurologic Clinics: Medical-Legal Issues Facing Neurologists. Neurol Clin 1999;17:307–313.
4. American Physical Therapy Association. Guide for Professional Conduct and Code of Ethics. Guide to Physical Therapy Practice. Phys Ther 2001;81:S689.
5. Swartz MH. The Clinical Record. In MH Swartz, Textbook of Physical Diagnosis: History and Examination. Philadelphia: W.B. Saunders, 1998;681–686.
6. Naumburg EH. Interviewing and the Health History. Philadelphia: Lippincott, 1999;35–39.

# I-B

# Acute Care Setting
*Michele P. West*

## Introduction

The physical therapist must have an appreciation for the distinct aspects of in-patient acute care. The purpose of this appendix is to briefly present information about the acute care environment, including safety and the use of physical restraints, the effects of prolonged bed rest, end-of-life issues, and some of the unique circumstances, conditions, or patient responses encountered in the hospital setting.

The acute care or hospital setting is a unique environment with protocols and standards of practice and safety that may not be applicable to other areas of health care delivery, such as an outpatient clinic or school system. Hospitals are designed to accommodate a wide variety of routine, urgent, or emergent patient care needs. The staff and medical-surgical equipment (see Appendices III-A, -B, and -C) reflect these needs. The nature of the hospital setting is to provide 24-hour care; thus, the patient, family, and caregivers are faced with the physical, psychological, and emotional sequelae of illness and hospitalization. This can include the response(s) to a change in daily routine; a lack of privacy and independence; or perhaps a response to a potential lifestyle change, medical crisis, critical illness, or long-term illness.

## Safe Caregiver and Patient Environment

Basic guidelines for providing a safe caregiver and patient environment include the following:

- Always following standard precautions, including thorough hand washing. Refer to Table 10-4 for a summary of infection prevention precautions, including contact, airborne, and droplet precautions.

- Knowledge of the facility's policy for accidental chemical, waste, or sharps exposure, as well as emergency procedures for evacuation, fire, and natural disaster. Know how to contact the employee health service and hospital security.

- Confirming the patient's name before physical therapy intervention by interview or identification bracelet. Notify the nurse if a patient is missing an identification bracelet.

- Reorienting a patient who is confused or disoriented. In general, patients who are confused are assigned rooms closer to the nursing station.

- Make recommendations to nursing for the use of bathroom equipment (e.g., tub bench or raised toilet seat) if the patient has functional limitations that may pose a safety risk.

- Elevating the height of the bed as needed to ensure proper body mechanics when performing a bedside intervention (e.g., stretching or bed mobility training).

- Leaving the bed or chair (e.g., stretcher chair) in the lowest position with wheels locked after physical therapy intervention is complete. Leave the top bed rails up for all patients.

- Always leaving the patient with the call bell or other communication devices within close reach. This includes eyeglasses and hearing aids.

- If applicable, using bed alarms so that the staff will know whether a patient has attempted to get out of bed alone.

- Keeping the patient's room as neat and clutter free as possible to minimize the risk of trips and falls. Pick up objects that have fallen on the floor. Secure electrical cords (e.g., for the bed or intravenous pumps) out of the way. Keep small-sized equipment used for physical therapy intervention (e.g., cuff weights) in a drawer or closet. Store assistive devices at the perimeter of the room when not in use. Do not block the doorway or pathway to and from the patient's bed.

• Providing enough light for the patient to move about the room or read educational materials.

• Only using equipment (e.g., assistive devices, recliner chairs, wheelchairs) that is in good working condition. If equipment is unsafe, then label it as such and contact the appropriate personnel to repair or discard it.

• Disposing of linens, dressings, and garbage according to the policies of the facility.

### Latex Allergy

A *latex allergy response* is defined as "the state in which an individual experiences an immunoglobulin E (IgE)–mediated response to latex" from tactile, inhaled, or ingested exposure to natural rubber latex.[1] Signs and symptoms of an allergic reaction to latex may range from swelling, itching, or redness of skin or mucous membranes to anaphylaxis.[1]

Natural rubber latex can be found in a multitude of products and equipment found in the acute care setting. Those products most commonly used by the physical therapist include gloves, stethoscopes, blood-pressure cuffs, Ambu bags, adhesive tape, electrode pads, and hand grips on assistive devices. If a patient has an allergy or hypersensitivity to latex, then it is documented in the medical record, nursing cardex or report, and at the patient's bedside. Hospitals will provide a special "latex-free kit," which consists of latex-free products for use with the patient.

Health care providers, including physical therapists, may be at risk for developing latex allergy from increased exposure to latex in the work setting. If there is a suspected latex hypersensitivity or allergy, then seek assistance from the employee health office or a primary care physician.

## Use of Restraints

The use of a restraint may be indicated for the patient who (1) is unconscious, (2) has altered mental status at risk for wandering or pulling out lines and tubes, (3) is unsafely mobile, (4) is physically aggressive, or (5) is so active or agitated that essential medical-surgical care cannot be completed.[2] The most common types of restraints in the acute care setting are wrist or ankle restraints, mitt restraints, or a vest restraint. An order from a physician, which must be updated approximately every 24–48 hours, is required to place a restraint on a patient.

General guidelines most applicable to the physical therapist for the use of restraints include

- Use a slipknot to secure a restraint rather than a square knot. This ensures that the restraint can be rapidly untied in an emergency.

- Do not secure the restraint to a moveable object (e.g., the bed rail), to an object that the patient is not lying or sitting on, or within the patient's reach.

- Ensure that the restraint is secure but not too tight. Place two fingers between the restraint and the patient to be sure circulation is not impaired.

- Always replace restraints after a physical therapy session.

- Be sure the patient does not trip on the ties or "tails" of the restraint during functional mobility training.

- Consult with the health care team to determine whether a patient needs to have restraints.

## Effects of Prolonged Bed Rest

The effects of short- (days to weeks) or long-term (weeks to months) bed rest can be deleterious and impact every organ system in the body. For the purposes of this discussion, bed rest incorporates immobilization, disuse, and recumbence with an end result of multisystem deconditioning. The physical therapist must recognize that a patient in the acute care setting is likely to have an alteration in physiology (i.e., a traumatic or medical-surgical disease or dysfunction) superimposed on bed rest, a second abnormal physiologic state.[3]

Most patients on bed rest have been in the intensive care unit (ICU) for many weeks with multisystem organ failure or hemodynamic instability requiring sedation and mechanical ventilation. Other clinical situations classically associated with long-term bed rest include severe burns and multi-trauma, including the need for skeletal traction, spinal cord injury, or grade IV non-healing wounds of the lower extremity or sacrum. It is beyond the scope of this text to discuss in detail the effects of prolonged bed rest; however, Table I-B.1 lists these major changes.

---

Clinical Tip

• Monitor vital signs carefully, especially during mobilization out of bed for the first few times.
• Progressively raise the head of the bed before or during a physical therapy session to allow blood pressure to regulate.
• A tilt table may be used if orthostatic hypotension persists despite volume repletion, medication, or therapeutic exercise.
• Time frames for physical therapy goals will likely be longer for the patient who has been on prolonged bed rest.
• Independent or family-assisted therapeutic exercise should supplement formal physical therapy sessions for a more timely recovery.
• Be aware of the psychosocial aspects of prolonged bed rest. Sensory deprivation, boredom, depression, and a sense of loss of control can occur.[4] These feelings may manifest as emotional lability or irritability, and caregivers may incorrectly perceive the patient to be uncooperative.
• As much as the patient wants to be off bed rest, the patient will likely be fearful the first time out of bed, especially if the patient has insight into his or her muscular weakness.
• Leave the patient with necessities or commonly used objects (e.g., the call bell, telephone, reading material, beverages, tissues) within reach to minimize the patient's feelings of being confined to bed.

---

# End-of-Life Issues

End-of-life issues are often complex moral, ethical, or legal dilemmas, or a combination of these, regarding a patient's vital physiologic func-

Table I-B.1. Systemic Effects of Prolonged Bed Rest

| Body System | Effects |
| --- | --- |
| Cardiac | Increased heart rate at rest and with submaximal exercise. Decreased stroke volume and left ventricular end-diastolic volume at rest. Decreased cardiac output, $\dot{V}o_2$max with submaximal and maximal exercise. |
| Hematologic | Decreased total blood volume, red blood cell mass, and plasma volume. Increased blood fibrinogen and risk of venous thrombosis. |
| Respiratory | Increased respiratory rate, forced vital capacity, and total lung capacity (slight). Increased risk of pulmonary embolism and possible ventilation-perfusion mismatch. |
| Gastrointestinal | Decreased appetite, fluid intake, bowel motility, and gastric secretion. |
| Genitourinary | Increased mineral excretion, calculus formation, difficulty voiding, postvoid residuals, and overflow incontinence. Decreased glomerular filtration rate. |
| Endocrine | Altered temperature and sweating responses, circadian rhythm, regulation of hormones, and impaired glucose intolerance. |
| Musculoskeletal | Muscle: increased muscle weakness (especially in antigravity muscles), atrophy, risk of contracture, weakened myotendinous junction, and altered muscle excitation. Bone: osteoporosis. Joints: degeneration of cartilage, synovial atrophy, and ankylosis. |
| Neurologic | Sensory and sleep deprivation. Decreased balance, coordination, and visual acuity. Increased risk of compression neuropathy. |
| Neurovascular | Orthostatic hypotension. |
| Body composition | Increased calcium, potassium, phosphorus, sulfur, and nitrogen loss; increased body fat and decreased lean body mass. |

$\dot{V}o_2$max = maximum oxygen uptake.
Source: Adapted from RM Buschbacher, CD Porter. Deconditioning, Conditioning, and the Benefits of Exercise. In RL Braddom (ed), Physical Medicine and Rehabilitation (2nd ed). Philadelphia: W.B. Saunders, 2000;704.

tions, medical-surgical prognosis, and quality of life as well as personal values and beliefs.[5] End-of-life issues facing patients, family, and caregivers include the following:

### Decision to Declare Resuscitation Status as Do Not Resuscitate or Do Not Intubate

Do not resuscitate (DNR) is the predetermined decision to decline cardiopulmonary resuscitation, including defibrillation and pharmacologic cardioversion in case of cardiorespiratory arrest. Do not intubate (DNI) is the predetermined decision to decline intubation for the purpose of subsequent mechanical ventilation in case of respiratory arrest. DNR or DNI status is officially documented in the medical record by the attending physician. The physical therapist must be aware of each patient's resuscitation or "code" status. DNR/DNI orders do not directly impact on the physical therapy plan of care.

### Withholding and Withdrawing Medical Therapies

Withholding support is not initiating a therapy for the patient, whereas withdrawing support is the discontinuation of a therapy (usually after it has proven unbeneficial to the patient).[6] Forgoing therapy is the combination of withholding and withdrawing support in which disease progression is allowed to take its course.[6] In the case of forgoing medical-surgical therapies, an order for "comfort measures only" (CMO) is written by the physician. The patient with comfort measures only status receives medications for pain control or sedation, or to otherwise eliminate distress. The patient on comfort measures only status does not receive physical therapy.

### Coma, Persistent Vegetative State, and Brain Death

The diagnosis of coma, persistent vegetative state, or brain death can be devastating. These conditions are very similar in that there is unconsciousness and absent self-awareness, but distinctions do exist in terms of neurologic function and recovery (Table I-B.2). Coma is characterized by a lack of responsiveness to verbal stimuli, variable responsiveness to painful stimuli, voluntary movement, and the potential for abnormal respiratory patterns and pupillary responses to light.[7] Characteristics of persistent vegetative state include the presence of sleep-

**Table I-B.2.** Comparison of Coma, Persistent Vegetative State (PVS), and Brain Death

| Condition | Sleep-Wake Cycle | Motor Control | Respiratory Control | EEG Activity | Cerebral Metabolism | Prognosis |
|-----------|------------------|---------------|---------------------|--------------|---------------------|-----------|
| Coma | Absent | Lacks purposeful movement | Present, variable, usually depressed | Present | Reduced by 50% or more | Usually recovers. Can progress to PVS or death in 2–4 wks. |
| PVS | Present | Lacks purposeful movement | Present, normal | Present | Reduced by 50% or more | Variable recovery. |
| Brain death | Absent | None or spinal reflex movements only | Absent | Absent | Absent | No recovery. |

EEG = electroencephalogram.
Source: Adapted from LA Thelan, LD Urden, ME Lough, KM Stacy (eds). Neurological Disorders. In Critical Care Nursing: Diagnosis and Management (3rd ed). St. Louis: Mosby, 1998;797.

wake cycles and partial or complete hypothalamic and autonomic brain stem functions but a lack of cerebral cortical function for longer than 1 month after acute traumatic or nontraumatic brain injury or metabolic or degenerative disorders.[8] The initial clinical criteria for *brain death* include coma and unresponsiveness, absence of brain stem reflexes, and cerebral motor responses to pain in all extremities, apnea, and hypothermia.[9] Brain death is usually confirmed by cerebral angiography, evoked potential testing, electroencephalography, or transcranial Doppler sonography.[9] Refer to Chapter 4 for more information on these neurologic diagnostic tests.

## Intensive Care Unit Setting

The ICU, as its name suggests, is a place of intensive medical-surgical care for those patients who require continuous monitoring, usually in conjunction with therapies such as vasoactive medications, sedation, circulatory assist devices, and mechanical ventilation. ICUs may be named according to the specialized care that they provide, such as the coronary care unit (CCU) or surgical ICU. The patient in the ICU requires a high acuity of care; thus, the nurse to patient ratio is one to one or one to two.

### Common Patient and Family Responses to the Intensive Care Unit

- Behavioral changes or disturbances can occur in the patient who is critically ill as a result of distress caused by physically or psychologically invasive, communication-impairing, or movement-restricting procedures.[10] When combined with the environmental and psychological reactions to the ICU, mental status and personality can be altered. Environmental stresses can include crowding, bright overhead lighting, strong odors, noise, and touch associated with procedures or from those the patient cannot see.[10] Psychological stresses can include diminished dignity and self-esteem, powerlessness, vulnerability, fear, anxiety, isolation, and spiritual distress.[10]

- *ICU psychosis* is a state of delirium that occurs between the third and seventh day in the ICU and is described as a "fluctuating state of consciousness characterized by features such as fatigue, confusion, distraction, anxiety, and hallucinations."[11] Delirium in the ICU, which is reversible, is thought to be caused by pain, the side effects of drugs, and the ICU environment.[11] Precipitants to delirium include a history of dementia, Alzheimer's disease, substance abuse, and chronic illness as well as advanced age, severe infection, fluid and electrolyte imbalance, hypoxia, and metabolic disorders.[12] Treatment for delirium consists of antipsychotic medications (e.g., haloperidol), the discontinuation of nonessential medications, proper oxygenation and hydration, and the company of family or others.[13]

- The patient's family is usually overwhelmed by the ICU. Family members may experience fear, shock, anxiety, helplessness, anger, hostility, guilt, withdrawal, or disruptive behaviors.[10] Like the patient, the family may be overwhelmed by the stimuli and technology of the ICU, as well as the stress of a loved one's facing a critical or life-threatening illness.

- The transfer of a patient from the ICU to a general floor can also be a stress to the patient and family. Referred to as *transfer anxiety*, the patient and family may voice concerns of leaving staff that they have come to recognize and know by name; they may have to learn to trust new staff,[10] or fear that the level of care is inferior to that in the ICU. To minimize this anxiety, the physical therapist may continue to treat the patient (if staffing allows), slowly transition care to another therapist, or reinforce with the patient and family that the general goals of physical therapy are unchanged.

### Critical Illness Polyneuropathy

*Critical illness polyneuropathy* is the acute or subacute onset of widespread symmetric weakness in the patient with critical illness, most commonly with sepsis or multisystem organ failure, or both.[14] The patient presents with distal extremity weakness, wasting, and sensory loss, as well as parasthesia and decreased or absent deep tendon reflexes.[15] The clinical features that distinguish it from other neuromuscular disorders (e.g., Guillain-Barré syndrome) are a lack of ophthalmoplegia, dysautonomia, and cranial nerve involvement and normal cerebrospinal fluid analysis.[14,15] Nerve conduction studies show decreased motor and sensory action potentials.[15] The specific pathophysiology of critical illness polyneuropathy is unknown; however, it is hypothesized to be related to drug, nutritional, metabolic, and toxic factors, as well as prolonged ICU stay, the number of invasive procedures, increased glucose level, decreased albumin level, and the severity of multisystem organ failure.[15]

### Critical Illness Myopathy

*Critical illness myopathy,* otherwise known as *acute quadriplegic myopathy* or *acute steroid myopathy,* is the acute or subacute onset of diffuse quadriparesis, respiratory muscle weakness, and decreased deep tendon reflexes[15] in the setting of exposure to short- or long-term high-dose corticosteroids and simultaneous neuromuscular blockade.[16] It is postulated that neuromuscular blockade causes a functional denervation that renders muscle fibers vulnerable to the catabolic effects of steroids.[16] Diagnostic tests demonstrate elevated serum creatine kinase levels at the onset of the myopathy, and, if severe, myoglobinuria or renal failure can ensue; a myopathic pattern with muscle fibrillation on electromyography; and a necrosis with dramatic loss of myosin (thick) filaments on muscle biopsy.[16]

### Sleep Pattern Disturbance

The interruption or deprivation of the quality or hours of sleep or rest can interfere with a patient's energy level, personality, and ability to heal and perform tasks. The defining characteristics of *sleep pattern disturbance* are difficulty falling or remaining asleep, with or without fatigue on awakening, dozing during the day, and mood alterations.[17]

In the acute care setting, sleep disturbance may be related to frequent awakenings related to a medical process (e.g., nocturia or pain) or the need for nursing intervention (e.g., vital sign monitoring), an inability to assume normal sleeping position, and excessive daytime sleeping related to medication side effects, stress, or environmental changes.[17]

The physical therapist should be aware of the patient who has altered sleep patterns or difficulty sleeping, as lack of sleep can impact a patient's ability to participate during a therapy session. The patient may have trouble concentrating and performing higher-level cognitive tasks. The pain threshold may be decreased, and the patient may also exhibit decreased emotional control.[17]

## Confusion

Confusion may be acute or chronic (e.g., related to a neurodegenerative process). Acute confusion frequently occurs in the acute care setting, especially in the elderly. *Acute confusion* is defined as "the state in which there is abrupt onset of a cluster of global, fluctuating disturbances in consciousness, attention, perception, memory, orientation, thinking, sleep-wake cycle, and psychomotor behavior."[18] Risk factors for confusion related to medications include the use of analgesics, polypharmacy, noncompliance, and inappropriate self-medicating.[19] Other risk factors include dehydration, electrolyte imbalance, hypoxia, infection, and poor nutrition. Acute or acute on chronic disease states can result in confusion, especially if metabolic in nature.

Additionally, a change in environment can exacerbate medical risks for confusion. This includes unfamiliar surroundings, noises, procedures, and staff or a change in daily routine, activity level, diet, and sleep.

## Substance Abuse and Withdrawal

The casual or habitual abuse of alcohol, drugs (e.g., cocaine), or medications (e.g., opioids) is a known contributor of acute and chronic illness, traumatic accidents, drowning, burn injury, and suicide.[20] The patient in the acute care setting may present with acute intoxication or drug overdose or with a known (i.e., documented) or unknown substance abuse problem.

The physical therapist is not initially involved in the care of the patient with acute intoxication or overdose until the patient is medically stable. However, the physical therapist may become secondarily involved when the patient presents with impaired strength, balance, coordination, and functional mobility as a result of chemical toxicity.

It is the patient with unknown substance abuse who is hospitalized for days to weeks who is a challenge to the hospital staff when withdrawal (commonly referred to as the DTs, for *delirium tremens*) occurs. It is beyond the scope of this text to list the symptoms of withdrawal of the many different types of drugs. For the purposes of this text, alcohol withdrawal will be discussed because of its relatively high occurrence.

*Alcohol withdrawal syndrome* is the group of signs and symptoms that occur when a heavy or prolonged user of alcohol (ethanol or ethyl alcohol) reduces alcohol consumption.[21] The signs and symptoms of alcohol withdrawal are the result of a hyperadrenergic state from increased central nervous system neuronal activity that attempts to compensate for the inhibition of neurotransmitters with chronic alcohol use.[20] The signs and symptoms of alcohol withdrawal syndrome, which begin 5–10 hours after alcohol use is decreased, are[21]

- Tachycardia and hypertension

- Nausea and vomiting

- Low-grade fever

- Hand tremor

- Anxiety, insomnia, agitation, or hallucinations

- Grand mal seizure or delirium (if severe)

Interventions to prevent or minimize alcohol withdrawal syndrome include hydration, adequate nutrition, reality orientation, thiamine, and the prophylactic use of benzodiazepines.

## References

1. Carpenito LJ. Latex Allergy Response. In Nursing Diagnosis: Application to Clinical Practice (8th ed). Philadelphia: Lippincott, 2000;553–557.
2. Smith SF, Duell DJ, Martin BC (eds). Restraints. Clinical Nursing Skills: Basic to Advanced Skills (5th ed). Upper Saddle River, NJ: Prentice Hall Health, 2000;139–146.
3. Downey RJ, Weissman C. Physiological Changes Associated with Bed Rest and Major Body Injury. In EG Gonzalez, SJ Myers, JE Edelstein, et al. (eds), Downey and Darling's Physiological Basis of Rehabilitation Medicine (3rd ed). Boston: Butterworth–Heinemann, 2001;449.
4. Buschbacher RM, Porter CD. Deconditioning, Conditioning, and the Benefits of Exercise. In RL Braddom (ed). Physical Medicine and Rehabilitation (2nd ed). Philadelphia: Saunders, 2000;716.
5. American Association of Critical-Care Nurses. Position Statement on Withholding and/or Withdrawing Life-Sustaining Treatment. In MR Kinney, SB Dunbar, J Brooks-Brunn, et al. (eds), AACN's Clinical Reference for Critical Care Nursing (4th ed). St. Louis: Mosby, 1998;1253–1254.
6. DeVita MA, Grenvik A. Forgoing Life-Sustaining Therapy in Intensive Care. In A Grenvick (ed), Textbook of Critical Care (4th ed). Philadelphia: Saunders, 2000;2110–2113.
7. Schnell SS. Nursing Care of Comatose or Confused Clients. In JM Black, E Matassarin-Jacobs (eds), Medical-Surgical Nursing: Clinical

Management for Continuity of Care (5th ed). Philadelphia: Saunders, 1997;743.

8. Thelan LA, Urden LD, Lough ME, Stacy KM (eds). Neurologic Disorders. In Critical Care Nursing: Diagnosis and Management (3rd ed). St. Louis: Mosby, 1998;795–798.

9. Sullivan J, Seem DL, Chabalewski F. Determining brain death. Critical Care Nurse 1999;19:37–46.

10. Urban N. Patient and Family Responses to the Critical Care Environment. In MR Kinney, SB Dunbar, J Brooks-Brunn, et al. (eds), AACN's Clinical Reference for Critical Care Nursing (4th ed). St. Louis: Mosby, 1998;145–162.

11. Hennemann AE. Preventing Complications in the Intensive Care Unit. In A Grenvick (ed), Textbook of Critical Care (4th ed). Philadelphia: Saunders, 2000;2035–2037.

12. Roberts BL. Managing delirium in adult intensive care patients. Critical Care Nurse 2001;21:48–55.

13. Wise MG, Cassem NH. Behavioral Disturbances. In JM Civetta, RW Taylor, RR Kirby (eds), Critical Care. Philadelphia: Lippincott–Raven, 1997;2022–2024.

14. Victor M, Ropper AH (eds). Diseases of the Peripheral Nerves. In Adams and Victor's Principles of Neurology (7th ed). New York: McGraw-Hill, 2001;1388.

15. Juel VC, Bleck PP. In Grenvik A (ed), Textbook of Critical Care (4th ed). Philadelphia: Saunders, 2001;1891–1892.

16. Victor M, Ropper AH (eds). The Metabolic and Toxic Myopathies. In Adams and Victor's Principles of Neurology (7th ed). New York: McGraw-Hill, 2001;1522.

17. Carpenito LJ. Sleep Pattern Disturbance. In Nursing Diagnosis: Application to Clinical Practice (8th ed). Philadelphia: Lippincott, 2000;858–865.

18. Carpenito LJ. Confusion. In Nursing Diagnosis: Application to Clinical Practice (8th ed). Philadelphia: Lippincott, 2000;230–239.

19. Prevost SS. Elder Responses. In MR Kinney, SB Dunbar, J Brooks-Brunn, et al. (eds), AACN's Clinical Reference for Critical Care Nursing (4th ed). St. Louis: Mosby, 1998;169–172.

20. Shaffer J. Substance Abuse and Withdrawal: Alcohol, Cocaine, and Opioids. In JM Civetta, RW Taylor, RR Kirby (eds). Critical Care. Philadelphia: Lippincott–Raven, 1997;1511–1514.

21. Greicus L. Alcohol Withdrawal. In HM Schell, KA Puntillo. Critical Care Nursing Secrets. Philadelphia: Hanley & Belfus, Inc., 2001;362–367.

# II

# Fluid and Electrolyte Imbalances
*Susan Polich and Jaime C. Paz*

Many causes and factors can alter a patient's fluid and electrolyte balance. These imbalances can result in a multitude of clinical manifestations, which in turn can affect a patient's functional mobility and activity tolerance. Recognizing the signs and symptoms of electrolyte imbalance is, therefore, an important aspect of physical therapy. Additionally, the physical therapist must be aware of which patients are at risk for these imbalances, as well as the concurrent pathogenesis, diagnosis, and medical management of these imbalances.

Maintaining homeostasis between intracellular fluid, extracellular fluid, and electrolytes is necessary to allow proper cell function. Proper homeostasis depends on the following factors:

- Concentration of intracellular and extracellular fluids
- Type and concentration of electrolytes
- Permeability of cell membranes
- Kidney function

## Fluid Imbalance

Fluid imbalance occurs when fluids are lost, either by loss of body water or failure to intake, or gained, either by fluid shift from the vasculature to the cell space or excessive intake without proper elimination.[1-3]

Loss of bodily fluid (hypovolemia) can occur from loss of blood (hemorrhage), loss of plasma (burns), or loss of body water (vomiting, diarrhea). Any of these situations can result in dehydration, hypovolemia, or shock in extreme cases. Clinical manifestations include decreased blood pressure, increased heart rate, changes in mental status, thirst, dizziness, hypernatremia, increased core body temperature, weakness, poor skin turgor, altered respirations, and orthostatic hypotension.[1-4] Clinical manifestations in children also include poor capillary refill, absent tears, and dry mucous membranes.[5]

Excessive bodily fluid (hypervolemia) can occur when there is a shift of water from the vascular system to the intracellular space. This can result from excessive pressure in the vasculature (ventricular failure), loss of serum albumin (liver failure), or fluid overload (excessive rehydration during surgery). Clinical manifestations of fluid overload include weight gain, pulmonary edema, peripheral edema, and bounding pulse. Clinical manifestations of this fluid shift may also resemble those of dehydration, as there is a resultant decrease in the intravascular fluid volume.[1-3] Table II-1 provides an overview of hypovolemia and hypervolemia.

---

### Clinical Tip

During casual conversation among physicians and nurses, patients who are hypovolemic are often referred to as being *dry*, whereas patients who are hypervolemic are referred to as being *wet*.

---

## Electrolyte Imbalance

Fluid imbalances are often accompanied by changes in electrolytes. Loss or gain of body water is usually accompanied by a loss or gain of electrolytes. Similarly, a change in electrolyte balance often

**Table II-1.** Fluid and Electrolyte Imbalances

| Imbalance | Definition | Contributing Factors | Clinical Manifestations | Diagnostic Test Findings |
|---|---|---|---|---|
| Hypovolemia | Fluid volume deficit | Vomiting, diarrhea, fever, blood loss, and uncontrolled diabetes mellitus | Weak, rapid pulse; decreased BP; dizziness; thirst; confusion; and muscle cramps | Increased hematocrit, BUN, serum sodium levels |
| Hypervolemia | Fluid volume excess | Renal failure, congestive heart failure, blood transfusions, and prolonged corticosteroid therapy | Shortness of breath, increased BP, bounding pulse, and presence of cough | Decreased hematocrit, BUN, and serum sodium levels |
| Hyponatremia | Sodium deficit (serum sodium level of <135 mEq/liter) | Diuretic therapy, renal disease, excessive sweating, hyperglycemia, NPO status, congestive heart failure, and SIADH | Lethargy, nausea, apathy, muscle cramps, muscular twitching, and confusion in severe states | Decreased urine and serum sodium levels |
| Hypernatremia | Sodium excess (serum sodium level of >145 mEq/liter) | Diabetes insipidus, diarrhea, hyperventilation, and excessive corticosteroid, sodium bicarbonate, or sodium chloride administration | Elevated body temperature; lethargy or restlessness; thirst; dry, flushed skin; weakness; irritability; tachycardia; hyper- or hypotension; oliguria; and pulmonary edema | Increased serum sodium and decreased urine sodium levels |

Table II-1. *Continued*

| Imbalance | Definition | Contributing Factors | Clinical Manifestations | Diagnostic Test Findings |
|---|---|---|---|---|
| Hypokalemia | Potassium deficit (serum potassium level of <3.5 mEq/liter) | Diarrhea, vomiting, chronic renal disease, gastric suction, polyuria, corticosteroid therapy, and digoxin therapy | Fatigue; muscle weakness; slow, weak pulse; ventricular fibrillation; paresthesias; leg cramps; and decreased blood pressure | ST depression or prolonged PR interval on ECG |
| Hyperkalemia | Potassium excess (serum potassium level of >5 mEq/liter) | Renal failure, Addison's disease, burns, use of potassium-conserving diuretics, and chronic heparin therapy | Vague muscle weakness, nausea, initial tachycardia followed by bradycardia, dysrhythmia, flaccid paralysis, paresthesia, irritability, and anxiety | ST depression; tall, tented T waves; or absent P waves on ECG |

BP = blood pressure; BUN = blood urea nitrogen; ECG = electrocardiogram; NPO = nothing by mouth; SIADH = syndrome of inappropriate antidiuretic hormone secretion.

Sources: Data from M Mulvey. Fluid and Electrolytes: Balance and Disorders. In SC Smeltzer, BG Bare (eds), Brunner and Suddarth's Textbook of Medical-Surgical Nursing (8th ed). Philadelphia: Lippincott, 1996;231; CC Goodman, TE Kelly Snyder. Problems Affecting Multiple Systems. In CC Goodman, WG Boissonnault. Pathology: Implications for the Physical Therapist. Philadelphia: Saunders,1998;72–82; and PJ Fall. Hyponatremia and hypernatremia: a systematic approach to causes and their correction. Postgrad Med 2000;107(5):75–82.

affects fluid balance. Cellular functions that are reliant on proper electrolyte balance include neuromuscular excitability, secretory activity, and membrane permeability.[6] Clinical manifestations will vary depending on the severity of the imbalance and can include those noted in Fluid Imbalance. In extreme cases, muscle tetany and coma can also occur. Common electrolyte imbalances are further summarized in Table II-1.

---

### Clinical Tip

Electrolyte levels are generally represented schematically in the medical record in a sawhorse figure, as shown in Figure II-1.

---

Medical management includes diagnosing and monitoring electrolyte imbalances via blood and urine tests. These tests include measuring levels of sodium, potassium, chloride, and calcium in blood and urine; arterial blood gases; and serum and urine osmolality. Treatment involves managing the primary cause of the imbalance(s), along with providing supportive care with intravenous or oral fluids, electrolyte supplementation, and diet modifications.

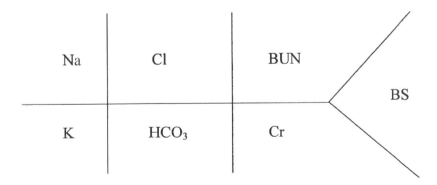

**Figure II-1.** *Schematic representation of electrolyte levels. (BUN = blood urea nitrogen; BS = blood sugar; Cl = chloride; Cr = creatinine; HCO$_3$ = bicarbonate; K = potassium; Na = sodium.)*

Clinical Tip

• Review the medical record closely for any fluid restrictions that may be ordered for a patient with hypervolemia. These restrictions may also be posted at the patient's bedside.

• Conversely, ensure proper fluid intake before, during, and after physical therapy intervention with patients who are hypovolemic.

• Slight potassium imbalances can have significant effects on cardiac rhythms; therefore, carefully monitor the patient's cardiac rhythm before, during, and after physical therapy intervention. If the patient is not on a cardiac monitor, then consult with the nurse or physician regarding the appropriateness of physical therapy intervention with a patient who has potassium imbalance.

• Refer to Chapter 1 for more information on cardiac arrhythmias.

• Refer to Chapter 9 for more information on fluid and electrolyte imbalances caused by renal dysfunction.

• Refer to Chapter 11 for more information on fluid and electrolyte imbalances caused by endocrine dysfunction.

# References

1. Rose BD (ed). Clinical Physiology of Acid-Base and Electrolyte Disorders (2nd ed). New York: McGraw-Hill, 1984.
2. Cotran RS, Kumar V, Robbins S, Schoes FJ (eds). Robbins Pathologic Basis of Disease. Philadelphia: Saunders, 1994.
3. Kokko J, Tannen R (eds). Fluids and Electrolytes (2nd ed). Philadelphia: Saunders, 1990.
4. McGee S, Abernethy WB III, Simel DL. Is this patient hypovolemic? JAMA 1999;281(11):1022–1029.
5. Gorelick MH, Shaw KN, Murphy KO. Validity and reliability of clinical signs in the diagnosis of dehydration in children. Pediatrics 1997;99(5): E6.
6. Marieb EN (ed). Human Anatomy and Physiology (2nd ed). Redwood City, CA: Benjamin Cummings, 1992;911.

# III-A

# Medical-Surgical Equipment in the Acute Care Setting
*Eileen F. Lang*

## Introduction

The purpose of this appendix is to (1) describe the various types of medical-surgical equipment commonly used in the acute care setting, including oxygen ($O_2$) therapy and noninvasive and invasive monitoring and management devices, and (2) provide a framework for the safe use of such equipment during physical therapy intervention.

Some equipment is used in all areas of the hospital, whereas other types of equipment are used only in specialty areas, such as the intensive care unit (ICU). The *ICU* is defined as "a place for the monitoring and care of patients with potentially severe physiological instability requiring technical and/or artificial life support."[1] The presence of certain types of equipment in a patient's room can provide the physical therapist with a preliminary idea of the patient's general medical condition and the appropriateness of therapeutic or prophylactic physical therapy intervention, or both. The physical therapist may initially be intimidated by the abundance of medical-surgical equipment (especially in the ICU); however, a proper orientation to such equipment allows the physical therapist to appropriately intervene with safety and confidence.

## Oxygen Therapy

The general indication for $O_2$ therapy is hypoxemia. Hypoxemia is considered to be present when the arterial oxyhemoglobin saturation ($Sao_2$) is less than 90%, corresponding to an arterial blood $O_2$ partial pressure ($Pao_2$) of less than 60 mm Hg.[2] Refer to Table 2-4 for the relation between $O_2$ saturation as measured by pulse oximetry ($Spo_2$) and $Pao_2$ and to Figure 2-7 for the oxyhemoglobin dissociation curve. The goal of $O_2$ therapy is to treat and prevent hypoxemia, excessive work of breathing, and excessive myocardial work by increasing the $Pao_2$.[3]

$O_2$ moves across the alveolar-capillary membrane by *diffusion*, the physiologic mechanism by which gas moves across a membrane from a region of higher to lower pressure and is driven by the partial pressure gradient of $O_2$ between alveolar air ($Pao_2$) and pulmonary capillary blood. To improve diffusion, a rise in $Pao_2$ can be attained by increasing the fraction of inspired $O_2$ ($Fio_2$) with supplemental $O_2$.[4]

Supplemental $O_2$ is delivered by variable performance (Table III-A.1) or fixed performance (Table III-A.2) systems. Each cannula or mask is designed to provide a range of $Fio_2$. A variable performance system should not be used if a *specific* $Fio_2$ is required. Variable performance systems are not intended to meet the total inspiratory requirements of the patient. The actual $Fio_2$ for a given flow rate in a variable system is dependent on a patient's tidal volume and respiratory rate, and the type, fit, and placement of the cannula or mask. If a specific $Fio_2$ is required, then a fixed performance system is indicated. Fixed performance systems deliver a specific $Fio_2$ despite the patient's respiratory rate and pattern.[4]

$O_2$ delivery devices with masks or reservoirs allow $O_2$ to collect about the nose and mouth during exhalation, which increases the availability of $O_2$ during inhalation. As the storage capacity of the mask or reservoir is increased, the $Fio_2$ for a given flow rate is also increased.[5]

The supplemental $O_2$ requirements of a patient may fluctuate with activity. Monitoring $Sao_2$ with pulse oximetry (identified as $Spo_2$) and subsequent titration (weaning) of $O_2$ may be indicated during exercise. The physician may order parameters for resting and exercise $Spo_2$ if a patient has a low activity tolerance or an abnormally low $Spo_2$ at baseline.

A patient with chronic obstructive pulmonary disease who has chronic carbon dioxide retention may become desensitized to the respiratory stimulant effects of carbon dioxide. In these patients, ventilation is driven by means of a reflex ventilatory response to a

**Table III-A.1.** Variable Performance Oxygen Delivery*

| Device/$Fio_2$ | Description | Clinical Implications |
|---|---|---|
| **Nasal cannula**<br>RA ≈ 21% $Fio_2$,<br>1 lpm ≈ 24% $Fio_2$,<br>2 lpm ≈ 28% $Fio_2$,<br>3 lpm ≈ 32% $Fio_2$,<br>4 lpm ≈ 36% $Fio_2$,<br>5 lpm ≈ 40% $Fio_2$,<br>6 lpm ≈ 44% $Fio_2$ | **Purpose:** delivers supplemental $O_2$ mixed with RA, usually 1–6 lpm. The maximum is 8 lpm.<br>**Consists of:** prongs, which are attached to an $O_2$ source via small-bore plastic tubing and are positioned in the patient's nose. The tubing is secured by placing it behind the patient's ears and under the patient's chin (Figure III.A.1). | • The rule of thumb for the cannula system is that $Fio_2$ is increased by 3–4% for each lpm of $O_2$.<br>• Mouth breathing does not necessarily indicate that a patient is not receiving supplemental $O_2$.<br>• If nasal passages are obstructed, $O_2$ is able to collect in the oral and nasal cavities and is drawn in on inspiration.<br>• Flow rates of greater than 8 lpm are unlikely to increase delivered $O_2$ further and may prove uncomfortable and lead to mucosa desiccation.<br>• Provide mobile patients with adequate lengths of extension tubing or a portable $O_2$ tank to enable functional mobility. Patients should be instructed to avoid tripping over or becoming tangled in the tubing.<br>• The tubing may lead to irritation or skin breakdown behind the ears of some patients. Soft gauze padding may be placed around the tubing to protect the patient's skin. |

**Table III-A.1.** *Continued*

| Device/$Fio_2$ | Description | Clinical Implications |
|---|---|---|
| **Nasopharyngeal catheter** <br> $Fio_2$ as Nasal cannula, above <br> RA ≈ 21% $Fio_2$, <br> 1 lpm ≈ 24% $Fio_2$, <br> 2 lpm ≈ 28% $Fio_2$, <br> 3 lpm ≈ 32% $Fio_2$, <br> 4 lpm ≈ 36% $Fio_2$, <br> 5 lpm ≈ 40% $Fio_2$, <br> 6 lpm ≈ 44% $Fio_2$ | **Purpose:** delivers supplemental $O_2$ into the patient's oropharynx, which acts as an anatomic reservoir. This method is sometimes used with pediatric patients, who may dislodge a nasal cannula. <br> **Consists of:** a soft tube with several distal holes, lubricated and inserted through a nare until its distal tip is visible just below the uvula. It is attached to an $O_2$ source via small-bore tubing and held in place with tape. | • The catheter is changed daily. |
| **Open face mask/tent** <br> $Fio_2$ ≈ 35–50% | **Purpose:** provides humidified, supplemental $O_2$ mixed with RA. <br> **Consists of:** a mask with straps under the chin, contacts the cheeks, and is open over the patient's nose. It is secured with an elastic strap around the patient's head. It connects to a humidified $O_2$ source with large-bore tubing (Figure III-A.2). | • A significant amount of mixing with RA occurs, although the capacity of the mask allows $O_2$ to collect about the nose and mouth. <br> • It may be more comfortable than a closed face mask for claustrophobic patients. <br> • Moisture may collect in the tubing and should be drained before moving the patient. <br> • The aerosol system is more cumbersome and may make mobilization of the patient more difficult than with nasal prongs. Collaborate with nursing to determine whether nasal prongs or a closed face mask can be used when mobilizing the patient. <br> • Titrate $O_2$ appropriately to maintain $O_2$ saturation as indicated. |

**Closed face mask**

5–6 lpm ≈ 40% $Fio_2$, 6–7 lpm ≈ 50% $Fio_2$, 7–8 lpm ≈ 60% $Fio_2$

**Purpose:** delivers supplemental $O_2$ mixed with RA. The mask has a small capacity but does allow for the collection of $O_2$ about the nose and mouth.

**Consists of:** a dome-shaped mask covering the nose and mouth with ventilation holes on either side. An elastic strap around the patient's head secures it in place. It is connected to an $O_2$ source via small-bore tubing (Figure III-A.3).

- The closed face mask interferes with coughing, talking, eating, and drinking and may be very drying and uncomfortable. Patients often remove the mask for these reasons. Educate the patient on the importance of keeping the mask in place.

**Transtracheal catheter**

1 lpm ≈ 28% $Fio_2$, 2 lpm ≈ 36% $Fio_2$, 3 lpm ≈ 44% $Fio_2$, 4 lpm ≈ 52% $Fio_2$, 5 lpm ≈ 60% $Fio_2$, 6 lpm ≈ 68% $Fio_2$

**Purpose:** used for long-term $O_2$ therapy. Provides continuous supplemental $O_2$ mixed with RA.

**Consists of:** a small-bore catheter, which is surgically inserted percutaneously between the second and third tracheal interspaces to provide $O_2$. It is held in place by a narrow strap or chain around the patient's neck. A low flow rate (approximately one-half with rest and two-thirds with exercise) is used instead of a nasal cannula system owing to the continuous enrichment of the anatomic dead space with $O_2$.

- Patients with severe bronchospasm, uncompensated respiratory acidosis (pH <7.3), or steroid use higher than 30 mg per day are excluded from the use of this device.
- The use of this device for $O_2$ delivery is delayed for 1 wk postoperatively because of the risk of subcutaneous emphysema.
- This device requires care and attention to hygienic maintenance. The most serious complication is tracheal obstruction resulting from the accumulation of mucus on the outside of the catheter, which can be avoided by routine secretion clearance multiple times per day.
- There is also a risk of infection around the catheter site and a risk of catheter dislodgement.

Table III-A.1. *Continued*

| Device/$Fio_2$ | Description | Clinical Implications |
|---|---|---|
| **Tracheostomy mask or collar** $Fio_2 \approx 25–70\%$ | **Purpose:** provides supplemental, humidified $O_2$ or air at a tracheostomy site. **Consists of:** a mask placed over a stoma or tracheostomy. It is held in place by an elastic strap around the patient's neck. Humidified $O_2$ is delivered by large bore tubing (Figure III-A.4). | • Significant mixing with RA occurs. • Humidification is particularly important for a patient with a tracheostomy, as the tracheostomy bypasses the natural humidification system. • Moisture may collect in the tubing and should be drained before moving the patient. • The mask can easily shift; re-position it over the site if necessary. • Gently pull the mask away from the patient to access the tracheostomy site for bronchopulmonary secretion clearance. |
| **Partial non-rebreather mask** $Fio_2 \approx 35–95\%$ | **Purpose:** provides a high $Fio_2$ to the patient while conserving the $O_2$ supply. **Consists of:** a closed face mask covering the nose and mouth with ventilation holes on either side, held in place with an elastic strap around the patient's head. A reservoir bag is attached at the base of the mask. The flow of $O_2$ is regulated to permit the initial one-third of the expired tidal volume ($O_2$-rich anatomic dead space) to distend the reservoir maximally, therefore allowing some rebreathing of air. The balance of expired air does not enter the reservoir and is vented out the sides of the mask. | • The partial non-rebreather mask is able to provide a similar $Fio_2$ to the non-rebreather mask at lower flow rates. • The closed face mask may interfere with talking, eating, and drinking. • High $O_2$ concentration may be drying and uncomfortable; however, humidification is not used with this method, because it interferes with $O_2$ delivery. |

| Non-rebreather face mask $Fio_2 \approx 80\text{--}95\%$ | **Purpose:** provides the patient with the highest concentration of supplemental $O_2$ available via a face mask in a variable performance system.<br>**Consists of:** a closed face mask covering the nose and mouth. It is attached to a reservoir bag, which collects 100% $O_2$. A one-way valve between the mask and bag allows $O_2$ to be inspired from the bag through the mask. Additional one-way valves on the side of the mask allow expired gases to exit the mask, thus preventing re-breathing of expired air (Figure III-A.5). | • See Partial non-rebreather mask, above.<br>• Physical therapy intervention is usually deferred if a patient requires this type of device to maintain oxygenation. However, bronchopulmonary hygiene may still be indicated. |

$Fio_2$ = fraction of inspired oxygen; lpm = liters per minute; $O_2$ = oxygen; RA = room air.

*Listed from least to most oxygen support.

Sources: Data from RR Kirby, RW Taylor, JM Civetta (eds). Handbook of Critical Care (2nd ed). Philadelphia: Lippincott–Raven, 1997; JM Rothstein (ed). The Rehabilitation Specialist's Handbook (2nd ed). Philadelphia: FA Davis, 1998; MR Kinney, SB Dunbar, JM Vitello-Cicciu, et al. (eds). AACN's Clinical Reference for Critical Care Nursing (4th ed). St. Louis: Mosby, 1998; JG Weg. Long-term oxygen therapy for COPD. Postgrad Med 1998;103:143–158; D Frownfelter, E Dean (eds). Principles and Practice of Cardiopulmonary Physical Therapy (3rd ed). St. Louis: Mosby, 1997; and EF Ryerson, AJ Block. Oxygen as a Drug: Clinical Properties, Benefits, Modes and Hazards of Administration. In GG Burton, JE Hodgkin (eds), Respiratory Care: A Guide to Clinical Practice (3rd ed). Philadelphia: Lippincott, 1991.

Table III-A.2. Fixed Performance Oxygen Delivery

| Device/Fio$_2$ | Description | Clinical Implications |
|---|---|---|
| **Air entrainment mask** (Venti mask, Venturi mask) Fio$_2$ ≈ 24–50% | **Purpose:** provides a specific concentration of supplemental O$_2$. **Consists of:** a high-flow system with a closed face mask over the nose and mouth and a jet mixing device located at the base of the mask, which forces 100% O$_2$ past an entrainment valve. The valve can be adjusted to entrain a specific percentage of RA to mix with the O$_2$, allowing precise control of Fio$_2$ (Figure III-A.6). | • The closed face mask interferes with coughing, talking, eating, and drinking and may be very drying and uncomfortable. Patients often remove the mask for these reasons. • Educate the patient on the importance of keeping the mask in place. • Humidification is not used with this method, because humidification will interfere with O$_2$ delivery. |
| **BiPAP** Fio$_2$ ≈ 21–100% | **Purpose:** provides positive inspiratory and positive end expiratory pressure without intubation to decrease the work of breathing by reducing the airway pressure necessary to generate inspiration throughout the respiratory cycle. May be used to avoid intubation and mechanical ventilation in cases of acute respiratory failure. Often used in the hospital or home setting for the management of obstructive sleep apnea. | • BiPAP may deliver supplemental O$_2$ at a specific concentration, or it may deliver RA. • Patients may feel claustrophobic owing to the tight fit of the mask. • The equipment may be noisy; thus, the therapist may need to speak loudly to communicate with the patient. • Abrasions on the bridge of the nose can occur and may be prevented with a dressing that provides padding to the area without interfering with the tight fit of the mask. • Depending on the patient's oxygen requirements, BiPAP may be turned off, and alternate methods of O$_2$ delivery may be used to allow the patient |

**Consists of:** a closed mask with a clear soft gasket around its border, placed over the nose to fit tightly against the patient's face. It is held firmly in place with straps around the top and back of the head.

to participate in functional activities or an exercise program. The unit may also be placed on a portable intravenous pole or cart for this purpose.

**T tube/piece**
$FiO_2 \approx 50$–$80\%$

**Purpose:** provides a specific concentration of supplemental $O_2$ to an intubated, spontaneously breathing patient while weaning from a ventilator.

**Consists of:** a T-shaped tube attached directly to an endotracheal or tracheostomy tube. Humidified $O_2$ is delivered through one end of the T, and expired gas exits the other end. The tubing acts as a reservoir for $O_2$, allowing a specific concentration of $O_2$ to be delivered.

• Patients who are weaning from a ventilator can tire easily. Consult with the medical-surgical team to determine whether the patient will tolerate ventilator weaning (i.e., the use of a T piece) and physical therapy intervention simultaneously, or whether the patient would benefit from bronchopulmonary hygiene to facilitate weaning.

BiPAP = bilevel positive airway pressure; $FiO_2$ = fraction of inspired oxygen; lpm = liters per minute; $O_2$ = oxygen; RA = room air.
Sources: Data from RR Kirby, RW Taylor, JM Civetta (eds). Handbook of Critical Care (2nd ed). Philadelphia: Lippincott–Raven, 1997; JM Rothstein (ed). The Rehabilitation Specialist's Handbook (2nd ed). Philadelphia: FA Davis, 1998: and EF Ryerson, AJ Block. Oxygen as a Drug: Clinical Properties, Benefits, Modes and Hazards of Administration. In GG Burton, JE Hodgkin (eds), Respiratory Care: A Guide to Clinical Practice (3rd ed). Philadelphia: Lippincott, 1991.

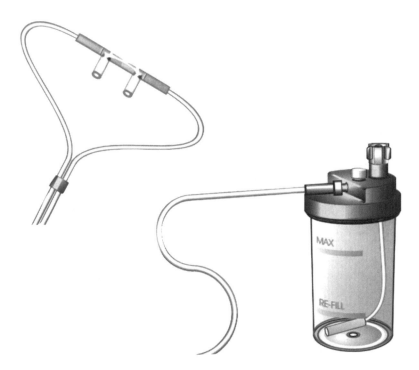

**Figure III-A.1.** *Nasal cannula with humidification. (Maersk Medical, Respiratory and Anesthesia Product Catalog, McAllen, TX.)*

decrease in $Pao_2$ originating in the aortic and carotid bodies.[6] In theory, providing supplemental $O_2$ may lead to a reduction in the hypoxic ventilatory drive. Apnea may result if chronic hypoxemia is reversed with higher flows of supplemental $O_2$. Potential respiratory depression should never contraindicate oxygen therapy in *severe* hypoxemia, however. If hypoventilation is a major problem, other support measures, including mechanical ventilation, can be used.[2]

## General Physical Therapy Considerations with Oxygen Therapy

- Note that a *green* label designates the $O_2$ supply on hospital walls. A similar gauge supplies pressurized air that is designated by a *yellow* label.

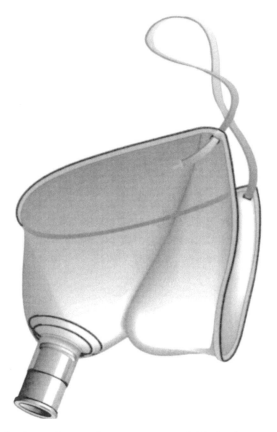

**Figure III-A.2.** *Open face mask or tent. (Maersk Medical, Respiratory and Anesthesia Product Catalog, McAllen, TX.)*

- Significant supplemental $O_2$ requirements usually indicate a respiratory compromise, which in turn may indicate the need to modify or defer physical therapy intervention.

- Observe the patient for clinical signs of hypoxemia: shortness of breath, use of accessory muscles of breathing, confusion, pallor, or cyanosis.

- The $Fio_2$ for a given system is dependent on its proper fit and application. Ensure that all connections are intact, that the $O_2$ is

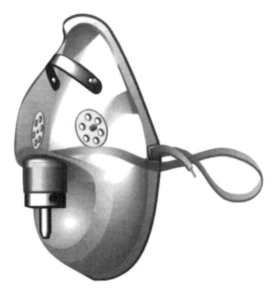

**Figure III-A.3.** *Closed face mask. (Maersk Medical, Respiratory and Anesthesia Product Catalog, McAllen, TX.)*

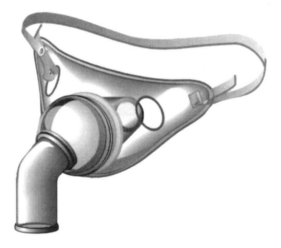

**Figure III-A.4.** *Tracheostomy mask or collar. (Maersk Medical, Respiratory and Anesthesia Product Catalog, McAllen, TX.)*

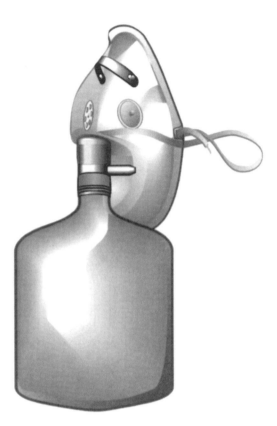

**Figure III-A.5.** *Nonrebreather mask. (Maersk Medical, Respiratory and Anesthesia Product Catalog, McAllen, TX.)*

flowing as indicated, and that the cannula or mask is properly positioned.

- The $O_2$ system may need added humidification, as supplemental $O_2$ may be drying to the nasal mucosa and lead to nosebleeds (epistaxis); however, added humidification is contraindi-cated in several systems, as indicated in Table III-A.1 and Table III-A.2.

- Provide extra lengths of $O_2$ tubing if functional mobility will occur farther than 5 or 6 ft from the bedside (i.e., the wall $O_2$ source).

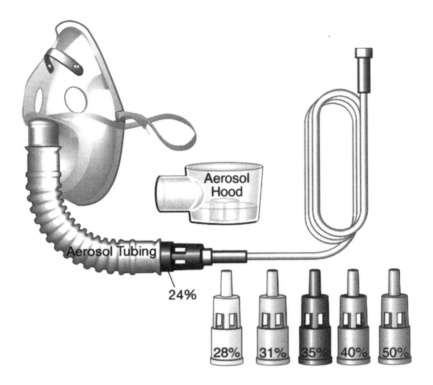

**Figure III-A.6.** *Air entrainment mask or venturi mask. (Maersk Medical, Respiratory and Anesthesia Product Catalog, McAllen, TX.)*

- Ensure that portable $O_2$ tanks are turned on and have sufficient levels of $O_2$ before use. Have back-up tanks available.

- Observe masks for the accumulation of mucus or clogging. Clear or change the cannula or mask if needed.

- Monitor the patient's skin for potential breakdown due to pressure from the cannula or mask. Provide appropriate padding without interfering with the fit of the cannula or mask.

- Document the type and amount of supplemental $O_2$ used during physical therapy intervention.

## Hemodynamic Monitoring

Monitoring hemodynamic events provides information about the adequacy of a patient's circulation, perfusion, and oxygenation of the tissues and organ systems. The goal of hemodynamic monitoring is to maintain the balance between oxygen demand and oxygen delivery.[7] Hemodynamic monitoring can be accomplished using noninvasive (Table III-A.3) or invasive (Table III-A.4) methods.

Noninvasive, or indirect, hemodynamic monitoring provides physiologic information without the risks of invasive monitoring and can be used in many settings; however, the accuracy of the data obtained is affected by the application of the device and the competence of the clinician gathering the data.[8]

Invasive, or direct, measurements are obtained by penetration of the skin and insertion of a cannula or catheter into a blood vessel, chamber of the heart, or both. The cannula or catheter is attached to a monitoring system, which consists of a transducer, amplifier, and oscilloscope for the display of the vascular waveforms and pressure measurements.[9] Direct monitoring can provide continuous, accurate data; however, thrombosis, infections, air embolisms, and trauma are potential complications.[8]

During invasive hemodynamic monitoring, the level of the right atrium is the standard zero reference point and is identified by the *phlebostatic axis*—the intersection of the midaxillary line and the fourth intercostal space (see Figure III-A.7).[10] The nurse will zero the system using a level to align the patient's phlebostatic axis with the transducer. Repositioning the patient may artificially alter waveforms by applying pressure to the catheter, shifting the catheter or stopcock, or shifting the phlebostatic axis relative to the transducer.[11]

## General Physical Therapy Considerations with Hemodynamic Monitoring

- Raising the level of the phlebostatic axis relative to the transducer gives false high readings; lowering the phlebostatic axis gives false low readings.[12]

- If a waveform changes during treatment, in the absence of other clinical signs, reposition the patient or limb (if an arterial line is in place) and reassess. If the waveform does not return to baseline, then notify the nurse.

Table III-A.3. Noninvasive Medical Monitoring

| Device | Description | Clinical Implications |
|---|---|---|
| **BP cuff** (sphygmomanometer) Normal adult values: systolic ≈ 100–140 mm Hg, diastolic ≈ 60–90 mm Hg | **Purpose:** indirectly measures arterial blood pressure. **Consists of:** an inflatable cuff, usually placed 2.5 cm proximal to the antecubital space, attached to a pressure monitoring device. Auscultate for Korotkoff's sounds (refer to Table 1-8) with a stethoscope over an artery, usually the brachial artery. | • Do not use a BP cuff on an extremity with an arterial line, lymphedema, AV fistula or graft, or blood clot, or in an extremity ipsilateral to a mastectomy. Try to avoid measuring BP in an extremity with a peripheral or central intra-venous line. Look for signs posted at the patient's bedside stating whether the use of a BP cuff on a particular extremity is contraindicated. • Use an appropriately sized cuff. The cuff bladder should be no less than 80% of limb circumference. A cuff that is too small overestimates BP. • The cuff may be placed on the upper extremity distal to the elbow with auscultation of the radial artery. • Alternative sites for measurement in the lower extremity are proximal to the popliteal space with auscultation of the popliteal artery or proximal to the ankle with auscultation of the posterior tibial artery. • Avoid contact between stethoscope tubing and the cuff tubing to minimize extraneous sounds. |

ECG

**Purpose:** continuous monitoring of heart rate and rhythm and respiratory rate (see Table 1-10).

**Consists of:** three to five color-coded electrodes placed on the chest, either hard wired to a monitor in a patient's room or monitored at a distant site (telemetry). Twelve electrodes are used for a formal ECG.

- Notify the nurse before physical therapy intervention, as many activities may alter the rate or rhythm or cause artifact (e.g., chest percussion).

- If an electrode(s) becomes dislodged, reconnect it. One way to remember electrode placement is *white is right* (white electrode is placed on the right side of the chest superior and lateral to the right nipple), *snow over grass* (the green electrode is placed below the white electrode on the anterolateral lower right rib cage), *smoke over fire* (the black electrode is placed on the upper left rib cage superior and lateral to the left nipple, and the red electrode is placed below the black one on the anterolateral left rib cage). The brown electrode is usually placed more centrally.

- Patients on telemetry should be instructed to stay in the area monitored by telemetry antennas.

- Collaborate with the nurse to determine whether patients who are "hard wired" to monitors in their room may be temporarily transferred to telemetry for ambulation activities or whether the monitor may be temporarily disconnected.

**Table III-A.3.** *Continued*

| Device | Description | Clinical Implications |
|---|---|---|
| **Pulse oximeter** Normal $SpO_2$ (at sea level) ≥ 93–94% | **Purpose:** a noninvasive method of measuring the percentage of hemoglobin saturated with $O_2$ in arterial blood. **Consists of:** a probe with an electro-optical sensor placed on a finger, toe, earlobe, or nose. The pulse oximeter emits two wavelengths of light to differentiate oxygenated from deoxygenated hemoglobin. | • $SpO_2$ ≤88% indicates the need for supplemental oxygen. • The waveform or pulse rate reading should match the ECG or palpated pulse. • Monitor changes in pulse oximetry during exercise and position changes. • Peripheral vascular disease, sunshine, or nail polish may lead to a false reading. • In low-perfusion states, such as hypothermia, hypotension, or vasoconstriction, pulse oximetry may understate oxygen saturation. • Small changes in the percentage of hemoglobin sites chemically combined (saturated) with oxygen ($SaO_2$) can correspond to large changes in the partial pressure of oxygen. Refer to Table 2-4 and Figure 2-7. |

AV = arteriovenous; BP = blood pressure; ECG = electrocardiography; $SaO_2$ = arterial oxyhemoglobin saturation; $SpO_2$ = measurement of $SaO_2$ with pulse oximetry.

Sources: Data from RR Kirby, RW Taylor, JM Civetta (eds). Handbook of Critical Care (2nd ed). Philadelphia: Lippincott–Raven, 1997; JM Rothstein (ed). The Rehabilitation Specialist's Handbook (2nd ed). Philadelphia: FA Davis, 1998; and MR Kinney, SB Dunbar, JM Vitello-Cicciu, et al. (eds). AACN's Clinical Reference for Critical Care Nursing (4th ed). St. Louis: Mosby, 1998.

**Table III-A.4.** Invasive Medical Monitoring

| Device/Normal Values | Description | Clinical Implications |
|---|---|---|
| **Arterial line (A-line)** Normal values: systolic, 100–140 mm Hg; diastolic, 60–90 mm Hg; MAP, 70–105 mm Hg | **Purpose:** to directly and continuously record arterial blood pressure, to obtain repeated arterial blood samples, or to deliver medications. **Consists of:** an arterial catheter. It is placed in the brachial, radial, or femoral artery. The catheter is usually connected to a transducer that converts a physiologic pressure into an electrical signal that is visible on a monitor. | • If the A-line is displaced, the patient can lose a significant amount of blood at the insertion site. If bleeding occurs from the line, immediately apply direct pressure to the site while calling for assistance.<br>• The normal A-line waveform is a biphasic sinusoidal curve with a sharp rise and a gradual decline (Figure III-A.8). A damped (flattened) waveform may indicate hypotension, or it may be due to pressure on the line.<br>• A patient with a femoral A-line is usually seen bedside. Hip flexion past 60–80 degrees is avoided. After femoral A-line removal, the patient is usually on strict bed rest for 60–90 mins, with a sandbag placed over the site.<br>• Upper-extremity insertion sites are usually splinted with an arm board to stabilize the catheter.<br>• The patient with a radial or brachial A-line can usually be mobilized out of bed, although the length of the line limits mobility to a few feet. The transducer may be taped to the patient's hospital gown at the level of the phlebostatic axis (see Figure III-A.7) during mobilization. |

Table III-A.4. *Continued*

| Device/Normal Values | Description | Clinical Implications |
|---|---|---|
| **Pacemaker** (temporary) | **Purpose:** to provide temporary cardiac pacing postoperatively, status post myocardial infarction, or before permanent pacemaker placement. Refer to Management in Chapter 1 for more information on pacemakers.<br><br>**Consists of:** pacing wires that connect to an external generator. There are three basic types.<br><br>*Epicardial*—the wires are placed after a heart surgery on the epicardium and exit through a mediastinal incision.<br><br>*Transvenous*—the wires are placed in the right ventricle via a central line.<br><br>*Transcutaneous*—large electrodes are placed on the skin over the anterior and posterior chest. | • The presence of a temporary pacemaker does not, in and of itself, limit functional mobility. However, the underlying indication for the pacemaker may limit the patient's activity level. Check for mobility restrictions.<br>• Temporary pacing wires should be kept dry.<br>• Be aware of the location of the generator and wires at all times, especially during mobility activities.<br>• If a temporary pacemaker is placed after a coronary artery bypass graft (CABG), the wires are usually removed 1–3 days after surgery. The patient is usually placed on bed rest for 1 hr after pacing wire removal, with vital sign monitoring every 15 mins. |
| **Pulmonary artery catheterization** (PA line, Swan-Ganz)<br>Normal values: PAP (mean), 10–20 mm Hg; PAWP (mean), 6–12 mm Hg; RAP, 0–8 mm Hg; core temperature, 98.2°–100.2°F (36.8°–37.9°C); | **Purpose:** to directly or indirectly measure PAP, PAWP, LAP, RAP, CVP, core body temperature, CI, and CO in cases of hemodynamic instability, heart failure, or cardiogenic shock. Provides access to mixed venous blood samples.<br><br>**Consists of:** a multilumen catheter inserted through an introducing sheath into a large vein, usually the subclavian, or the | • The patient with a PA line is usually on bed rest. Avoid head and neck (for subclavian access) or extremity movements that could disrupt the PA line at the insertion site, including the line dressing.<br>• PAWP is an indirect measure of LAP.<br>• PAP is equal to right ventricle pressure.<br>• RAP is equal to CVP.<br>• CO equals stroke volume (SV) × heart rate (HR). |

CO, 4–5 lpm; CI (CO/ body surface area), 3 lpm/ m² for an average 150-lb man

brachial, femoral, or internal jugular vein (Figure III-A.9). The catheter is directed by blood flow into various locations of the heart and pulmonary artery, with proper placement confirmed by x-ray.

The catheter is connected to a transducer to allow for continuous monitoring.

The proximal lumen opens into the right atrium to measure RAP and CO, and for the delivery of fluids or medications.

The distal lumen opens into the pulmonary artery to measure PAP and PAWP.

To obtain a PAWP measurement, a balloon at the end of the distal lumen is temporarily inflated. It follows the blood flow from the right ventricle into the pulmonary artery to a distal branch of the pulmonary artery, where it is "wedged" for a short time (up to 15 secs).

A-line = arterial line; CI = cardiac index; CO = cardiac output; CVP = central venous pressure; LAP = left atrial pressure; lpm = liters per minute; MAP = mean arterial pressure; PAP = pulmonary artery pressure; PAWP = pulmonary artery wedge pressure; RAP = right atrial pressure.
Sources: Data from RR Kirby, RW Taylor, JM Civetta (eds). Handbook of Critical Care (2nd ed). Philadelphia: Lippincott–Raven, 1997; MR Kinney, SB Dunbar, JM Vitello-Cicciu, et al. (eds). AACN's Clinical Reference for Critical Care Nursing (4th ed). St. Louis: Mosby, 1998; EK Daily, JP Schroeder. Clinical Management Based on Hemodynamic Parameters. In EK Daily, JP Schroeder (eds), Techniques in Bedside Hemodynamic Monitoring (5th ed). St. Louis: Mosby, 1994; and EJ Bridges. Monitoring pulmonary artery pressures: just the facts. Crit Care Nurse 2000;21(16):67.

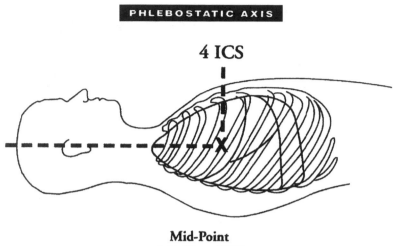

Figure III-A.7.  *The phlebostatic axis at the intersection of the fourth intercostal space (ICS) and the midpoint of the anterior (A) and posterior (P) chest wall. (Reprinted with permission from Edwards Lifesciences LLC.)*

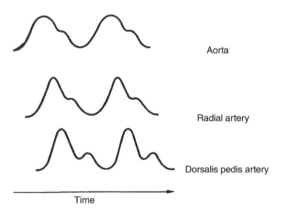

Figure III-A.8.  *Arterial line tracing from different sites. (Reprinted with permission from SM Yentis, NP Hirsh, GB Smith [eds], Anaesthesia and Intensive Care A–Z. An Encyclopedia of Principles and Practice [2nd ed]. Oxford, UK: Butterworth–Heinemann, 2000;45.)*

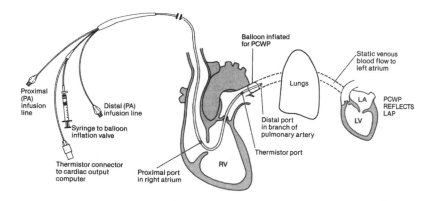

**Figure III-A.9.** *Pulmonary artery (PA) catheter (four lumen model) in a branch of a PA with the balloon inflated; the pulmonary capillary wedge pressure (PCWP) reflects left atrial pressure (LAP). (LA = left atrium; LV = left ventricle; RV= right ventricle.) (Reprinted with permission from LD Kersten [ed]. Comprehensive Respiratory Nursing: A Decision-Making Approach. Philadelphia: Saunders, 1989;758.)*

## Intracranial Pressure Monitoring

Intracranial pressure (ICP) and cerebral perfusion pressure may be measured in a variety of ways, depending on how urgently ICP values are needed and the patient's neurologic or hemodynamic stability. Refer to Intracranial and Cerebral Perfusion Pressure in Chapter 4 for a description of these terms, Table 4-20 for a description of the early and late signs of increased ICP, and Table 4-21 for a list of treatment options to decrease ICP.

Table III-A.5 describes the different types of ICP monitors. For some ICP monitors, such as the intraventricular catheter, the sensor and the transducer must be level. Often, the zero point for the transducer is at the *tragus*, or the top of the ear. A normal ICP waveform has a triphasic sinusoidal waveform and should correspond to heart rate.

## General Physical Therapy Considerations with Intracranial Pressure Monitoring

- As with hemodynamic monitoring, be aware of the ICP value and the corresponding waveform on the monitor. The waveform may change shape (plateau wave) if cerebral hypoxia or ischemia occurs.[13]

**Table III-A.5.** Intracranial Pressure (ICP) Monitors

| Device | Description | Clinical Implications |
|---|---|---|
| Epidural sensor | **Purpose:** to monitor ICP.<br>**Consists of:** a fiberoptic sensor. It is placed in the epidural space (i.e., superficial to the dura) and connects to a transducer and monitor. | • The transducer does not need to be adjusted (releveled) with position changes.<br>• Fair reliability. |
| Subarachnoid/<br>subdural bolt | **Purpose:** to directly monitor ICP and provide access for CSF sampling.<br>**Consists of:** a bolt or screw placed in the subarachnoid or subdural space through a burr hole. | • The physician will determine the level to which the transducer should be positioned. This is documented in the chart and posted at the bedside.<br>• The transducer must be repositioned to the appropriate level with position changes.<br>• Poor reliability. |
| Intraventricular<br>catheter<br>(ventriculostomy) | **Purpose:** to directly monitor ICP and provide access for the sampling and drainage of CSF. Occasionally used to administer medications.<br>**Consists of:** a small catheter that is placed in the anterior horn of the lateral ventricle through a burr hole. The catheter connects to a transducer and to a drainage bag, where CSF collects. | • The nondominant hemisphere is the preferable insertion site.<br>• There are two different types of drainage systems: intermittent and continuous.<br>• The intermittent system allows the nurse to drain CSF for 30–120 secs by momentarily opening a stopcock when the ICP exceeds the parameters set by the physician.<br>• A continuous system allows the drainage of CSF to occur against a pressure gradient when the collection bag is positioned (leveled) above the foramen of Monro. This is usually 15 cm above the external auditory meatus. |

| Fiberoptic transducer tipped catheter | **Purpose:** to monitor ICP. Can also monitor intraparenchymal pressure (if the catheter is placed in the parenchyma). <br><br> **Consists of:** a fiberoptic transducer-tipped catheter. It is placed in the ventricle, within the parenchyma, or in the subarachnoid or subdural space. | • The transducer must be repositioned to the appropriate level with position changes. <br> • Very reliable. <br> • The transducer does not need to be adjusted (releveled) with position changes. <br> • Very reliable. |

CSF = cerebrospinal fluid.

Sources: Data from AE Davis, TL Briones. Intracranial Disorders. In MR Kinney, SB Dunbar, JM Vitello-Cicciu, et al. (eds), AACN's Clinical Reference Manual for Critical Care Nursing (4th ed). St. Louis: Mosby, 1998; and LA Thelan, KM Stacy, LD Urden, ME Lough (eds). Neurologic Therapeutic Management, Critical Care Nursing: Diagnosis and Management (3rd ed). St. Louis: Mosby, 1998.

- Momentary elevations in ICP will normally occur. It is a *sustained* elevation in ICP that is of concern and should be reported to the nurse.

- Patients with elevated ICP are often positioned with the head of the bed at 30 degrees, which maximizes venous blood flow from the brain to help decrease ICP.[14] Therefore, be aware that lowering the head of the bed may increase ICP. Other positions that increase ICP are the Trendelenburg position, lateral neck flexion, and extreme hip flexion.

- Additional conditions that increase ICP are the Valsalva maneuver, noxious stimuli, pain, and coughing.

## Medical-Surgical Management Devices

Different lines, tubes, catheters, and access devices comprise the wide variety of medical-surgical equipment used in the acute care setting. In general, these devices may be peripheral or central, for short- or long-term use, and inserted or applied at the bedside in a special procedure (e.g., under fluoroscopic guidance) or in the operating room. Table III-A.6 describes the medical-surgical management devices most commonly encountered in the acute care setting.

## General Physical Therapy Considerations with Medical-Surgical Management Devices

The following clinical tips apply to medical-surgical equipment, as well as to the $O_2$ therapy and noninvasive, invasive, and ICP monitoring equipment previously discussed.

---

### Clinical Tip

- Before entering a patient's room, review the medical record, particularly new orders, recent progress notes, and test results. Review graphic sheets for vital signs, noting trends or variations from the norms.
- Note whether any particular precautions protecting the patient or the caregiver from specific pathogens are in

Table III-A.6.  Medical Management Devices*

| Device | Description | Clinical Implications |
|---|---|---|
| **Antithrombolytic boots** (pneumatic compression stockings/Venodyne boots) | **Purpose:** provides intermittent pressure to the lower extremities to promote venous return and prevent deep vein thrombosis secondary to prolonged or postoperative bed rest.<br><br>**Consists of:** inflatable sleeves, applied to the lower legs, which intermittently inflate and deflate. In some cases, the sleeve is applied to the leg from the ankle to midthigh. | • Usually worn when the patient is in bed, but can be worn when sitting in a chair.<br>• Reapply when patient returns to bed.<br>• Discontinued when the patient is ambulating on a regular basis. |
| **AV graft or AV fistula** | **Purpose:** provides access for hemodialysis.<br><br>**Consists of:** The *graft* is an artificial blood vessel, usually made of Gore-Tex or Dacron, used to join an artery and vein when a patient's own vessels are not viable for an AV fistula. The *fistula* is the surgical joining of an artery and vein, allowing arterial blood to flow directly to a vein. Usually located in the forearm. | • Elevate and avoid weight bearing on the involved extremity for 24 hrs after surgical procedure.<br>• Do not use blood pressure cuff on the involved extremity.<br>• Avoid pressure over the site.<br>• Palpable turbulence is normal in the graft or fistula, which will have a raised, rope-like appearance. |
| **Central (venous) line**<br>Normal value,<br>CVP = 0–8 mm Hg | **Purpose:** provides vascular access for up to 2–4 wks for TPN, repeated blood sampling, or administration of drugs or fluid. May measure CVP (see Pulmonary artery catheterization in Table III-A.4). May be used to place a temporary pacemaker or a vena cava filter or for hemodialysis.<br><br>**Consists of:** a single- or multiple-lumen intravenous line placed in the subclavian, basilic, jugular, or femoral vein, terminating in the right atrium. | • Do not use a blood pressure cuff on an extremity with a central line. |

**Table III-A.6.** *Continued*

| Device | Description | Clinical Implications |
|---|---|---|
| **Chest tube** | **Purpose:** removes and prevents the re-entry of air (pneumothorax) or fluid (hemothorax, pleural effusion, empyema, or chylothorax) from the pleural space or mediastinal space and provides negative intrapleural pressure.<br><br>**Consists of:** tube(s) placed in the pleural or mediastinal space that exit the chest and are usually connected to a drainage system (**Figure III-A.10**). The placement of the tubes is determined by indication. Mediastinal chest tubes, placed to drain the pericardium after surgery, exit the chest directly below the sternum. Apical chest tubes drain air, which typically collects in the apices of the pleural spaces. Fluid tends to collect near the bases; in these cases, tubes are placed more inferiorly near the fluid collection.<br><br>Postoperatively, tubes often exit the chest through the surgical incision. If chest tubes are placed in a nonsurgical situation, they are often placed along the midaxillary line at the appropriate level. Tubes usually connect to a drainage system with three compartments: the drainage collection chamber, the water seal chamber with a one-way valve that prevents air or fluid from re-entering the drainage collection chamber; and the suction chamber, which decreases excess pressure in the pleural space.<br><br>Tubes may be connected to a small one-way valve (Heimlich valve) that allows air or fluid to escape from the pleural space while preventing re-entry. | • Chest tubes may cause discomfort, which may inhibit a cough, deep breath, or mobility.<br>• The patient may benefit from premedication for pain before treatment.<br>• The drainage system should be below the level of chest tube insertion.<br>• Avoid tipping the collection reservoir. The reservoir may be hung from the side of the bed or taped to the floor to prevent tipping.<br>• If the reservoir is overturned, return the drainage container to the upright position and notify the nurse.<br>• If the chest tube itself becomes dislodged, stop activity and notify the nurse immediately. If possible, place the patient in an upright sitting position, and monitor the patient's breath sounds, vital signs, and respiratory rate and pattern for possible signs of tension pneumothorax.<br>• Prevent kinks in the line. |

- The presence of a chest tube should not, in and of itself, limit activity. Position changes and mobility can facilitate drainage.
- Ask the nurse or doctor whether the chest tube may be temporarily disconnected from suction during mobility activities. If the suction must remain connected, additional lengths of tubing may be added, or a portable suction device may be used during mobility activities.
- The occlusive dressing, usually a petrolatum gauze dressing to prevent the influx of air, should remain intact. Do not apply pressure over the insertion site.
- Patients with this device are typically very ill and unable to participate in mobility activities.

**Esophagogastric tamponade tube** (Blakemore tube, Sengstaken-Blakemore tube, Minnesota tube)

**Purpose:** to compress hemorrhaging esophageal varices. The tube, which is passed by mouth through the esophagus into the stomach, has a proximal (esophageal) cuff, which compresses esophageal varices, and a distal (gastric) cuff, which compresses gastric varices. Channels allow aspiration of gastric contents. The balloons typically remain in place for up to 24–72 hrs, as longer duration may cause tissue necrosis or ulceration.

Table III-A.6. *Continued*

| Device | Description | Clinical Implications |
|---|---|---|
| **Lumbar drainage device (LDD)** | **Purpose:** continuous drainage of CSF from the subarachnoid space in the lumbar spine. For the treatment of CSF leaks or shunt infections or to reduce intracranial pressure. <br> **Consists of:** a spinal catheter inserted in L4-5 subarachnoid space, advanced to an appropriate level, and connected to a sterile closed CSF collection system. | • The position of the patient, the position of the transducer (if any), and the position of the collection bag are determined by the rationale for the LDD intervention. <br> • Changes in the patient's position, in the level of the collection bag, or in the intrathecal pressure impact the amount and rate of drainage. <br> • Note any restrictions in the medical record or posted in the patient's room. <br> • Patients are usually on bed rest while the drain is in place. <br> • Patients are often instructed to avoid coughing while practicing post-operative deep breathing exercises. <br> • Over-drainage or under-drainage complications include tension pneumocranium, central herniation of the brain, compression of the brain stem, and subdural hematoma. <br> • Monitor the patient for any changes in neurologic status. Notify nursing immediately if any changes are noted. |

| Midline catheter | **Purpose:** delivers i.v. medications or fluids for up to 4–6 wks. Cannot be used to draw blood.<br>**Consists of:** a 3- to 8-in. peripheral catheter placed via the antecubital fossa into the basilic or cephalic vein. | • Do not use blood pressure cuff on the involved extremity. |
| --- | --- | --- |
| **Nasoenteric feeding tube** (Dobbhoff tube) | **Purpose:** placed for enteral feedings when patients are unable to take in adequate nutrition by mouth.<br>**Consists of:** a small-diameter, ~26 mm or No. 7–10 French, tube inserted via the nostril, through the esophagus into the stomach or duodenum, and held in place with tape across the nose. | • The position of the tube in the nostril and the back of the throat can be irritating to the patient and may inhibit a cough.<br>• The tube often hangs in front of the patient's mouth and may also hinder airway clearance.<br>• The patient may be more comfortable if the tube is positioned away from his or her mouth and taped to the forehead or cheek.<br>• The tube can be dislodged easily. Check that the tape is secure. Notify the nurse if the tube becomes dislodged.<br>• Patients may be on aspiration precautions.<br>• Place feedings on hold when the head of the bed is flat to minimize the risk of regurgitation or aspiration. |

Table III-A.6. *Continued*

| Device | Description | Clinical Implications |
|---|---|---|
| Nasogastric tube (NGT) | **Purpose:** keeps the stomach empty after surgery and rests the bowel by preventing gastric contents from passing through the bowels. Some NGTs allow access to the stomach for medications or tube feedings (see Nasoenteric feeding tube). **Consists of:** a tube inserted *via* the nostril, through the esophagus, and into the stomach. Often attached to low-level suction pressure. Held in place with tape across the nose. | • This small-diameter tube can clog easily; some facilities require that feeding tubes be flushed with water when placed on hold for >15 mins to minimize the risk of clogging.<br>• See above (Nasoenteric feeding tube) for positioning tips.<br>• Ask the nurse if the tube may be disconnected from suction for mobilization of the patient.<br>• When disconnected from suction, cap the open end. |
| Nebulizer | **Purpose:** delivers inhaled medications, usually bronchodilators and mucolytics. **Consists of:** a hand-held chamber with a mouthpiece through which pressurized air aerosolizes medications that are then inhaled. May deliver medications through ventilator or tracheostomy tubing. | • Treatment time is usually 10–20 mins; however, the medications are usually effective for 3–6 hrs.<br>• Patients may be better prepared for mobility activities or airway clearance after nebulizer treatments.<br>• These treatments are often referred to as *nebs.* |
| Percutaneous endoscopic gastronomy/ jejunostomy tube (PEG/PEJ) tube | **Purpose:** provides long-term access for nourishment to patients who are unable to tolerate food by mouth. May be used to supplement nutrition taken by mouth. **Consists of:** a feeding tube placed by endoscopy into the stomach or jejunum through the abdominal wall. | • Place tube feedings on hold when the head of the bed is flat to minimize the risk of regurgitation/aspiration.<br>• PEJ tube is considered postpyloric; therefore, the risk of aspiration from regurgitation is minimized. |

- This small-diameter tube can clog easily; some facilities require that feeding tubes be flushed with water when placed on hold for >15 mins to minimize the risk of clogging.

**Percutaneous sheath introducer** (Cordis)

**Purpose:** dilates a vein to provide a channel for introduction of pulmonary catheter.

**Consists of:** a Teflon sheath that often has a port for i.v. access.

- The patient may be mobilized with the sheath in place once the pulmonary catheter has been removed.

- A secure dressing should cover the sheath during any mobilization, as the large bore opening of the sheath can allow air into the venous system if the sheath is dislodged.

**Peripheral intravenous line**

**Purpose:** provides temporary access for delivery of medications, fluids or blood transfusions. Cannot be used to draw blood.

**Consists of:** a short catheter, 0.75–1.00 in. long, inserted into a small peripheral vein.

- Avoid using blood pressure cuff on the involved extremity.

- Watch i.v. tubing for kinks or occlusions.

- Position the patient to avoid occluding flow.

- Observe the patient for signs of infiltrated i.v. or phlebitis: localized pain, edema, erythema, or tenderness. Notify the nurse if signs are present.

**Table III-A.6.** *Continued*

| Device | Description | Clinical Implications |
|---|---|---|
| **Peripherally inserted central venous catheter (PICC)** | **Purpose:** provides long-term administration of TPN, medications or fluid.<br>**Consists of:** a catheter placed via the cephalic or basilic veins, terminating in the superior vena cava. This is the only central line placed by a nurse. | • Wait for x-ray results before mobilizing the patient to confirm proper placement of the line.<br>• Improper placement can break the line; cause a hematoma; pierce the lung, causing a pneumothorax; or terminate in a vessel other than the vena cava.<br>• Do not use a blood pressure cuff on the involved extremity.<br>• Encourage range of motion of the involved extremity.<br>• Use of axillary crutches may be contraindicated. |
| **Rectal pouch/tube** | **Purpose:** temporarily collects bowel drainage and protects fragile skin from contact with feces.<br>**Consists of:** a pouch placed externally or a tube placed internally in the rectum. | • Both are easily dislodged.<br>• Use a draw sheet when moving the patient in bed.<br>• Keep the collection bag below the level of insertion. |
| **Suprapubic catheter** | **Purpose:** drains the bladder temporarily after some bladder surgeries, or permanently in cases of blocked urethra due to a tumor, periurethral abscess, or a severe voiding dysfunction.<br>**Consists of:** a catheter placed in the bladder through a surgical incision in the lower abdominal wall. | • Keep the collection bag below the level of the bladder.<br>• The collection tubing may be taped to the patient's thigh.<br>• Avoid pressure over the insertion site. |

**Surgical drain**

**Purpose:** removes blood or fluid from a surgical site that would otherwise collect internally.

Surgical drains are of two basic types: passive or active. *Passive drainage* is accomplished by gravity or capillary action. Drainage is further facilitated by transient increases in intra-abdominal pressure, as with coughing. Passive surgical drains include Penrose, Foley, Malecot, and Word catheters. *Active drainage* is accomplished by suction from a simple bulb device or a suction pump. These systems may be closed, like the Hemovac and Jackson-Pratt (JP) drains.

- Be aware of the location of the drain when moving the patient.
- The tubing may be taped or pinned to the patient's skin or clothing to prevent tugging.
- Check with the nurse before disconnecting a drain from suction.

**Texas catheter**

**Purpose:** noninvasively drains and collects urine from the penis.

**Consists of:** a condom-like flexible sheath that fits over the penis to drain urine into a collection bag. This noninvasive method of collecting urine has a much lower risk of infection and irritation than does an indwelling catheter and is often the preferred method of managing male urinary incontinence.

- It is easily dislodged.
- It may be held in place with a Velcro strap.
- The drainage bag should always be below the level of the bladder to allow drainage by gravity.
- Keep the collection bag off the floor.
- Secure the collection bag or catheter tubing to patient's leg, clothing, or assistive device to prevent the patient from tripping or becoming tangled in the tubing during mobility activities.

**Table III-A.6.** *Continued*

| Device | Description | Clinical Implications |
|---|---|---|
| **Totally implantable intravascular device** (Port-A-Cath, MediPort) | **Purpose:** surgically implanted catheter used for long-term chemotherapy, TPN, or other long-term infusion therapy. **Consists of:** a completely implanted catheter, usually placed in the subclavian or jugular vein, terminating in the superior vena cava. Access to the catheter is obtained through a tunneled portion attached to a port that is implanted in a subcutaneous pocket in the chest wall, usually below the clavicle. The subcutaneous titanium, plastic, or stainless steel port has a reservoir with a self-sealing septum that is accessed by a special noncoring needle through intact skin. The tunneled portion is anchored to a muscle or subcutaneous tissue with sutures. | • Once healed, physical activity is not limited. <br> • Patients can usually swim or bathe without limitation. |
| **Tunneled central venous catheter** (Hickman, Broviac, Groshong, Silastic, and Quinton catheters) | **Purpose:** surgically implanted catheter used for long-term chemotherapy, TPN, or other long-term infusion therapy. May be used for months to years. Very similar to the totally implantable intravascular device (previously described); however, access is obtained through a "tailed" portion, which exits the skin from the anterior chest wall superior to the nipple. A Dacron cuff surrounds the tunneled portion just inside the exit site. The cuff causes a subcutaneous inflammatory reaction to occur after insertion, which, when healed, provides fixation and a barrier to infection within 1 to 2 wks of implantation. | • The tailed portion should be taped down to prevent dislodging. <br> • Do not perform manual techniques directly over the tail. <br> • Patients are allowed to shower once the insertion site is healed; however, tub bathing and swimming are usually limited. |

**Urinary catheter**
**(Foley catheter)**

**Purpose:** temporarily drains and collects urine from bladder. It allows accurate measurement of urine output.
**Consists of:** a tube inserted through the urethra into the bladder that drains into a collection bag. It is held in place internally by an inflated cuff.

- Be aware of the position of the catheter.
- The collection bag should always be below the level of the bladder to allow drainage by gravity.
- Secure the collection bag or tubing to the patient's leg, clothing, or assistive device to prevent the patient from tripping or becoming tangled in the tubing during mobility activities.
- The collection bag should be kept off the floor.

**Ventriculoperitoneal shunt (VP)**
**Ventriculoatrial shunt (VA)**

**Purpose:** drains excess CSF from the brain into the abdominal cavity or heart.
**Consists of:** a shunt, tunneled under the skin, from the cerebral ventricles to the collection cavity.

- The patient may be on bed rest for 24 hrs after placement.
- The shunt can often be palpated under the skin.
- Avoid excess pressure over the shunt.

**Yankauer suction**

**Purpose:** clears secretions from the oral cavity or the oropharynx.
**Consists of:** a hand-held clear rigid tube attached to wall suction via tubing. The suction pressure is usually 120–150 mm Hg.

- Some patients use this independently; if so, place within the patient's reach.
- Patients with a decreased cough reflex or dysphagia or on ventilator support may collect secretions in the mouth or in the back of the throat. Gentle Yankauer suctioning before rolling or other mobility may prevent aspiration of the collected secretions.

Table III-A.6. *Continued*

| Device | Description | Clinical Implications |
|---|---|---|
| | | • Yankauer suctioning may stimulate a cough and help clear secretions in patients who are unable to clear secretions independently.<br>• If a patient bites down on the Yankauer, do not attempt to pull on the device. Wait for the patient to relax, then gently slide the Yankauer from the patient's mouth. |

AV = arteriovenous; CSF = cerebrospinal fluid; CVP = central venous pressure; TPN = total parenteral nutrition.

*Listed in alphabetical order.

Sources: Data from RR Kirby, RW Taylor, JM Civetta (eds). Handbook of Critical Care (2nd ed). Philadelphia: Lippincott–Raven, 1997; F Halderman. Selecting a vascular access device. Nursing 2000;11:59–61; DF Colixxa. Actionstat: dislodged chest tube. Nursing 1995;25–33; HJ Thompson. Managing patients with lumbar drainage devices. Crit Care Nurse 2000;20:60–68; and Guidelines for intensive care unit admission, discharge, and triage. Task Force of the American College of Critical Care Medicine, Society of Critical Care Medicine. Crit Care Med 1999;27:633–638.

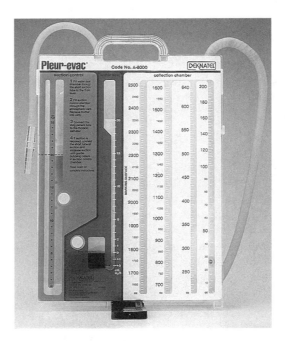

**Figure III-A.10.** *A chest drainage system has three main compartments from left to right: (1) the suction control, (2) the water seal, (3) the collection chamber. (Reprinted with permission from Genzyme Biosurgery.)*

place (e.g., contact precautions). Refer to Table 10-4 for a summary of infection prevention precautions.

• Practice universal precautions. The likelihood of encountering bodily fluids is increased in the acute care setting, especially in the ICU.

• Discuss your planned intervention with the nurse. Scheduled procedures may take precedence over this intervention, or it may coordinate well with another planned procedure.

• On entering the patient's room, *take inventory*. Observe the patient's appearance and position. Systematically observe the patient and verify the presence of all documented lines. Develop a consistent method of surveying the room: left to right, or top of bed to bottom of bed, to ensure that all lines and equipment are observed and considered in your treatment plan. Take note of all readings on the monitors before intervention.

• Anticipate how your intervention may change the patient's vital signs and how this will likely appear on the monitors. Be aware of which readings may change artificially owing to relative position change.

• Using appropriate precautions, gently trace each line from the patient to its source. Ask for assistance, if needed, to untangle any lines or to free any lines that might be under the patient.

• Ensure that there is no tension on each line before attempting to move the patient.

• Never attempt to free a line that cannot be completely visualized!

• Discuss with the nurse whether any lines can be removed or temporarily disconnected from the patient before your treatment.

• Ask for appropriate assistance when mobilizing the patient.

• Most invasive monitoring systems have two alarm controls: one to silence or discontinue the alarm for a few minutes, and another to disable or turn off the alarm. Do not silence or disable an alarm without permission from the nurse!

• On completion of your treatment, ensure that all appropriate alarms are turned on and that the patient is positioned with the appropriate safety and communication measures in place. Notify the nurse of any change in the patient's status.

# References

1. Anonymous. Guidelines for intensive care unit admissions, discharge, and triage. Task Force of the American College of Critical Care Medicine, Society of Critical Care Medicine. Crit Care Med 1999;27(3):633–638.
2. Kirby RR, Taylor RW. Oxygen Therapy. In RR Kirby, RW Taylor, JM Civetta (eds), Handbook of Critical Care (2nd ed). Philadelphia: Lippincott–Raven, 1997;254,260.

3. Kacmarek RM. Oxygen Therapy. In RM Kacmarek, CW Mack, S Dimas (eds), The Essentials of Respiratory Care (3rd ed). St. Louis: Mosby, 1990;408.
4. Scanlan CL, Heur A. Medical Gas Therapy. In DF Egan, CL Scanlan (eds), Egan's Fundamentals of Respiratory Care (7th ed). St. Louis: Mosby, 1999;738,748.
5. Ryerson EF, Block AJ. Oxygen as a Drug: Clinical Properties, Benefits, Modes and Hazards of Administration. In GG Burton, JE Hodgkin (eds), Respiratory Care: A Guide to Clinical Practice (3rd ed). Philadelphia: Lippincott, 1991;325–326.
6. Kacmarek RM. Neurologic Control of Ventilation. In RM Kacmarek, CW Mack, S Dimas (eds), The Essentials of Respiratory Care (3rd ed). St. Louis: Mosby, 1990;80.
7. Daily EK, Schroeder JP. Clinical Management Based on Hemodynamic Parameters. In EK Daily, JP Schroeder (eds), Techniques in Bedside Hemodynamic Monitoring (5th ed). St. Louis: Mosby, 1994;235.
8. Whalen DA, Kelleher RM. Cardiovascular Patient Assessment. In MR Kinney, SB Dunbar, JM Vitello-Cicciu, et al (eds), AACN's Clinical Reference for Critical Care Nursing (4th ed). St. Louis: Mosby, 1998;303.
9. Smith RN. Concepts of Monitoring and Surveillance. In MR Kinney, SB Dunbar, JM Vitello-Cicciu, et al (eds), AACN's Clinical Reference for Critical Care Nursing (4th ed). St. Louis: Mosby, 1998;19.
10. Bridges EJ. Monitoring pulmonary artery pressures: just the facts. Crit Care Nurse 2000;20:67.
11. Daily EK, Schroeder JP. Principles and Hazards of Monitoring Equipment. In EK Daily, JP Schroeder (eds), Techniques in Bedside Hemodynamic Monitoring (5th ed). St. Louis: Mosby, 1994;37.
12. Bridges EJ, Woods SL. Pulmonary artery pressure measurement: state of the art. Heart Lung 1993;22:99.
13. Hickey JV. Theory and Management of Increased Intracranial Pressure. In JV Hickey (ed), The Clinical Practice of Neurological and Neurosurgical Nursing (4th ed). Philadelphia: Lippincott, 1997;316.
14. Boss BJ. Nursing Management of Adults with Common Neurologic Problems. In PG Beare, JL Myers (eds), Adult Health Nursing (3rd ed). St. Louis: Mosby, 1998;917–924.

# III-B

# Mechanical Ventilation
*Sean M. Collins*

Mechanical ventilatory support provides positive pressure to inflate the lungs. Patients with acute illness, serious trauma, exacerbation of chronic illness, or progression of chronic illness may require mechanical ventilation.[1]

The following are physiologic objectives of mechanical ventilation[2]:

- Support or manipulate pulmonary gas exchange

- Increase lung volume

- Reduce or manipulate the work of breathing

The following are clinical objectives of mechanical ventilation[2]:

- Reverse hypoxemia and acute respiratory acidosis

- Relieve respiratory distress

- Reverse ventilatory muscle fatigue

- Permit sedation, neuromuscular blockade, or both

- Decrease systemic or myocardial oxygen consumption and intracranial pressure

- Stabilize the chest wall

- Provide access to tracheal-bronchial tree for pulmonary hygiene

- Provide access for delivery of an anesthetic, analgesic, or sedative medication

The following are indications for mechanical ventilation[2]:

- Partial pressure of arterial oxygen of less than 50 mm Hg with supplemental oxygen

- Respiratory rate of more than 30 breaths per minute

- Vital capacity less than 10 liters per minute

- Negative inspiratory force of less than 25 cm $H_2O$

- Protection of airway from aspiration of gastric contents

- Reversal of respiratory muscle fatigue[3]

## Process of Mechanical Ventilation

### Intubation

*Intubation* is the passage of an artificial airway (tube) into the patient's trachea (Figure III-B.1), generally through the mouth (*endotracheal tube* intubation) or occasionally through the nose (*nasotracheal* intubation). Intubation is considered for four reasons: (1) the presence of upper airway obstruction, (2) inability to protect the lower airways from aspiration, (3) inability to clear pulmonary secretions, and (4) the need for positive pressure ventilation.[4] The process of removing the artificial airway is called *extubation*.

When patients require ventilatory support for a prolonged time period, a tracheostomy is considered. According to one author, it is best to allow 1 week of endotracheal intubation; then, if extubation seems unlikely during the next week, tracheostomy should be considered.[1] However, a patient can also be intubated for many weeks without tracheostomy, depending on the clinical situation. A *trache-*

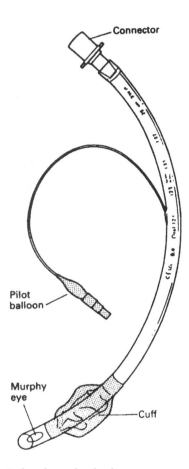

Connector

Pilot
balloon

Murphy
eye

Cuff

Figure III-B.1. *A typical endotracheal tube.*

*ostomy tube* is inserted directly into the anterior trachea below the vocal cords, generally performed in the operating room. Benefits of tracheostomy include (1) reduced laryngeal injury, (2) improved oral comfort, (3) decreased airflow resistance, (4) increased effectiveness of airway care, and (5) feasibility of oral feeding and vocalization.[4] If the patient is able to be weaned from ventilatory support, humidified oxygen can be delivered through a tracheostomy mask (Table III-A.1).

## Cuff

Approximately 0.5 in. from the end of an endotracheal or tracheal tube is a *cuff* (balloon). The cuff is inflated to (1) ensure that all of the supplemental oxygen being delivered by the ventilator via the artificial airway enters the lungs and (2) help hold the artificial airway in place. Cuff inflation pressure should be adequate to ensure that no air is leaking around the tube; however, cuff pressures should not exceed 20 mm Hg. High cuff pressures have been linked to tracheal damage and scarring, which can cause tracheal stenosis.

---

### Clinical Tip

- A cuff leak should be suspected if the patient is able to phonate or audible sounds come from his or her mouth.
- Cuff leaks can occur if the endotracheal tube is shifted (positional leak) or if the pressure changes in the cuff.
- If a cuff leak is suspected, then the respiratory therapist or nurse should be notified. (Physical therapists who specialize in critical or cardiopulmonary care may be able to add air to the cuff according to the facility's guidelines.)

---

### Positive Pressure Ventilators

Positive pressure ventilators are classified based on the method used to stop the inspiratory phase and allow expiration (cycling method) to occur.[4] There are three basic cycling methods: (1) pressure cycled, (2) volume cycled, and (3) time cycled.

*Pressure-cycled ventilators* stop inspiration at a preset pressure, *volume-cycled ventilators* stop inspiration at a preset volume, and *time-cycled ventilators* stop inspiration at a preset time interval. Although these methods allow for increased control of certain variables during inspiration, holding only one variable constant for the termination of positive pressure inhalation allows other factors to affect inspiration and potentially cause barotrauma or reduced inspiratory volumes. These factors include position changes and manual techniques.

For example, with a volume-cycled ventilator, a preset volume will be delivered regardless of the patient's position, and reductions in chest wall expansion owing to a patient's position (e.g., side lying) may increase the pressure placed on the dependent lung tissue and result in barotrauma. Conversely, in the same scenario, if a patient is on a pressure-cycled ventilator, then pressure will be delivered to the predetermined level, but because the patient's position may hinder chest expansion, a resultant lower volume of inspired air may be delivered, because the preset pressure limit was reached. Many newer ventilators provide the clinician with more than one cycling option, and certain modes of ventilation allow for more than one parameter to determine the inspiratory phase (as discussed throughout this appendix).

---

### Clinical Tip

• Being aware of the cycling method, the therapist can pay attention to changes in the pressure or tidal volume ($V_T$) associated with his or her interventions.
• Wide bore plastic tubing is used to create the mechanical ventilator's circuit. The terminal end of this circuit directly connects to an endotracheal or tracheal tube or, less commonly, to a face mask.[4] Some ventilator circuits have an extra port at their terminal end for an "in-line" suction catheter, which allows for suctioning without the removal of the ventilator circuit from the patient.[4]

---

## Modes of Ventilation

Modes of ventilation can range from providing total support (no work performed by the patient) to minimal support (near-total work performed by the patient). Modes of ventilation are geared toward allowing the patient to do as much of the work of breathing as is physiologically possible, while meeting the intended objectives of ventilatory support. Even short periods (11 days) of complete dependence on positive pressure ventilation can lead to respiratory muscle atrophy and concomitant reductions in diaphragm strength (25%) and endurance (36%).[5] Figure III-B.2 provides a schematic of the conventional modes of ventilation based on the amount of support they provide. Characteristics of conventional and alternative modes of ventilation are presented in Tables III-B.1 and III-B.2, respectively.

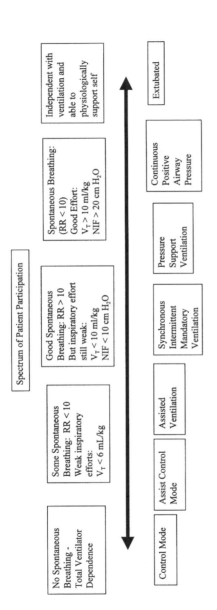

**Figure III-B.2.** *Schematic of mechanical ventilator modes: the ability of patients to participate in the process of ventilation and oxygenation in part determines the mode of ventilation. Parameters used to determine the patient's ventilatory effort include the presence of spontaneous breaths, the number of breaths per minute he or she initiates (respiratory rate [RR]), the volume of those breaths per breath (tidal volume [$V_T$]), and the negative inspiratory force (NIF) generated with those breaths. The values indicated above are examples of patient characteristics along the spectrum from complete ventilatory dependence to independence. The effectiveness of the patient's efforts needs to be assessed based not only on the above parameters, but on "outcome" variables, such as oxygenation ($Pa_{O_2}$, oxygen saturation as measured by pulse oximetry), ventilation ($Pa_{CO_2}$), and overall status (hemodynamic stability, symptoms).*

**Table III-B.1.**  Conventional Modes of Ventilation

| Modes | Characteristics |
|---|---|
| CV | Total control of the patient's ventilation: preset rate; $Fio_2$; $V_T$; flow rate; I:E ratio. |
| | Patients may be sedated or pharmacologically paralyzed. |
| | No active respiratory muscle activity is necessary. |
| AV | Patient controls respiratory pattern and rate; breath initiated by patient creates negative airway pressure in circuit; once initiated, the volume is delivered with either a preset volume or pressure and flow rate; respiratory muscles are still working. |
| | Patient can trigger RRs that are too high, leading to respiratory alkalosis or auto PEEP (see text). |
| Assist/ control ventilation | Combination of CV and AV; delivers breath of predetermined tidal volume with the patient's inspiratory effort. |
| | If the patient does not initiate a breath within a specified time period, the ventilator will deliver a breath to maintain preset RR. |
| IMV | Delivers breaths intermittently at preset time intervals with a preset RR, $V_T$, and flow rate. |
| | Patient is allowed to breathe spontaneously through a separate circuit between machine-delivered breaths. |
| | Different from AV in that attempts to breathe by the patient are not assisted by the ventilator. |
| | Patient may "fight" the ventilator if patient tries to exhale during the mechanical inspiratory phase, leading to dyssynchrony; this mode has largely been abandoned— replaced by SIMV. |
| SIMV | Similar to IMV: Mandatory breaths are delivered with a preset RR, $V_T$, and flow; however, like AV, it will assist a patient-initiated breath. |
| | Mandatory breaths are only delivered when the patient is not initiating enough breaths to allow a preset minute ventilation. |
| Pressure- supported ventilation | Patient-initiated breaths are augmented with a preset flow of gas from the ventilator to maintain constant inspiratory pressure; when the inspiratory flow drops to a preset value, the flow of gas terminates. |
| | Patient controls RR, inspiratory time, and flow; patient and ventilator determine $V_T$ and minute ventilation. |
| | The $V_T$ received from the machine is related not only to the patient's effort but also to the amount of pressure provided by the ventilator. |

Table III-B.1. *Continued*

| Modes | Characteristics |
|---|---|
| Continuous positive airway pressure | Intended to decrease work of breathing by reducing the airway pressure necessary to generate inspiration throughout the respiratory cycle while the patient is spontaneously breathing.<br>Positive pressure is constantly maintained above atmospheric pressure.<br>Most commonly used during weaning from the mechanical ventilator or in an attempt to postpone intubation (can be delivered via an endotracheal tube or a specially designed face mask, respectively).<br>Commonly used at night for the treatment of sleep apnea. |

AV = assisted ventilation; CV = controlled ventilation; $F_{IO_2}$ = fraction of inspired oxygen; I:E ratio = inspiratory time to expiratory time ratio; IMV = intermittent mandatory ventilation; PEEP = positive end-expiratory pressure; RR = respiratory rate; SIMV = synchronous IMV; $V_T$ = tidal volume.
Sources: Data from P Marino. The ICU Book (2nd ed). Philadelphia: Lea & Febiger, 1998; AS Slutsky. Mechanical ventilation. American College of Chest Physicians' Consensus Conference [see comments]. Chest 1993;104:1833; and SF Howman. Mechanical ventilation: a review and update for clinicians. Hospital Physician 1999;December: 26–36.

## Ventilatory Settings

Ventilatory settings are parameters established to provide the necessary support to meet the patient's individual ventilatory and oxygenation needs.[3,6] Establishment of the ventilatory settings is dependent on the patient's (1) arterial blood gas levels, (2) vital signs, (3) airway pressures, (4) lung volumes, and (5) pathophysiologic condition, including the patient's ability to spontaneously breathe.[3,6] Ventilator settings, subdivided into those that influence oxygenation and those that influence ventilation, are presented in Table III-B.3.

## Complications of Mechanical Ventilation

### Auto Positive End-Expiratory Pressure

Auto positive end-expiratory pressure (PEEP) occurs when lung volumes fail to return to functional residual capacity before the onset of the next inspiration. The process leading to auto PEEP is referred to

**Table III-B.2.**  Alternative Modes of Ventilation

| Mode | Characteristics |
|---|---|
| Pressure control ventilation | Delivers a preset airway pressure for a predetermined inspiratory time interval. |
| | Inspiratory time is usually prolonged, and patients are generally sedated because of discomfort due to the prolonged mechanical inspiration. |
| | $V_T$ is determined by lung compliance; useful in cases in which barotrauma is thought to exacerbate the acute lung injury (ARDS); now also available in ACV or SIMV modes. |
| High-frequency oscillation ventilation | A relatively rare technique of ventilation that is administered with frequencies of 100–3,000 breaths per minute and consequently small tidal volumes of 1–3 ml/kg. |
| | Primary advantage is dramatic reduction of airway pressure and has shown beneficial results in neonates and adults with ARDS. |
| Inverse ratio ventilation | A rarely used technique involving the use of an inspiratory to expiratory ratio of more than 1 to 1; can be delivered as a pressure-controlled or volume-cycled mode. |
| | The proposed benefit is the recruitment of a greater number of lung units during the respiratory pause and longer inspiration. |
| | Potential risk of generating auto PEEP and dynamic hyperinflation (see text). |
| Mandatory minute ventilation | Only set parameter is the minute ventilation; if spontaneous, unassisted breaths do not meet that minute ventilation, the ventilator makes up the difference by supplying mechanical breaths. |
| Noninvasive positive pressure ventilators (NIPPV) | Delivery of ACV, SIMV, and PSV modes of ventilation via a nose or face mask to reduce the need for intubation. |
| | Shown to be useful in reducing in-hospital mortality in COPD patients and long-term use in patients with neuromuscular diseases. |
| Negative pressure ventilators | Exposes the chest wall to subatmospheric pressure during inspiration to reduce intrapleural pressure, thereby allowing air to enter the lungs. |
| | Efficacy has not been demonstrated in patients with COPD and is unproven for acute respiratory failure. |

Table III-B.2. *Continued*

| Mode | Characteristics |
|---|---|
| Airway pressure release ventilation (APRV) | Lungs are kept inflated with a preset airway pressure, and exhalation occurs during cyclic reductions in pressure.<br>Advocated for protecting the lung from high peak airway pressures, although no benefit has been demonstrated over conventional methods. |
| High-frequency jet ventilation | Uses a nozzle and injector to deliver jets of gas directly into the lung at high rates.<br>Attempts to reduce mean airway pressure; however, no benefits have been identified. |
| Partial liquid ventilation | Uses perfluorocarbon liquids (does not mix with surfactant and has a high solubility for $O_2$ and $CO_2$). Lungs are filled with the liquid to approximately functional residual capacity; then, standard mechanical ventilation is attempted.<br>Has not demonstrated benefits above conventional ventilator modes. |

ACV = assist/control ventilation; ARDS = adult respiratory distress syndrome; COPD = chronic obstructive pulmonary disease; I:E ratio = inspiratory time to expiratory time ratio; PEEP = positive end-expiratory pressure; PSV = pressure supported ventilation; SIMV = synchronous intermittent mandatory ventilation; $V_T$ = tidal volume.
Sources: Data from P Marino. The ICU Book (2nd ed). Philadelphia: Lea & Febiger, 1998; AS Slutsky. Mechanical ventilation. American College of Chest Physicians' Consensus Conference [see comments]. Chest 1993;104:1833; and SF Howman. Mechanical ventilation: a review and update for clinicians. Hospital Physician 1999;December: 26–36.

as *dynamic hyperinflation*.[2,3] The primary consequence of dynamic hyperinflation is increased air trapping, which results in physiologic dead space due to pulmonary shunting (perfusion is delivered to alveolar units that are not receiving fresh ventilation), which decreases gas exchange. Ultimately, this leads to an increased work of breathing owing to higher respiratory demand, as well as altered length-tension relationships of the inspiratory muscles. Auto PEEP and concomitant air trapping can occur when the minute ventilation or respiratory rate is too high, the inspiratory-expiratory ratios are not large enough, or the endotracheal tube is too narrow or kinked, when there is excess water condensation in the tubing, or in patients with obstructive lung disease. A combination of the aforementioned factors can increase the likelihood of auto PEEP. In patients with chronic obstructive pulmo-

**Table III-B.3.** Ventilator Settings

| Purpose | Setting | Characteristic |
|---------|---------|----------------|
| Oxygen-ation | Fraction of inspired oxygen ($Fio_2$) | The percentage of inspired air that is oxygen; at normal respiratory rate (RR), tidal volume ($V_T$), and flow rates, an $Fio_2$ of 21% (ambient air) yields a normal oxygen partial pressure of 95–100 mm Hg; an increase in the percentage of oxygen delivered to the alveoli results in a greater $Pao_2$ and therefore a greater driving force for the diffusion of oxygen into the blood. $Fio_2$ of 60% has been set as the threshold value to avoid toxicity with prolonged use. |
| | Positive end-expiratory pressure (PEEP) | The pressure maintained by the mechanical ventilator in the airways at the end of expiration; normal physiologic PEEP (maintained by sufficient surfactant levels) is considered to be 5 cm $H_2O$. Settings are adjusted as needed to maintain functional residual capacity above closing capacity to avoid closure of alveoli. Closure of alveoli can result in shunting of blood past the alveoli without gas exchange, which results in decreased oxygenation. |
| Ventilation | RR | Set according to the amount of spontaneous ventilatory efforts by the patient; different ventilatory modes, described in Table III-B.1, are prescribed according to the patient's needs; patients who are unable to generate any spontaneous breaths are fully ventilated at respiratory rates of 12–20 breaths per minute. This rate is decreased accordingly for those who are able to generate spontaneous breaths. |
| | $V_T$ | The amount of volume delivered with each breath is adjusted with respiratory rate to control partial pressure of arterial carbon dioxide ($Paco_2$). Excessive volume leads to increased airway pressures, and therefore pressures are routinely monitored to prevent barotrauma. At times, hypercapnia is allowed to prevent high lung pressures due to the delivered volume and noncompliance of lung tissue, termed *permissive hypercapnia*. |

**Table III-B.3.** *Continued*

| Purpose | Setting | Characteristic |
|---|---|---|
| | Inspiratory flow rate | Set to match the patient's peak inspiratory demands; if this match is not correct, it can cause the patient discomfort while breathing with the ventilator. |
| | | High flow rates deliver greater volume in less time and therefore allow longer expiratory times (prevents hyperinflation); however, this also leads to greater peak airway pressure and the possibility of barotrauma. |
| | | If the rate is too slow, the patient may attempt to continue to inhale against a closed circuit, resulting in respiratory muscle fatigue. |
| | Inspiratory to expiratory ratio | The inspiratory to expiratory ratio is set with the goal of allowing the ventilator to be as synchronous as possible with the patient's respiratory ratio. |
| | | For patients who are not spontaneously breathing, this ratio is set according to what is required to maintain adequate ventilation and oxygenation. |
| | Sensitivity | Pressure change is required in the airway to trigger an ACV or PSV breath; typically −1 to −3 cm $H_2O$. |
| | | If mechanical sensors respond poorly, then respiratory muscle fatigue can occur. |
| | | If the sensors are too sensitive, then hyperventilation can develop. |

ACV = assist/control ventilation; $Pao_2$ = oxygen saturation as measured by pulse oximetry; PSV = pressure-supported ventilation.

Sources: Data from P Marino. The ICU Book (2nd ed). Philadelphia: Lea & Febiger, 1998; AS Slutsky. Mechanical ventilation. American College of Chest Physicians' Consensus Conference [see comments]. Chest 1993;104:1833; and SF Howman. Mechanical ventilation: a review and update for clinicians. Hospital Physician 1999;December:26–36.

nary disease who are on ventilator modes that allow them to initiate ventilator-assisted breaths (assisted ventilation, assist/control ventilation, synchronous intermittent mandatory ventilation [SIMV], pressure-supported ventilation [PSV]), the therapist should realize that activity could increase the patient-generated respiratory rate. Some modes will then, given the initiation of a breath, provide a set volume of air (assisted ventilation, assist/control ventilation, SIMV) that could increase the likelihood of hyperinflation owing to auto PEEP. This can also happen in modes that do not deliver a set volume of air (PSV), because inspiration is assisted with positive pressure.

### Barotrauma

*Barotrauma* refers to damage to the lungs caused by excessive airway pressure. Many of the alternative modes of ventilation are geared toward reducing this complication (see Table III-B.2). In the normal lung, spontaneous inhalation without ventilatory support takes place because of negative pressure. The volume of inhaled air is limited by the return of intrapulmonary pressure back to atmospheric pressure in the lungs during inhalation. Because mechanical ventilation is predominantly delivered with positive inspiratory pressure, these normal physiologic mechanisms for preventing such trauma are bypassed, and pressures in the lung exceed normal pressures. Another consideration is that many of the lung conditions requiring mechanical ventilation do not uniformly affect the lungs (adult respiratory distress syndrome, pneumonia). Inhalation volumes are delivered to those areas that are still normal, which can overdistend (causing high pressure) as a result. This can produce stress fractures in the walls of the alveoli, thus exacerbating the acute lung condition.[7,8] Infants who are mechanically ventilated are five times more likely to develop bronchopulmonary dysplasia than are infants who are not mechanically ventilated.[9] It is thought that barotrauma exacerbates the acute lung injury associated with adult respiratory distress syndrome.[1] Other complications associated with barotrauma include pneumothorax and subcutaneous emphysema.[3]

The following are other possible complications of mechanical ventilation[2,3,6]:

- Improper intubation can result in esophageal or tracheal tears. If the artificial airway is mistakenly placed in the esophagus and is not detected, gastric distention can occur with the initiation of positive pressure.

• Oxygen toxicity: Oxygen levels that are too high and maintained for a prolonged time can result in (1) substernal chest pain that is exacerbated by deep breathing, (2) dry cough, (3) tracheal irritation, (4) pleuritic pain with inspiration, (5) dyspnea, (6) nasal stiffness and congestion, (7) sore throat, and (8) eye and ear discomfort.

• Cardiovascular: High positive pressures can result in decreased cardiac output from compression of great vessels by over-inflated lungs.

## Weaning from Mechanical Ventilation

The process of decreasing or discontinuing mechanical ventilation in a patient is referred to as the *weaning process*.[6] A contributing factor to a successful wean from ventilatory support is the resolution or stability of the condition that led to the need for ventilatory support. The patient criteria for an attempt at weaning from mechanical ventilation include

• Spontaneous breathing

• Fraction of inspired oxygen <50% and PEEP <5 cm $H_2O$ with oxygen saturation as measured by pulse oximetry >90%

• Negative inspiratory force >20 cm $H_2O$

• Respiratory rate <35

• Respiratory rate/$V_T$ ratio of <105 (a respiratory rate/$V_T$ >105 indicates shallow and rapid breathing and is a powerful predictor of an unsuccessful wean)[10]

Examples of weaning methods include

• IMV or SIMV: Decreasing the number of breaths per minute that the ventilator provides requires the patient to increase his or her spontaneous breaths. This is commonly used after surgery, while patients are waking up from anesthesia. These patients typically have not been on support for an extended period of time and do not usually have a lung condition that required them to be intubated in the first place. As soon as respiratory drive and spontaneous breathing return, it is expected that the patient can be removed from ventilatory support.

• T-piece: Breathing off of the ventilator, while still intubated, for increasing periods of time. This technique is sort of an all-or-none method. Patients need to have the respiratory drive to breathe spontaneously and the capability to generate adequate $V_T$ to attempt this weaning process. The process aims to improve respiratory muscle strength and endurance with prolonged time periods of independent ventilation.

• PSV: The patient spends periods of time with decreased pressure support to increase his or her spontaneous ventilation. Two factors can be manipulated with PSV: (1) to increase the strength load on the respiratory muscles, PSV can be reduced, and (2) to increase the endurance requirement on the respiratory muscles, the length of time that PSV is reduced can be increased.

Recently, it was demonstrated that the T-piece and PSV methods of weaning were superior to the IMV or SIMV methods.[11]

Five major factors to consider during a patient's wean follow[6]:

1. Respiratory demand (the need for oxygen for metabolic processes and the need to remove carbon dioxide produced during metabolic processes) and the ability of the neuromuscular system to cope with the demand

2. Oxygenation

3. Cardiovascular performance

4. Psychological factors

5. Adequate rest and nutrition

The following are signs of increased distress during a ventilator wean[3,6]:

• Increased tachypnea (more than 30 breaths per minute)

• Drop in pH to less than 7.25–7.30 associated with an increasing $Pa_{CO_2}$

• Paradoxical breathing pattern (refers to a discoordination in movements of the abdomen and thorax during inhalation) (Refer to Chapter 2.)

• Oxygen saturation as measured by pulse oximetry less than 90%

- Change in heart rate of more than 20 beats per minute
- Change in blood pressure more than 20 mm Hg
- Agitation, panic, diaphoresis, cyanosis, angina, arrhythmias

## Physical Therapy Considerations

A patient who is mechanically ventilated may require ventilatory support for a prolonged period of time. Patients who require prolonged ventilatory support are at risk for developing pulmonary complications, skin breakdown, joint contractures, and deconditioning from bed rest. Physical therapy intervention, including bronchopulmonary hygiene and functional mobility training, can help prevent or reverse these complications despite mechanical ventilation.

### Bronchopulmonary Hygiene

Patients on ventilatory support are frequently suctioned as part of their routine care. Physical therapists working with patients on their bronchopulmonary hygiene and airway clearance should use suctioning as the last attempt to remove secretions. Encouraging the process of huffing and coughing during treatment will improve or maintain cough effectiveness (huffing is performed without glottis closure, which cannot be achieved when intubated), owing to activation of the expiratory muscles. If patients have difficulty with a deep inspiration for an effective huff or cough, then the use of manual techniques, postural changes, or assistive devices, such as an adult manual breathing unit (AMBU bag), can be used to facilitate depth of inspiration.

### Weaning from Ventilatory Support

During the weaning process, the physical therapist can play a vital role on an interdisciplinary team responsible for coordinating the wean. Physical therapists offer a combined understanding of the respiratory difficulties faced by the patient, the biomechanics of ventilation, the principles of exercise (weaning is a form of exercise), and the general energy requirements of functional activities. Physical therapists can work with the multidisciplinary team to optimize the conditions under which the patient attempts each wean (time of day, activities before and after the wean, position during the wean) and parameters to be manipulated during the wean (frequency, intensity, duration). Patients should be placed in a position that facilitates the biomechanics of their ventilation.[12] For many patients, this is seated and may also include the ability to sit forward with the arms supported.

Biofeedback to increase $V_T$ and relaxation has been shown to improve the effectiveness of weaning and reduce time on the ventilator.[13] Inspiratory muscle resistive training has also been shown to increase respiratory muscle strength and endurance to facilitate the weaning success.[14]

## References

1. Marino P. The ICU Book (2nd ed). Philadelphia: Lea & Febiger, 1998.
2. Slutsky AS. Mechanical ventilation. American College of Chest Physicians' Consensus Conference [see comments]. Chest 1993;104:1833.
3. Howman SF. Mechanical ventilation: a review and update for clinicians. Hospital Physician 1999;December:26–36.
4. Sadowsky HS. Thoracic Surgical Procedures, Monitoring, and Support Equipment. In EA Hillegass, HS Sadowsky (eds), Essentials of Cardiopulmonary Physical Therapy (2nd ed). Philadelphia: Saunders, 2001; 464–469.
5. Anzueto A, Peters JI, Tobin MJ, et al. Effects of prolonged mechanical ventilation on diaphragmatic function in healthy adult baboons. Crit Care Med 1997;25:1187–1190.
6. Gerold KB. Physical therapists' guide to the principles of mechanical ventilation. Cardiopul Phys Ther 1992;3:8.
7. Costello ML, Mathieu-Costello O, West JB. Stress fracture of alveolar epithelial cells studied by scanning electron microscopy. Am Rev Respir Dis 1992;145:1446–1455.
8. Mathieu-Costello O, West JB. Are pulmonary capillaries susceptible to mechanical stress? Chest 1994;105(Suppl):102S–107S.
9. Heimler R, Huffman RG, Starshak RJ. Chronic lung disease in premature infants: A retrospective evaluation of underlying factors. Crit Care Med 1988;16:1213–1217.
10. Yang KL, Tobin MJ. A prospective study of indexes predicting the outcome of trials of weaning from mechanical ventilation. N Engl J Med 1991;324:1446–1495.
11. Dries DJ. Weaning from mechanical ventilation. J Trauma 1997; 43:372–384.
12. Shekleton ME. Respiratory muscle condition and the work of breathing-a critical balance in the weaning patient. AACN Clin Issues Crit Care 1991;2:405–414.

13. Holliday JE, Hyers TM. The reduction of wean time from mechanical ventilation using tidal volume and relaxation biofeedback. Am Rev Respir Dis 1990;141:1214–1220.
14. Aldrich TK, Karpel JP, Uhrlass RM, et al. Weaning from mechanical ventilation: adjunctive use of inspiratory muscle resistive training. Crit Care Med 1989;17:143–147.

# III-C

# Circulatory Assist Devices
*Jaime C. Paz*

The purpose of this appendix is to describe the following circulatory assist devices: (1) intra-aortic balloon pump (IABP), (2) ventricular assist device (VAD), and (3) extracorporal membrane oxygenation (ECMO). These devices are primarily used with a patient who has severe cardiac pump dysfunction, with or without concurrent pulmonary pump dysfunction.

## Intra-Aortic Balloon Pump

The main function of the IABP is to lessen the work (decreased myocardial oxygen demand) of the heart by decreasing afterload in the proximal aorta. The IABP also improves coronary artery perfusion (increased myocardial oxygen supply) by increasing diastolic pressure in the aorta.[1,2]

The IABP consists of a catheter with a sausage-shaped balloon at the end of it, all of which is connected to an external pump-controlling device. The catheter is inserted percutaneously or surgically into the femoral artery and is threaded antegrade until it reaches the proximal descending thoracic aorta. Figure III-C.1 illustrates the balloon

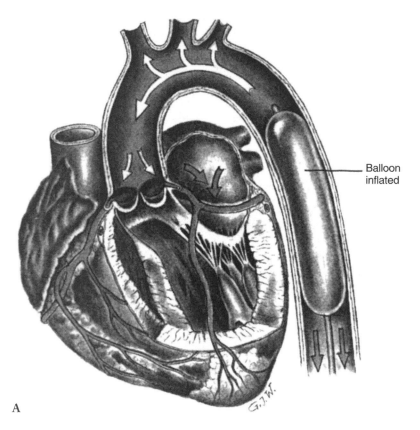

A

**Figure III-C.1.** *Mechanisms of action of intra-aortic balloon pump.* **A.** *Diastolic balloon inflation augments coronary blood flow.* **B.** *Systolic balloon deflation decreases afterload.* *(Reprinted with permission from LA Thelan [ed]. Critical Care Nursing: Diagnosis and Management [2nd ed]. St. Louis: Mosby, 1994.)*

inflating during ventricular filling (diastole) and deflating during ventricular contraction (systole). The deflation of the balloon just before aortic valve opening decreases afterload and therefore reduces resistance to the ejection of blood during systole. The blood in the aorta is then propelled forward into the systemic circulation. The inflation of the balloon during diastole assists with the perfusion of the coronary and cerebral vessels. This process is referred to as *counterpulsation*, because the inflation and deflation of the balloon occur opposite to the contraction and relaxation of the heart.[1,2]

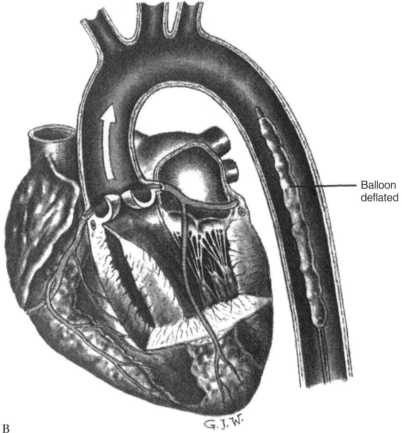

Balloon deflated

B

Indications for IABP include the following:

- Acute left ventricular failure
- Unstable angina
- Status post acute myocardial infarction
- Cardiogenic shock
- Papillary muscle dysfunction with resultant mitral valve regurgitation
- Ventricular septal defect

- Refractory ventricular dysrhythmias

- Anticipated heart transplantation

The ratio of heart beats to counterpulsations of the IABP indicates the amount of circulatory support an individual requires (e.g., 1 to 1 is one counterpulsation to one heart beat; 1 to 4 is one counterpulsation to every fourth heart beat; a ratio of 1 to 1 provides maximum circulatory support). Weaning from IABP involves gradually decreasing the number of counterpulsations to heart beats, with the goal being one counterpulsation for every fourth heart beat, as tolerated, before discontinuing the IABP. Although weaning from the IABP is generally performed by decreasing the number of counterpulsations, weaning can also be performed by gradually decreasing the amount of inflation pressure of the balloon in the aorta.[1,2]

The following are complications of IABP:

- Ischemia of the involved limb secondary to occlusion of femoral artery from compression or from thrombus formation

- Slippage of the balloon, resulting in occlusion of subclavian or renal arteries

---

### Clinical Tip

- During IABP, the lower extremity in which femoral access is obtained cannot be flexed at the hip, and the patient's head cannot be raised higher than 40 degrees in bed.
- Depending on the amount of time spent on the pump, the patient may require active-assistive range of motion exercises for hip flexion after the IABP is removed.

---

## Ventricular Assist Device

A VAD is a mechanical pump that provides prolonged circulatory assistance in patients who have ventricular failure from myocardial infarction or are awaiting transplantation because of severe cardiomyopathy. The mechanical pump can be internal or external to the patient. An internal VAD consists of a pump that is surgically placed extraperitoneally within the patient's abdominal cavity with access lines leading to an external control device. An external VAD consists of a pump that is completely external to the patient, but with access lines shunting blood from the heart to the great vessels.[2,3]

Figures III-C.2 and III-C.3 illustrate an example of an internal VAD and an external VAD, respectively. Generally, the left ventricle is most commonly assisted (left VAD [LVAD]), but occasionally, the

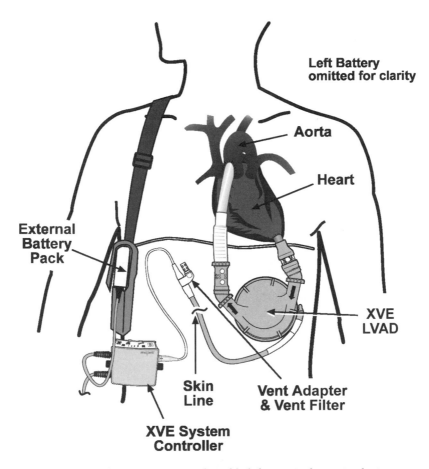

Figure III-C.2. *The HeartMate implantable left ventricular assist device (LVAD). (XVE = extended lead vented electric.) (Reprinted with permission from Thoratec Corporation, Woburn, MA.)*

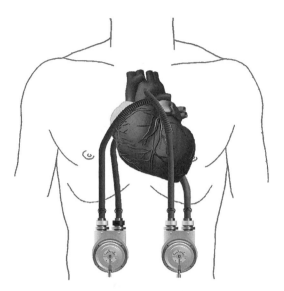

**Figure III-C.3.** *The Thoratec paracorporeal ventricular assist device. (Reprinted with permission from Thoratec Corporation, Woburn, MA.)*

right ventricle also needs assistance (right VAD). In more severe situations, both ventricles need to be assisted (biventricular assist device). The various types and general characteristics of internal and external VADs are described briefly in Table III-C.1. It is beyond the scope of this appendix to describe in detail all the aspects of each type of VAD; however, physical therapists working with patients on a VAD need to be familiar with the type of machine that the patient is on, as well as the safety features of the VAD.

Weaning from VAD involves a gradual decrease in flow rates, which allows the patient's ventricle to contribute more to total systemic circulation. Complications of VAD include thrombosis, bleeding, and infection at or near the insertion sites of the access lines.

The combination of technological advancements and a lack of donor organs has increased the use of VADs in patients with cardiomyopathy. Therefore, physical therapists are more likely to encounter this equipment in the hospital. Research has demonstrated that patients with a VAD can be mobilized safely in the hospital and that their exercise tolerance can be improved while awaiting transplantation.[4–6]

Table III-C.1.  Ventricular Assist Devices (VADs)

| Pump Name | Pump Mechanism | Use |
|---|---|---|
| Internal VADs | | |
| HeartMate | Pneumatic or electric | Left ventricle |
| Novacor | Electric | Left ventricle |
| Symbion/CardioWest totally artificial heart | Pneumatic | Both ventricles |
| External VADs | | |
| Bio-Medicus | Centrifugal | Right or left ventricle, or both |
| Thoratec | Pneumatic | Right or left ventricle, or both |
| Hemopump | Axial flow | Left ventricle |
| Abiomed BVAD 5000 | Pneumatic | Right or left ventricle, or both |

Sources: Data from EF Bond, J Dax. Nursing Management Critical Care. In SM Lewis, MM Heitkemper, SR Dirksen (eds), Medical Surgical Nursing: Assessment and Management of Clinical Problems (5th ed). St. Louis: Mosby, 2000;1926–1927; and NG Smedira, RL Vargo, PM McCarthy. Mechanical Support Devices for End-Stage Heart Failure. In DL Brown (ed), Cardiac Intensive Care. Philadelphia: Saunders, 1998;697–703.

The following are general considerations for the physical therapist working with a patient on a VAD:

• The patient's native heart is still contracting (albeit ineffectively) and, therefore, the patient's electrocardiogram will reflect the native heart's electrical activity. However, because the VAD is performing a majority of the patient's cardiac output, the patient's peripheral pulse is indicative of the rate set on the VAD.[4]

• The rate on a VAD can be fixed or automatic. VADs that have automatic rates are able to adjust their rate according to the patient's needs (i.e., increase with exercise).[3,4]

• Patients typically complain of pain at the insertion site of access lines in the abdomen and may need appropriate premedication with analgesics before therapy.[5]

• Certain VADs have a manual mechanical pump feature in case the VAD malfunctions. Therapists working with these patients need to be trained on how to use this critically important safety feature.[4]

• A patient who demonstrates the following hemodynamic variables should have physical therapy deferred until he or she is more stable[4]:

a. LVAD rate <50 beats per minute

b. LVAD volumes <30 ml

c. LVAD flows <3.0 liters per minute

d. Systolic blood pressure <80 mm Hg

e. Heart rate (native) >150 beats per minute

f. Sustained ventricular tachycardia or ventricular fibrillation

## Extracorporal Membrane Oxygenation

ECMO involves the use of a device external to the body for direct oxygenation of blood, assistance with the removal of carbon dioxide, or both. The primary indication for ECMO is cardiac or respiratory failure that is not responding to maximal medical therapy. The pediatric population with respiratory failure seems to benefit from this therapy the most; however, the successful use of ECMO in the adult population is improving.[7–9]

Patient situations that are likely to require ECMO include the following:

• Postcardiotomy cardiac or pulmonary support

• Cardiac arrest

• Cardiogenic shock

• Primary respiratory failure

• The period after lung or heart transplantation or LVAD placement

The ECMO system consists of a venous drainage cannula, a reservoir for blood, a pumping device that uses a centrifugal or a roller system, an oxygenator, and an arterial or a second venous return cannula.[7] The pumping device is used to help a failing ventricle circulate blood, whereas the oxygenator device assists the failing respiratory system to fully oxygenate the patient. Patients who have respiratory failure require concurrent mechanical ventilation to prevent atelectasis while on ECMO. However, less positive pressure is required to oxygenate blood when on ECMO, resulting in a decreased incidence of barotrauma.[2,7]

The system that uses the venous drainage to arterial return cannula (V-A mode) is primarily performed on patients who require cardiac or cardiorespiratory support. The V-A mode can be achieved in three ways[7]:

1. Femoral vein to the ECMO system back to the femoral artery

2. Right atrium to the ECMO system back to the ascending aorta

3. Femoral vein to the ECMO system back to the ascending aorta

The system that uses the venous drainage to venous return cannula (V-V mode) is primarily used for patients who only have respiratory failure. The V-V mode can be achieved in two ways[7]:

1. Internal jugular vein to the ECMO system back to the common femoral vein

2. Common femoral vein drainage to the ECMO system back to the contralateral common femoral vein

Patients who are on V-A mode ECMO are typically anticoagulated with heparin and may require the use of IABP to further assist the ventricle. Patients on the V-V mode may require sedation and or medical paralysis to help improve oxygenation to organs and tissues by minimizing the metabolic demands of an awake person.[7]

Complications of ECMO include lower limb ischemia, thrombocytopenia, thromboembolism, and failure of the oxygenator device.[9]

## General Physical Therapy Considerations

• Patients requiring the use of circulatory assist devices are typically on bed rest, and physical therapy usually consists of bronchopulmonary hygiene and airway clearance, along with the prevention of secondary complications of bed rest, such as joint contracture and skin breakdown.

• Special care should be taken to avoid disruption of the tubes associated with these devices.

• Range-of-motion exercises should not be performed on extremities with ECMO catheters unless otherwise cleared by the physician.

• Patients with an internal or external VAD who are allowed out of bed should progress their activity very gradually with careful monitoring of vital signs and Borg's rating of perceived exertion.

## References

1. Mahaffey KW, Kruse KR, Ohman EM. Intra-aortic Balloon Pump Counterpulsation: Physiology, Patient Management, and Clinical Efficacy. In DL Brown (ed), Cardiac Intensive Care. Philadelphia: Saunders, 1998;647–653.
2. Bond EF, Dax J. Nursing Management; Critical Care. In SM Lewis, MM Heitkemper, SR Dirksen (eds), In Medical Surgical Nursing: Assessment and Management of Clinical Problems (5th ed). St. Louis: Mosby, 2000;1926–1927.
3. Smedira NG, Vargo RL, McCarthy PM. Mechanical Support Devices for End-Stage Heart Failure. In DL Brown (ed), Cardiac Intensive Care. Philadelphia: Saunders, 1998;697–703.
4. Humphrey R, Buck L, Cahalin L, Morrone T. Physical therapy assessment and intervention for patients with left ventricular assist devices. Cardiopulmonary Phys Ther 1998;9(2):3–7.
5. Buck LA. Physical therapy management of three patients following left ventricular assist device implantation: a case report. Cardiopulmonary Phys Ther 1998;9(2):8–14.
6. Morrone TM, Buck LA, Catanese KA, et al. Early progressive mobilization of patients with left ventricular assist devices is safe and optimizes recovery before heart transplantation. J Heart Lung Transplant 1996;15:423–429.
7. Kaplon RJ, Smedira NG. Extracorporeal Membrane Oxygenation in Adults. In DJ Goldstein, MC Oz (eds), Cardiac Assist Devices. Armonk, NY: Futura Publishing, 2000;263–273.
8. Mulroy J. Acute Respiratory Distress Syndrome. In L Bucher, S Melander (eds), Critical Care Nursing. Philadelphia: Saunders, 1999; 457–458.
9. Copeland JG, Smith RG (eds). Bridge to Transplantation with Mechanical Assist Devices. New York: McGraw-Hill, 2000.

# IV

# Pharmacologic Agents
*Jaime C. Paz and Michele P. West*

## Pharmacologic Agents

The purpose of this appendix is to provide an overview of the pharmaco-logic agents that are commonly prescribed as an adjunct to the medical-surgical management of a wide variety of diseases and disorders. The medications in this appendix are organized according to drug class in the following index. A description of the indication(s), mechanism of action, and common side effects is included for each type of medication.

Note that some pharmacologic agents are listed in another chapter or appendix, as referenced below.

## Pharmacologic Agents Index

| Drug Class | Location | Page Number |
|---|---|---|
| Genitourinary medications | See genitourinary disorders in Chapter 9 | 557 |
| Human immunodeficiency virus infection medications | See Human Immunodeficiency Virus Infection in Chapter 10 and Table 10-5 | 614, 635 |
| Immunosuppressive drugs used in organ transplantation | Table 12-1 | 704 |
| Intranasal steroids | Table IV-21 | 864 |
| Lipid lowering agents | Table IV-22 | 865 |
| Mucolytics | Table IV-23 | 865 |
| Nitrates | Table IV-24 | 866 |
| Nutritional agents for anemia | Table IV-25 | 866 |
| Osmotic diuretics | Table IV-26 | 867 |
| Pain medications | See Appendix VI | 879–884 |
| Positive inotropes | Table IV-27.A–B | 867 |
| Cardiac glycosides | Table IV-27.A | 867 |
| Sympathomimetics | Table IV-27.B | 867 |
| Skeletal muscle relaxants | Table IV-28 | 868 |
| Thrombolytic agents (fibrinolytics) | Table IV-29 | 868 |
| Topical agents commonly used for the treatment of burns | See Table 7-8 | 460 |
| Vasodilators | Table IV-30 | 869 |

**Table IV-1.** Adrenocortical Steroids (Glucocorticoids)*

Indications: To decrease cerebral edema or inflammation in neoplastic or inflammatory diseases, or both

Mechanism of action: Prevent the accumulation of inflammatory cells at the infection site, inhibit lysosomal enzyme release and chemical mediators of inflammatory response, reduce capillary dilatation and permeability

General side effects: Headache, vertigo, diaphoresis, nausea, vomiting, congestive heart failure in susceptible patients, euphoria, insomnia, seizure, muscle weakness, cushingoid features, osteoporosis, dermatitis, decreased wound healing, thromboembolism, aggravation of hypertension

Generic name (trade name): Dexamethasone (Decadron, Dexone, Hexadrol), dexamethasone sodium phosphate (Cortastat, Dalalone, Decadron Phosphate, Decaject, Dexone, Hexadrol Phosphate, Solurex), methylprednisolone (Medrol), prednisone (Deltasone, Meticorten, Orasone, Panasol-S, Prednicen-M, Sterapred), prednisolone (Delta-Cortef, Prelone), prednisolone acetate (Key-Pred, Predcor, Predalone), prednisolone sodium phosphate (Hydeltrasol, Key-Pred-SP, Pediapred)

*For neuroscience patients.
Sources: Data from Drug Facts and Comparisons 2000 (54th ed). St. Louis: Wolters Kluwer, 2000; and Drug Facts and Comparisons 2001 (55th ed). St. Louis: Wolters Kluwer, 2001.

**Table IV-2.** Angiotensin-Converting Enzyme Inhibitors

Indication: Heart failure

Mechanism of action: Inhibit conversion of angiotensin I to angiotensin II and therefore act to decrease excess water and sodium retention while also preventing vasoconstriction

General side effects: Edema, cough, hypotension, skin rash, renal failure, taste disturbances

Generic (trade name): Captopril (Capoten), enalapril (Vasotec), lisinopril (Prinivil, Zestril)

Source: Data from K Grimes, M Cohen. Cardiac Medications. In EA Hillegass, HS Sadowsky (eds), Essentials of Cardiopulmonary Physical Therapy (2nd ed). Philadelphia: Saunders, 2001;537–585.

**Table IV-3.** Antiarrhythmic Drugs

---

Indications: Arrhythmia, ischemia, hypertension
Mechanism of action
  *Class I:* Sodium channel blockers—slow the fast sodium channels, thereby
    controlling rate of depolarization
    *General side effects:* Gastrointestinal or urinary retention, or both,
    central nervous system abnormality
  *Class II:* Beta blockers—block sympathetic stimulation of cardiac muscle
    *General side effects:* Smooth muscle spasm, exaggeration of therapeutic
    actions (bradycardia), fatigue, insomnia, masking hypoglycemic
    symptoms in diabetics, impaired glucose tolerance, decreased high-
    density lipoprotein cholesterol
  *Class III:* Refractory period alterations—prolong refractory period of
    cardiac tissue
    *General side effects:* May transiently increase pacemaker (sinoatrial
    node) activity
  *Class IV (calcium channel blockers):* Block slow calcium channels
    *General side effects:* Negative inotrope at high doses
Sodium channel blockers (generic name [trade name]): Disopyramide
  (Norpace, Rythmodan), encainide (Enkaid), flecainide (Tambocor),
  lidocaine (Xylocaine), mexiletine (Mexitil), moricizine (Ethmozine),
  phenytoin (Dilantin), procainamide (Pronestyl), propafenone (Rhythmol),
  quinidine (Biquin, Cardioquin), tocainide (Tonocard)
Beta blockers: Refer to Table IV-12
Refractory period alterations: Amiodarone (Cordarone), bretylium tosylate
  (Bretylol), ibutilide fumarate (Corvert)
Calcium channel blockers: Refer to Table IV-14

---

Source: Data from K Grimes, M Cohen. Cardiac Medications. In EA Hillegass, HS
Sadowsky (eds), Essentials in Cardiopulmonary Physical Therapy (2nd ed). Philadelphia: Saunders, 2001;562.

Table IV-4. Anticoagulants

| | |
|---|---|
| Low-molecular-weight heparin, enoxaparin sodium (Lovenox), dalteparin sodium (Fragmin), ardeparin sodium (Normiflo) | Indications: Prophylaxis or treatment of thromboembolic complications after surgery; for ischemic complications of unstable angina, NQWMI, or cardiovascular accident; prophylaxis of DVT after total knee replacement.* <br><br> Mechanism of action: Enhances inhibition of factor Xa and thrombin by binding to and accelerating antithrombin III activity. <br><br> General side effects: Bleeding from gastrointestinal, genitourinary, respiratory, or other tracts; thrombocytopenia. |
| Danaparoid sodium (Orgaran) | Indication: Prophylaxis of DVT after total hip replacement. <br><br> Mechanism of action: See Low-molecular-weight heparin. <br><br> General side effects: Bleeding from gastrointestinal, genitourinary, respiratory, or other tracts; thrombocytopenia; fever; nausea. |
| Heparin sodium | Indications: Prophylaxis or treatment of venous thrombosis, PE, peripheral arterial embolism, atrial fibrillation, acute myocardial infarction, disseminated intravascular coagulopathy. <br><br> Mechanism of action: Prolongs clotting time by inhibiting the conversion of prothrombin to thrombin. <br><br> General side effects: Bleeding from gastrointestinal, genitourinary, respiratory, or other tracts; hemorrhage; thrombocytopenia. |
| Lepirudin (Refludan) | Indication: Thrombus prophylaxis in heparin-induced thrombocytopenia. <br><br> Mechanism of action: Directly inhibits thrombin. <br><br> General side effects: Bleeding from gastrointestinal, genitourinary, respiratory, or other tracts; anemia; hematoma. |

| Warfarin sodium (Couma-din), anisindione (Mira-don) | Indications: Long-term prophylaxis and treatment of venous thrombosis, PE, atrial fibrillation, or with prosthetic heart valve. Mechanism of action: Interferes with synthesis of vitamin K–dependent clotting factors that decrease prothrombin. General side effects: Bleeding from gastrointestinal, genitourinary, respiratory, or other tracts; dyspnea; headache; chest or abdominal pain; systemic cholesterol microembolism (purple toe syndrome). Additional side effects of anisindione are hemorrhage and dermatitis. |
|---|---|

DVT = deep vein thrombosis; NQWMI = non-Q wave myocardial infarction; PE = pulmonary embolism.
*Ardeparin sodium only.
Sources: Data from Drug Facts and Comparisons 2000 (54th ed). St. Louis: Wolters Kluwer, 2000; and Anticoagulant, Antiplatelet, and Thrombolytic Drugs. In RA Lehne (ed), Pharmacology for Nursing Care (4th ed). Philadelphia: Saunders, 2001.

Table IV-5. Anticonvulsant Agents*

Indication: To decrease seizure activity.
Mechanism of action: Exact mechanism is unclear; however, electrical impulses from the cerebral motor cortex are decreased in frequency and voltage.
General side effects: Headache, nausea, vomiting, dizziness, vertigo, confusion, agitation, fatigue, visual hallucinations, diplopia, tremor, hyperreflexia, hypo- or hypertension, arrhythmia, congestive heart failure, edema, urinary frequency or retention.
Generic name (trade name): Carbamazepine (Atretol, Carbatrol, Epitol, Tegretol), clonazepam (Klonopin), clorazepate dipotassium (Gen-Xene, Clorazepate), diazepam (Diastat, Valium), ethosuximide (Zarontin), ethotoin (Peganone), felbamate (Felbatol), gabapentin (Neurontin), lamotrigine (Lamictal), magnesium sulfate, methsuximide (Celontin), Phensuximide (Milontin), phenytoin, primidone (Mysoline), tiagabine hydrochloride (Gabitril Filmtabs), topiramate (Topamax), valproic acid (Depacon, Depakene, Depakote).

*Consists of multiple drug categories, including barbiturates, hydantoins, succinimides, and benzodiazepines.
Sources: Data from Drug Facts and Comparisons 2000 (54th ed). St. Louis: Wolters Kluwer, 2000; and Drug Facts and Comparisons 2001 (55th ed). St. Louis: Wolters Kluwer, 2001.

**Table IV-6.**  Antiemetic Agents

Indications: Control symptoms of nausea and vomiting associated with chemotherapy, radiation treatment, or both.

Mechanism of action: Depressive effects on central nervous system that can result in decreased nausea and vomiting, particularly if these symptoms are associated with anxiety during chemotherapy.

| Family Name | Generic Name (Trade Name) | Side Effects |
|---|---|---|
| Phenothiazines | Chlorpromazine (Thorazine) | Extrapyramidal reactions, sedation, tardive dyskinesia, pseudoparkinsonism, orthostatic hypotension, arrhythmias, blurred vision, electrocardiographic changes |
| | Prochlorperazine (Compazine) | Extrapyramidal reactions, sedation, blurred vision, pseudoparkinsonism |
| | Promethazine (Phenergan) | Sedation, drowsiness, confusion, hypotension, nausea, dry mouth, agranulocytosis |
| Butyrophenones | Haloperidol (Haldol) | Severe extrapyramidal reaction, tardive dyskinesia, blurred vision, neuroleptic malignant syndrome |
| | Droperidol (Inapsine) | Drowsiness, hypotension, extrapyramidal reaction, orthostatic hypotension |
| Cannabinoids | Tetrahydrocannabinol (marijuana) | Impaired psychomotor performance, altered sensory perception, tachycardia, paresthesia, tinnitus |
| Antihistamines | Diphenhydramine (Benadryl) | Drowsiness, nausea, dry mouth, vertigo, palpitations, confusion, headache |
| Corticosteroids | Dexamethasone (Decadron, Hexadrol, Dexone) | Insomnia, hypertension, edema, muscle weakness, hyperglycemia |
| Benzodiazepines | Lorazepam (Ativan) | Drowsiness, lethargy, restlessness, transient hypotension, visual disturbances |

| Family Name | Generic Name (Trade Name) | Side Effects |
|---|---|---|
| | Metoclopra-mide (Reglan) | Restlessness, anxiety, drowsiness, dizziness, extrapyramidal symptoms, tardive dyskinesia, dystonic reactions, transient hypertension |
| Other | Trimethobenza-mide (Tigan) | Drowsiness, hypotension, diarrhea, hepatotoxicity |

Sources: Data from C Ciccone (ed). Cancer Chemotherapy. Philadelphia: FA Davis, 1996; D Moreau (ed). Nursing '96 Drug Handbook. Springhouse, PA: Springhouse, 1996; and LM Tierney, SJ McPhee, MA Papadakis (eds). Current Medical Diagnosis and Treatment. New York: McGraw-Hill, 2000.

**Table IV-7.** Antihistamines

Indications: To decrease inflammation and bronchoconstriction associated with hypersensitivity reactions, such as allergic rhinitis

Mechanism of action: Reduce or prevent the physiologic effects of histamine by competing for histamine binding sites

General side effects: Drowsiness, dizziness, decreased coordination, orthostatic hypotension, hypotension, hypertension, palpitations, bradycardia, tachycardia, epigastric distress, urinary frequency, thickening of bronchial secretions, dry mouth

Generic name (trade name): Astemizole (Claritin), azatadine maleate (Optimine), azelastine hydrochloride (Astelin), chlorpheniramine maleate (Aller-Chlor, Allergy, Chlo-Amine, Chlor-Pro, Chlor-Trimeton, clemastine fumarate (Anti-hist 1, Tavist), dexchlorpheniramine maleate, diphenhydramine hydrochloride (AllerMax, Benadryl, Banophen, Diphenhist, Siladryl, Tusstat), promethazine hydrochloride (Anergan, Phenergan)

Source: Data from Drug Facts and Comparisons 2000 (54th ed). St. Louis: Wolters Kluwer, 2000.

Table IV-8.A. Aminoglycosides (Anti-Infective Agents)

Indications: Used for short-term treatment of infections of susceptible bacteria, for suspected gram-negative infections, for staphylococcus infections for which penicillin is contraindicated, as part of a multidrug treatment regimen for *Mycobacterium* complex (common in patients with acquired immunodeficiency syndrome)

Mechanism of action: Inhibit protein synthesis in susceptible strains of gram-negative bacteria and disrupts the functional integrity of bacterial cell membrane

General side effects: Ototoxicity, confusion, depression, fever, nausea, vomiting, diarrhea, leukopenia, electrolyte disturbances, palpitations, hyper- or hypotension, thrombocytopenia, anemia, nephrotoxicity, hepatic toxicity

Generic name (trade name): Amikacin sulfate (Amikin), gentamicin (Garamycin, Apogen), kanamycin (Kantrex), neomycin (Neo-Rx, Mycifradin), tobramycin (Tobex, Tobi, Tobrex)

Sources: Data from AM Karch. Lippincott's Nursing Drug Guide. Philadelphia: Lippincott–Raven, 2001;13; and Mosby's GenRX. The Complete Reference for Generic and Brand Drugs. St. Louis: Mosby,1999;85, 1030, 1257, 1597, 2156.

Table IV-8.B. Cephalosporins

Indications: Pharyngitis, tonsillitis, urinary tract infection, gonorrhea, septicemia, meningitis, bone and joint infections

Mechanism of action: Inhibit synthesis of bacterial cell wall, resulting in cell death

General side effects: Headache, dizziness, lethargy, nausea, vomiting, diarrhea, bone marrow suppression (decreased white blood cells, red blood cells, platelets), rash, fever, nephrotoxicity

Generic names (trade names)

First generation: Cefadroxil (Ultracef, Duricef), cefazolin (Ancef), cephalexin (Keflex, Keflet), cephapirin (Cefadyl), cephradine (Velosef, Anspor)

Second generation: Cefaclor (Ceclor), cefamandole (Mandol), cefoxitin (Mefoxin), cefonicid (Monocid), cefotetan (Cefotan), cefprozil (Cefzil), cefpodoxime (Vantin), cefuroxime (Zinacef), loracarbef (Lorabid)

Third generation: Cefepime (Maxipime), cefixime (Suprax), cefoperazone (Cefobid), cefotaxime (Claforan), ceftazidime (Fortaz), ceftibuten (Cedax), ceftizoxime (Cefizox), ceftriaxone (Rocephin)

Sources: Data from AM Karch (ed). Lippincott's Nursing Drug Guide. Philadelphia: Lippincott–Raven, 1999;48; and Mosby's GenRX. The Complete Reference for Generic and Brand Drugs (9th ed). St Louis: Mosby, 1999;360–430, 1351.

Table IV-8.C.  Macrolides

Indications: Acute infections, including upper and lower respiratory tract infections, skin and soft tissue infections, prophylaxis against alpha-hemolytic streptococcal endocarditis in dental and surgical procedures

Mechanism of action: Bind to cell membranes and causes changes in protein function, leading to bacteria cell death

General side effects: Reversible hearing loss, confusion, anorexia, diarrhea, vomiting, edema, dermatitis, rash, burning, itching

Generic name (trade name): Amoxicillin (Amoxil), aspirin (Fiorinal), chlorzoxazone (Paraflex), dirithromycin (Dynabac), erythromycin (Ilotycin), lincomycin (Lincocin), tacrolimus (Prograf), troleandomycin (Tao)

Sources: Data from AM Karch (ed). Lippincott's Nursing Drug Guide. Philadelphia: Lippincott–Raven, 2001;40; and Mosby's GenRX. The Complete Reference for Generic and Brand Drugs (9th ed). St Louis: Mosby, 1999;114, 164, 473, 726, 814, 1333, 2079, 2237.

Table IV-8.D.  Penicillins

Indications: Moderate to severe infections caused by sensitive organisms, including streptococci, pneumococci, and staphylococci; also syphilis and gonococcal infections and Lyme disease

Mechanism of action: Inhibit cell wall synthesis of sensitive organisms, resulting in cell death

General side effects: Lethargy, hallucinations, gastritis, nausea, vomiting, diarrhea, anemia, thrombocytopenia, leukopenia, rash, fever, protein-uria, hematuria

Generic name (trade name): Amoxicillin (Amoxil), ampicillin (Omnipen-N, Totacillin-N), bacampicillin (Spectrobid), carbenicillin (Miostat), cloxacillin (Tegopen), dicloxacillin (Pathocil), mezlocillin (Mezlin), nafcillin (Nafcil, Nallpen, Unipen), oxacillin (Bactocill, Prostaphlin), penicillin G, potassium (Pen-G, Pentids), penicillin V (V-cillin K), piper-acillin (Pipracil), ticarcillin (Ticar)

Sources: Data from AM Karch (ed). Lippincott's Nursing Drug Guide. Philadelphia: Lippincott–Raven, 2001;48; and Mosby's GenRX. The Complete Reference for Generic and Brand Drugs (9th ed). St. Louis: Mosby, 1999;114, 128, 211, 342, 553, 669, 1495, 1566, 1676, 1726, 1779, 2138.

Table IV-8.E.  Sulfonamides

Indications: Ulcerative colitis, Crohn's disease, otitis, conjunctivitis, meningitis, toxoplasmosis, urinary tract infections, rheumatoid arthritis, collagenous colitis

Mechanism of action: Antagonize para-aminobenzoic acid, which is essential for folic acid synthesis, causing cell death in gram-negative and grampositive bacteria

General side effects: Headache, peripheral neuropathy, ataxia, convulsions, vertigo, drowsiness, nausea, diarrhea, anorexia, impaired folic acid absorption, thrombocytopenia, crystalluria, proteinuria, photosensitivity, alopecia, skin eruptions, dermatitis

Generic name (trade name): Sulfadiazine Sodium (Microsulfon), sulfamethizole (Gantanol), sulfamethoxazole (Urobiotic-250), sulfasalazine (Azulfidine) sulfisoxazole (Gantrisin)

Sources: Data from AM Karch (ed). Lippincott's Nursing Drug Guide. Philadelphia: Lippincott–Raven, 2001;53; and Mosby's GenRX. The Complete Reference for Generic and Brand Drugs. St. Louis: Mosby, 1999;1692, 2050, 2058, 2060.

Table IV-8.F.  Tetracyclines

Indications: Various susceptible pathogens, including rickettsiae, and infections of eye and gastrointestinal and genitourinary tracts; also used in treatment of acne

Mechanism of action: Inhibit protein synthesis and prevents cell replication of susceptible bacteria

General side effects: Discoloring of teeth, anemia, leukopenia, phototoxic reactions, increased intracranial pressure, dermatitis, local irritation

Generic name (trade name): Demeclocycline (Declomycin), doxycycline (Vibramycin), minocycline (Minocin), oxytetracycline (Terramycin), tetracycline (Achromycin, Topicycline)

Sources: Data from AM Karch. Lippincott's Nursing Drug Guide. Philadelphia: Lippincott–Raven, 2001;75; and Mosby's GenRX. The Complete Reference for Generic and Brand Drugs (9th ed). St Louis: Mosby, 1999;619, 769, 1510, 1690, 2112.

**Table IV-9.** Antiparkinsonian Agents

Indications: To decrease bradykinesia, rigidity, and tremor (as in parkinsonian disorders).

Mechanism of action: Anticholinergics suppress central cholinergic activity and may inhibit reuptake and storage of dopamine. Dopaminergics increase dopamine content in the brain via an unknown mechanism.

General side effects: Headache, blurred vision, confusion, restlessness, agitation, muscle weakness, heaviness of limbs, tachycardia, palpitations, orthostatic hypotension, flushing, urinary retention.

Generic name (trade name): Anticholinergics include benztropine mesylate (Cogentin), biperiden (Akineton), diphenhydramine, procyclidine (Kemadrin), trihexyphenidyl hydrochloride (Artane, Trihexy). Other agents include amantadine hydrochloride (Symmetrel), carbidopa (Lodosyn), ethopropazine (Parsidol), levodopa-carbidopa (Sinemet), pramipexole (Mirapex), ropinirole HCL (Requip), selegiline hydrochloride (Carbex, Eldepryl).

Sources: Data from Drug Facts and Comparisons 2000 (54th ed). St. Louis: Wolters Kluwer, 2000; and Drug Facts and Comparisons 2001 (55th ed). St. Louis: Wolters Kluwer, 2001.

**Table IV-10.** Antiplatelet Agents

| | |
|---|---|
| Clopidogrel (Plavix) | Indication: Reduction of atherosclerotic events in the patient with recent CVA or myocardial infarction, or established PVD<br>Mechanism of action: Platelet aggregation inhibitor (inhibits ADP-mediated aggregation)<br>General side effects: Gastrointestinal and genitourinary tract or intracranial bleeding; headache, dizziness, hypertension, dyspnea, TTP, allergic reaction |
| Ticlopidine hydrochloride (Ticlid) | Indication: To decrease risk of CVA in patients experiencing stroke precursors<br>Mechanism of action: See Clopidogrel<br>General side effects: Gastrointestinal and genitourinary tract or intracranial bleeding; gastrointestinal disturbances, neutropenia, TTP |
| Tirofiban (Aggrastat) | Indications: ACS and PTCI<br>Mechanism of action: Glycoprotein IIb/IIIa inhibitor (inhibits fibrinogen and von Willebrand's factor from binding to IIb/IIIa receptor site to inhibit platelet aggregation).<br>General side effects: Gastrointestinal and genitourinary tract or intracranial bleeding; dizziness, bradycardia, pelvic pain |

Table IV-10.  *Continued*

| | |
|---|---|
| Eptifibatide (Integrelin) | Indications: Angina, ACS, PTCI<br>Mechanism of action: See Tirofiban<br>General side effects: See Tirofiban |
| Abciximab (ReoPro) | Indications: For use with heparin for ACS, PTCI<br>Mechanism of action: See Tirofiban<br>General side effects: See Tirofiban |
| Anagrelide hydrochloride (Agrylin) | Indication: Essential thrombocytopenia<br>Mechanism of action: Unknown<br>General side effects: Headache, palpitations, edema, diarrhea, abdominal pain |
| Dipyridamole (Persantine) | Indication: For use with warfarin to decrease thromboembolic complications after cardiac valve replacement<br>Mechanism of action: Platelet adhesion inhibitor, with exact mechanism unknown<br>General side effect: Hypotension |

ACS = acute coronary syndrome; ADP = adenosine diphosphate; CVA= cerebrovascular accident; PTCI = percutaneous transluminal coronary intervention; PVD = peripheral vascular disease; TTP = thrombotic thrombocytopenic purpura.
Sources: Data from Drug Facts and Comparisons 2000 (54th ed). St. Louis: Wolters Kluwer, 2000; and Anticoagulant, Antiplatelet, and Thrombolytic Drugs. In RA Lehne (ed), Pharmacology for Nursing Care (4th ed). Philadelphia: Saunders, 2001.

Table IV-11.  Antitussives*

Indications: Suppression of cough induced by chemical or mechanical irritation of the respiratory tract
Mechanism of action: Act centrally on the cough center in the medulla or anesthetize stretch receptors in the respiratory tract
General side effects: Drowsiness, dizziness, headache, sedation, nausea, vomiting, orthostatic hypotension, tachycardia, palpitations, sweating, chills, oliguria
Generic name (brand name): Benzonatate (Tessalon Perles), codeine (codeine sulfate), dextromethorphan hydrobromide (Benylin, Creo-Terpin, Delsym, Diabetes CF, Drixoral, Hold DM, Pertussin, Robitussin, Suppress, Sucrets, Silphen, Trocal), diphenhydramine hydrochloride (Bydramine, Diphen Cough, Tusstat, Uni-Bent Cough)

*Narcotic and non-narcotic forms.
Source: Data from Drug Facts and Comparisons 2000 (54th ed). St. Louis: Wolters Kluwer, 2000.

Table IV-12.  Beta Blockers

Indications: Ischemia, hypertension, arrhythmias
Mechanism of action: Decreases myocardial oxygen demand by decreasing
  sympathetic input to myocardium, therefore decreasing heart rate and
  contractility
General side effects: Smooth muscle spasm (bronchospasm), exaggeration of
  therapeutic cardiac actions (bradycardia), fatigue, insomnia, masking of
  hypoglycemic symptoms in diabetics, impaired glucose tolerance,
  decreased high-density lipoprotein cholesterol
Selective agents
  Beta 1 selective*: Acebutolol (Sectral), alprenolol, atenolol (Tenormin),
    esmolol (Brevibloc), metoprolol (Lopressor)
  Beta 2 selective*: Alpha and beta antagonists—labetalol (Normodyne,
    Trandate), butoxamine, carvedilol (Coreg)
Nonselective agents: Carteolol (Cartol), labetalol (Normodyne), nadolol
  (Corgard), pindolol (Visken), propanolol (Inderal), timolol (Blocadren)

*Selective refers to blockade of beta-1, beta-2, or alpha receptors. Nonselective means
not selective in blocking receptors.
Source: Data from K Grimes, M Cohen. Cardiac Medications. In EA Hillegass, HS
Sadowsky (eds), Essentials of Cardiopulmonary Physical Therapy (2nd ed). Philadelphia: Saunders, 2001;537–585.


Table IV-13.  Bronchodilators

Indications: To relieve bronchospasm associated with obstructive pulmonary
  disease, including exercise-induced bronchospasm
Mechanism of action: Smooth muscle relaxation of the bronchi or
  bronchioles
General side effects: Headache, dizziness, irritability, nervousness, tremor,
  tachycardia, dysrhythmia, hypotension
Generic name (trade name): Sympathomimetics—albuterol (Airet, Proventil,
  Ventolin, Volmax), bitolterol mesylate (Tornalate), ephedrine sulfate, epinephrine (Adrenaline chloride, Ana-Guard, AsthmaHaler Mist, AsthmaNe-
  frin, microNefrin, Primatene Mist, Sus-Phrine), isoetharine hydrochloride,
  levalbuterol hydrochloride (Xopenex), metaproterenol sulfate (Alupent), pir-
  buterol acetate (Maxair), salmeterol (Serevent), terbutaline sulfate (Brethaire,
  Brethine, Bricanyl); xanthine derivatives—aminophylline (Phyllocontin, Tru-
  phylline), dyphylline (Dilor, Lufyllin), oxtriphylline (Choledyl SA), theophyl-
  line (Accurbron, Aquaphyllin, Asmalix, Bronkodyl, Elixomin, Elixophyllin,
  Lanophyllin, Quibron-T/SR Dividose, Respbid, Slo-bid, Slo-Phyllin, Sustaire,
  Theobid, Theostat, Theovent, Theo-Dur, T-Phyl, Uni-Dur, Uniphyl)

Source: Data from Drug Facts and Comparisons 2000 (54th ed). St. Louis: Wolters
Kluwer, 2000.

**Table IV-14.** Calcium Channel Blockers

Indications: Ischemia, arrhythmias, hypertension
Mechanism of action: Decrease myocardial oxygen demand and increase supply of myocardial oxygen by slowing down transport of calcium on smooth muscle and myocardial cells, therefore reducing contractility and afterload
General side effects: Negative inotrope at high doses, orthostatic hypotension, peripheral edema, dizziness, gastrointestinal upset, headache
Generic name (trade name): Amlodipine (Lotrel, Norvasc), bepridil (Vascor), diltiazem (Cardizem), felodipine (Plendil), isradipine (DynaCirc), nicardipine (Cardene), nifedipine (Procardia, Adalat), nimodipine (Nimotop), nisoldipine (Sular), verapamil (Isoptin, Calan)

Source: Data from K Grimes, M Cohen. Cardiac Medications. In EA Hillegass, HS Sadowsky (eds), Essentials of Cardiopulmonary Physical Therapy (2nd ed). Philadelphia: Saunders, 2001;537–585.

**Table IV-15.A.** Alkylating Agents (Chemotherapy Agents)

Indications: Malignant neoplasms, metastatic disease
Mechanism of action: Inhibit DNA function and replication

| Generic Name (Trade Name) | Side Effects |
| --- | --- |
| Busulfan (Myleran) | Myelosuppression, pulmonary fibrosis, anemia, leukopenia, thrombocytopenia, fatigue, weight loss |
| Carboplatin (Paraplatin) | Myelosuppression, nausea, vomiting, neurotoxicity |
| Carmustine (BiCNU) | Nausea; vomiting; pain; tissue necrosis; pulmonary, renal, and hepatotoxicity |
| Chlorambucil (Leukeran) | Nausea, vomiting, stomatitis, thrombocytopenia, myelosuppression, neutropenia, anemia, interstitial pneumonitis, exfoliative dermatitis, hyperuricemia |
| Cisplatin (Platinol) | Peripheral neuritis, tinnitus, nausea, vomiting, leukopenia, thrombocytopenia, anemia, renal toxicity |
| Cyclophosphamide (Cytoxan) | Cardiotoxicity, leukopenia, thrombocytopenia, anemia, pulmonary fibrosis |
| Dacarbazine (DTIC-Dome) | Nausea, leukopenia, thrombocytopenia, fever, malaise |

| Generic Name (Trade Name) | Side Effects |
|---|---|
| Ifosfamide (Ifex) | Lethargy, somnolence, confusion, depressive psychosis, ataxia, coma, seizures, nausea, vomiting, hemorrhagic cystitis, hematuria, leukopenia, thrombocytopenia, myelosuppression, alopecia |
| Lomustine (CeeNU) | Nausea, vomiting, anemia, leukopenia, thrombocytopenia |
| Mechlorethamine (Mustargen, Nitrogen Mustard) | Headache, weakness, tinnitus, nausea, vomiting, myelosuppression, metallic taste in the mouth |
| Melphalan (Alkeran) | Thrombocytopenia, agranulocytosis, pneumonitis, pulmonary fibrosis, anaphylaxis |
| Procarbazine | Nausea; vomiting; pain; tissue necrosis; pulmonary, renal, and hepatotoxicity |
| Streptozocin (Zanosar) | Nausea, vomiting, diarrhea, anemia, leukopenia, thrombocytopenia, anemia, hyperglycemia |
| Thiotepa (Thiotepa) | Headache, dizziness, nausea, leukopenia, thrombocytopenia, anemia |
| Uracil mustard | Irritability, nervousness, nausea, thrombocytopenia, anemia, hyperpigmentation of skin |

Sources: Data from C Ciccone (ed). Cancer Chemotherapy. Philadelphia: FA Davis, 1996; and D Moreau (ed). Nursing '96 Drug Handbook. Springhouse, PA: Springhouse, 1996; and LM Tierney, SJ McPhee, MA Papadakis (eds). Current Medical Diagnosis and Treatment. New York: McGraw-Hill, 2000.

**Table IV-15.B.**  Antibiotics (Chemotherapy Agents)

Indications: Malignant neoplasms, metastatic disease
Mechanism of action: Disrupt the DNA and RNA synthesis

| Generic Name (Trade Name) | Side Effects |
|---|---|
| Bleomycin (Blenoxane) | Nausea, vomiting, fever, chills, anaphylaxis, alopecia, stomatitis, erythema, pulmonary toxicity (interstitial pneumonitis), general weakness and malaise, headache, leukocytosis, pulmonary fibrosis, joint swelling |
| Dactinomycin (Cosmegen) | Nausea, vomiting, myelosuppression, tissue necrosis, alopecia, mucositis |

**Table IV-15.B.** *Continued*

| Generic Name (Trade Name) | Side Effects |
|---|---|
| Daunorubicin (Cerubidine) | Nausea, vomiting, myelosuppression, tissue necrosis, stomatitis, alopecia, cardiotoxicity |
| Doxorubicin (Adriamycin) | Nausea, vomiting, myelosuppression, tissue necrosis, stomatitis, alopecia, cardiotoxicity |
| Mitomycin (Mutamycin) | Nausea, vomiting, myelosuppression, tissue necrosis, stomatitis, pulmonary and renal toxicity |
| Mitoxantrone (Novantrone) | Myelosuppression, cardiotoxicity (congestive heart failure, arrhythmias), nausea, vomiting, diarrhea, abdominal pain, hepatic dysfunction, seizures |
| Plicamycin (Mithracin) | Myelosuppression, central nervous system and renal toxicity, nausea, vomiting, coagulation abnormalities, tissue necrosis, weakness, malaise |

Sources: Data from C Ciccone (ed). Cancer Chemotherapy. Philadelphia: FA Davis, 1996; and D Moreau (ed). Nursing '96 Drug Handbook. Springhouse, PA: Springhouse, 1996.

**Table IV-15.C.** Antimetabolite Agents (Chemotherapy Agents)

Indications: Malignant neoplasms, metastatic disease
Mechanism of action: Interfere with normal metabolites during DNA and RNA biosynthesis

| Generic Name (Trade Name) | Side Effects |
|---|---|
| Cladribine (2-chlorodeoxyadenosine) | Neutropenia, anemia, leukopenia, nausea, rash, chills, diaphoresis, arthralgia, myalgia, malaise |
| Cytarabine (Cytosar-U) | Neurotoxicity, ataxia, nystagmus, keratitis, nausea, vomiting, thrombocytopenia, flulike syndrome |
| Floxuridine (FUDR) | Anorexia, stomatitis, cramps, ataxia, vertigo, nystagmus, seizures, nausea, vomiting, diarrhea, bleeding, leukopenia, anemia, thrombocytopenia, erythema, alopecia, hiccups, jaundice |
| 5-Fluorouracil (Adrucil) | Ataxia, weakness, malaise, stomatitis, nausea, vomiting, diarrhea, anorexia, leukopenia, thrombocytopenia, anemia, alopecia, dermatitis, erthema, pain, burning, scaling, pruritus, confusion, disorientation |

| Generic Name (Trade Name) | Side Effects |
|---|---|
| Hydroxyurea (Hydrea) | Anorexia, vomiting, diarrhea, leukopenia, thrombocytopenia, anemia, nausea, myelosuppression, skin rash, renal and neurotoxicity |
| Mercaptopurine (Purinethol) | Nausea, vomiting, anorexia, thrombocytopenia, anemia, jaundice, hepatic necrosis, rash, leukopenia |
| Methotrexate (Folex, Mexate, Rheumatrex) | Pharyngitis, nausea, anemia, leukopenia, pulmonary fibrosis |
| Thioguanine (Lanvis) | Leukopenia, anemia, thrombocytopenia, hepatotoxicity, nausea |

Sources: Data from C Ciccone (ed). Cancer Chemotherapy. Philadelphia: FA Davis, 1996; D Moreau (ed). Nursing '96 Drug Handbook. Springhouse, PA: Springhouse, 1996; and LM Tierney, SJ McPhee, MA Papadakis (eds). Current Medical Diagnosis and Treatment. New York: McGraw-Hill, 2000.

**Table IV-15.D.** Hormones (Chemotherapy Agents)

Indications: Malignant neoplasms, metastatic disease
Mechanism of action: Inhibit growth of neoplasm; usually combined with other chemotherapy agents

| | Generic Name (Trade Name) | General Side Effects |
|---|---|---|
| Antiestrogens | Tamoxifen (Nolvadex) | Nausea, vomiting, transient fall in white blood cell and platelet counts |
| | Toremifene | Occasional fluid retention, rare thrombosis, weight gain |
| Estrogens | Chlorotrianisene (TACE) | Nausea, leg cramps, thromboembolism, cerebrovascular accident, pulmonary embolism, myocardial infarction |
| | Diethylstilbestrol (DES) | Nausea, leg cramps, thromboembolism, cerebrovascular accident, pulmonary embolism, myocardial infarction |
| | Estradiol (Oestradiol, Valerate) | Thromboembolism, nausea, leg cramps |
| | Medroxyprogesterone | Occasional fluid retention, rare thrombosis, weight gain |

**Table IV-15.D.** *Continued*

| | Generic Name (Trade Name) | General Side Effects |
|---|---|---|
| Adrenocortico-steroids | Prednisone (Del-tasone, Ora-sone) | Euphoria, insomnia, muscle weakness, osteoporosis, congestive heart failure, hypertension, delayed wound healing |
| | Prednisolone (Delta-Cortef) | Euphoria, insomnia, muscle weakness, osteoporosis, congestive heart failure, hypertension, delayed wound healing |
| Androgens | Fluoxymesterone (Android-F) | Edema, nausea, vomiting, thrombo-cytopenia |
| Antiandrogens | Flutamide (Eulexin) | Drowsiness, confusion, numbness, diarrhea, nausea, vomiting, hot flashes |
| | Anastrazole | Occasional fluid retention, rare throm-bosis, weight gain |
| Aromatase inhibitor | Aminoglute-thimide | Skin rash, weight gain, fluid retention, leg cramps, jaundice |
| Gonadotropin-releasing hormone drugs | Leuprolide (Lupron) | Hot flashes, pulmonary embolism, arrhythmia, angina, myocardial infarction |
| | Goserelin acetate | Hot flashes, pulmonary embolism, arrhythmia, angina, myocardial infarction |
| | Goserelin (Zoladex) | Lethargy, pain, arrhythmia, congestive heart failure, hypertension, myocardial infarction, chronic obstructive pulmonary disease, upper respiratory tract infections |
| | Megestrol (Megace) | Hypertension, edema, thrombo-phlebitis, nausea, vomiting, carpal tunnel syndrome |
| Anticachetics | Megestrol acetate | Occasional fluid retention, rare throm-bosis, weight gain |

Sources: Data from C Ciccone (ed). Cancer Chemotherapy. Philadelphia: FA Davis, 1996; D Moreau (ed). Nursing '96 Drug Handbook. Springhouse, PA: Springhouse, 1996; and LM Tierney, SJ McPhee, MA Papadakis (eds). Current Medical Diagnosis and Treatment. New York: McGraw-Hill, 2000.

Table IV-15.E.  Plant Alkaloids (Chemotherapy Agents)

Indications: Malignant neoplasms, metastatic disease
Mechanism of action: Disrupt the mitotic apparatus and cause death of the
cancerous cell

| Generic Name (Trade Name) | General Side Effects |
|---|---|
| Etoposide (VePesid) | Myelosuppression, anemia, leukopenia, thrombocytopenia, nausea, vomiting, hypotension, anaphylaxis, alopecia, headache, peripheral neuropathy, central nervous system toxicity, fever, chills |
| Teniposide (VM-26) | Myelosuppression, tissue necrosis, fever, hypotension, anaphylaxis, alopecia |
| Vinblastine (Velban, Alkaban) | Myelosuppression, leukopenia, nausea, vomiting, stomatitis, alopecia, central and peripheral neuropathy, tissue necrosis |
| Vincristine (Oncovin, Vincasar) | Myelosuppression, nausea, vomiting, tissue necrosis, peripheral neuropathy, constipation |

Sources: Data from C Ciccone (ed). Cancer Chemotherapy. Philadelphia: FA Davis,
1996; D Moreau (ed). Nursing '96 Drug Handbook. Springhouse, PA: Springhouse,
1996; and LM Tierney, SJ McPhee, MA Papadakis (eds). Current Medical Diagnosis
and Treatment. New York: McGraw-Hill, 2000.


Table IV-15.F.  Interferons (Chemotherapy Agents)

Indications: Malignant neoplasms, metastatic disease
Mechanism of action: Provide antiviral and antineoplastic properties

| Name | General Side Effects |
|---|---|
| Interferon alfa-2a | Fever, chills, malaise, dizziness, anorexia, bronchospasm, leukopenia, hepatitis |
| Interferon alfa-2b | Fever, chills, malaise, dizziness, anorexia, leukopenia, hepatitis |

Sources: Data from C Ciccone (ed). Cancer Chemotherapy. Philadelphia: FA Davis,
1996; D Moreau (ed). Nursing '96 Drug Handbook. Springhouse, PA: Springhouse,
1996; and LM Tierney, SJ McPhee, MA Papadakis (eds). Current Medical Diagnosis
and Treatment. New York: McGraw-Hill, 2000.

Table IV-15.G. Colony-Stimulating Factors (Chemotherapy Agents)

Indications: Malignant neoplasms, metastatic disease.
Mechanism of action: Colony-stimulating factors stimulate the production of white blood cells and accelerate the recovery of bone marrow.

| Generic Name (Trade Name) | Side Effects |
|---|---|
| Filgrastim (Neupogen) | Medullary bone pain, nausea, vomiting, skeletal pain, diarrhea |
| Sargramostim (Leukine, Prokine) | Fever, malaise, nausea, diarrhea, anorexia, gastrointestinal upset, edema, alopecia, rash, dyspnea |

Sources: Data from C Ciccone (ed). Cancer Chemotherapy. Philadelphia: FA Davis, 1996; D Moreau (ed). Nursing '96 Drug Handbook. Springhouse, PA: Springhouse, 1996; and LM Tierney, SJ McPhee, MA Papadakis (eds). Current Medical Diagnosis and Treatment. New York: McGraw-Hill, 2000.

Table IV-15.H. Other Antineoplastic Agents (Chemotherapy Agents)

Indications: Malignant neoplasms, metastatic disease
Mechanism of action:
  Aminoglutethimide—inhibits production of steroid hormones from adrenal glands
  Aldesleukin—affects leukocyte function
  Procarbazine—inhibits growth of cancer cells and blocks monoamine oxidase in the central nervous system

| Generic Name (Brand Name) | General Side Effects |
|---|---|
| Aminoglutethimide (Cytadren) | Drowsiness, dizziness, tachycardia, hypotension, myalgia |
| Aldesleukin (IL-2) | Hypoglycemia, anemia |
| Procarbazine (Matulane) | Nausea, vomiting, myelosuppression, hallucinations, pleural effusion, central nervous system and renal toxicity |

Sources: Data from C Ciccone (ed). Cancer Chemotherapy. Philadelphia: FA Davis, 1996; D Moreau (ed). Nursing '96 Drug Handbook. Springhouse, PA: Springhouse, 1996; and LM Tierney, SJ McPhee, MA Papadakis (eds). Current Medical Diagnosis and Treatment. New York: McGraw-Hill, 2000.

**Table IV-16.**  Corticosteroids (Inhaled)

Indication: Stabilize and limit the inflammatory response (bronchoconstriction) in the respiratory tract
Mechanism of action: Unknown (may decrease the number and activity of inflammatory cells, inhibit bronchoconstriction mechanisms, or directly relax smooth muscle)
General side effects: Hypotension, hypertension, tachycardia, immunosuppression, osteoporosis, decreased healing
Generic name (trade name): Beclomethasone (Beclovent, Vanceril), budesonide (Pulmicort), flunisolide (AeroBid), fluticasone propionate (Flovent), triamcinolone acetonide (Azmacort)

Source: Data from Drug Facts and Comparisons 2000 (54th ed). St. Louis: Wolters Kluwer, 2000.

**Table IV-17.**  Diuretics

Indications: Heart failure, hypertension
Mechanism of action: Reduce preload and vascular volume
General side effects: Volume reduction, hypotension, arrhythmias, hyper- or hypokalemia (Only potassium-sparing diuretics can lead to hyperkalemia, all others generally lead to hypokalemia.)
Thiazides (generic name [trade name]): Bendrofluazide (Aprinox, Centyl), bendroflumethiazide (Naturetin), benthiazide (Exna, Hydrex), chlorothiazide (Diuril), chlorthalidone (Hygroton), cyclothiazide (Anhydron), cyclopenthiazide (Navidrex), hydrochlorothiazide (Esidrex, HydroDIURIL), hydroflumethiazide (Diucardin, Saluron), indapamide (Lozol, Natrilix), methyclothiazide (Enduron, Aquatensen), metolazone (Mykrox, Diulo, Zaroxolyn), polythiazide (Renese), quinethazone (Hydromox), trichlormethiazide (Metahydrin, Naqua)
Loop (generic [trade name]): Bumetanide (Bumex), ethacrynic acid (Edecrin), furosemide (Lasix, Furoside), frusemide (Frusetic, Frusid), piretanide (Arlix)
Potassium sparing (generic [trade name]): Amiloride (Midamor), potassium canrenoate (Spiroctan-M), spironolactone (Aldactone), triamterene (Dyrenium)
Carbonic anhydrase inhibitors (generic [trade name]): Acetazolamide (Diamox), dichlorphenamide (Daranide), methazolamide (Neptazane)

Source: Data from K Grimes, M Cohen. Cardiac Medications. In EA Hillegass, HS Sadowsky (eds), Essentials of Cardiopulmonary Physical Therapy (2nd ed). Philadelphia: Saunders, 2001;537–585.

**Table IV-18.** Expectorants

Indication: To facilitate bronchopulmonary secretion removal
Mechanism of action: Reduce adhesiveness and surface tension of
  respiratory tract fluid to enhance expectoration
General side effects: Nausea, vomiting, headache, rash
Generic name (brand name): Guaifenesin (Anti-Tuss, Breonesin, Fenesin,
  Genatuss, Glycotuss, Humibid, Organidin, Pneumomist, Robitussin),
  iodinated glycerol (Iophen, Par Glycerol, R-Gen)

Source: Data from Drug Facts and Comparisons 2000 (54th ed). St. Louis: Wolters
Kluwer, 2000.

**Table IV-19.A.** Antacids

Indications: Peptic ulcer disease, reflux esophagitis, gastritis, hiatal hernia
Mechanism of action: Neutralize gastric acidity (increases pH), decrease the
  rate of gastric emptying, strengthen gastric mucosal barrier, and increase
  esophageal sphincter tone
General side effects: Constipation, osteomalacia, encephalopathy, headache,
  irritability, diarrhea, nausea, abdominal pain
Generic name (trade name): Aluminum carbonate (Basaljel), aluminum
  hydroxide (AlternaGEL, Alu-Cap, Aluminum Hydroxide Gel, Alu-Tab,
  Amphojel, Dialume), calcium carbonate (Alka-Mints, Amitone, Cal-sup,
  Dicarbosil, Maalox Antacid Caplets, Rolaids Calcium Rich, Tums, Tums E-
  X, Tums Ultra), magaldrate (Lowsium, Riopan), magnesium oxide (Mag-
  Ox 400, Uro-Mag)

Sources: Data from CD Ciccone. Gastrointestinal Drugs. In CD Ciccone (ed), Pharma-
cology in Rehabilitation (2nd ed). Philadelphia: FA Davis, 1996;390; Nursing 2001
Drug Handbook (21st ed). Springhouse PA: Springhouse, 2001;643–648, 684–694; and
L Skidmore-Roth (ed). Mosby's Nursing Drug Reference. St. Louis: Mosby, 2001;3.

**Table IV-19.B.** Antiulcer Medications

$H_2$-receptor blockers
  Indications: Primarily duodenal ulcers, but can also be used for gastric
    ulcer and Zollinger-Ellison syndrome
  Mechanism of action: Inhibit action of $H_2$ receptor sites of the parietal
    cells, resulting in decreased acid secretion
  General side effects: Headache, dizziness, mild nausea, diarrhea, or
    constipation

Generic name (trade name): Cimetidine (Tagamet, Tagamet HB), cimetidine hydrochloride (Tagamet HCL), famotidine (Pepcid, Pepcid AC, Pepcidine ), nizatidine (Axid, Axid AR, Tazac), ranitidine bismuth citrate (Tritec), ranitidine hydrochloride (Apo-Ranitidine, Zantac)

Proton-pump inhibitors

Indications: Active duodenal ulcer, gastroesophageal reflux disease

Mechanism of action: Inhibit acid production

General side effects: Diarrhea, nausea, abdominal pain, back pain, constipation, dizziness, headache

Generic name (trade name): Lansoprazole (Prevacid, Zoton), omeprazole (Losec, Prilosec), rabeprazole sodium (Aciphex)

Miscellaneous antiulcer drugs

Indication: Prevention of nonsteroidal anti-inflammatory drug–induced gastric ulcer

Mechanism of action: Replace gastric prostaglandins depleted by nonsteroidal anti-inflammatory drug therapy with a synthetic prostaglandin analogue

General side effects: Headache, diarrhea, abdominal pain, constipation

Generic name (trade name): Misoprostol (Cytotec)

Sources: Data from CD Ciccone. Gastrointestinal Drugs. In CD Ciccone (ed), Pharmacology in Rehabilitation (2nd ed). Philadelphia: FA Davis, 1996;390; Nursing 2001 Drug Handbook (21st ed) Springhouse PA: Springhouse, 2001;643–648, 684–694; and L Skidmore-Roth (ed). Mosby's Nursing Drug Reference. St. Louis: Mosby, 2001;3.

**Table IV-20.A.** Antidiarrheal Medications

Indication: Diarrhea

Mechanism of action: Decrease water absorption, inhibit peristaltic activity, increase smooth muscle tone

General side effects: Nausea, abdominal discomfort, constipation, drowsiness, fatigue, dizziness, arrhythmia, tachycardia or bradycardia

Generic name (trade name): Attapulgite (Diasorb, Donnagel, Fowler's, Kaopectate, K-Pek Parepectolin, Rheaban Maximum Strength), bismuth subsalicylate (Bismatral, Pepto-Bismol, Pink Bismuth), diphenoxylate hydrochloride and atropine sulfate (Logen, Lomanate, Lomotil, Lonox), loperamide (Imodium, Kaopectate II Caplets, Maalox Antidiarrheal Caplets, Pepto Diarrhea Control), octreotide acetate (Sandostatin), opium tincture

Sources: Data from CD Ciccone. Gastrointestinal Drugs. In CD Ciccone (ed), Pharmacology in Rehabilitation (2nd ed). Philadelphia: FA Davis, 1996;393; and Nursing 2001 Drug Handbook (21st ed) Springhouse, PA: Springhouse, 2001;653–672.

Table IV-20.B. Laxatives

Indications: Constipation; preparation of bowel for examination, surgery, or both

Mechanism of action: Increase water retention in the stool to increase bulk, promote peristalsis

General side effects: Nausea, cramps, spastic colitis, diarrhea, fluid and electrolyte imbalances (e.g., hypokalemia), dehydration

Generic name (trade name): Bisacodyl (Bisacolax, Bisalax, Bisco-Lax, Dulcagen, Dulcolax, Durolax, Fleet Bisacodyl, Fleet Laxative), calcium polycarbophil (Equalactin, Fiberall, FiberCon, Fiber-Lax, Mitrolan), castor oil (Emulsoil, Fleet Flavored Castor Oil, Purge), docusate calcium (DC softgels, Pro-Cal-Sof, Sulfa-lax Calcium, Surfak), docusate sodium (Colace, Coloxyl, Diocto, Dioctyl, Dioeze, Diosuccin, Disonate, Di-Sosul, DOS, D-S-S, Duosol, Fletcher's Enemette, Modane Soft, Norgalax, Micro-enema, Pro-Sof, Regulax SS, Regulex ), glycerin (Fleet Babylax, Sani-Supp), lactulose (Constilac, Constulose, Chronulac, Cephulac, Cholac, Duphalac, Enulose, Evalose, Heptalac, Lactulax), magnesium citrate (Citroma, Citromag), magnesium hydroxide (Milk of Magnesia), magnesium sulfate (Epsom salts), methylcellulose (Citrucel, Cologel), mineral oil (Agoral, Nujol, Fleet Enema Mineral Oil, Kondremul, Lansoyl, Liqui-Doss, Milkinol, Neo-Cultol, Petrogalar Plain), psyllium (Fiberall, Genfiber, Hydrocil, Metamucil, Restore, Serutan, Siblin, Syllact, Unilax, V-Lax), senna (Senokot, Black-Draught, Fletcher's Castoria), phenolphthalein (Correctol, Ex-Lax, Feen-a-Mint), sodium phosphate (Fleet Enema, Fleet Phospho-Soda)

Sources: Data from CD Ciccone. Gastrointestinal Drugs. In CD Ciccone (ed), Pharmacology in Rehabilitation (2nd ed). Philadelphia: FA Davis, 1996;393; and Nursing 2001 Drug Handbook (21st ed) Springhouse, PA: Springhouse, 2001;653–672.

Table IV-21. Intranasal Steroids

Indication: Relief of seasonal or perennial rhinitis

Mechanism of action: Unknown, although inhibit cell (e.g., neutrophils) and mediator (e.g., histamine) action in allergic and nonallergic inflammation

General side effects: Headache, dizziness, nervousness, nausea, vomiting, throat or nasal soreness and dryness

Generic name (trade name): Beclomethasone dipropionate (Beconase, Vancenase), budesonide (Rhinocort), fluticasone propionate (Flonase), mometasone furoate monohydrate (Nasonex), triamcinolone acetonide (Nasacort)

Source: Data from Drug Facts and Comparisons 2000 (54th ed). St. Louis: Wolters Kluwer, 2000.

Table IV-22.  Lipid-Lowering Agents

Indication: Lipid disorders
Mechanism of action: Decrease levels of low-density lipoproteins,
 triglycerides, or both
General side effects: Constipation, diarrhea, nausea, liver function
 abnormalities, skin rashes, increased bleeding time
Anion exchange resins/bile acid sequestrants (generic name [trade name]):
 Cholestyramine (Questran), colestipol (Colestid)
Fibric acid derivatives: Clofibrate (Atromid-S), gemfibrozil (Lopid)
HMG-CoA reductase inhibitor/statins: Lovastatin (Mevacor), pravastatin
 (Pravachol), simvastatin (Zocor), fluvastatin (Lescol), atorvastatin
 (Lipitor), cerivastatin (Baycol)
Nicotonic acid: Niacin
Fish oils: Omega-3 fatty acid (SuperEPA, many other over-the-counter
 varieties)

HMG-CoA = hepatic 3-methylglutaryl coenzyme A.
Source: Data from K Grimes, M Cohen. Cardiac Medications. In EA Hillegass, HS
Sadowsky. Essentials in Cardiopulmonary Physical Therapy (2nd ed). Philadelphia:
Saunders, 2001;570.


Table VI-23.  Mucolytics

Indication: Viscous bronchopulmonary secretions associated with chronic
 bronchopulmonary diseases
Mechanism of action: Act directly to split molecular mucoprotein
 molecular complexes, resulting in a depolymerization and viscosity
General side effects: Nausea, vomiting, fever, drowsiness, bronchoconstriction
Generic name (trade name): Acetylcysteine (Mucomyst, Mucosil), dornase
 alpha (Pulmozyme)

Source: Data from Drug Facts and Comparisons 2000 (54th ed). St. Louis: Wolters
Kluwer, 2000.

**Table IV-24.**  Nitrates

Indication: Ischemia

Mechanism of action: Decrease myocardial oxygen demand and increase myocardial oxygen supply; venodilation by promoting smooth muscle relaxation on both the venous and arterial side and therefore reducing preload and afterload

General side effects: Headache, hypotension

Generic name (trade name; route of entry): Amyl nitrite (Aspirol, Vaporole; inhalation), nitroglycerin (Nitro-Bid, Nitrostat; sublingual, spray, percutaneous ointment, oral, sustained release, i.v.) (Nitro-Dur, Transderm-Nitro, Nitrodisc; transdermal patch), isosorbide dinitrate (Isordil, Sorbitrate; sublingual, oral, chewable), isosorbide mononitrate (ISMO), pentaerythritol tetranitrate (Peritrate; sublingual, pentrinitrol, Pentafin; oral Vasitol; sustained release), erythrityl tetranitrate (Tetranitrol, Erythrol tetranitrate; oral) (Cardilate; sublingual)

Source: Data from K Grimes, M Cohen. Cardiac Medications In EA Hillegass, HS Sadowsky (eds), Essentials of Cardiopulmonary Physical Therapy. Philadelphia: Saunders, 2001;493.

**Table IV-25.**  Nutritional Agents for Anemia

Indication: Iron deficiency anemia

General side effects: Nausea, vomiting, constipation, dark stools

Generic name (brand name): Ferrous fumarate (Femiron, Feostat, Hemocyte, Ircon, Nephro-Fer, Vitron C), ferrous gluconate (Fergon), ferrous sulfate (ED-IN-SOL, Fe50, Feosol, Fer-gen-sol, Fer-In-Sol, Fer-Iron, Feratab), iron dextran (Imferon)*

Indication: Vitamin $B_{12}$ deficiency anemia

General side effects: Itchy skin or rash, pain at injection site, diarrhea, pulmonary edema, congestive heart failure, peripheral vascular thrombosis

Generic name (brand name): Cyanocobalamin crystalline (Crystamine, Crysti 1000, Cyanoject, Cyomin, Rubesol-1000), hydroxocobalamin (Hydro-Cobex, Hydro-Crysti-12, LA-12)

Indication: Folic acid anemia

General side effects: Mild allergic reaction, otherwise nontoxic

Generic name (trade name): Folic acid (Folacin, Folvite), leucovorin (Wellcovorin)

*For severe iron deficiency anemia.
Sources: Data from Drug Facts and Comparisons 2000 (54th ed). St. Louis: Wolters Kluwer, 2000; and Drug Facts and Comparisons 2001 (55th ed). St. Louis: Wolters Kluwer, 2001.

**Table IV-26.**  Osmotic Diuretics

Indication: To reduce intracranial pressure by reducing cerebral edema and interstitial pressure
Mechanism of action: Increase plasma osmolarity of the glomerular filtrate, thus hindering tubular reabsorption of water
General side effects: Headache, nausea, vomiting, fever, confusion, blurred vision, tachycardia, hypo- or hypertension, congestive heart failure, electrolyte imbalance
Generic name (brand name): Mannitol (Osmitrol), glycerin (Osmoglyn), urea (Ureaphil)

Source: Data from Drug Facts and Comparisons 2000 (54th ed). St. Louis: Wolters Kluwer, 2000.

**Table IV-27.A.**  Positive Inotropes: Cardiac Glycosides (Digitalis)

Indication: Heart failure
Mechanism of action: Increase contractility
General side effects: Decreased heart rate, conduction delay, digitalis toxicity
Generic name(trade name): Digitoxin (Crystodigin), digoxin (Lanoxin), deslanoside (Cedilanid-DIV)

Source: Data from K Grimes, M Cohen. Cardiac Medications. In EA Hillegass, HS Sadowsky (eds), Essentials of Cardiopulmonary Physical Therapy (2nd ed). Philadelphia: Saunders, 2001;537–585.

**Table IV-27.B.**  Positive Inotropes: Sympathomimetics

Indication: Heart failure
Mechanism of action: Increase contractility by mimicking the effects of the sympathetic nervous system
General side effects: Smooth muscle dilation (bronchodilation and vasodilation), prolonged use may decrease sensitization of beta receptors (decreased inotropism). Bipyridines may exacerbate ischemia, may worsen ectopy.
Beta 1-selective: Generic name (trade name)—dobutamine (Dobutrex), prenalterol
Nonselective: Epinephrine (Adrenaline Chloride), isoproterenol (Isuprel)
Dopaminergic: Dopamine (Intropin, Dopastat)
Mixed alpha and beta: Norepinephrine (Levophed)
Bipyridines: Amrinone (Inocor)

Source: Data from K Grimes, M Cohen. Cardiac Medications. In EA Hillegass, HS Sadowsky (eds), Essentials of Cardiopulmonary Physical Therapy (2nd ed). Philadelphia: Saunders, 2001;537–585.

**Table IV-28.** Skeletal Muscle Relaxants

Indication: To decrease muscle spasticity

Mechanism of action: Depress mono- and polysynaptic afferent spinal reflex activity or alter calcium ion activity within muscle

General side effects: Nausea, vomiting, fatigue, drowsiness, weakness, insomnia, ataxia, confusion, hypotension, hyperglycemia, urinary frequency

Generic name (brand name): Baclofen (Lioresal), dantrolene sodium (Dantrium), diazepam (Valium), tizanidine hydrochloride (Zanaflex)

Source: Data from Drug Facts and Comparisons 2000 (54th ed). St. Louis: Wolters Kluwer, 2000.

**Table IV-29.** Thrombolytic Agents (Fibrinolytics)

| | |
|---|---|
| Alteplase (Activase), reteplase (Retavase) | Indications: Acute MI,* ischemic CVA, or massive PE <br> Mechanism of action: Tissue plasminogen activator; binds to fibrin in a thrombus and converts plasminogen to plasmin to degrade (fibrinolysis) the fibrin matrix of a thrombus <br> General side effects: Alteplase—bleeding of gastrointestinal, genitourinary, or respiratory tracts, or intracranial bleeding; cerebral edema (in the setting of CVA), reperfusion arrhythmia; reteplase—bleeding and arrhythmia as above, heart failure, myocardial reinfarction, hypotension |
| Anistreplase (Eminase), streptokinase (Kabikinase, Streptase), urokinase (Abbokinase) | Indications: Anistreplase—acute MI; streptokinase—evolving MI, PE, deep vein thrombosis, occluded arteriovenous cannula; urokinase—acute massive PE, evolving MI, intravenous catheter clearance <br> Mechanism of action: Thrombolytic enzyme; acts with plasminogen to convert it to plasmin to degrade the fibrin matrix of a thrombus <br> General side effects: See Alteplase; hypotension, fever, allergic reactions |

CVA = cerebrovascular accident; MI = myocardial infarction; PE = pulmonary embolism.
*The only indication for reteplase.
Source: Data from Drug Facts and Comparisons 2000 (54th ed). St. Louis: Wolters Kluwer, 2000; and Anticoagulant, Antiplatelet, and Thrombolytic Drugs. In RA Lehne (ed), Pharmacology for Nursing Care (4th ed). Philadelphia: Saunders, 2001.

**Table IV-30.**  Vasodilators

---

Indications: Heart failure, hypertension

Mechanism of action: Venodilators reduce preload, arteriodilators reduce afterload, combined venodilators and arteriodilators reduce both preload and afterload

General side effects: Headache, hypotension, compensatory sympathetic reflex causing increased heart rate, vasoconstriction, and elevated plasma renin (usually avoided with combination of medications that includes a sympathetic inhibiting agent)

Venodilators: Refer to Table IV-24 Nitrates

Arteriodilators (generic name [trade name]): diazoxide (Hyperstat i.v.), hydralazine (Apresoline), minoxidil (Loniten), milrinone (Primacor), nifedipine (Procardia)

Combined venodilators and arteriodilators: Sodium nitroprusside (Nipride)

---

Source: Data from K Grimes, M Cohen. Cardiac Medications. In EA Hillegass, HS Sadowsky (eds), Essentials of Cardiopulmonary Physical Therapy (2nd ed). Philadelphia: Saunders, 2001;537–585.

# V

# Effects of Anesthesia
*Michele P. West*

The recovery period after surgery is characterized as a time of physiologic alteration as a result of the operative procedure and the effects of anesthesia.[1] On transport from the operating room, a patient is transferred to a postanesthesia care unit (PACU) (after general anesthesia) or to an ambulatory surgery recovery room (after regional anesthesia), both of which are located near the operating room for continuous nursing care. During this immediate postoperative phase, the priorities of care are to assess recovery from anesthesia and the status of the surgical site, to determine the patient's physiologic status and trends, and to identify actual or potential postsurgical problems.[2] A patient who is able to be aroused, is oriented and comfortable, and has stable vital signs for at least 1 hour, meets the criteria for discharge from the PACU.[3] The criteria for discharge from the ambulatory recovery room are similar to that of the PACU and include recovery from sedation or nerve block.[3]

The physical therapist should be aware of common postoperative complications (and the protocols and procedures to address them) to intervene as safely as possible, prioritize the physical therapy plan of care, and modify treatment parameters.

I.   The major systemic effects of general anesthesia are the following:

A.   Neurologic effects. Anesthetic agents decrease cortical and autonomic function.

B.   Cardiovascular effects. Anesthetic agents create the potential for arrhythmia, decreased blood pressure, myocardial contractility, and peripheral vascular resistance.[4]

C.   Respiratory effects[5,6]

1.   Anesthesia has multiple effects on the lung, including decreased or altered

a.   Arterial oxygenation

b.   Response to hypercarbia or hypoxia

c.   Vasomotor tone and airway reflex

d.   Respiratory pattern

e.   Minute ventilation

f.   Functional residual capacity

g.   Mucociliary function

h.   Surfactant

2.   The shape and motion of the chest are altered secondary to decreased muscle tone, which causes the following[1]:

a.   Decreased anteroposterior diameter

b.   Increased lateral diameter

c.   Increased cephalad position of the diaphragm

3.   Other factors that affect respiratory function and increase the risk of postoperative pulmonary complications (e.g., atelectasis, pneumonia, lung collapse) include the following:

a.   Underlying pulmonary disease

b.   Incisional pain, especially if there is a thoracic or abdominal incision

    c.   Smoking history

    d.   Obesity

    e.   Increased age

    f.   The need for large intravenous fluid administration intraoperatively

    g.   Prolonged operative time

II.   During the postsurgical phase, the patient is monitored for the proper function and return of all of the major body systems. The most common postoperative complications include the following[2,3]:

    A.   Neurologic complications

        1.   Delayed arousal, agitation, or altered consciousness

        2.   Cerebral edema, seizure, or stroke

        3.   Peripheral muscle weakness or altered sensation

    B.   Cardiovascular and hematologic complications

        1.   Hypotension, shock, or both

        2.   Hypertension

        3.   Dysrhythmia

        4.   Myocardial infarction

        5.   Hemorrhage

        6.   Deep vein thrombosis

        7.   Pulmonary embolism

    C.   Respiratory complications

        1.   Airway obstruction

        2.   Hypoxemia

        3.   Hypercapnia

        4.   Aspiration of gastric contents

        5.   Hypoventilation

        6.   Pulmonary edema

D. Renal complications

   1. Acute renal failure

   2. Urine retention

   3. Urinary infection

E. Gastrointestinal complications

   1. Nausea and vomiting

   2. Hiccups

   3. Abdominal distention

   4. Paralytic ileus

F. Integumentary complications

   1. Wound infection

   2. Wound dehiscence, evisceration, or both

   3. Hematoma

G. Other complications

   1. Hypothermia

   2. Sepsis

   3. Hyperglycemia

   4. Fluid overload or deficit

   5. Electrolyte imbalance

   6. Acid-base disorders

The development of these conditions in the immediate (up to 12 hours postoperatively) or secondary (the remainder of the hospital stay) postsurgical phase determines further medical-surgical management and treatment parameters. A review of the anesthesia and surgical notes can provide information about the patient's surgical procedure(s) and findings, hemodynamic and general surgical status, unexpected anesthetic effects, operative time, position during surgery, vital signs, electrocardiographic changes, and degree of blood loss.

# References

1. Litwack K. Immediate Postoperative Care: A Problem-Oriented Approach. In JS Vender, BD Spiess (eds), Post-Anesthesia Care. Philadelphia: Saunders, 1992;1.
2. Litwack K. Postoperative Patient. In SM Lewis, MM Heitkemper, SR Dirksen (eds), Surgical Nursing: Assessment and Management of Clinical Problems. St. Louis: Mosby, 2000;390–399.
3. Feeley TW, Macario A. The Postanesthesia Care Unit. In RD Miller (ed), Anesthesia, Vol. 2 (5th ed). Philadelphia: Churchill Livingstone, 2000;2302–2322.
4. Wilson RS. Anesthesia for Thoracic Surgery. In AE Baue, AS Geha, GL Hammond, et al. (eds), Glenn's Thoracic and Cardiovascular Surgery (96th ed). Stamford, CT: Appleton & Lange, 1996;23.
5. Conrad SA, Jayr C, Peper EA. Thoracic Trauma, Surgery, and Perioperative Management. In DB George, RW Light, MA Matthay, RA Matthay (eds), Chest Medicine: Essentials of Pulmonary and Critical Care Medicine (3rd ed). Baltimore: Williams & Wilkins, 1995;629.
6. Benumof JL. Anesthesia for Thoracic Surgery (2nd ed). Philadelphia: Saunders, 1995;94.

# VI

# Pain Management
*Jaime C. Paz*

In the acute care setting, physical therapists encounter patients who are experiencing pain for a variety of reasons, most commonly from surgical intervention. This appendix provides information on tools to evaluate and manage pain that can facilitate the therapist's ability to provide care for a patient.

## Evaluation

The subjective complaint of pain is often difficult to objectify in the clinical setting. However, an effective pain treatment plan depends on an accurate evaluation of the patient's pain.[1,2] Each evaluation requires a complete physical and diagnostic examination of the patient's pain. The goal for evaluation should be toward individualization while maintaining consistency among patients. To assist with this process, various pain rating tools have been developed. Table VI-1 describes some of the pain rating tools that are used in the acute care setting, with the visual analogue and numeric rating scales being the most commonly used.[1,3,4]

Table VI-1. Pain Assessment Tools

| Tool | Description |
| --- | --- |
| Verbal descriptor scales | The patient describes pain by choosing from a list of adjectives representing gradations of pain intensity. |
| Numeric rating scale | The patient picks a number from 0 to 10 to rate his or her pain, with 0 indicating no pain, and 10 indicating the worst pain possible. |
| Visual analog scales | |
| Line scale | The patient marks his or her pain intensity on a 10-cm line, with one end labeled "no pain," and the other end labeled "worst pain possible." |
| Faces scale | The patient chooses one of six faces, portrayed on a scale that depicts graduated levels of distress, to represent his or her pain level. |
| Pain diary | A daily log is kept by the patient denoting pain severity, by using the numeric rating scale, during activities of daily living. |
| | Medication and alcohol use (if out of the hospital), along with emotional responses, are also helpful pieces of information to record. |

Sources: Data from KP Kittelberger, AA LeBel, D Borsook. Assessment of Pain. In D Borsook, AA LeBel, B McPeek (eds), The Massachusetts General Hospital Handbook of Pain Management. Boston: Little Brown, 1996;27; and Carey SJ, Turpin C, Smith J, et al. Improving pain management in an acute care setting: the Crawford Long Hospital of Emory University experience. Orthop Nurs 1997;16(4):29.

---

### Clinical Tip

• The validity of these scales may be improved by asking the patient about his or her current level of pain, rather than asking the patient to speculate about "usual" or "previous" levels of pain.[5]
• The patient's self-reporting of pain is the most accurate indicator of the existence or intensity of his or her pain, or both.[6]

- Be sensitive and respectful to how different cultures perceive pain, as certain cultures may be very stoic about their pain, whereas others are very demonstrative.

## Physical Therapy Considerations for Pain Evaluation

- Be aware of the nonverbal indicators of pain, such as behavior changes, facial expressions, and body language, in patients who have an impaired ability to communicate their pain, as with an unconscious patient or an adult with dementia.

- Monitoring vital signs during the pain evaluation may provide insight into the sympathetic tone of the patient, which can be indicative of their level of pain. This can be performed easily in the intensive care setting, because the patient's hemodynamic status is being continuously monitored.

- The physical therapist should recognize when the patient is weaning from pain medication (e.g., transitioning from intravenous to oral administration), as the patient may complain of increased pain with a concurrent reduced activity tolerance during this time period.

- To optimize consistency in the health care team, the physical therapist should use the same pain rating tool as the medical-surgical team to determine adequacy of pain management.

- Often the best way to communicate the adequacy of a patient's pain management to the nurses or physicians is in terms of the patient's ability to complete a given task or activity (e.g., the patient is effectively coughing and clearing secretions).

## Management

Nonsteroidal anti-inflammatory drugs (Table VI-2) and systemic opioids (Table VI-3) are the most common pharmacologic agents prescribed for postoperative pain. Aspirin and acetaminophen (Tylenol) are also common medications prescribed for pain relief and are categorized as non-narcotic analgesic and antipyretic drugs.[7,8] Alterna-

**Table VI-2.** Nonsteroidal Anti-Inflammatory Drugs

Indications:
  Used as the sole therapy for mild to moderate pain
  For patients with osteoarthritis, rheumatoid arthritis, and dysmenorrhea
  Used in combination with opioids for moderate postoperative pain, especially
    when weaning from stronger medications
  Useful in children younger than 6 mos of age
  Contraindicated in patients undergoing anticoagulation therapy, with peptic
    ulcer disease, or with gastritis
Mechanism of action:
  Accomplish analgesia by inhibiting prostaglandin synthesis, which leads to anti-
    inflammatory effects (Prostaglandin is a potent pain-producing chemical.)
  A useful alternative or adjunct to opioid therapy
General side effects:
  Platelet dysfunction and gastritis, nausea, abdominal pain, anorexia,
    dizziness, and drowsiness
  Severe reactions include nephrotoxicity (dysuria, hematuria) and cholestatic
    hepatitis
Medications: Generic name (trade name)
  Celecoxib (Celebrex)
  Diclofenac potassium (Cataflam)
  Diclofenac sodium (Voltaren, Voltarol)
  Etodolac (Lodine, Lodine XL)
  Fenoprofen calcium (Fenopron, Nalfon)
  Flurbiprofen (Ansaid, Apo-Flurbiprofen, Froben, Ocufen, Opthalmic)
  Ibuprofen (Motrin, Advil, Excedrin, Medipren, Nuprin, Pamprin, Nurofen,
    Pedia Profen, Rafen, Saleto-200, 400, and 600, Trendar)
  Indomethacin (Apo-Indomethacin, Indocin)
  Ketoprofen (Actron, Apo-Keto, Novo-Keto, Orudis, Rhodis)
  Ketorolac tromethamine (Toradol)
    Nabumetone (Relafen, Relifex)
  Naproxen (Naprosyn)
  Naproxen sodium (Aleve)
  Oxaprozin (Daypro)
  Piroxicam (Apo-Piroxicam, Feldene, Novo-Pirocam, Pirox)
  Rofecoxib (Vioxx)
  Sulindac (Aclin, Apo-Sulin, Clinoril, Novo-Sundac, Saldac)
  Tolmetin (Tolectin)

Sources: Data from JC Ballantyne, D Borsook. Postoperative Pain. In D Borsook, AA LeBel, B McPeek (eds), The Massachusetts General Hospital Handbook of Pain Management. Boston: Little, Brown, 1996;247; Nursing 2001 Drug Handbook (21st ed). Springhouse, PA: Springhouse Corporation, 2001;346–367; and L Skidmore-Roth (ed), Mosby's Nursing Drug Reference. St. Louis: Mosby, 2001;56–57, 924.

tives to oral, intravenous, or intramuscular drug delivery for pain are described in Tables VI-4–VI-6. Communication among therapists, nurses, physicians, and patients on the effectiveness of pain management is essential to maximize the patient's comfort. This includes a thorough review of the patient's medical history and the doctor's orders by the physical therapist before prescribing any modalities or therapeutic exercises.

**Table VI-3.** Systemic Opioids

Indication:
    Moderate to severe postoperative pain, can also be used preoperatively
Mechanism of action:
    Blocks transmission of pain from the spinal cord to the cerebrum by interacting with opioid receptors
    Can be administered orally, intravenously, intramuscularly, subcutaneously, and intrathecally
General side effects:
    Decreased gastrointestinal motility, nausea, vomiting, and cramps
    Mood changes and sedation
    Pruritus (itching)
    Urinary retention
    Respiratory and cough depression
    Pupillary constriction
Medications: Generic name (trade name)
    Alfentanil hydrochloride (Alfenta, Rapifen)
    Buprenorphine (Buprenex, Temgesic)
    Butorphanol (Stadol)
    Codeine (Paveral)
    Dezocine (Dalgan)
    Fentanyl (Sublimaze)
    Fentanyl transdermal (Duragesic)
    Hydromorphone (Dilaudid, CD Palladone)
    Levorphanol (Dromoran, Levorphan)
    Meperidine (Demerol, CD Pamergan, CD Pethidine)
    Methadone (Dolophine, Methadose, Physeptone)
    Morphine (MS Contin, Roxanol, Anamorph, Astramorph, Morcap, Duramorph, Epimorph, Infumorph, Oramorph, Rescudose, Statex)
    Nalbuphine (Nubain)
    Naloxone (Narcan)
    Oxycodone (Roxicodone, Supeudol, Endodan, Tylox, Percocet, Percodan)
    Oxymorphone (Numorphan)
    Pentazocine (Fortral, Talwin)

**Table VI-3.** *Continued*

Propoxyphene (Darvon, Dolene, Doloxene, Novo-Propoxyn)
Remifentanil (Ultiva)
Sufentanil citrate (Sufenta)
Tramadol hydrochloride (Ultram, Zamadol, Zydol)

Sources: Data from JC Ballantyne, D Borsook. Postoperative Pain. In D Borsook, AA LeBel, B McPeek (eds), The Massachusetts General Hospital Handbook of Pain Management. Boston: Little, Brown, 1996;249; and HL Fields (ed). Pain. New York: McGraw-Hill, 1987;253; Nursing 2001 Drug Handbook (21st ed). Springhouse, PA: Springhouse Corporation, 2001;368–392; and L Skidmore-Roth (ed). Mosby's Nursing Drug Reference. St. Louis: Mosby, 2001;58–59.

**Table VI-4.** Epidural Catheters

Indications:
  Surgeries of the thorax or upper and lower abdomen, especially in patients
    with significant pulmonary disease
  Surgery of the lower extremity, especially when early mobilization is important
  Vascular procedures of the lower extremity, when sympathetic blocks are used
Mechanism of action:
  Prevent transmission of pain signals to the cerebrum at the spinal level with a
    catheter that is placed in the epidural space.
  A mixture of opioids and local anesthetics is often used. This drug combin-
    ation provides a synergistic effect for pain relief with a decreased incidence
    of side effects.
  If patients do experience adverse side effects, nonsteroidal anti-inflammatory
    drugs can be added to the mixture, and the dosages of the opioids or local
    anesthetics are reduced.
General side effects:
  Epidural opioids
    Pruritus (itching), nausea, sedation and respiratory depression, decreased
      gastrointestinal motility
  Local anesthetics
    Hypotension, temporary lower-extremity weakness, urine retention,
      local anesthetic toxicity (ringing in the ears, metallic taste, slow
      speech, irritability, cardiac arrhythmias, and seizures)
Medications: Generic (trade name)
  Epidural opioids
    Morphine, fentanyl, sufentanil, alfentanil, hydromorphone (Dilaudid),
      and meperidine (Demerol)

Local anesthetics
  Bupivacaine, ropivacaine (Naropin), or articaine combined with
    epinephrine
Nonsteroidal anti-inflammatory drugs
  Acetaminophen, ketorolac (Toradol), or ibuprofen

Sources: Data from JC Ballantyne, D Borsook. Postoperative Pain. In D Borsook, AA
LeBel, B McPeek (eds), The Massachusetts General Hospital Handbook of Pain Management. Boston: Little, Brown, 1996;252; C Pasero, M McCaffery. Providing epidural
analgesia. Nursing 1999;29(8):34; and WM Davis, MC Vinson. New drug approvals
of 2000, part 2. Drug Topics 2001;145(5):89.

**Table VI-5.** Patient-Controlled Analgesia

---

Indication:
  Used for moderate to severe postoperative pain in patients who are capable
    of properly using the pump
Mechanism of action:
  A microprocessor pump that controls infusion of pain medicine,
    usually through an intravenous line.
  Dosage, dosage intervals, maximum dosage per set time, and background
    (basal) infusion rate can be programmed.
  Patient is provided with a button that allows for self-dosing of pain
    medication as needed.
Considerations:
  Preoperative education of the patient on the use of patient-controlled
    analgesia
  Ensuring that only the patient doses him- or herself
General side effects:
  Similar to those of opioids (Table VI-3)
Medications: Generic (trade name)
  Morphine is the drug of choice.
  Dilaudid or meperidine (when morphine is contraindicated or has failed to
    relieve pain).

---

Sources: Data from JC Ballantyne, D Borsook. Postoperative Pain. In D Borsook, AA
LeBel, B McPeek (eds), The Massachusetts General Hospital Handbook of Pain Management. Boston: Little, Brown, 1996;254; CL White, RP Pokrupa, MH Chan. An
evaluation of the effectiveness of patient-controlled analgesia after spinal surgery. J
Neurosci Nurs 1998;30(4):225; and K Hoare, KH Sousa, L Person, et al. Comparing
three patient controlled analgesia methods. Medsurg Nurs 2000;9(1):33.

Table VI-6.  Implanted Pump

---

Indication:
  For patients with chronic pain, as a last resort before ablative surgery
Mechanism of action:
  A pump, approximately the size of a hockey puck, is surgically implanted
  into the subcutaneous tissue in the lower right or left abdominal quadrant.
  A catheter, which is placed in the epidural or intrathecal space, is tunneled
  subcutaneously along the flank and connected to the pump.
  Pumps are programmable or nonprogrammable and require refilling every 2–
  12 wks.
Consideration:
  Generally performed as an outpatient procedure, but patients may remain in
  the hospital for several days for observation
General side effects:
  Similar to systemic opioids (Table VI-3)
Medications: Generic (trade name)
  Morphine or hydromorphone (Dilaudid)

---

Sources: Data from L Valentino, KV Pillay, J Walker. Managing chronic nonmalignant pain with continuous intrathecal morphine. J Neurosci Nurs 1998;30(4):233; and M York, JA Paice. Treatment of low back pain with intraspinal opioids delivered via implanted pumps. Orthop Nurs 1998;17(3);61.

## Physical Therapy Considerations for Pain Management

• The physical therapist should be aware of the patient's pain medication schedule and the duration of the effectiveness of different pain medications when scheduling treatment sessions. (Pharmacist, nurse, physician, and medication reference books are good resources.)

• The physical therapist should also use a pillow, blanket, or his or her hands to splint or support a painful area, such as an abdominal or thoracic incision or rib fractures when the patient coughs or performs functional mobility tasks, such as going from side-lying to sitting at the edge of the bed.

• The physical therapist can also use a corset, binder, or brace to support a painful area during intervention sessions that focus on functional mobility.

• The physical therapist should instruct the patient not to hold his or her breath during mobility, because doing so increases pain.

# References

1. Kittelberger KP, LeBel AA, Borsook D. Assessment of Pain. In D Borsook, AA LeBel, B McPeek (eds), The Massachusetts General Hospital Handbook of Pain Management. Boston: Little, Brown, 1996;26.
2. Cristoph SD. Pain assessment: the problem of pain in the critically ill patient. Crit Care Nurs Clin N Am 1991;3(1):11–16.
3. Carey SJ, Turpin C, Smith J, et al. Improving pain management in an acute care setting: the Crawford Long Hospital of Emory University experience. Orthop Nurs 1997;16(4):29.
4. Haggell P. Pain management. J Neurosci Nurs 1999;31(4):251.
5. Turk DC, Okifuji A. Assessment of patients' reporting of pain: an integrated perspective. Lancet 1999;353(9166):1784.
6. Acello B. Meeting JCAHO standards for pain control. Nursing 2000;30(3):52–54.
7. Nursing 2001 Drug Handbook (21st ed). Springhouse, PA: Springhouse Corporation, 2001;337–342.
8. Skidmore-Roth L (ed). Mosby's Nursing Drug Reference. St. Louis: Mosby, 2001;70, 135.

# VII

# Amputation

*Jason D. Rand and Jaime C. Paz*

## Introduction

This appendix describes the most common types of lower- and upper-extremity amputations. The etiology of these amputations and the physical therapy management that is pertinent to the acute care setting are described. Although the incidence of upper-extremity (UE) amputation is quite low compared to lower-extremity (LE) amputation, it is important that the acute care physical therapist have an understanding of all types of amputations to properly plan for the evaluation and treatment of the patient.

## Lower-Extremity Amputation

Peripheral vascular disease accounts for approximately 85–90% of LE amputations in the developed world, with 25–50% of this percentage resulting from diabetes mellitus.[1] Refer to Chapter 11 for more information on the complications of diabetes mellitus. Trauma is the second highest cause of amputation in developed countries and is the primary cause in developing parts of the world.[1] Traumatic amputation often results from environmental injury or land mines in various parts of the world.[1] The various locations of LE amputation are shown in Figure VII-1 and are described in Table VII-1.

## Upper-Extremity Amputation

UE amputation is most often the result of trauma, such as automobile or industrial accidents.[1] Disease and congenital limb deficiency are also major causes of UE amputation.[2] Despite peripheral vascular disease being a major cause of LE amputation, it often does not create the need for UE amputation.[1] The various locations of UE amputations are shown in Figure VII-1 and are described in Table VII-2.

## Physical Therapy Intervention for Patients with an Amputation

The focus of physical therapy intervention in the acute care setting is on preprosthetic evaluation and training. Prosthetic training, if appropriate, most often occurs in the subacute or home setting. The primary components of the evaluation for a patient who is status post amputation in the acute care setting are the following[3]:

- The onset and type of amputation
- Premorbid lifestyle and functional mobility
- Current level of functional mobility
- Discharge plans

Table VII-3 outlines general physical therapy considerations and treatment suggestions for the care of patients who experience UE or LE amputations. Table VII-4 outlines specific clinical concerns for these patients.

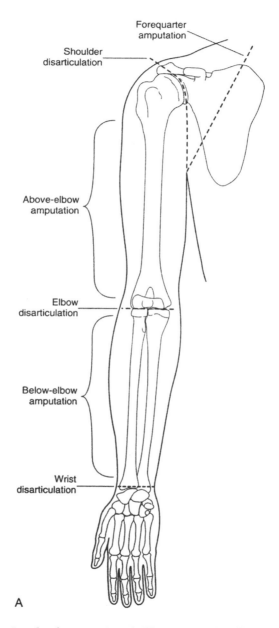

**Figure VII-1.**  *Levels of amputation. A. Upper extremity. (Reprinted with permission from AB Maher, SW Salmond, TA Pellino [eds]. Orthopaedic Nursing [2nd ed]. Philadelphia: Saunders, 1998;724.)*

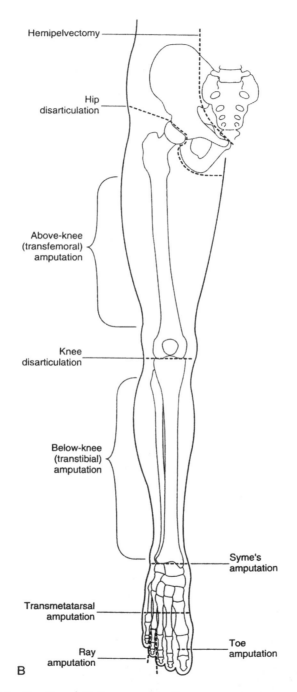

Figure VII-1. *Continued. B. Lower extremity.*

Table VII-1. Types of Lower-Extremity Amputations*

| Type | Description |
|------|-------------|
| Ray | Single or multiple rays can be amputated depending on the patient's diagnosis. If the first ray is amputated, balance is often affected, as weight is transferred to the lateral border of the foot, which may also cause ulceration and skin break down. Postoperative weight-bearing status will range from non-weight bearing to partial weight bearing according to the physician's orders. |
| Transmetatarsal | The metatarsal bones are transected with this procedure as compared to other types of partial foot amputations, which may disarticulate the metatarsals from the cuboid and cuneiform bones. Balance is maintained with a transmetatarsal amputation, because the residual limb is symmetric in shape and major muscles remain intact. An adaptive shoe with a rocker-bottom is used to help facilitate push-off in gait. |
| Syme's amputation (ankle disarticulation) | Often performed with traumatic and infectious cases, this type of amputation is preferred to more distal, partial foot amputations (Ray and transmetatarsal) because of the ease of prosthetic management at this level. Patients may ambulate with or without a prosthesis. |
| Below the knee (transtibial) | Ideal site for amputation for patients with a variety of diagnoses. Increased success rate with prosthetic use. In cases with vascular compromise, the residual limb may be slow to heal. Residual limb length ranges from 12.5 cm to 17.5 cm from the knee joint. |
| Through-the-knee (disarticulation) | Often performed on elderly and young patients. Maximum prosthetic control can be achieved with this procedure because of the ability to fully bear weight on the residual limb. Also, a long muscular lever arm and intact hip musculature contribute to great prosthetic mobility. The intact femoral condyles, however, leave a cosmetically poor residual limb. |
| Above the knee (transfemoral) | Traditional transfemoral amputation preserves 50–66% of femoral length. Prosthetic ambulation with an artificial knee joint requires increased metabolic demand. |
| Hip disarticulation (femoral head from acetabulum) | Often performed in cases of trauma or malignancy. The pelvis remains intact; however, patients may experience slow wound heeling and may require secondary grafting to fully close the amputation site. |

**Table VII-1.** *Continued*

| Type | Description |
| --- | --- |
| Hemipelvectomy (half of the pelvis is removed along with the entire lower limb) | Also indicated in cases of malignancy. A muscle flap covers the internal organs. |

*Unless otherwise stated, the etiology of these amputations is from peripheral vascular disease.
Sources: Data from A Thompson, A Skinner, J Piercy (eds). Tidy's Physiotherapy (12th ed). Oxford, UK: Butterworth–Heinemann, 1992;260; B Engstrom, C Van de Ven (eds). Therapy for Amputees (3rd ed). Edinburgh, UK: Churchill Livingstone, 1999;208, 187–188, 149–150; B May (ed). Amputations and Prosthetics: A Case Study Approach. Philadelphia: FA Davis, 1996;62–63; G Sanders (ed). Lower Limb Amputations: A Guide to Rehabilitation. Philadelphia: FA Davis, 1986;101–102; M Lusardi, C Nielsen (eds). Orthotics and Prosthetics in Rehabilitation. Boston: Butterworth–Heinemann, 2000; 370–373; and JE Edelstein. Prosthetic Assessment and Management. In SB O'Sullivan, TJ Schmitz (eds), Physical Rehabilitation; Assessment and Treatment (4th ed). Philadelphia: FA Davis, 2001;645–673.

**Table VII-2.** Types of Upper-Extremity Amputations*

| Type | Description |
| --- | --- |
| Transmetacarpal | Only the affected regions are removed; remaining digits are preserved to spare as much function as possible. With amputations of the fifth metacarpal, hand function is seriously compromised, especially for tasks such as grasping. |
| Wrist disarticulation | Distal radial ulnar joint function is often retained to maintain rotation of the radius. |
| Transradial | Optimum residual limb length for eventual prosthetic fitting is 8 cm above the ulnar styloid. Active prosthetic devices are operated by elbow extension and shoulder flexion, shoulder girdle protraction, or both. |
| Elbow disarticulation | Not a choice location for amputation secondary to the poor cosmetic look created and decreased postsurgical function of the prosthesis. |

| Type | Description |
|------|-------------|
| Transhumeral | Often performed as a result of primary malignancy or metastatic disease. Optimum residual limb length for eventual prosthetic fitting is 10 cm above the elbow joint. |
| Shoulder disarticulation | Often performed as a result of primary maligancy or metastatic disease. The head of humerus is maintained, or the acromion process and clavicle are trimmed to create a rounded appearance. |
| Forequarter | Often performed as a result of primary malignancy or metastatic disease. Consists of removal of the patient's clavicle, scapula, and arm. |

*Unless otherwise stated, the etiology of these amputations is from trauma.
Sources: Data from B Engstrom, C Van de Ven (eds). Therapy for Amputees (3rd ed). Edinburgh, UK: Churchill Livingstone, 1999;243–257; M Lusardi, C Nielsen (eds). Orthotics and Prosthetics in Rehabilitation. Boston: Butterworth–Heinemann, 2000;573; SN Banerjee (ed). Rehabilitation Management of Amputees. Baltimore: Williams & Wilkins, 1982;30–33; and R Ham, L Cotton (eds). Limb Amputation: From Aetiology to Rehabilitation. London: Chapman & Hall, 1991;136–143.

**Table VII-3.** General Physical Therapy Considerations and Treatment Suggestions

| Considerations | Treatment Suggestions |
|----------------|-----------------------|
| Psychological impact of amputation | Patients who undergo an amputation, especially of the upper extremity, often experience psychological changes during the acute stage of their care. Patients may experience grief, anger, denial, and sadness. It is important to establish a rapport with the patient based on trust and respect. To help the patient regain his or her self-esteem, encourage him or her to take an active role in the therapy session, and highlight successes in therapy. The physical therapist should request a psychiatric or social service consult if the patient's psychosocial issues are interfering with physical therapy intervention. |
| Residual limb edema | Physical therapy techniques may involve the use of ace wraps, shrinker socks, rigid dressings (lower extremity), or a combination of these according to the patient's needs along with the physician's or facility's protocols. |

Table VII-3. *Continued*

| Considerations | Treatment Suggestions |
| --- | --- |
| | Safe residual limb wrapping involves the use of a figure eight or angular pattern, anchoring turns around the most proximal joint, increased distal pressure, and a smooth or wrinkle-free application. |
| | The physical therapist should elevate the residual limb in a position that prevents joint contracture formation. |
| | In patients with upper-extremity amputation, a sling may be used to help manage edema. |
| Phantom limb pain | Often described as a cramping, squeezing, shooting, or burning pain felt in the part of the extremity that has been removed. The physical therapist may use desensitizing techniques (e.g., massaging the residual limb), exercise, hot and cold therapy, electrical stimulation, or other modalities when phantom limb pain is determined as the cause of the patient's pain. |
| Hypersensitivity | Patient should be encouraged to rub the residual limb with increasing pressure as tolerated. |
| Skin condition | Ensure stability of new incision(s) before, during, and after physical therapy intervention. Examine the incision for any changes in the appearance (size, shape, open areas, color), temperature, and moisture level. Instruct patient and nursing staff on importance of frequent position changes to prevent skin breakdown. Implement out-of-bed activities as soon as possible. Instruct patient in active movements and bed mobility activities such as bridging, rolling, and moving up and down in the bed. |

Sources: Data from B Engstrom, C Van de Ven (eds). Therapy for Amputees (3rd ed). Edinburgh, UK: Churchill Livingstone, 1999;27–37, 43–45; B May (ed). Amputations and Prosthetics: A Case Study Approach. Philadelphia: FA Davis, 1996;73, 86–88; and SN Banerjee (ed). Rehabilitation Management of Amputees. Baltimore: Williams & Wilkins, 1982;30–33, 255–258.

**Table VII-4.**  Specific Considerations and Treatment Suggestions for
Patients with Upper- or Lower-Extremity Amputation

| Consideration | Treatment Suggestions |
|---|---|
| Joint contracture | Upper extremity<br>Physical therapy should consist of active movements of all of the joints above the level of the amputation, including movements of the scapula. Patients who use upper-extremity slings to fixate the arm in elbow flexion and shoulder internal rotation should be examined regularly for contractures.<br>Lower extremity<br>The physical therapist should provide the patient and members of the nursing staff with education on residual limb positioning, proper pillow placement, and the use of splint boards.<br>Patients with a below-the-knee amputation will be most susceptible to knee flexion contraction. A pillow should be placed under the tibia rather than under the knee to promote extension.<br>Patients with above-the-knee amputations or disarticulations will be most susceptible to hip flexor and abductor contractures.<br>The physical therapist should begin active range-of-motion exercises and provide passive stretching as indicated. |
| Decreased functional mobility | Upper extremity<br>During ambulation, patients tend to flex their trunk toward the side of the amputation and maintain a stiff gait pattern that lacks normal arm swing. Patients often need gait, balance, posture retraining, or a combination of these.<br>It is important to work on active movements, specifically the movements that might be used for powering a prosthesis, such as in the following:<br>Transradial body powered prosthesis: elbow extension, shoulder flexion, shoulder girdle protraction, or a combination of these<br>Transhumeral body powered prosthesis: elbow flexion, shoulder extension, internal rotation, abduction and shoulder girdle protraction and depression. |

**Table VII-4.** *Continued*

| Consideration | Treatment Suggestions |
| --- | --- |
| | Lower extremity<br>Techniques should range from bed mobility training to transfer training to ambulation or wheelchair mobility. Patients with bilateral above-knee amputations will need a custom wheelchair that places the rear axle in a more posterior position to compensate for the alteration in the patient's center of gravity when sitting. |

Sources: Data from LA Karacoloff, FJ Schneider (eds). Lower Extremity Amputation: A guide to Functional Outcomes in Physical Therapy Management. Rockville, MD: Aspen, 1985; B Engstrom, C Van de Ven (eds). Therapy for Amputees (3rd ed). Edinburgh, UK: Churchill Livingstone, 1999;27–37, 43–45, 243–257; B May (ed). Amputations and Prosthetics: A Case Study Approach. Philadelphia: FA Davis, 1996;86–88; SN Banerjee (ed). Rehabilitation Management of Amputees. Baltimore: Williams & Wilkins, 1982;30–33, 255–258; and R Ham, L Cotton (eds). Limb Amputation: From Aetiology to Rehabilitation. London: Chapman & Hall, 1991;136–143.

# References

1. Engstrom B, Van de Ven C (eds). Therapy for Amputees (3rd ed). Edinburgh, UK: Churchill Livingstone, 1999;27–37, 43–45, 149–150, 187–188, 208.
2. Karacoloff LA, Schneider FJ (eds). Lower Extremity Amputation: A Guide to Functional Outcomes in Physical Therapy Management. Rockville, MD: Aspen, 1985.
3. Thompson A, Skinner A, Piercy J (eds). Tidy's Physiotherapy (12th ed). Oxford, UK: Butterworth–Heinemann, 1992;260.

# VIII

# Postural Drainage
*Michele P. West*

Postural drainage is the positioning of a patient with an involved lung segment as close to perpendicular to the floor as possible to facilitate the drainage of bronchopulmonary secretions.[1] Figure VIII-1 demonstrates the various postural drainage positions most applicable in the acute care setting. The use of postural drainage as an adjunct to other techniques (mainly breathing and coughing exercises, vibration, shaking, and percussion) can be highly effective for mobilizing retained secretions and maximizing gas exchange. The physical therapist should note that there are many clinical contraindications and considerations for postural drainage that may require position modification to maximize patient safety, comfort, and tolerance.

The contraindications for the use of Trendelenburg (placing the head of the bed in a downward position) include the following[2,3]:

- Patients in which an increase in intracranial pressure should be avoided
- Uncontrolled hypertension
- Uncontrolled or unprotected airway with a risk of aspiration
- Recent gross hemoptysis

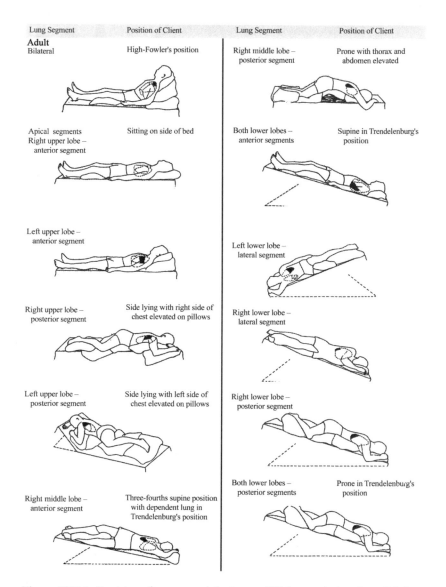

| Lung Segment | Position of Client | Lung Segment | Position of Client |
|---|---|---|---|
| **Adult**<br>Bilateral | High-Fowler's position | Right middle lobe –<br>posterior segment | Prone with thorax and<br>abdomen elevated |
| Apical segments<br>Right upper lobe –<br>anterior segment | Sitting on side of bed | Both lower lobes –<br>anterior segments | Supine in Trendelenburg's<br>position |
| Left upper lobe –<br>anterior segment | | Left lower lobe –<br>lateral segment | |
| Right upper lobe –<br>posterior segment | Side lying with right side of<br>chest elevated on pillows | Right lower lobe –<br>lateral segment | |
| Left upper lobe –<br>posterior segment | Side lying with left side of<br>chest elevated on pillows | Right lower lobe –<br>posterior segment | |
| Right middle lobe –<br>anterior segment | Three-fourths supine position<br>with dependent lung in<br>Trendelenburg's position | Both lower lobes –<br>posterior segments | Prone in Trendelenburg's<br>position |

**Figure VIII-1.** *Positions for postural drainage. (With permission from PA Potter, AG Perry. Fundamentals of Nursing [5th ed]. St. Louis: Mosby, 2001; 1165.)*

- Recent esophageal surgery

- Significantly distended abdomen

- Orthopnea

The contraindications for reverse Trendelenburg (placing the head of the bed in an upward position) include the following[3]:

- Hypotension

- Use of vasoactive medications

The following are contraindications for postural drainage in conjunction with other bronchopulmonary hygiene techniques.[2,3] In some conditions, such as pleural effusion, postural drainage in the upright sitting position may be acceptable. *The use of postural drainage with or without other bronchopulmonary techniques should be considered on the severity of the condition on an individual patient basis.*

- Acute hemorrhage with hemodynamic instability

- Acute hemoptysis

- Unstabilized head or neck injury

- Intracranial pressure greater than 20 mm Hg

- Unstable cardiac dysrhythmia

- Bronchopleural fistula

- Large pleural effusion

- Unstable pneumothorax

- Subcutaneous emphysema (air in the subcutaneous tissue)

- Pulmonary embolism

- Pulmonary edema or congestive heart failure

Physical therapy considerations and clinical tips for the use of postural drainage include the following:

- The timing of postural drainage after pain medication or bronchodilators can improve its effectiveness.

• Monitor vital signs with position changes to evaluate patient tolerance, especially for critically ill patients or those status post cardiothoracic surgery with a history of blood pressure and heart rate changes when turned to one side.

• Modify the position of the patient if anxiety, pain, skin breakdown, abnormal posture, decreased range of motion, or positioning restrictions exist.

• To improve patient tolerance of postural drainage, consider modifying the time spent in each position, the angle of the bed, or patient position.

• Provide time for the patient to rest or become acclimated to position changes if necessary.

• Use pillows, blankets, foam rolls, or wedges to maximize comfort or provide pressure relief.

• Bed mobility training can be incorporated during position changes with patients who have decreased independence with rolling or supine-to-sit transfers.

• Have a good working knowledge of the controls on the patient's bed that are needed to position the patient for postural drainage. Each bed model, especially pressure relief or rotating beds, has different controls, locks, and alarms.

## References

1. Starr JA. Chronic Pulmonary Dysfunction. In B O'Sullivan, TJ Schmitz (eds), Physical Rehabilitation: Assessment and Treatment. Philadelphia: FA Davis, 2001;461.
2. Downs AM. Physiological Basis for Airway Clearance Techniques. In D Frownfelter, E Dean (eds), Principles and Practice of Cardiopulmonary Physical Therapy (3rd ed). St. Louis: Mosby, 1996;330–331.
3. Hess DR, Branson RD. Chest Physiotherapy, Incentive Spirometry, Intermittent Positive-Pressure Breathing, Secretion Clearance, and Inspiratory Muscle Training. In RD Branson, DR Hess, RL Chatburn (eds), Respiratory Care Equipment (2nd ed). Philadelphia: Lippincott Williams & Wilkins, 1999;340.

# IX

# Functional Tests
*Jennifer A. Silva and Jaime C. Paz*

## Introduction

The purpose of this appendix is to describe various objective measures that can be used to determine the functional levels of various patient populations in the acute care setting. The timed "up and go" test, Berg balance scale (BBS), Tinetti performance oriented mobility assessment (POMA), functional reach test, and the 6-minute walk test will be reviewed here. These functional tests were selected because of their ease of use, reliable and valid test results, and the population that can use these tests in the acute care setting. All of these tests showed high inter-rater (tested by different therapists) and intrarater (retested over time by a single therapist) reliability.[1] These tests also show high content,* construct,† and predictive‡ validity unless otherwise noted in the respective description of each test.

---

*Content validity*: Degree in which a test actually measures what it was designed for.[1]

†*Construct validity*: Degree to which a theoretical construct is measured against the test.[1]

‡*Predictive validity*: Ability of a test to predict future performance.[1]

## Berg Balance Scale

The BBS is a 56-point scale that evaluates 14 tasks. Katherine Berg developed this test to assess the level of function and balance in various patient populations.[2]

### Procedure

The patient is evaluated and graded on a sequence of balance activities, such as sitting unsupported with arms folded, rising, standing, and transferring between one surface and another, reaching forward in standing, picking up objects off the floor, turning around in a full circle, and standing on one leg.[2] Figure IX-1 outlines the evaluation form for this test. Table IX-1 describes the appropriate population, required equipment, completion time, reliability, and validity of the BBS.

Scoring for each task ranges from 0 to 4. A score of 0 indicates that the patient is unable to complete a particular task. A score of 4 indicates that the patient can completely carry out the task.[2]

### Interpretation of Results

A total score of less than 45 predicts that the patient is at risk for falls.[3,4] In contrast, higher scores on the BBS indicate greater independence and better ability to balance.[5]

## Timed "Up and Go" Test

The "get up and go" test was originally developed in 1986 to serve as a clinical measure of balance in elderly people.[6] The original test used a numeric scoring system to determine a patient's level of balance but was later modified to a timed version by Posiadlo and Richardson in 1991.[7] The timed "up and go" test uses a time score to assess gait and balance in the elderly population[8] and is summarized in Table IX-2.

### Procedure

The patient is timed during a five-part mobility task from start to finish. The task consists of the following[9]:

1. Rising from an armchair

2. Walking 3 m

3. Turning around

# BALANCE SCALE

Name_____    Date_____

Location_____    Rate_____

Item    Description                                    Score (0–4)

1. Sitting to standing                                 _____
2. Standing unsupported                                _____
3. Sitting unsupported                                 _____
4. Standing to sitting                                 _____
5. Transfers                                           _____
6. Standing with eyes closed                           _____
7. Standing with feet together                         _____
8. Reaching forward with outstretched arm              _____
9. Retrieving object from floor                        _____
10. Turning to look behind                             _____
11. Turning 360 degrees                                _____
12. Placing alternate foot on stool                    _____
13. Standing with one foot in front                    _____
14. Standing on one foot                               _____

                                            Total      _____

## GENERAL INSTRUCTIONS

Please demonstrate each task and/or give instructions as written. When scoring, please record the lowest response category that applies for each item. In most items, the subject is asked to maintain a given position for a specific time. Progressively more points are deducted if the time or distance requirements are not met, if the subject's performance warrants supervision, or if the subject touches an external support or receives assistance from the examiner. Subjects should understand that they must maintain their balance while attempting the tasks. The choices of which leg to stand on or how far to reach are left to the subject. Poor judgment will adversely influence the performance and the scoring.

Figure IX-1. *Berg Balance Scale. Reprinted with permission of Katherine Berg. (Data from S Wood-Dauphinee, K Berg, G Bravo, JI Williams. The balance scale: responding to clinically meaningful changes. Can J Rehabil 1997;10:35–50; K Berg, S Wood-Dauphinee, JI Williams. The balance scale: reliability assessment for elderly residents and patients with an acute stroke. Scand J Rehab Med 1995;27:27–36; K Berg, B Maki, JI Williams, et al. A comparison of clinical and laboratory measures of postural balance in an elderly population. Arch Phys Med Rehabil 1992;73:1073–1083; K Berg, S Wood-Dauphinee, JI Williams, B Maki. Measuring balance in the elderly: validation of an instrument. Can J Public Health 1992;[suppl 2]:S7–S11; and K Berg, S Wood-Dauphinee, JI Williams, D Gayton. Measuring balance in the elderly: preliminary development of an instrument. Physiother Can 1989;41:304–311.)*

Equipment required for testing are a stopwatch or watch with a second hand, and a ruler or other indicator of 2, 5, and 10 in. (5, 12.5, and 25 cm). Chairs used during testing should be of reasonable height. Either a step or a stool (of average step height) may be used for item #12.

1. **Sitting to Standing**
   Instructions: Please stand up. Try not to use your hands for support.
   ( ) 4 able to stand without using hands and stabilize independently
   ( ) 3 able to stand independently using hands
   ( ) 2 able to stand using hands after several tries
   ( ) 1 needs minimal aid to stand or to stabilize
   ( ) 0 needs moderate or maximal assist to stand

2. **Standing Unsupported**
   Instructions: Please stand for 2 minutes without holding.
   ( ) 4 able to stand safely 2 minutes
   ( ) 3 able to stand 2 minutes with supervision
   ( ) 2 able to stand 30 seconds unsupported
   ( ) 1 needs several tries to stand 30 seconds unsupported
   ( ) 0 unable to stand 30 seconds unassisted
   *If a subject is able to stand 2 minutes unsupported, score full points for sitting unsupported. Proceed to item #4.*

3. **Sitting with Back Unsupported But Feet Supported on Floor or on a Stool**
   Instructions: Please sit with arms folded for 2 minutes.
   ( ) 4 able to sit safely and securely 2 minutes
   ( ) 3 able to sit 2 minutes under supervision
   ( ) 2 able to sit 30 seconds
   ( ) 1 able to sit 10 seconds
   ( ) 0 unable to sit without support 10 seconds

4. **Standing to Sitting**
   Instructions: Please sit down.
   ( ) 4 sits safely with minimal use of hands
   ( ) 3 controls descent by using hands
   ( ) 2 uses back of legs against chair to control descent
   ( ) 1 sits independently but has uncontrolled descent
   ( ) 0 needs assistance to sit

5. **Transfers**
   Instructions: Arrange chair(s) for a pivot transfer. Ask subject to transfer one way toward a seat with armrests and one way toward a seat without armrests. You may use two chairs (one with and one without armrests) or a bed and a chair.

**Figure IX-1.** *Continued*

( ) 4 able to transfer safely with minor use of hands
( ) 3 able to transfer safely definite need of hands
( ) 2 able to transfer with verbal cueing and/or supervision
( ) 1 needs one person to assist
( ) 0 needs two people to assist or supervise to be safe

6.  **Standing Unsupported with Eyes Closed**
Instructions: Please close your eyes and stand still for 10 seconds.
( ) 4 able to stand 10 seconds safely
( ) 3 able to stand 10 seconds with supervision
( ) 2 able to stand 3 seconds
( ) 1 unable to keep eyes closed 3 seconds but stays steady
( ) 0 needs help to keep from falling

7.  **Standing Unsupported with Feet Together**
Instructions: Place your feet together and stand without holding.
( ) 4 able to place feet together independently and stand 1 minute safely
( ) 3 able to place feet together independently and stand for 1 minute with
supervision
( ) 2 able to place feet together independently and to hold for 30 seconds
( ) 1 needs help to attain position but able to stand 15 seconds feet
together
( ) 0 needs help to attain position and unable to hold for 15 seconds

8.  **Reaching Forward with Outstretched Arm while Standing**
Instructions: Lift arm to 90 degrees. Stretch out your fingers and reach
forward as far as you can. (Examiner places a ruler at end of fingertips when
arm is at 90 degrees. Fingers should not touch the ruler while reaching
forward. The recorded measure is the distance forward that the fingers reach
while the subject is in the most forward lean position. When possible, ask
subject to use both arms when reaching to avoid rotation of the trunk.)
( ) 4 can reach forward confidently >25 cm (10 in.)
( ) 3 can reach forward >12.5 cm safely (5 in.)
( ) 2 can reach forward >5 cm safely (2 in.)
( ) 1 reaches forward but needs supervision
( ) 0 loses balance while trying, requires external support

9.  **Pick Up Object from the Floor from a Standing Position**
Instructions: Pick up the shoe/slipper that is placed in front of your feet.
( ) 4 able to pick up slipper safely and easily
( ) 3 able to pick up slipper but needs supervision
( ) 2 unable to pick up but reaches 2–5 cm (1–2 in.) from slipper and
keeps balance independently
( ) 1 unable to pick up and needs supervision while trying
( ) 0 unable to try, needs assist to keep from losing balance or falling

**10. Turning to Look Behind Over Left and Right Shoulders while Standing**

Instructions: Turn to look *directly* behind you over left shoulder. Repeat to the right.

Examiner may pick an object to look at directly behind the subject to encourage a better twist turn.

( ) 4 looks behind from both sides and weight shifts well
( ) 3 looks behind one side only, other side shows less weight shift
( ) 2 turns sideways only but maintains balance
( ) 1 needs supervision when turning
( ) 0 needs assist to keep from losing balance or falling

**11. Turn 360 Degrees**

Instructions: Turn completely around in a full circle. Pause. Then turn a full circle in the other direction.

( ) 4 able to turn 360 degrees safely in 4 seconds or less
( ) 3 able to turn 360 degrees safely one side only in 4 seconds or less
( ) 2 able to turn 360 degrees safely but slowly
( ) 1 needs close supervision or verbal cueing
( ) 0 needs assistance while turning

**12. Placing Alternate Foot on Step or Stool while Standing Unsupported**

Instructions: Place each foot alternately on the step/stool. Continue until each foot has touched the step/stool four times.

( ) 4 able to stand independently and safely and complete 8 steps in 20 seconds
( ) 3 able to stand independently and complete 8 steps >20 seconds
( ) 2 able to complete 4 steps without aid with supervision
( ) 1 able to complete >2 steps, needs minimal assist
( ) 0 needs assistance to keep from falling, unable to try

**13. Standing Unsupported with One Foot in Front**

Instructions: (demonstrate to subject)

Place one foot directly in front of the other. If you think that you cannot place your foot directly in front, try to step far enough ahead that the heel of your forward foot is ahead of the toes of the other foot. (To score 3 points, the length of the step should exceed the length of the other foot and the width of the stance should approximate the subject's normal stride width.)

( ) 4 able to place foot tandem independently and hold 30 seconds
( ) 3 able to place foot ahead of other independently and hold 30 seconds
( ) 2 able to take small step independently and hold 30 seconds
( ) 1 needs help to step but can hold 15 seconds
( ) 0 loses balance while stepping or standing

Figure IX-1. *Continued*

---

**14. Standing on One Leg**

Instructions: Stand on one leg as long as you can without holding.

( ) 4 able to lift leg independently and hold >10 seconds
( ) 3 able to lift leg independently and hold 5–10 seconds
( ) 2 able to lift leg independently and hold ≥3 seconds
( ) 1 tries to lift leg unable to hold 3 seconds but remains standing
    independently
( ) 0 unable to try or needs assist to prevent fall

**(  ) Total Score (maximum = 56)**

---

Table IX-1. Overview of the Berg Balance Scale

| Population | Equipment | Time | Reliability | Validity |
|---|---|---|---|---|
| Elderly patients who have sustained acute cerebrovascular accident and/or are in a rehabilitation setting | Ruler Stopwatch Chair Step stool Flat surface | 10–20 mins required to complete test | Inter-rater reliability: ICC = 0.98 rs = 0.88 Intrarater reliability: ICC = 0.98 Internal consistency: Cronbach's alpha = 0.96 | Concurrent validity: Tinetti, r = 0.91 Get up and go, r = –0.76 Predictive validity: <45 score predicts falls |

ICC = intraclass correlation coefficient; r = correlation coefficient; rs = Spearman's rank correlation coefficient.

Sources: Data from S Whitney, J Poole, S Cass. A review of balance instruments for older adults. Am J Occup Ther 1998;52(8):666–671; KO Berg, SL Wood-Dauphinee, JI Williams, B Maki. Measuring balance in the elderly: validation of an instrument. Can J Public Health 1992;83:S7–S11; L Thorbahn, R Newton. Use of the Berg Balance Test to predict falls in elderly persons. Phys Ther 1996;76(6):576–583; and K Berg, S Wood-Dauphinee, JI Williams, D Gayton. Measuring balance in the elderly: preliminary development of an instrument. Physiotherapy Can 1989;41:304.

Table IX-2. Overview of the Timed "Up and Go" Test

| Population | Time | Equipment | Reliability | Validity |
|---|---|---|---|---|
| Geriatric population with various diagnoses | 1–3 mins to complete test | Armchair Stopwatch Assistive device* | Inter-rater reliability: r = 0.99 Intrarater reliability: r = 0.99 ICC = 0.99 | Content validity: none reported Concurrent validity: Berg balance scale (r = −0.81) Predictive validity: none reported |

ICC = intraclass correlation coefficient; r = correlation coefficient.
*If necessary, an assistive device may be used while performing this test.
Sources: Data from S Whitney, J Poole, S Cass. A review of balance instruments for older adults. Am J Occup Ther 1998;52(8):666–671; D Posiadlo, S Richardson. The Timed "Up and Go": a test of basic functional mobility for frail elderly persons. J Am Geriatr Soc 1991;39:142–148; LG Portney, MP Watkins (eds). Foundations of Clinical Research Applications to Practice. Norwalk, CT: Appleton & Lange, 1993; and KO Berg, SL Wood-Dauphinee, JI Williams, B Maki. Measuring balance in the elderly: validation of an instrument. Can J Public Health 1992;83:S7–S11.

4.  Walking 3 m back to the armchair

5.  Sitting down

It is important to instruct the patient to walk at a comfortable and normal pace to maintain safety throughout the test. It is appropriate to provide assistance for the patient if it is needed. Documenting the level of assistance (i.e., assistive device, contact guard) is essential in demonstrating progress when performing the test over time.

### Interpretation of Results

Test completion in fewer than 20 seconds indicates that the patient is independent with functional mobility.[9] The time needed to complete the test may improve for many reasons, including (1) altering the use of an assistive device, (2) actual change in function, and (3) increased familiarity of the test, or a combination of these. Therefore, it is important to periodically perform this test over the course of a patient's physical therapy intervention to allow for comparison to their baseline results.

As described in Table IX-2, when compared to other functional tests (i.e., BBS), with regards to balance testing, the timed up and go is a consistent test of the balance characteristics in this population.

When used in an acute care setting, this test can objectively demonstrate improvements in balance and ambulation. Over the course of therapy, it is expected that the time the patient takes to complete the timed "up and go" test will decrease as the patient improves.[8]

## Functional Reach Test

The functional reach test was developed to assess the risk for falls in the elderly population and is a dynamic measure of stability during a self-initiated movement.[10] The functional reach test evaluates balance by measuring the maximum distance an elderly person can reach forward, backward, and sideward while standing on the floor at a fixed position.[5]

### Procedure

The procedure involves a series of three trials of the distance a patient is willing to reach from a fixed surface.[5] After every reach, distance is measured with a yardstick attached to the wall at shoulder level. The difference in inches between a person's arm length and maximal forward, backward, and sideward reach with the shoulder flexed to 90 degrees while maintaining a fixed base of support in standing is then recorded.[6,11] Refer to Table IX-3 for a summary of the functional reach test.

### Interpretation of Results

The functional reach in inches correlates with the patients relative risk for falling.[10]

- A reach of greater than 10 in. indicates that the subject being tested is not likely to fall.[10]

- A reach between 6 and 10 in. indicates the subject is two times more likely to fall.[10]

Table IX-3. Overview of the Functional Reach Test

| Population | Equipment | Time | Reliability | Validity |
|---|---|---|---|---|
| Elders who are community ambulators Population limitation, excluding patients with dementia, extreme spinal deformities, severely restricted upper extremity function, frail elders, and nursing home residents. | Yardstick Level Assistive device* | <5 mins to complete test | Test-retest reliability: r = 0.89 Interrater reliability: ICC = 0.99 | Concurrent validity: Walking speed, r = 0.71 Tandem walk, r = 0.71 Center of pressure, r = 0.71 Predictive validity: >10 in.: not likely to fall 6–10 in.: two times more likely to fall 1–6 in.: four times more likely to fall 0 in.: 28 times more likely to fall |

ICC = intraclass correlation coefficient; r = correlation coefficient.
*An assistive device may be used while performing this test if it is necessary.
Sources: Data from LG Portney, MP Watkins (eds). Foundations of Clinical Research Applications to Practice. Norwalk, CT: Appleton & Lange, 1993; PW Duncan, DK Weiner, J Chandler, S Studenski. Functional reach: A new clinical measure of balance. J Gerontol 1990;45: M192–M197; and PB Thapa, P Gideon, RL Fought, et al. Comparison of clinical and biomechanical measures of balance and mobility in elderly nursing home residents. J Am Geriatr Soc 1994;42:493–500.

- Reaching between 1 and 6 in. indicates that the subject is four times more likely to fall.[10]

- If the subject is unwilling to reach, they are 28 times more likely to fall.[10]

When working with an elderly patient in an acute care setting, this test may be an objective way to quickly gauge balance abilities and determine the need for balance treatment, an assistive device, or both. It is important to remember that there are limitations to the population that can participate in this test. Elders who are frail, demented, or both, are excluded, because participation in this test may lead to unnecessary injury or falls.

## Tinetti Performance Oriented Mobility Assessment

The Tinetti POMA is a performance test of balance and gait maneuvers used during normal daily activities.[12] This test has two subscales of balance and gait, as described in Table IX-4. There are 13 maneuvers in the balance portion and nine maneuvers in the gait portion. The balance subscale, the performance oriented assessment of balance (POAB), can be used individually as a separate test of balance.

### Procedure

The balance maneuvers are graded on an ordinal scale as normal (2 points), adaptive (1 point), or abnormal (0 points). The gait maneuvers are graded as normal or abnormal, with the exception of a few items (see Table IX-4). A combination of the total points for the balance and gait portions are summed together to determine the final score.[6,13] A summary of the Tinetti POMA can be found in Table IX-5.

### Interpretation of Results

A total combined score on the balance and gait subscales of the Tinetti POMA correlates with the patient's relative risk of falling.[14]

- A combined score of 18 or less on the Tinetti POMA is a predictor of a high fall risk.[14]

**Table IX-4.** Performance Oriented Mobility Assessment I

Balance
Instructions: Subject is seated in hard, armless chair. The following
maneuvers are tested.
1. Sitting balance
    2 = steady, stable
    1 = holds onto chair to keep upright
    0 = leans, slides down in chair
2. Arising from chair
    2 = able to rise in a single movement without use of arms
    1 = uses arms (on chair or walking aid) to pull or push up; and/or
    moves forward in chair before attempting to arise
    0 = multiple attempts required or unable without human assistance
3. Immediate standing balance (first 5 secs)
    2 = steady without holding onto walking aid or other object for
    support
    1 = steady, but uses walking aid or other object for support
    0 = any sign of unsteadiness
4. Standing balance
    2 = steady, able to stand with feet together without holding object
    for support
    1 = steady, but cannot put feet together
    0 = any sign of unsteadiness regardless of stance or holds onto object
5. Balance with eyes closed (with feet as close together as possible)
    2 = steady without holding onto any object with feet together
    1 = steady with feet apart
    0 = any sign of unsteadiness or needs to hold onto an object
6. Turning balance (360 degrees)
    2 = no grabbing or staggering; no need to hold onto any objects;
    steps are continuous (turn is a flowing movement)
    1 = steps are discontinuous (patient puts one foot completely on
    floor before raising other foot)
    0 = any sign of unsteadiness or holds onto an object
7. Nudge on sternum (patient standing with feet as close together as
    possible, examiner pushes with light even pressure over sternum
    three times)
    2 = steady, able to withstand pressure
    1 = needs to move feet, but able to maintain balance
    0 = begins to fall, or examiner has to help maintain balance

8. Neck turning (patient asked to turn to side and look up while standing with feet as close together as possible)

   2 = able to turn head at least half way side to side and able to bend head back to look at ceiling; no staggering, grabbing, or symptoms of lightheadedness, unsteadiness, or pain

   1 = decreased ability to turn side to side or to extend neck, but no staggering, grabbing, or symptoms of lightheadedness, unsteadiness, or pain

   0 = any sign of unsteadiness or symptoms when turning head or extending neck

9. One leg standing balance

   2 = able to stand on one leg for 5 secs without holding object for support

   1 = some staggering, swaying, or moves foot slightly

   0 = unable

10. Back extension (ask patient to lean back as far as possible, without holding onto object)

    2 = good extension without holding object or staggering

    1 = tries to extend, but decreased range of motion (compared with other patients of same age) or needs to hold object to attempt extension

    0 = will not attempt or no extension seen or staggers

11. Reaching up (have patient attempt to remove an object from a shelf high enough to require stretching or standing on toes)

    2 = able to take down object without needing to hold onto other object for support and without becoming unsteady

    1 = able to get object but needs to steady self by holding onto something for support

    0 = unable or unsteady

12. Bending down (patient is asked to pick up small objects [e.g., a pen] from the floor)

    2 = able to bend down and pick up the object and is able to get up easily in single attempt without needing to pull self up with arms

    1 = able to get object and get upright in single attempt but needs to pull self up with arms or hold onto something for support

    0 = unable to bend down or unable to get upright after bending down or takes multiple attempts to become upright

13. Sitting down

    2 = able to sit down in one smooth movement

    1 = needs to use arms to guide self into chair or movement is not smooth

    0 = falls into chair, misjudges distances (lands off center)

**Table IX-4.** *Continued*

Gait

Instructions: Subject stands with examiner, then walks 15 ft down a premeasured hallway, turns, and walks back to starting point. Subject should use customary walking aid as necessary.

1. Initiation of gait (patient asked to begin walking down hallway)

    1 = begins walking immediately without observable hesitation; initiation of gait is single, smooth motion

    0 = hesitates; multiple attempts; initiation of gait is not a smooth motion

2. Step height (begin observing after first few steps; observe one foot, then the other; observe from side)

    1 = swing foot completely clears floor but by no more than 1–2 in.

    0 = swing foot is not completely raised off floor (may hear scraping) or is raised too high (>2 in.)

3. Step length (observe distance between toe of stance foot and heel of swing foot; observe from side; do not judge first few or last few steps; observe one side at a time)

    1 = at least the length of individual's foot between the stance toe and swing heel (step length usually longer but foot length provides basis for observation)

    0 = step length less than the individual's foot

4. Step symmetry (observe the middle part of walking, not the first or last steps; observe from side; observe distance between heel of each swing foot and toe of each stance foot)

    1 = step length same or nearly same on both sides for most step cycles

    0 = step length varies between sides or patient advances with same foot with every step

5. Step continuity

    1 = begins raising heel of one foot (toe off) as heel of other foot touches the floor (heel strike); no breaks or stops in stride; step lengths equal over most cycles

    0 = places entire foot (heel and toe) on floor before beginning to raise other foot; or stops completely between steps; or step length varies over cycles

6. Path deviation (observe from behind; observe one foot over several strides; observe in relation to line on floor [e.g., tiles] if possible; difficult to assess if patient uses a walker)

    2 = foot follows close to straight line as patient advances

    1 = foot deviates from side to side or toward one direction or patient uses a walking aid

    0 = marked deviation from straight line

7. Trunk stability (observe from behind; side to side motion of trunk may be a normal gait pattern, need to differentiate this from instability)

2 = trunk does not sway; knees or back are not flexed; arms are not abducted in effort to maintain stability

1 = no sway but flexion of knees or back or spreads arms out while walking

0 = any of the preceding features are present

8. Walk stance (observe from behind)

1 = feet should almost touch as one passes the other

0 = feet apart with stepping

9. Turning while walking

2 = no staggering or use of a walking aid; turning is continuous with walking; and steps are continuous while turning

1 = steps are discontinuous but no staggering, or uses walking aid

0 = staggers; unsteady; stops before initiating turn

Sources: Data from ME Tinetti. Performance-oriented assessment of mobility problems in elderly patients. J Am Geriatr Soc 1986;34:119–126; ME Tinetti, TF Williams, R Mayewski. Fall index for elderly patients based on number of chronic disabilities. Am J Med 1986;80:429–434; and SB O'Sullivan. Assessment of Motor Function. In SB O'Sullivan, TJ Schmitz (eds), Physical Rehabilitation: Assessment and Treatment (4th ed). Philadelphia: FA Davis, 2000;196, 205, 210–211.

- Scores ranging between 19 and 23 indicate a moderate risk for falls.[14]

- Scores of 24 or higher indicate a low risk for falls.[14]

This functional test is an effective and objective measure to predict falls in elderly and adult population, as well as assist in determining progress over time in therapy.

## Six-Minute Walk Test

The 6-minute walk test is a symptom-limited measure of functional capacity in which a patient walks as far as possible on a premeasured course for 6 minutes. This test evolved from the 12-minute walk test, originally designed to assess disability levels in patients with chronic bronchitis. The 6-minute walk test was found to provide similar measures of exercise tolerance and therefore was adopted by clinicians for its convenience.[15,16]

**Table IX-5.** Overview of the Tinetti Performance Oriented Mobility Assessment

| Population | Equipment | Time | Reliability | Validity |
|---|---|---|---|---|
| Balance portion: adult or geriatric population with a wide variety of diagnoses | Chair Stopwatch | 10–15 mins to complete test | Inter-rater reliability: 85% = ±10% agreement Balance portion | Concurrent validity: Berg, r = 0.91 Predictive validity: ≤18 total score predicts high fall risk |

r = correlation coefficient.
Sources: Data from JYM Wee, SD Bagg, A Palepu. The Berg Balance Scale as a predictor of length of stay and discharge destination in an acute stroke rehabilitation setting. Arch Phys Med Rehabil 1999;80(4):448–452; DM Nakamura, MB Holm, A Wilson. Measures of balance and fear of falling in the elderly: a review. Phys Occup Ther Geriatr 1998;15(4):17–32; M Tinetti. Performance oriented assessment of mobility problems in elderly patients. J Am Geriatr Soc 1986;41:479; MB King, JO Judge, R Whipple, L Wolfson. Reliability and responsiveness of two physical performance measures examined of a functional training intervention. Phys Ther 2000;80(1):8–16; W Anemaet, M Moffa-Trotter. Functional tools for assessing balance and gait impairments. Top Geriatr Rehabil 1999;15(1):66–83; and ME Tinetti, TF Williams, R Mayewski. Fall index for elderly patients based on number of chronic disabilities. Am J Med 1986;80:429–434.

## Procedure

The patient is instructed to walk as far as possible for 6 minutes within a designated test area of a premeasured distance. The patient is instructed to report if he or she experiences shortness of breath, muscular pain, dizziness, or anginal symptoms, at which time the test is terminated. The patient is also instructed to rest whenever necessary during the test but asked to continue as soon as he or she is able. Timing begins when the tester states "go" or "start." During the test, the tester should walk alongside the patient and offer appropriate guarding as needed. (Walking behind or ahead of the patient influences his or her pace.) Vital signs should be taken at rest, one or two times during the test, and immediately at the end of the 6 minutes or on completion of the test. If the patient is unable to complete the full 6 minutes, then the distance covered on termination is measured along with establishing the reason for termination by the patient.

Table IX-6. Overview of the Six-Minute Walk Test

| Population | Equipment | Time | Reliability | Validity |
|---|---|---|---|---|
| Patients with cardiac and/or pulmonary disease and osteo-arthritis of knee. | Chair Stopwatch Pulse oximeter Portable blood pressure cuff Rate of per-ceived exer-tion scale Visual pain analog scale Measuring wheel | 10–15 mins to complete test | Test-retest reliability: ICC = 0.93 | Responsive-ness index validity: 0.6 |

ICC = intraclass correlation coefficient.

Sources: Data from MB King, JO Judge, R Whipple, L Wolfson. Reliability and respon-siveness of two physical performance measures examined of a functional training inter-vention. Phys Ther 2000;80(1):8–16; MA Woo, DK Moser, LW Stevenson, WG Stevenson. Six-minute walk test and heart rate variability: lack of association in advanced stages of heart failure. Am J Crit Care 1997;6(5):348–354; GH Guyatt, MJ Sullivan, PJ Thompson, et al. The 6-minte walk: new measure of exercise capacity in patients with chronic heart failure. Can Med Assoc J 1985;132:919–923; GH Guyatt, SO Pugsley, MJ Sullivan, et al. Effect of encouragement on walking test performance. Thorax 1994;39:818–822; T Kavanaugh, MG Myers, RS Baigrie, et al. Quality of life and cardiorespiratory function in chronic heart failure: effects of 12 months aerobic training. Heart 1996;76:42–49; and PA Kovar, JP Allegrante, CR MacKenzie, et al. Supervised fitness walking in patients with osteoarthritis of the knee: a randomized con-trolled trial. Ann Intern Med 1992;116:529–534.

## Interpretation of Results

Many studies have examined the usefulness of the 6-minute walk test in specific populations (Table IX-6) and have found it to be effective in predicting oxygen consumption and determining the efficacy of surgical intervention on functional mobility.[15–18] No standards, however, have been established for the average distance a "normal" or nondiseased individual should walk in 6 minutes. Therefore, the test is most useful to physical therapists as a means of prescribing exercise intensity and measuring progress in patients' functional activity tolerance.

## Conclusion

The use of functional tests is becoming more common among physical therapists in the acute care setting. With the profession moving into an era of evidence-based practice, it is important to become aware of some effective, objective measures that can be used to determine the functional level of various patient populations. The functional tests described in this appendix offer objective, reliable, and valid measurement options that examine the functional mobility of varying populations. In the current health care system, evidence-based practice is required to survive the ongoing changes in insurance reimbursement. These tests are quick, effective measures that can objectively demonstrate fall risk and progress with functional mobility in the acute care setting.

## References

1. Portney LG, Watkins MP (eds). Foundations of Clinical Research Applications to Practice. Norwalk, CT: Appleton & Lange, 1993;680,689.
2. Wee JYM, Bagg SD, Palepu A. The Berg Balance Scale as a predictor of length of stay and discharge destination in an acute stroke rehabilitation setting. Arch Phys Med Rehabil 1999;80(4):448–452.
3. Berg KO, Wood-Dauphinee SL, Williams JI, Maki B. Measuring balance in the elderly: validation of an instrument. Can J Public Health 1992;83:S7–S11.
4. Berg K, Wood-Dauphinee S, Williams JI, Gayton D. Measuring balance in the elderly: preliminary development of an instrument. Physiother Can 1989;41:304.
5. Nakamura DM, Holm MB, Wilson A. Measures of balance and fear of falling in the elderly: a review. Phys Occup Ther Geriatr 1998;15(4):17–32.
6. Whitney S, Poole J, Cass S. A review of balance instruments for older adults. Am J Occup Ther 1998;52(8):666–671.
7. Posiadlo D, Richardson S. The timed "Up and Go": a test of basic functional mobility for frail elderly persons. J Am Geriatr Soc 1991;39:142–148.
8. Thompson M, Medley A. Performance of community dwelling elderly on the Timed Up and Go test. Phys Occup Ther Geriatr 1995;13(3):17–30.
9. White, J. Functional assessment tools—use them! Phys Ther Case Rep 2000;3(4):188–189.
10. Duncan PW, Weiner DK, Chandler J, Studenski S. Functional reach: a new clinical measure of balance. J Gerontol 1990;45:M192–M197.

11. Newton R. Reach in four directions as a measure of stability in older adults. Phys Ther 1996;76:S23.
12. Umphred DA (ed). Neurological Rehabilitation (3rd ed.). St. Louis: Mosby, 1995;808–809, 812, 816–817, 822–823, 828–829.
13. Tinetti M. Performance oriented assessment of mobility problems in elderly patients. J Am Geriatr Soc 1986;41:479.
14. Tinetti ME, Williams TF, Mayewski R. Fall index for elderly patients based on number of chronic disabilities. Am J Med 1986;80:429–434.
15. McGavin CR, Gupta SP, McHardy GJR. Twelve-minute walking test for assessing disability in chronic bronchitis. BMJ 1976;1:822.
16. Butland RJ, Pang J, Gross ER, et al. Two-, six-, and twelve-minute walking tests in respiratory disease. BMJ 1982;284:1607.
17. Cahalin LP, Mathier MA, Semigran MJ, et al. The six-minute walk test predicts peak oxygen uptake and survival in patients with advanced heart failure. Chest 1996;110:310.
18. Laupacis A, Bourne R, Rorabeck C, et al. The effect of elective total hip replacement on health-related quality of life. J Bone Joint Surg [Am] 1993;75:1619.

# X

# Physical Therapy Considerations for Patients Who Complain of Chest Pain

*Michele P. West*

The purpose of this appendix is to discuss the different etiologies of cardiogenic and noncardiogenic chest pain and provide a means of taking an efficient history when a patient complains of chest pain. Chest pain is a common complaint for which many patients seek medical attention.

Cardiogenic chest pain may be ischemic or nonischemic. Ischemic chest pain may be caused by atherosclerosis, coronary spasm, systemic or pulmonary hypertension, aortic stenosis, hypertrophic cardiomyopathy, severe anemia or hypoxia, or polycythemia.[1] Nonischemic chest pain may be owing to aortic dissection or aneurysm, pericarditis, mitral valve prolapse, or myocarditis.[1] (Refer to Figure 1-8 for the possible clinical courses of patients admitted with cardiogenic chest pain.)

Noncardiogenic chest pain can arise from a wide range of diseases and disorders as described in Table X-1, each with its own distinctive associated signs and symptoms. Refer to Table 8-1 for gastrointestinal pain referral patterns. Very commonly, the patient rationalizes chest pain as a gastrointestinal disturbance rather than angina.

**Table X-1.** Possible Etiologies and Associated Signs of Noncardiogenic Chest Pain

| Origin | Possible Etiology | Signs and Symptoms |
|---|---|---|
| Pulmonary | Pneumonia<br>Pulmonary embolism<br>Tuberculosis | Abnormal breath sounds and respiratory rate, presence of cough or hemoptysis |
| Pleural | Pleuritis<br>Pneumothorax<br>Mediastinitis | Pain with respiration, pleural rub, abnormal breath sounds and respiratory rate |
| Gastrointestinal | Hiatal hernia<br>Esophagitis<br>Esophageal reflux<br>Acute pancreatitis | Nausea, vomiting, burping, abdominal pain |
| Musculoskeletal | Muscle strain<br>Repetitive coughing<br>Rib fracture(s) | Reproduction of pain with palpation and pain with respiration or cough |

Sources: Data from NH Holmes, M Foley, PH Thompson (eds). Professional Guide to Signs and Symptoms (3rd ed). Springhouse, PA: Springhouse, 1997;153; and RL Wilkins, SJ Krider, RL Sheldon (eds). Clinical Assessment in Respiratory Care (3rd ed). St. Louis: Mosby, 1995;28.

Chest pain can present with signs and symptoms other than the classic angina pectoris owing to myocardial ischemia. The mnemonic *OLD CART* can be used as a rapid survey for the differential diagnosis of chest pain during a physical therapy session[1-3]:

Onset—Sudden versus insidious, with exertion or stress versus rest? (Cardiogenic chest pain is usually of sudden onset.)

Location—Substernal or on the left side of the chest? (Cardiogenic chest pain typically occurs in this location, but can also present in any area above the waist.)

Duration—Lasts longer than 20 minutes? (Cardiogenic chest pain typically lasts 2–20 minutes.)

Characteristics—Pressure, tightness, or heaviness versus other feelings, such as sharpness, or with inspiration? (Cardiogenic chest pain is usually described as a deep visceral sensation.)

Accompanying symptoms—Associated with diaphoresis, dyspnea, or light-headedness versus a lack of these symptoms? (Cardiogenic chest pain is typically associated with one or more of these accompanying symptoms.)

Radiation—Does the pain radiate to the arm(s), shoulder(s), neck, jaw, or teeth? (Cardiogenic chest pain can radiate widely.)

Treatment—Relieved by rest, oxygen, or nitroglycerin? (Cardiogenic chest pain is usually relieved by these interventions.)

As this information is ascertained, the physical therapist should discontinue the activity (if not resting) and determine the need for seated or supine rest, observe the patient for signs of altered cardiac output (decreased blood pressure), take vital signs, and monitor telemetry as appropriate. If the chest pain appears cardiogenic, the physical therapist must determine whether it is stable or unstable. Refer to Myocardial Ischemia and Infarction in Chapter 1 for a description of stable, unstable, and variant (Prinzmetal's) angina.

During an episode of unstable angina, an electrocardiograph may reveal ST segment elevation or depression with or without T-wave inversion that reverses when anginal pain decreases.[4] These electrocardiograph changes are depicted in Figure X-1. Vital sign findings include the following:

- Hypotension or hypertension
- Bradycardia or tachycardia
- Irregular pulse

If the patient presents with one or more of these unstable anginal findings, the therapist should stop or defer treatment and immediately notify the nurse.

Regardless of the etiology of the patient's complaint of chest pain, the physical therapist must be prepared to expedite a reliable chest pain description and respond accordingly for prompt medical therapies or for further investigation of the cause of noncardiogenic chest pain.

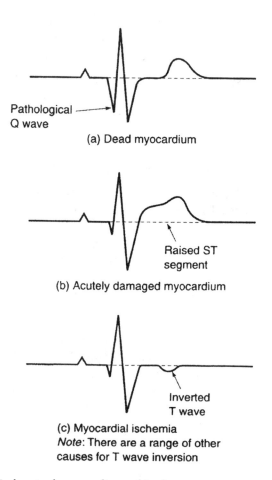

Figure X-1. *Ischemic electrocardiographic changes.*

# References

1. Becker RC (ed). Chest Pain. Boston: Butterworth–Heinemann, 2000;40.
2. McAvoy JA. Cardiac pain: discover the unexpected. Nursing 2000; 30:34.
3. Pathophysiology of Coronary Artery Disease. In FJ Brannon, MW Foley, JA Starr, MG Black (eds), Cardiopulmonary Rehabilitation: Basic Theory and Application (2nd ed). Philadelphia: FA Davis, 1993;82.
4. Chandra NC. Angina Pectoris. In LR Barker, PD Burton, PD Ziere (eds), Principles of Ambulatory Medicine (4th ed). Baltimore: Williams & Wilkins, 1995;691.

# Index

Note: Page numbers followed by *f* indicate figures;
numbers followed by *t* indicate tables.